Pathology and Epidemiology of Aquatic Animal Diseases for Practitioners

Pathology and Epidemiology of Aquatic Animal Diseases for Practitioners

Edited by

Laura Urdes
University of Agricultural Sciences and Veterinary Medicine of Bucharest
Bucharest
Romania

Chris Walster
The Island Veterinary Associates
Stafford
UK

Julius Tepper
Long Island Fish Hospital
NY, US

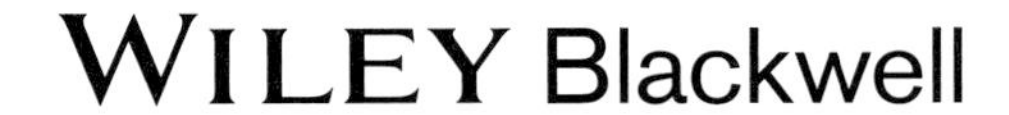

This edition first published 2023

Registered Offices
John Wiley & Sons, Inc., 111 River Street, Hoboken, NJ 07030, USA
John Wiley & Sons Ltd, The Atrium, Southern Gate, Chichester, West Sussex, PO19 8SQ, UK

Editorial Office
9600 Garsington Road, Oxford, OX4 2DQ, UK
For details of our global editorial offices, customer services, and more information about Wiley products visit us at www.wiley.com.

Wiley also publishes its books in a variety of electronic formats and by print-on-demand. Some content that appears in standard print versions of this book may not be available in other formats.

Library of Congress Cataloging-in-Publication Data
Names: Urdes, Laura, editor. | Walster, Christopher, editor. | Tepper, Julius, editor.
Title: Pathology and epidemiology of aquatic animal diseases for practitioners / edited by Laura Urdes, Chris Walster, Julius Tepper.
Other titles: Fundamentals of aquatic veterinary medicine.
Description: Hoboken, NJ : Wiley-Blackwell, 2023. | "This book is intended to complement the Fundamentals of aquatic veterinary medicine textbook"–ECIP galley. | Includes bibliographical references and index.
Identifiers: LCCN 2022052874 (print) | LCCN 2022052875 (ebook) | ISBN 9781119839675 (paperback) | ISBN 9781119839705 (adobe pdf) | ISBN 9781119839712 (epub)
Subjects: MESH: Aquatic Organisms | Animal Diseases | Fish Diseases | Amphibians | Reptiles | Invertebrates
Classification: LCC SF997.5.A65 (print) | LCC SF997.5.A65 (ebook) | NLM SF 997.5.A65 | DDC 636.089–dc23/eng/20230120
LC record available at https://lccn.loc.gov/2022052874
LC ebook record available at https://lccn.loc.gov/2022052875

Cover Design: Wiley
Cover Images: Courtesy of Alex Hall (Left and top left); Laura Urdes (Histogram); Pádraig Duignan (Seal); María J. Forzán (Frog)

Set in 9.5/12.5pt STIXTwoText by Straive, Pondicherry, India

Printed in Singapore
M118880_270223

Contents

List of Contributors

Acacia Alcivar-Warren
Environmental Genomics Inc.
Southborough, MA,
United States

Ellen Ariel
James Cook University
Townsville
Queensland, Australia

Kelly Bateman
World Organisation for Animal Health
Collaborating Centre for Emerging Aquatic
Animal Diseases
Centre for Environment
Fisheries and Aquaculture Sciences
Weymouth, UK

Wes Arend Baumgartner
University of Illinois Urbana
IL, USA

Morag Clinton
University of Alaska
Fairbanks
Alaska, USA

Pádraig Duignan
Marine Mammal Center
Sausalito
California, USA

María J. Forzán
College of Veterinary Medicine
Long Island University
Brookville, New York
New York, USA

Leo Foyle
James Cook University
Townsville
Queensland, Australia

Marius Hangan
University of Agricultural Sciences and
Veterinary Medicine of Bucharest
Bucharest, Romania

Karina Jones
Murdoch University
Murdoch, Perth
Western Australia, Australia

Gregory Lewbart
College of Veterinary Medicine
North Carolina State University Raleigh
North Carolina, USA

Richmond Loh
Perth, Australia

Nicole M. Nemeth
Southeastern Cooperative Wildlife
Disease Study
Department of Pathology
University of Georgia Athens
Georgia, USA

Julius Tepper
Long Island Fish Hospital Manorville
New York, USA

Laura Urdes
University of Agricultural Sciences and
Veterinary Medicine of Bucharest
Bucharest, Romania

Chris Walster
The Island Veterinary Associates
Stafford, UK

Foreword

Complimenting the *Fundamentals of Aquatic Veterinary Medicine*, which provides veterinarians with essential knowledge of aquatic veterinary medicine, this book moves on to further describe the pathology of aquatic animal diseases, together with practical epidemiological and economic concepts.

Aimed at clinicians, the book is divided into two sections. The first section discusses the pathology of aquatic animal disease by taxonomic grouping, both in the wild and captivity; invertebrates, fish, amphibians, reptiles, mammals, and birds, and has been written by leading authors in their field. Each section has an introduction to the manifestation of disease and the major pathogens in each grouping. The discussion then extends to genus and major species with each section providing a list of references and further reading to compliment the text.

Intended to be used as a practical, concise reference for daily use, there are comprehensive tables of clinical signs useful for differential diagnosis.

The second section discusses practical usage of epidemiological principles, as well as the basic concepts for animal health economics, which will aid the clinician in interpretation of test results, formulating a biosecurity plan and discussion of suitable treatments, and so on.

Working spreadsheet templates are included to allow clinicians to put into practice the concepts discussed using their computer, tablet or phone, emphasizing how the book can be used on a daily basis.

Preface

The knowledge base of aquatic veterinary medicine is continuing to expand and includes the treatment of several classes of animals, fish, birds, reptiles, amphibians, and mammals. This book builds on the introduction provided in *Fundamentals of Aquatic Veterinary Medicine* and completes the coverage of the diseases of the major aquatic animal classes. It provides concise, practical information on the most common diseases seen in aquatic animals, their causes, symptoms, and treatment. It also provides insight into how to use epidemiological and economics principles to decide on the right treatment or design a biosecurity plan for a facility.

Written by some of the leading veterinary experts in their field, Part I of the book devotes a chapter to each class and discusses common diseases their signs, symptoms, diagnostic tests, and treatment. At the end of each chapter are tables of differential diagnoses which can be used as a "quick reference" by the clinician, based on signs and symptoms seen to aid in diagnosis.

Part II provides a refresher of epidemiological terms and statistics with which the clinician should be familiar. This is followed by chapters discussing how the clinician can use these subjects to better determine such things as the likelihood of a new outbreak of disease, or what is the right treatment decision based on likely costs and outcomes, to deciding on the requirement, the resources required, and possible benefits of a biosecurity plan. Spreadsheets and the formula to use are provided throughout. The final chapter in this section discusses the principles of animal health economics, again providing formulae and spreadsheets the reader can use to determine the cost benefit to a business and determining whether the business can provide the necessary resources.

The book is aimed at all clinicians but is also useful for students or someone wishing to become more familiar with the knowledge available in aquatic veterinary medicine. It is intended to be concise enough to use in the field, and some previous knowledge or training, in the subject matter, may be necessary to fully understand the concepts demonstrated and to use them effectively.

Acknowledgments

The editors would like to acknowledge Alex Hall Bsc BVetMed CertAqV MRCVS for his knowledge and expertise in the preparation of Diseases of Coral in Cultivation and Aquaria in Chapter One, and Wes Arend Baumgartner PhD DVM for helping with the clinical tables in Part I.

Part I

Pathology of Aquatic Animal Species

Introduction to the Manifestation of Disease and Major Pathogens

1

Aquatic Invertebrates

Acacia Alcivar-Warren, Kelly Bateman, Morag Clinton, Leo Foyle, Gregory Lewbart, Richmond Loh, and Julius Tepper

Porifera (sponges)
Coelenterates: • Cnidarians (Hydrozoa, Scyphozoa/jellyfish, Anthozoa/anemones and corals) • Mollusca - Bivalves (oysters, clams, mussels, scallops, cockles) - Cephalopod (Nautiloidea, Coleiodea; Decapodiformes/cuttlefish and squid, Octopodiformes/octopus) Gastropods: - Prosobranchia (limpets, abalone, cowries, conch, winkles, snails, whelks) - Opistobranchia (sea hares, sea slugs) - Pulmonata (snails) • Crustaceans: - Shrimp - Lobsters - Crabs - Crayfish • Echinoderms: - Crinoidea (crinoids, sea lilies, feather stars) - Asteroidea (sea stars/starfish) - Ophiuroidea (brittle stars, basket stars) - Echinoidea (sea urchins, sand dollars) - Holothuroidea (sea cucumbers) - Concentrocycloidea • Urochordates: - Ascidians (sea squirts) - Thalaceans (salps, doliolids) - Larvacians

Pathology and Epidemiology of Aquatic Animal Diseases for Practitioners, First Edition.
Edited by Laura Urdes, Chris Walster, and Julius Tepper.

Porifera (Sponges)

Overview

The phylum Porifera is a diverse group of ancient and anatomically undifferentiated animals commonly referred to as sponges. Until the middle of the 18th century, sponges were classified as plants (Ruppert et al., 2004). Sponges occur in the fossil record back to the Precambrian era (over 600 million years ago) and were the most important contributors to reefs during the Paleozoic and Mesozoic eras (Hooper and Van Soest, 2002). All members lack defined organs, with differentiated connective tissue cells performing necessary biologic functions. A unique system of water canals facilitates transport of food, gametes, and waste products. Nearly all species are sessile, and most are marine. Of the approximately 8300 species belonging to over 680 genera, only about 3% occur in freshwater (Hooper and Van Soest, 2002; Ruppert et al., 2004). Sponges are normally found on firm substrates in shallow water, although some occur on soft bottoms, or at great depth.

Despite their being termed "primitive" or "simple" in form and function, Srivastava et al. (2010) discovered that at least one species shares over 70% of its DNA with humans. This finding may lead to further use of sponges in biomedical research, where they are already making important contributions in the areas of embryology, pharmacology, and toxicology. Sponges are highly sensitive to water quality and flow changes, including suspended sediments. Zinc and copper may be toxic to some species. Infectious diseases are not well characterized. Bacterial and algal microbiota, and occasionally protozoa have been implicated.

Clinical Signs

- Sudden death – toxicity, trauma, extreme sedimentation.
- Poor growth – water pollution, sedimentation, inadequate food supply, loss of symbiotic bacteria.

A listing of outbreaks of the major disease syndromes of sponges is given in Table 1.1. A list of the etiology of the major disease syndromes of sponges can be found in Appendix 1.1.

Coelenterates

Taxonomic Overview

This large phylum is made up of the cnidarians, including scyphozoans (jellyfishes), anthozoans (stony corals, soft corals, sea anemones) and hydrozoans (hydras, fire coral, Portuguese Man-o-War) and the ctenophores (comb jellies). This is an economically important group for research, environmental monitoring, public and private display, and tourism. Jellyfish exhibits are now some of the most popular displays in public aquariums and upscale restaurants throughout the world. Coral reefs collectively are one of the most beautiful, diverse, and fragile ecosystems on the planet. Investigations on the diseases of corals are some of the most active areas of research for any aquatic animal group.

Key Points

- Some diseases of hard and soft corals have been well documented, but etiologies are often an enigma. The nomenclature for many of the infectious diseases is in the process of standardization.

Table 1.1 Miscellaneous disease outbreaks in invertebrates – Porifera (sponges).

Outbreak	Species	Ecological description	Microbiological description
Indian Ocean, 1884	*Ircinia*	Unknown	Fungal filaments destroy sponge body leaving a crust of spongin fibers
Florida, 1895	*Commercials*	Loss of commercial sponges	Internal tissue completely eroded
Tunisia, 1906	*Hippospongia equina*	Attributed to shallow water and low water exchange	Dermal cortex covered in white, gray or green liquid
Caribbean, 1938	*Hippospongia*	Heavy mortality	Fungi always present
Florida Keys, 1939	Commercials	70–95% mortality	Unidentified fungal filaments in diseased tissue
Cuba, 1939	Commercials	70–95% mortality	Unidentified fungal filaments in diseased tissue
British Honduras, 1939	Commercials	Unseasonably high temperature and salinity	Unbranched fungal filaments between live and dead tissue
Panama, 1984–1995	*Iotrochota, Amphimedon compressa, Aplysina fulva, Callyspongia vaginalis, Niphates, Xestospongia, Verongula rigida, Ircinia*	Disease symptoms evident over multiple census periods. Cross species contact infections unsuccessful. Excision of diseased tissue often successful as a treatment	Spreading lesions. *I. birotulata*: dulling of surface tissue, tissue loss and white discoloration. *A. compressa*: glossing of surface and advancing narrow brown band. *Ap. fulva*: glossing of surface tissue and a narrow brown band progression, exposure of skeletal fibers
Belize, 1985	*Geodia papyracea*	Mutualism changed to disease in high water temperature	Extensive tissue decay caused by proliferation of cyanobacterial symbiont
Mediterranean, 1986–1990	*Hippospongia, Spongia*	Devastated commercial sponge populations and more prevalent in shallow, warm water. Spread rapidly	Rapidly spreading white spots, brittle skeletons, putrefied tissue, white veil (Oscillatoria?). Unidentified bacteria tunnel through skeleton
Sicily and Ligurian coast, 1986–1995	*Spongia* and *Hippospongia* spp., *Petrosia ficiformis, Ircinia variabilis, Anchinoe paupertas*	Disappearance of *Spongia officinalis* in Marsala Lagoon; 60% of commercial specimens affected in 1987, 5% in 1988 and 20% in 1989. Recolonization by 1995	White patches observed on the surface of affected sponges. Ovoid bacteria filled the canaliculi of exposed skeletal fibers
Libya, 1987	Commercial	Pollution, environmental conditions, and neglect of fishery	Unknown

(*Continued*)

Table 1.1 (Continued)

Outbreak	Species	Ecological description	Microbiological description
North Wales, 1988–1989	*Haliclona oculate, Halichondria panicea*	A number of individuals affected in 1988–1989 but no disease detected since	Brown decaying patches in *H. oculata* (possibly algal overgrowth) and decayed patches in *H. panicea* covered in white bacterial film
Mediterranean, 1994–1996	*Ircinia spinosula, Ircinia*	Massive mortality in 1994 Decay of spongin fibers	No excavation of spongin fibers. Putative agent unknown
Belize, 1996	*Xestospongia muta*	No data	Not performed
Great Britain, 1998	*Rhopaloeides odorabile*	Soft and fragile tissue with portions of pinacoderm eroded away to reveal the skeletal fibers	Bacteria observed burrowing through the spongin fibers. Causative agent identified as an alpha-proteobacterium
Mediterranean, 1994–1996	*Ircinia spinosula, Ircinia*	Massive mortality in 1994 Decay of spongin fibers	No excavation of spongin fibers. Putative agent unknown
Papua New Guinea, 1996–2000	*Ianthella basta*. Diseased specimens of *Jaspis* and *Xestospongia*	Decline in health and abundance of *I. basta*. Brown lesions with rotted tissue, large holes and brown biofilm	Five bacterial strains within the *Bacillus* and *Pseudomonas* genera were strongly correlated with disease
Curacao, 2000	*Xestospongia muta*	White holes with brittle dead tissue around perimeter of lesions	Not performed
Greece, 2001	*Aplysina aerophoba*	Massive necrosis associated with temperature increase. Suspected bacterial pathogen	Not performed
Antarctica, 2002	*Cinachyra antarctica, Inflatella belli, Isodictya setifera*	Discolored and fragile tissue in *I. belli* and *Is. setifera*. Putrefaction of tissue in *C. antarctica*	Not performed
Bahamas, 2004	*Aplysina cauliformis*	*Aplysina* red band syndrome. Rust -colored leading edge, necrosis	Cyanobacteria responsible for coloration but etiological agent uncertain
Florida Keys, 2005	*Xestospongia muta*	Orange band between healthy and bleached tissue	No environmental trigger identified; putative agent unknown
Great Britain, 2006	*Coscinoderma, Rhopaloeides odorabile*	Pinacoderm eroded away to reveal skeletal fibers	Not performed
Mexico, 2004–2005	*Xestospongia muta, Geodia, Ircinia, Xestospongia gigantea, Callyspongia plicifera*	100% of *X. muta* populations affected by disease. White with brittle dead tissue around perimeter of lesions	Not performed
Mediterranean, 2006	*Spongia officinalis* and others	Significant mortality and necrosis	Not performed
Lake Baikal, 2017	11 different	Decreased thriftiness	Not performed

- Many coelenterates, especially the sessile hard and soft corals, are important indicators of ecosystem health and can be sentinels for environmental changes and problems.
- Trauma and "eversion syndrome" are major concerns when keeping captive jellyfish.
- A variety of therapeutic compounds have been used in this phylum, almost exclusively on an empirical basis, and with mixed results.
- Our overall knowledge of coelenterate medicine and surgery is growing steadily.
- Fragging is a term used to describe "surgical propagation" of hard and soft corals using a variety of instruments, adhesives, and substrates. This technique is important for propagation of corals for conservation, scientific study, and captive display.

Clinical Signs

- Jellyfish (scyphozoans): a listing of the etiology of the major disease syndromes of jellyfish and anemones (Actinaria) is found in Appendix 1.1.

Clinical Signs: Corals (Anthozoans)

- Sudden death – toxicity, trauma, predation, extreme water-quality parameters. White film, excessive mucus, when draped over the coral, appears like a white film. White film can be a response to chemical irritation, rough handling, or areas of anaerobic decay.
- Poor growth – inadequate nutritional quality, inadequate food supply, loss of symbiotic bacteria, water pollution, interspecific competition.

Clinical signs for the major disease syndromes of corals are listed in Appendix 1.1.

Diseases of Coral in Cultivation and Aquaria

- Clinical signs – as with naturally occurring reefs; specific lesions due to parasites.
  Major diseases:
  - Trauma – induced by parasitic copepods, flatworms, coral eating fish, fragging, extreme water current. Healing and regeneration are possible if water conditions are stabilized.
  - Toxicity – Heavy metals like copper are known to be toxic to coral (Patel and Bielmyer-Fraser, 2015). Some species are much more susceptible to toxicity, such as *Acropora*. Coral is very sensitive to ammonia. Fluctuations in calcium and alkalinity will kill many stony coral species.
  - Inadequate environment – different species require different amount of current and lighting for optimal health. Generally, soft corals are the most tolerant and small polyp stony corals are the more exigent.

Diseases of Small Polyp Stony Coral

Acropora-Eating Flatworm

Species:	*Amakusaplana acroporae*
Host:	*Acropora* spp.
Diagnostics:	Visual inspection of eggs and feeding mark (the actual flatworm is difficult to see)
Eggs:	Orange-reddish brown
Adult:	Brown, clear brown spots (difficult to see)
Feeding marks:	Small, diffuse, circular, lighter in color

Treatment 1: Flatworm eXit™ (Salifert) Read the treatment sheet for the dosage. There are reports of both success and failure with this product; use at your own risk. Other species of *Acropora*-eating flatworm (AEFW) should be treated the same way.

Treatment 2: Egg Removal The eggs are resistant to treatment and are best manually removed (Figure 1.1). If possible, remove the infected colony from the display and place in a separate container. Generally (AEFW) lay their eggs at the base of or underneath the coral (Figure 1.2). Many egg clusters can be found at the junction of live tissue and coral skeleton. The eggs laid on dead coral skeleton adjacent to live tissue, so once the larva hatch their first meal is nearby (Figures 1.3, 1.4 and 1.5).

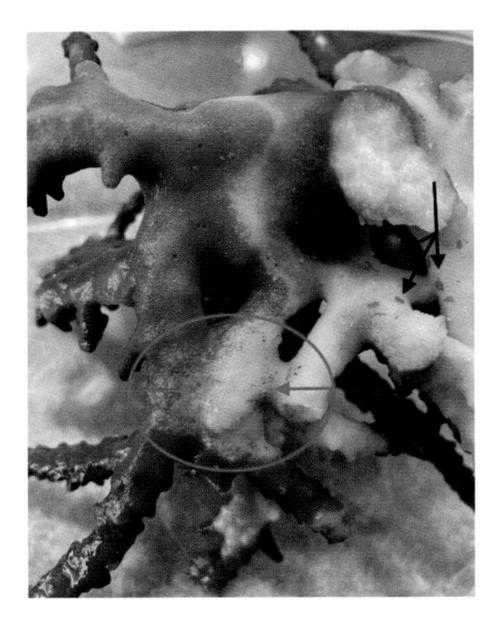

Figure 1.1 Egg clusters (black arrows) and larval migration (red circle) of *Amakusaplana acroporae*.

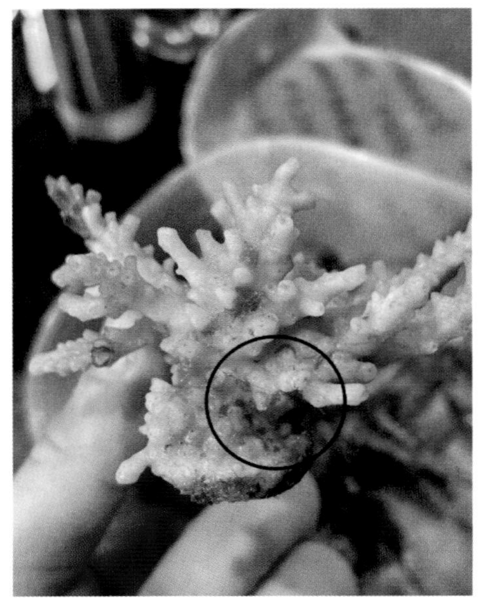

Figure 1.2 Large quantities of *Amakusaplana acroporae* egg clusters under the branches of a dead *Acropora* species.

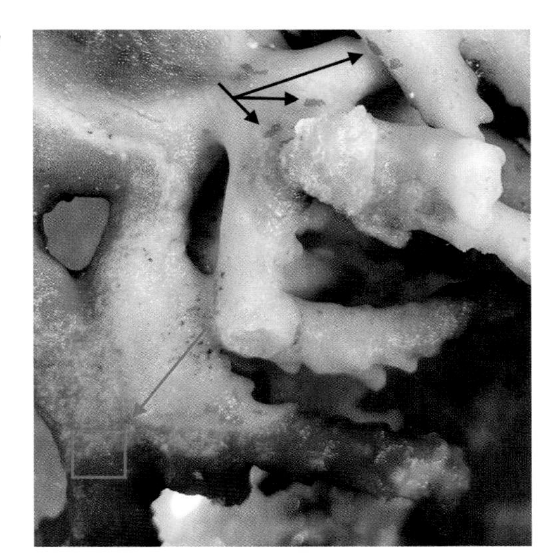

Figure 1.3 Egg clusters (black arrows) of *Amakusaplana acroporae*. Eggs hatch and then the larva migrate to the junction where the dead and alive tissues meet, where they begin to feed (red arrow to box).

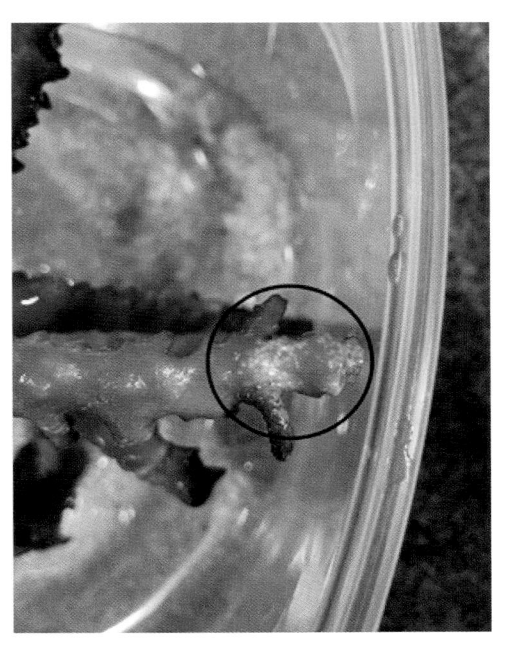

Figure 1.4 Circular feeding marks induced by *Acropora*-eating flatworms (circle). It is often easier to see these marks than the adults themselves.

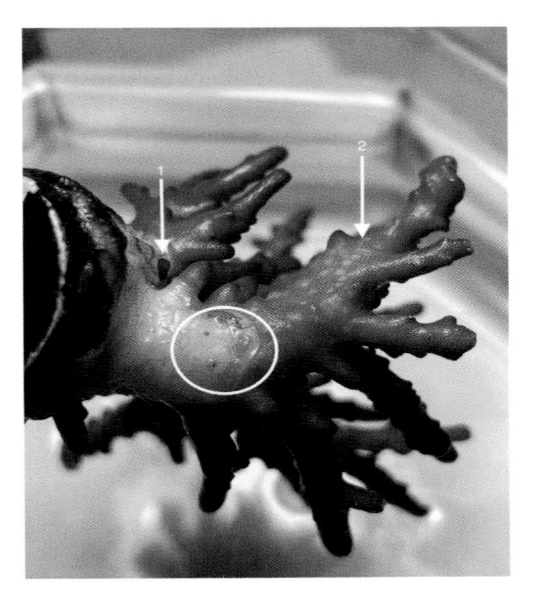

Figure 1.5 *Acropora*-eating flatworms. Arrows: 1 – Adult. 2: Feeding marks. Circle – egg clusters.

Using a toothbrush thoroughly brush the base of the skeleton. Try to remove as many egg capsules as possible. Be careful at the junction between the live tissue and bare skeleton. Make sure this area is thoroughly cleaned. Be gentle, as the toothbrush bristles can irritate the already stressed tissue.

Treatment 3: Biological Control Some wrasses will tend to eat these flatworms like sixline and melanurus wrasses. However, these fish do not eat the eggs; they only eat adult AEFWs. This may be a means to control a chronic AEFW infestation but will never be curative. As a result, the worms may continue to spread with time. There are also reports of blue velvet nudibranch eating these flatworms.

Treatment 4: Dip Treatment New corals should always be dipped before being added to a reef, especially *Acropora*. There are various dips that can be used, such as ReVive Coral Cleaner™ (Two Little Fishies) and iodine, but no firm data on efficacy have been established. These dips are not guaranteed to remove or kill these worms and the coral should always be carefully inspected before addition into the tank.

Parasitic Copepods/Amphipods

Species:	Tegastes acropranus ("red bug") is one of the most common parasites infesting *Acropora* in the home aquarium, as fragments of infected coral can easily be passed from one aquarist to another (Figures 1.6 and 1.7).
Host:	*Acropora* spp.
Diagnostics:	Visual inspection, low magnification
Treatment:	milbemycin oxime (0.1% otic solution)
Dosage:	0.167 μg/l
Duration:	Treat twice weekly for three weeks.
Notes:	0.25-ml tubes can be applied at a rate of 1 tube/1500 l During treatment, carbon and other filtration modalities should be turned off for at least 6 hours. Perform a 20% water change after each treatment.

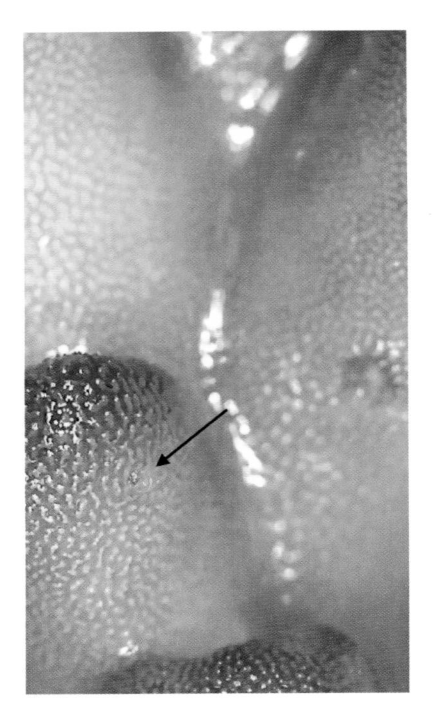

Figure 1.6 *Tegastes acroporanus* on the surface of an Acropora species.

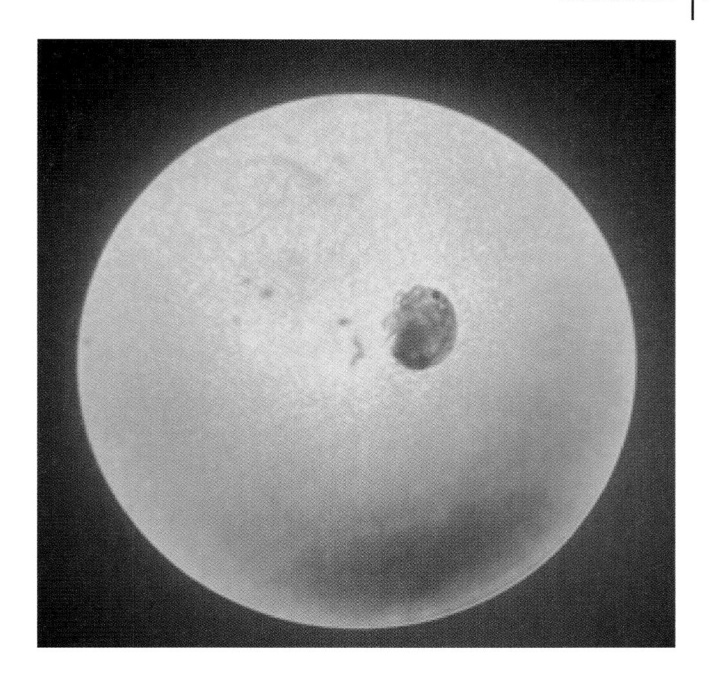

Figure 1.7 *Tegastes acroporanus* (40× magnification).

Milbemycin oxime is toxic to some invertebrates. Certain species of crabs, shrimp, and copepods are extremely susceptible. If the infestation is caught early enough, it is recommended to remove the infected colonies and treat via dip.

For other species of parasitic copepods/amphipod the dose may vary slightly. Published milbemycin oxime dose range is 0.167 μg/l to 0.625mg/l (Christie and Raines, 2016).

Ciliates

Species: *Heterotrich* (Figures 1.8 and 1.9), *Acropora* ciliates.
Host: *Acropora* spp.
Diagnostics: Visual inspection, low magnification
Treatment: No known treatment.
Notes: *Halofolliculina corallasia*, a heterotrich ciliate, has been identified as the probable causal agent of skeletal eroding band syndrome (Figure 1.10).

Metronidazole has been reported to kill similar protozoa; however, the coral succumbs to secondary bacterial infection (Sweet et al., 2014). Infected branches should be immediately removed from the tank.

Montipora-Eating Nudibranch

Species: *Phestilla* (Figure 1.11)
Host: *Montipora* spp.
Diagnostics: Visual identification, light microscopy

Treatment 1: Manual Removal The eggs are resistant to treatment and are best manually removed. If possible, remove the infected colony from the display and place in a separate container. Generally, *Phestilla* lay their eggs at the base of or underneath the coral. The eggs laid on dead coral skeleton adjacent to live tissue, so once the larva hatch, they begin feeding nearby.

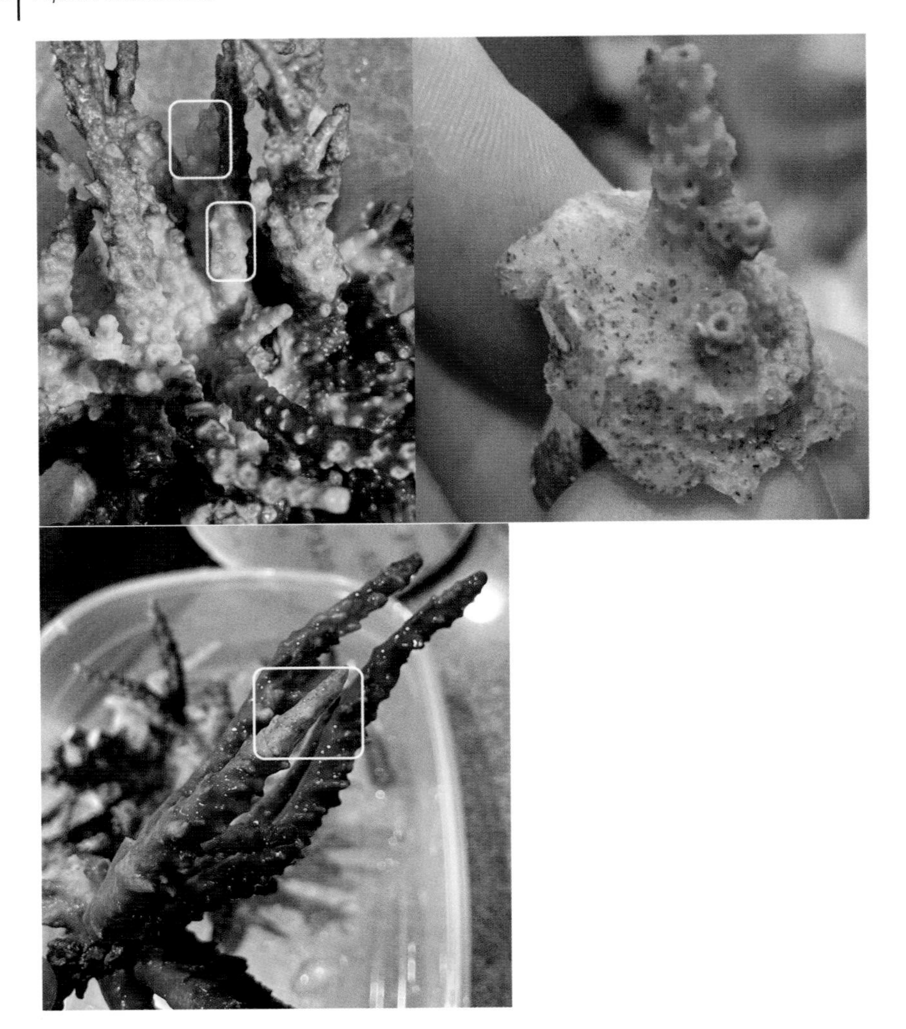

Figure 1.8 Skeletal eroding band syndrome. Note the black/green protozoa embedded in the coral skeleton.

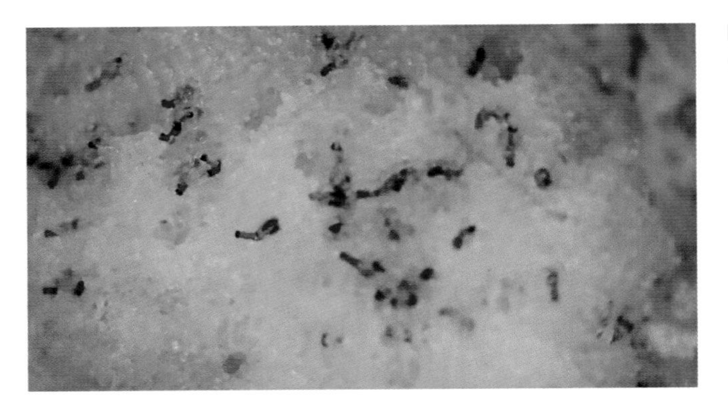

Figure 1.9 *Heterotrich* spp. (2.5× magnification).

If possible, remove the colony and remove all visible adults. If removal is not an option, use a powerhead or turkey baster to blow the adults off to be eaten by predatory wrasses. Consistently removing the adults may help to limit the infestation, but the coral may still struggle to thrive. Chemical treatment is risky as more stress is put on the dying coral.

Treatment 2: Iodine Iodine dips for one hour will kill most adults (but not the eggs).

Treatment 3: Potassium Permanganate Remove the colony and treat in an external tank.

Dosage: 50 mg/l for 30–90 minutes (Borneman, 2007)

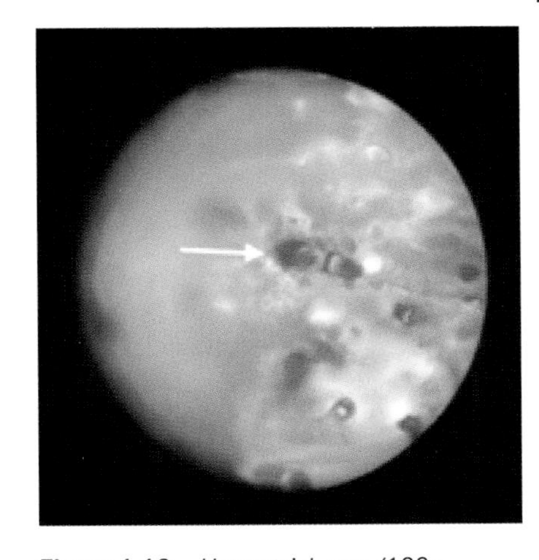

Figure 1.10 *Heterotrich* spp. (100× magnification).

Diseases of Large Polyp Stony Corals

Euphyilla Flatworms

Species:	*Polyclad* (Figure 1.12)
Host:	*Euphyilla spp.* (Figure 1.13)
Diagnostics:	Visual inspection, microscopy.
Note:	Once a polyp is infected, it will close with the worms inside, making it nearly impossible to identify the disease while the infected coral is still in the tank. Remove a closed but not a dead polyp, and leave in the open air for around five minutes; the flatworms should begin to come to the surface (Figure 1.14).

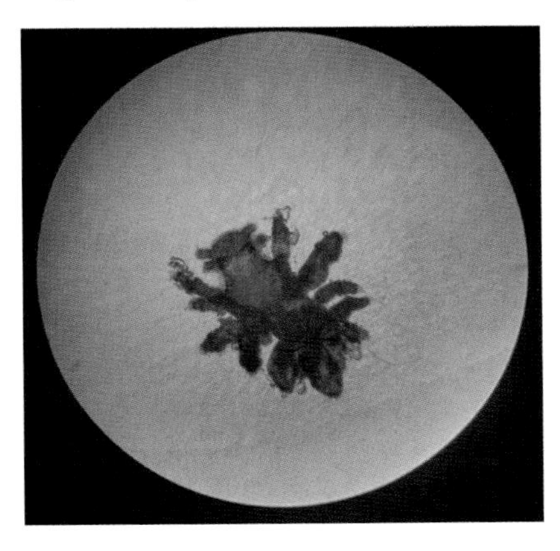

Figure 1.11 *Phestilla* spp. (10× magnification).

Treatment Polyclad species are notoriously hard to treat and the risk of collateral damage is high when treating chemically. While in the tank, the flatworms are resistant to chemical treatment since they are protected inside the closed polyp. If the colony cannot be removed from the tank, using a turkey baster, apply current directly into the center of the closed polyp to dislodge the flatworms. By doing this multiple times a day, a few hours apart, it may be possible to mitigate damage. This method of dislodgement should be applied in combination with all attempted chemical treatments.

Chemical Treatment

- Treatment 1: Several over the counter treatments are available. Efficacy is still debated, and dose unestablished. Treatment may cause stress to small polyp stony species.
- Treatment 2: Levamisole; the optimal dose is unestablished. This treatment should only be used in a separate tank if the coral can be removed from the display.

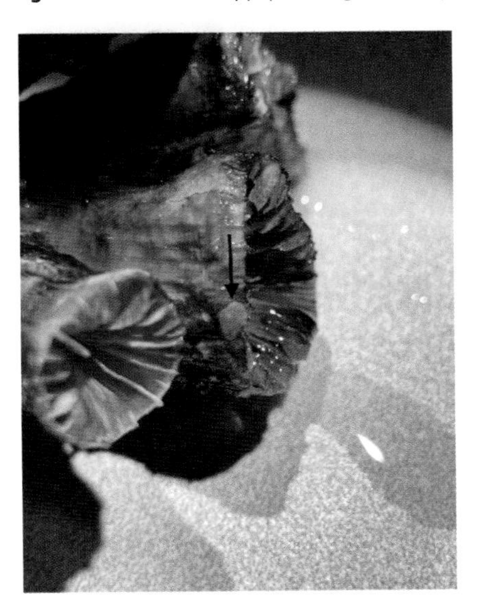

Figure 1.12 *Polyclad* species remaining on a dead *Euphyilla* polyp.

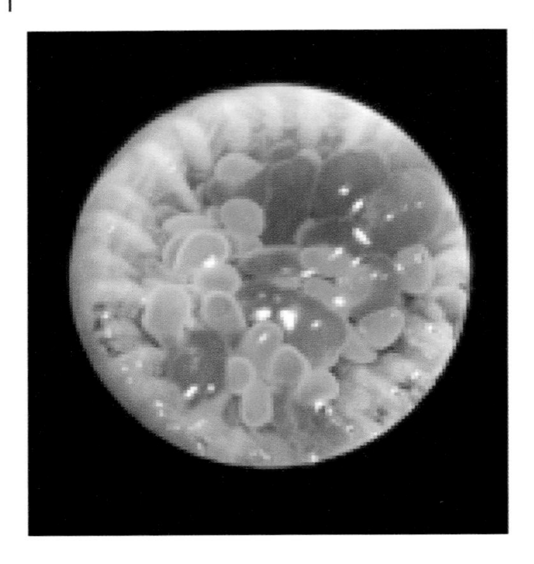

Figure 1.13 Euphilia flatworms under low-level magnification (< 2.5×).

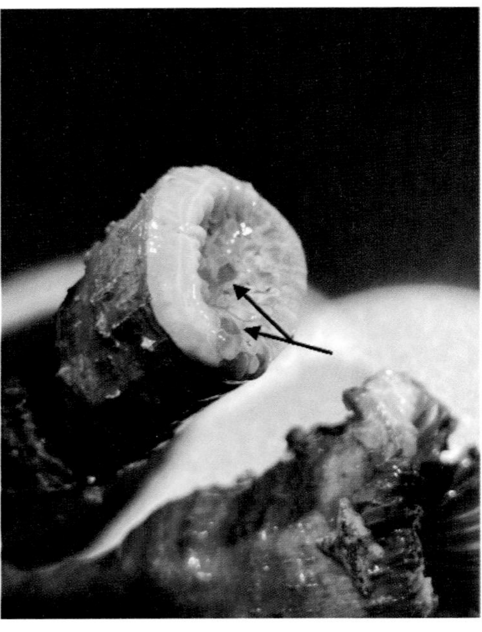

Figure 1.14 *Polyclad* species emerging from an infected polyp after being removed from the water (arrows).

- Treatment 3: Iodine immersion. Place the infected colony in a small bucket of saltwater, apply iodine until a "dark tea" is achieved. Leave the colony submerged for 10–15 minutes. After the bath, in a new bucket containing saltwater only, vigorously shake the colony under the water to dislodge the remaining flatworms.

Dendrophilia-Eating Nudibranch

Species:	*Phestilla melanobrachia*
Host:	*Dendrophylliidae*
Diagnostics:	Visual inspection. These nudibranchs look extremely similar to the coral polyp they consume! Look for horizontal movement of the mimicked "polyp."
Treatment:	Manual removal. They are not very prolific, so it is possible to clear the infection.

Diseases of Zoanthids

Zoanthid-Eating Nudibranch

Species: Unknown
Host: *Zoanthid* spp.
Diagnostics: Visual inspection. Zoanthid-eating nudibranch (Figure 1.15) will glow under blue light, typically green, but other colors are possible.
Treatment: Manual removal of the eggs is necessary as they are resistant to chemical treatment. Some predatory wrasses may consume adults. Use a moderate current created by a power head and systematically blow out the colony to dislodge adults, making them easier for fish to eat.

Zoanthid Sea Spider

Species: *Pycnogonida* (Figure 1.16)
Host: *Zoanthid* spp.
Diagnostics: Visual inspection; look for the legs hanging out from the closed polyp.
Treatment: They must be manually removed with a forceps as they are protected from chemical treatment while they are inside the polyp.

Other Parasites

Red Planaria (*Convolutriloba retrogemma*) (Figure 1.17)

Diagnostics: Visual inspection, low magnification

Pathogenicity The pathogenicity of these worms comes from their ability to proliferate and an internal toxin. These flatworms can proliferate out of control if unregulated, resulting in two problems. The worms do not eat coral but they do irritate the coral tissues, resulting in less polyp

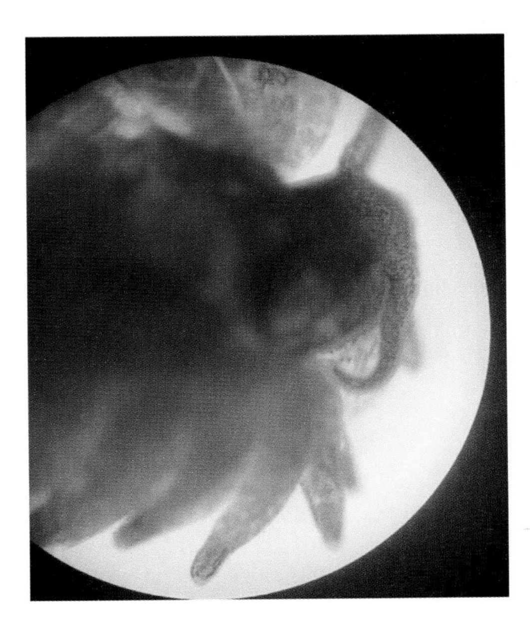

Figure 1.15 Zoanthid-eating nudibranch (10× magnification).

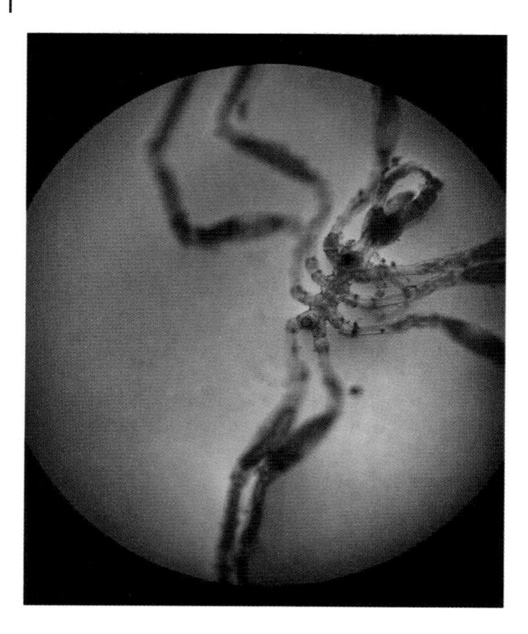

Figure 1.16 Pycnogonida species (10× magnification).

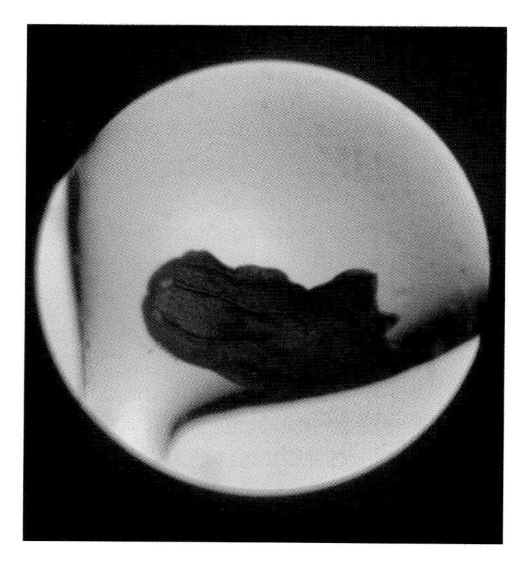

Figure 1.17 *Convolutriloba retrogemma* (10× magnification).

extension and unnecessary stress. If uninterrupted, these flatworms will proliferate until the population is too large for the environment to support them (Figure 1.18). This can result in a mass death of the flatworms and the release of their internal toxin. This toxin in a high enough concentration can cause a tank "crash." To prevent this toxic crash event, if you have red planaria it is imperative to be running fresh activated carbon, which has the ability to absorb the toxin that may be released into the water.

Treatment 1: Manual Removal Manual removal will be one of the biggest components of red planaria management. These flatworms proliferate at a tremendous rate. For the other treatment

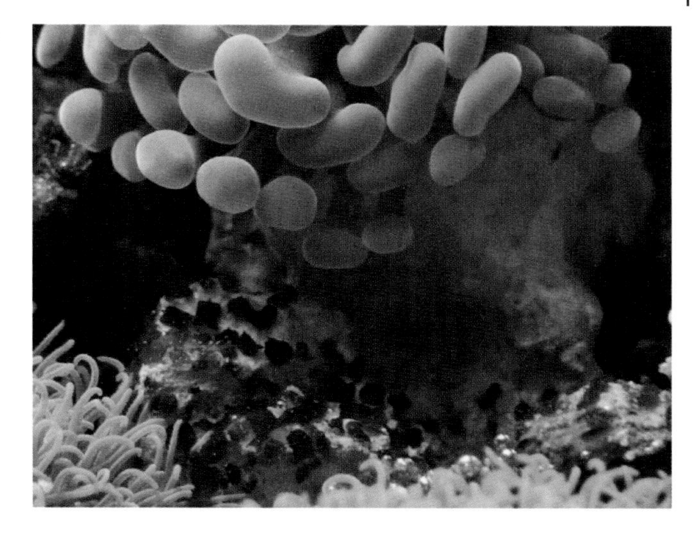

Figure 1.18 There is a large amount of planaria around the base of this *Euphyilla.*

modalities to be effective, they must be accompanied by manual removal of the worms. Methods of removal include:

1) Vacuuming the sand bed. These flatworms tend to stay towards the lower portions of the tank and the sand bed. Vacuuming the sand bed can remove a massive quantity of them.
2) Airline syphon. These flatworms have few adhesive properties and are easily knocked off their substrate. A gentle syphon with an airline manually moved over the rocks will easily suck the flatworms out of the tank.
3) Refugium cleaning. These worms can accumulate in massive quantities in a tanks refugium. Freshwater washes of hardy macroalgae can be very effective at flatworm removal.

Treatment 2: Biological Control These flatworms contain an unappetizing toxin, which deters natural predators. Thus, some of the usual flatworm consuming fish tend to ignore this species. Melanarus wrasses (*Halichoeres melanurus*) and sixline wrasses (*Pseudocheilinus hexataenia*) may be able to control minor infestations of red planaria. Alternatively, blue velvet nudibranch (*Chelidonura varians*) have a diet consisting of flatworms of various species.

Treatment 3: Chemical Control (Risky) Treatment of these worms chemically without collateral damage has proven to be challenging. There are several over the counter products labeled to treat these flatworms with uncertain efficacy.

Conclusion: As always, prevention and good biosecurity are always more effective than treatment.

Vermetidae Infestation

Species: *Vermetidae* spp.
Host: Any solid surface
Diagnostics: Visual inspection. Sometimes they are easier to spot after feeding as their mucus nets will be full of particulate.

These snails can grow on any hard surface, generally on the rock or near glass, near but not directly on growing corals (Figure 1.19). These worms release a mucus net to catch food. However, this mucus is extremely irritating to most species of coral, causing prolonged closure. Since these

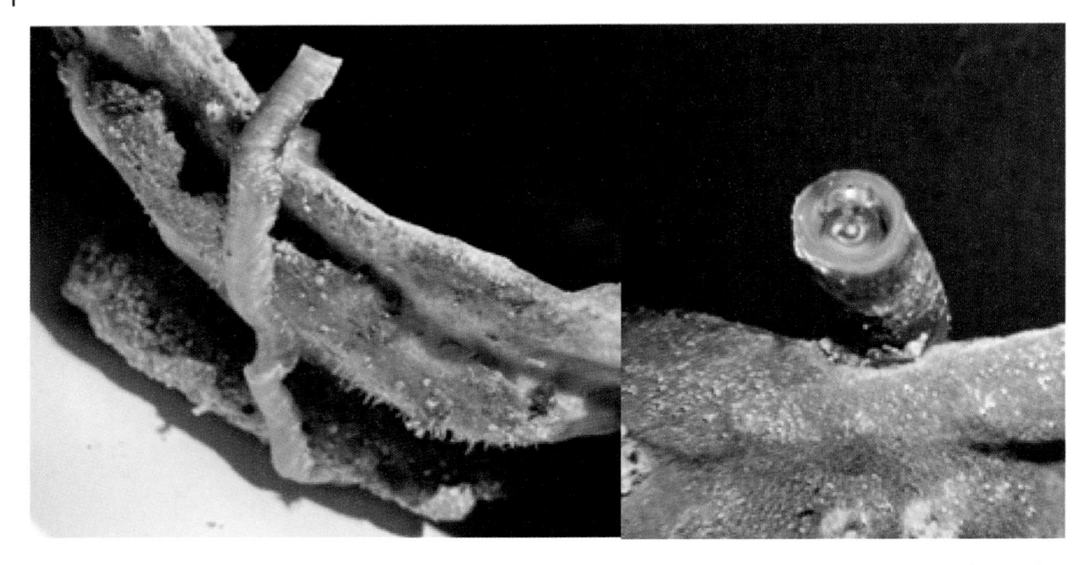

Figure 1.19 Vermentid snails can attach to any hard substrate. In this example, the sessile snail is growing off a Turbinaria species. Make sure to remove the bottom of the snail, as they will survive if only the top is crushed.

worms do not move their location, this persistent mucus will eventually kill nearby corals. Use bone cutters to crush the shell and remove the snail from its substrate.

Class Hydrozoa

Hydrozoans are the hydras, colonial hydroids, and colonial pelagic jellies like *Physalia physalis* (the Portuguese Man-of-War). Little is known about their pathology and diseases.

- Phylum Ctenophora: These are the comb jellies. Little is known about their pathology and diseases.
- Subphylum Urochordata: These are the tunicates (sea squirts) and a few other less well-known taxa (e.g. Salps). There are some economically important diseases that affect this group.

Introduction

The urochordates or tunicates make up an evolutionarily important group. They bridge invertebrates and vertebrates, making them interesting and valuable to researchers in a variety of disciplines. Many research facilities maintain cultures of urochordates or their cell lines. There is also some demand for these animals as human food or display in aquaria. There is relatively little information available on the diseases or treatments of these animals, but a few important disease problems are reviewed here.

Infectious Diseases

Secondary invasion of bacteria occurs as a result of injury or decomposition of dead epibiota. The latter is more common among aquarium animals, a function of deteriorating tissue remaining on the host as opposed to removal by scavengers in nature (Monniot, 1990).

Urochordate large body cavities with extensive water circulation make them good parasitic and commensal hosts, but there are few reports of pathogen-induced morbidity (Monniot, 1990; Moiseeva et al., 2004). The line between organisms being parasitic or commensal is often not clear in the literature. Metazoan commensals and parasites of urochordates are numerous and varied. Amphipods, annelids, barnacles, bivalves, bryozoans, cephalopods, cnidarians, copepods, ctenophores, decapods, fish, gastropods, isopods, nemerteans, and turbellarians have also been widely identified (Monniot, 1990). Appendix 1.1 lists the major disease syndromes of Urochordata.

Mollusks (Bivalves)

Mollusks represent a large phylum of invertebrates abundant in aquatic environments. Organisms within this grouping are highly diverse, including but not limited to bivalves (hinge-shelled mollusks such as mussels, oysters, scallops, and clams), cephalopods (squids, octopus, cuttlefish) and gastropods (slugs, snails, limpets). Discussion of the structure, life strategies, and diseases of all mollusks is out of the scope of this text. However, an effort has been made to present the basic assessment and differential diagnoses of a number of important aquacultured species from across the world, focused on bivalves.

Wild fisheries of bivalves farm such species as abalone, razor clams, scallops, and geoducks. Also harvested are gastropods such as winkles and whelks, sea urchins, and the cephalopods. In addition to fisheries, bivalves represent important aquaculture species in many countries, and are the focus of much research into their health for optimized production. Although many species are cultured for aquaria or display, this chapter focuses on two commonly cultured mollusks for human consumption: oysters and mussels. Cultured mussel species include blue or edible mussels (*Mytilus edulis*), as well as many other *Mytilus* and *Perna* species. Cultured oysters include the American oyster (*Crassostrea virginica*), European flat oyster (*Ostrea edulis*), and Pacific oysters (*Crassostrea gigas*). Other commercially important bivalves such as blood clams and Palourde clams are not covered here.

Bivalves vary greatly in their anatomy and life strategies. Sessile bivalves like mussels and oysters attach themselves to hard substrate using cement or byssal threads, forming large colonies in tidal or deeper water environments. The life cycles of bivalves vary between species, but a "standard" model involves external fertilization of released eggs, development to free-swimming larvae, and growth to spat and juvenile stages with shell development. Stage of settlement varies with species, but both mussels and oysters require a substrate for growth. Aquaculture of these organisms is then performed in different ways. Mussels produced using aquaculture can be cultured in various systems, including on longline ropes, rafts, or posts (Bouchot), whereas oysters are often grown in container systems. Both freshwater and marine mussel production occurs, although the majority are cultured in the marine environment.

Anatomy and Clinical Features

Shared anatomy of bivalves includes complete enclosure of organisms within the two valves of a shell, hinged by a ligament of elastic protein and held closed by adductor muscles. Food and oxygen are obtained from the aquatic environment when the shell is 'open' via filter feeding across bivalve gills, with inhaled and exhaled products often passed via siphons. Starvation and water quality are therefore important initial avenues of exploration in investigation of apparent pathology in bivalves. As with fish, uniform mortalities are suggestive of an environmental or husbandry issue, whereas less uniform patterns of impact suggest an infectious etiology.

Bivalves are problematic to assess clinically in open water. This is due partially to the presence of some organisms beneath substrate, or in non-tidal zones, but also due to their limited clinical signs. It is possible to assess larval feeding and behavior, however, and the behavior of gaping or

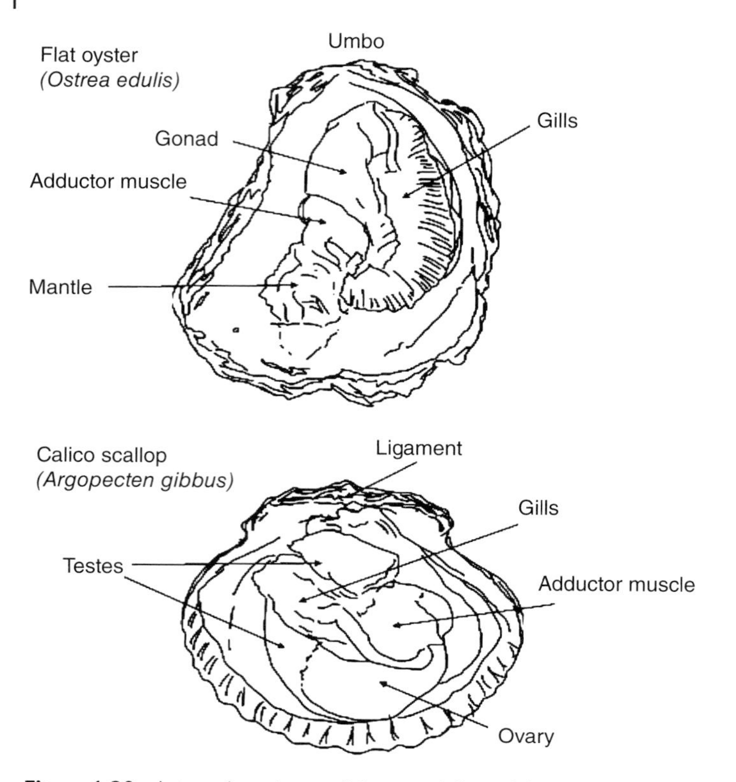

Figure 1.20 Internal anatomy of *Ostrea edulis* and *Argopecten gibbus* immediately on removal of one side shell valve.

delayed closer in adults is a useful indicator of impaired health. Further behavioral indices such as mobility can be assessed for a number of groups; scallops swim, clams burrow, and abalone graze. Signs are unfortunately mainly non-specific, and further investigation is often required.

When assessing the gross anatomy of bivalves, assessment should begin externally with the shell. The shell should then be opened carefully to avoid damaging soft internal structures (Figure 1.20). Visceral organs within can be described as firm/fat, medium, or of poor condition. Poor condition bivalves have limp, watery flesh that sinks away from shell edges and is often translucent in appearance. Mantle retraction is considered a common sign of poor health. Condition can also be quantitively measured using a tissue condition index (dry tissue/shell weight) or shell condition index (dry tissue weigh × 100/shell length). Overall, it should be noted that condition varies seasonally with events such as spawning, but poor conditions can also be a useful indicator of infectious pathology within animals.

Diagnostic interventions in the treatment of bivalves are similar to those available in the veterinary care of fish, including collection of samples for histology, molecular workup, and hemolymph (the bivalve equivalent to blood) for smears. Hemolymph is often obtained from the adductor muscle of bivalves. This can be done destructively or in live animals. Live sampling is performed through insertion of a needle between the shell valve opening, simply performed in some species such as *Mya arenaria* where valves do not tightly oppose. Other bivalves require a small notch to be made in the shell to allow access. Squash or smear preparations of tissue are useful initial diagnostic techniques too, particularly for protozoan organisms. A number of protozoans within bivalves are identified as notifiable diseases by the World Organisation for Animal Health (WOAH). Histology and molecular diagnostics thus often represent confirmatory diagnosis. When submitting samples for histology or molecular diagnostics, guidance is available from the Food and Agriculture Organization regarding totally sample number requirements to ensure detection of pathogens of different prevalence within a population. Davidson's fixative is recommended for bivalve tissue sections for histology.

For hobbyists and commercial producers, water quality is paramount for optimized bivalve health. Flow dynamics are also crucial for these organisms, in both environmental and recirculating settings. Nitrogenous waste buildup and availability of food are also important points to cover when taking a history for aquaria-reared bivalves. In addition to the infectious and production diseases that can impact bivalves, their method of filter feeding can lead to bioaccumulation of contaminants, algal toxins, and pathogens such as Norovirus or bacteria. If contamination is suspected, specialised sampling must be conducted in line with regional guidelines and legislation to ensure food safety.

Although contaminants such as algal toxins can induce altered gene expression within tissue, clinical indicators of exposure are often not observable. Specialised testing is therefore essential. Infectious diseases of concern for bivalve production largely differ from those of concern from a public health or zoonotic viewpoint. Some indicators used in public health surveillance can be informative though in exploring pathology observed within a population, such as assessment of levels of metallothionein as an indicator of level of heavy metal exposure, or mixed function oxygenase as indicator of organic xenobiotic compound (hydrocarbons, pesticides) exposure.

Clinical Differentials

Clinical presentation is hard to discern for living bivalves beyond determining if the organism is alive, responsive or motile (where relevant). A healthy mussel, for example, will be either closed or the shell partially opened with the siphon extended for feeding. Gently touching an open mussel should lead to the shell closing. A "gaping" shell is suggestive of death, and a delayed closure response might be considered lethargy. The remainder of mollusk anatomy is not externally visible. Assessment of the shell can though provide useful insight into bivalve health. In addition to any visible shell lesions or fouling, appraisal of the shell can give an indication of previous stresses. Expected growth rate of mussels varies between species and with environmental parameters (with selectively bred aquaculture mussels tending to grow faster than their wild counterparts, and slower growth occurring in winter months). With a good understanding of the life history of the bivalve in question, however, growth rings on the shell can be a valuable indicator of patterns of stress or periods of reduced growth. Shell is deposited sequentially throughout the life of bivalves, so a closer pattern of ridges indicates periods of slower growth. A disrupted pattern might indicate a stress event or pathological condition that impaired growth or calcium metabolism. Calcareous shell tissue is also laid down internally to wall off damage or the attempted ingress of parasites to the viscera. These shell nodules are often described as "blisters" and can be mud filled. Generally, however, holes in the shell are of little consequence unless full-thickness perforation has occurred – in which case this can lead to further pathogen ingress. Biofouling on the inner shell can also indicate general weakness of the bivalve.

In addition to the causative agents of clinical signs described below, incidental findings might be reported from diagnostic workups. Ciliates, parasitic copepods, and lipofuscin pigment accumulation (associated with pollution exposure and other stresses, but a common finding in older mussels) are usually of little consequence in health screens. A strong smell when handling freshly obtained bivalves can indicate a soft tissue pathology, is also suggestive of less than fresh samples.

Gaping or moribund bivalves should be avoided in sample collection where possible. One shocking but occasional finding can be the expulsion of red liquid on shucking of a bivalve. This is usually due to release of pigmented algae in seawater from a closed shell. Algal presence is of little concern unless associated with toxic algal blooms.

Specific Diseases

Of the major economically significant diseases in oysters and mussels, many are WOAH notifiable. Detailed description of the diagnosis and control of these conditions and the other notifiable diseases of mollusks are available in the WOAH *Manual of Aquatic Animal Disease*. The conditions of concern for other aquaculture mollusks including diseases of razor clams, scallops, limpets, and other clams are not covered in this chapter, but do present essential reading in understanding the breadth of infectious disease in shellfish.

Reported diseases of importance in abalone include abalone viral ganglioneuritis (abalone herpes virus) and the notifiable condition withering syndrome (*Xenophaliotis californiensis*). Brief details of some of the major pathologies of concern in oysters and mussels are given here; however, this list is not exhaustive, and further reading of texts listed in the bibliography are recommended.

Ostreid Herpes Virus

Brief overview: Ostreid herpes virus (OsHV-1) is a viral disease with a number of variants identified within a different mollusk species.

Host range and distribution: It is documented as causing mortalities primarily in the larvae and juvenile life states of *Crassostrea gigas* and *Crassostrea angulate*. Other variants can have different host species.

Transmission: Transmission is considered to be host to host by shedding from adjacent infected individuals. Latently infected individuals, as well as actively diseased stock, are thought to transmit viral particles.

Signs/diagnosis: High mortality (up to 100%) is the main indicator of active infection within a population, often occurring during the summer (temperatures exceeding 16°C). A reduction in swimming and feeding behavior of larvae can be seen, whereas adults present as gaping and slow to close when stimulated to do so, however none of these signs are pathognomonic. Definitive diagnosis can only be reached using molecular techniques such as polymerase chain reaction and sequencing.

Differentials: Diseases that present similarly include other viral pathologies, as well as systemic bacterial infections, and the major protozoan infections of bivalves. Samples should be collected for molecular as a priority, as well as histopathology and electron microscopy.

Treatment: No treatment is currently available for OsHV-1.

Management: Biosecurity is paramount. Quarantine procedures and hygiene such as filtration and ultraviolet treatment of water are recommended.

Bonamia

Brief overview: *Bonamia ostrea* and *Bonamia exitosa* are protozoan parasites within the Haplosporidian phylum that cause lethal disease in bivalve oysters (Figure 1.21).

Host range and distribution: Transmission: *B. ostrea* is known to infect Australian mud oyster (*O. angasi*), Chilean flat oyster (*Ostrea chilensis*), Olympia flat oyster (*Ostrea conchaphila*), Asiatic oyster (*Ostrea denselammellosa*), European flat oyster (*O. edulis*) and Argentinian oysters (*Ostrea puelchana*). *B. exitosa* infects *Ostrea stenina*, European flat oysters, Australian mud oysters, and Chilean flat oysters. Transmission occurs both vertically and horizontally through released infective particles, hypothesized to be via the gills. These are ingested by oysters and infective particles are phagocytosed by hemocytes where they are infective. Older individuals appear more susceptible to disease. *B. ostreae*, *C. gigas*, and *Mytilus edulis* appear resistant to infection.

Signs/diagnosis: Clinical indicators are non-specific. Mass mortalities within a population can be observed, with infection late autumn/winter and deaths peaking in spring of *B. ostrea*. Infected individuals can also be clinically normal. Previously reported gross changes include yellow to black discoloration, lesions such as ulcers in the connective tissues of the gills, mantle, and digestive gland (Comps et al., 1980). These gross signs are not pathognomonic for infection with *B. ostrea* and most infected oysters appear normal. Gill imprints and histology are both useful in diagnosing infection with this parasite (Figure 1.21a). Transmission electron microscopy can help differentiate *Bonamia* organisms. Specific PCR represents an option for confirmatory information, as well as diagnosis from larvae.

Differentials: High mortalities can occur due to a number of infectious and non-infectious challenges to oysters. Tissue ulceration when present is not unique to *B. ostrea* infection, and discoloration can be caused by other protozoal infections, as well as viral, bacterial and fungal infections. Gill erosions can occur as well with OsHV-1 infections.

Treatment: There is currently no treatment available for *B. ostrea* or *B. exitosa* infection in oysters.

Management: General husbandry practices should be implemented to avoid stressing a population.

Perkinsus

Brief overview: *Perkinsus* species (previously referred to as *Dermocystidium*) infect mollusks globally. *Perkinsus olensi marinus* is the causative agent of 'dermo' disease in oysters, and although *P. olensi* infects primarily clams, it is also a concern in oysters.

Host range and distribution: *P. marinus* infects *Crassostrea virginica* (the most susceptible species), *Crassostrea gigas*, *Crassostrea ariakensis*, *Crassostrea rhizophorae*, and *Crassostrea corteziensis* oysters, as well as the mollusks *Mya arenaria* and *Macoma balthica*. Infection can be lethal or may persist throughout life. *P. olseni* is primarily a pathogen of venerid clams, although it does also infect *C. virginica*.

Transmission: All *Perkinsus* life stages are infective and are acquired through horizontal transmission in host feces or disrupted diseased tissue, with uptake by feeding.

Signs/diagnosis: Infection is often eventually lethal. Oysters can be infected for one to two years prior to mortality, with deaths coinciding with high water temperatures. Infection presents as a chronic wasting condition, with *P. martinus* infection leading to pale, poor-condition tissue. Macroscopic nodules in tissue are also reported. Multifocal lesions containing *Perkinsus* cells and infiltrated haemocytes can be observed in histopathology sections, with definitive diagnosis achieved using molecular techniques.

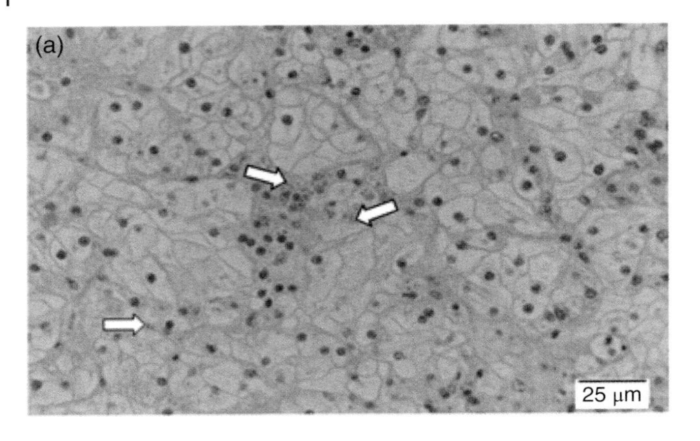

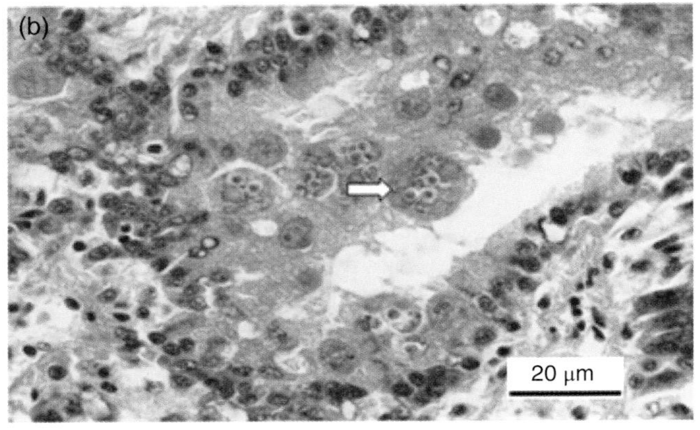

Figure 1.21 *Bonamia ostrea* and *Marteilia refringens* in oyster tissues. Scale bar 25μm. Hematoxylin and eosin stain. a) *B. ostrea* parasites (arrows) within connective tissue cells of European flat oyster *Ostrea edulis*. Scale bar 20μm. Hematoxylin and eosin stain. b) *M. refrigens* parasites within the digestive gland of European flat oyster, *O. edulis*. Note the cell within cell arrangement of the cells (arrow). Scale bar = 20 micrometers/Hematoylin and eosin stain.

Differentials: Similar wasting conditions are reported with viral infections such as hemocyte infection virus, or even seasonal changes associated with spawning or over stocking. Prolonged *Marteilia* infection presents similarly with poor condition and mantle retractions.

Treatment: Bacitracin, cycloheximide and freshwater treatments have been demonstrated to reduce *P. marinus* load in hosts. N-halamine compounds kill *P. marinus* cells without impacting larvae, indicating a use in disinfection of contaminated eggs and larvae.

Marteilia

Brief overview: *Marteilia* parasites are thought to have an indirect life cycle with suggested intermediate hosts including nematodes, copepods and cnidaria. *Marteilia refringens* infects both mussels and oysters as the final host, although geographical distribution is thus far limited mainly to Europe and Northern Africa.

Host range and distribution: Oyster and mussel species in which *Marteilia* have been observed include *Ostrea edulis*, *Crassostrea virginica*, *Mytilus edulis*, *Mytilus galloprovincialis*, *Xenostrobus secures*, *Ostrea chilensis*, *Ostrea puelchana*, *Ostrea angasi*, *Ostrea denselamellosa*, and *Ostrea stentina*. *M. refringens* also impacts the clams *Solen marginatus*, *Chamelea gallina*, *Ruditapes decussatus*, *Ruditapes philippinarum*, *Tapes rhomboides*, *Tapes pullastra*, *Ensis minor*, *Ensis siliqua*, and cockles (*Cerastoderma edule*).

Transmission: Juveniles and adults can become infected by horizontal transmission of shed propagules in feces. The impact on oysters is much greater from this infection, which can last over a lifetime.

Signs/diagnosis: Wild populations of *O. edulis* and mussels can present without obvious clinical impact, but naïve populations can also see very high mortalities. Infection in oysters can also be lethal. Deaths coincide with parasite sporulation in late summer/autumn (water temperature 17°C). Gross changes include pale, poor-condition flesh with watery viscera and mantle retraction. Reduced growth rate is reported in oysters and mussels from impaired uptake ability of nutrition and storage, with impaired gonad development also reported for infected mussels.

Histopathology is considered diagnostic in infected juveniles and adults (Figure 1.21b). Tissue imprints can also provide initial diagnosis, with confirmatory diagnosis as ever achieved using molecular techniques such as PCR and sequencing.

Differentials: Chronic wasting in this condition presents similarly to *Perkinsus* infection, as well as viral conditions and starvation.

Mikrocytos mackini

Brief overview: *Mikrocytos mackini* infection (sometimes referred to as Denman Island disease) is a condition that appears ubiquitous to some regions of Western North America, but is not found and therefore of great importance if isolated elsewhere.

Host range and distribution: *Crassostrea gigas*, *Crassostrea virginica*, *Ostrea edulis* and *Ostrea lurida* oysters are all susceptible to infection.

Transmission: Transmission appears to be horizontal open death of the initial host, and through feeding uptake by the next.

Signs/diagnosis: Infection at cooler temperatures (10°C for 3–4 months) is considered essential for disease development. Mortalities occur therefore in the spring, and infections appear otherwise to be subclinical. Moribund individuals gape and are slow to close. Foci of pustules (up to 5 mm in diameter) are seen in the body wall, adductor or on the mantle and labial palps due to hemocyte accumulation. Pustules typical of this disease are usually green but can range from yellow–brown to colorless.

Differentials: Other conditions can cause high mortality in the spring. Pustules appear similar to conditions such as systemic bacterial disease, *Bonamia* infection and Pacific oyster nocardiosis (*Nocardia crassostreae*).

Treatment: There are no currently available treatments, vaccinations, or decontamination protocols for this pathogen.

Management: New stock should not be seeded at low tide or prior to June. Mature stock should be harvested within three years and before February.

Haplosporidia

Overview: Haplosporidia are organisms of importance as major marine epizootics not only in bivalves but also crustaceans. They are a concern for both cultured and wild populations, with consequences for aquaculture, food security, and ecosystem health.

Host range: Research is continuing to characterise the diversity of these organisms. *Haplosporidium nelson* and *Haplosporidium costale* infect Pacific oysters such as *Crassostrea virginica* and *Crassostrea gigas*. Recently reclassified, *Haplosporidium amoricana* infects mussels such as *Ostrea edulis* as well as crab species, and recently described *Haplosporidium pinnae* is linked with disease in *Pinna nobilis* (fan mussel). Parasite abundance is linked with seasonal changes, including warm temperatures and high salinity.

Transmission: It is suspected that an intermediate host acts in transmission.

Signs/diagnosis: Infection of *H. nelson* and *H. costale* can manifest as slow growth or deformities within a population, or with altered environmental conditions, mass mortalities can occur. Brown discoloration to the gill and mantle have been previously described for all species. Diagnosis is achieved by histology and molecular techniques.

Differentials: Brown discoloration presents similarly to changes with bacteria disease, and phaeohyphomycosis. The majority of notifiable pathologies can cause high mortalities, and deformities can be induced by any number of stressed.

Treatment: There are currently no treatment options available for these organisms.

Management: Filtration and ultraviolet radiation of influent water in hatcheries seems to be effective in prevention.

Other Pathologies

Although not covered here, a number of important pathologies impact other commercially important bivalves. Resources are provided at the end of the section to assist in understanding the health of these additional species.

In addition to pathologies caused by viruses, bacteria, fungi, and parasites, a number of additional factors can impact bivalve health. Infectious neoplastic conditions of unknown etiology appear important in large-scale mortality events of various oyster and mussel species for example, and bacterial disease are frequently reported, either as systemic infections or due to endotoxic effects. Of major consideration are environmental and non-infectious impacts on health. Temperature, pH, and salinity are important to bivalve growth and survival, as are presence of toxic algae, pollutants, and suspended solids. High inorganic suspended solids can impair feeding in bivalves, and bioaccumulation of aquatic contaminants has been linked to many instances of reduced production and even failure of stocks. Die-off can occur from as simple a reason as altered water parameters, so environmental factors must always be considered when exploring suspected disease in bivalves.

Zoonoses

Handling shellfish often leads to cuts or mild abrasions of the skin because of their sharp shells. Systemic infection leading to sepsis is rare but not unheard of. An important consideration for bivalves and public health specifically is their adaptation for filter feeding, and the potential to bioaccumulate toxic products of phytoplankton. Shellfish toxins and infectious agents like Norovirus and various bacterial pathogens from bivalves are a food safety concern, causing poisoning in humans. Even with proper cooking, toxic algae and viral pathologies can cause severe disease, and in some extreme cases, death. Care should therefore be taken in harvesting bivalves during seasonal peaks of algal blooms. Commonly held knowledge is that bivalves are unsafe to eat when gaping (which is true); however, those that do not gape can also pose a risk to public health.

Abalone

Abalone are herbivorous marine gastropods. Common species of abalone are listed; those with asterisks are commercially grown in aquaculture: brownlip abalone (*Haliotis conicopora*), greenlip abalone (*Haliotis laevigata*), Roe's abalone (*Haliotis roei*), blacklip abalone (*Haliotis rubra*), "tiger" abalone (hybrid of *H. laevigata* and *H. rubra*), diversicolor or jiukong abalone (*Haliotis diversicolor*). The anatomy and function of abalone are illustrated in Figures 1.22 and 1.23).

Culture Methods

- Land-based raceway: Long, shallow ponds are situated adjacent to the sea for access to seawater. Hides to provide habitats and parallel ridges along the base of tanks are positioned to allow periodic flushing of detritus down the channels. Abalone are fed a pelleted diet.
- Ranch: Habitats made of large concrete blocks anchored to a sandy seabed are placed in the ocean. Abalone stay in their habitats and do not escape since they dislike travelling across the sand substrate. Ocean currents deliver detached seaweed to the hides.

Breeding

Broodstock may be harvested from the wild or are line bred. Spawning is by adding peroxide to the water to simulate stormy weather that creates free radicals in the water. Larvae are grown on plastic sheets with a lawn of algae.

Anesthetics

Various anesthetics have been used for handling, grading, or transferring animals, and all have depressive effects on growth rates. However, benzocaine has the fewest adverse effects.

Environmental Requirements

Temperature:

- Greenlip: growth 12–22°C (prefer 18°C)
- Blacklip: growth 10–22°C (prefer 16–18°C)
- Roe's: growth 14–26°C
- Donkey ear: growth 20–32°C (prefer 28°C)
- Diurnal variations may also impact growth rates.

pH:

- Greenlip: 7.78-8.77
- Blacklip: 7.93-8.46
- Hazardous if < 7.16 or > 9.01.

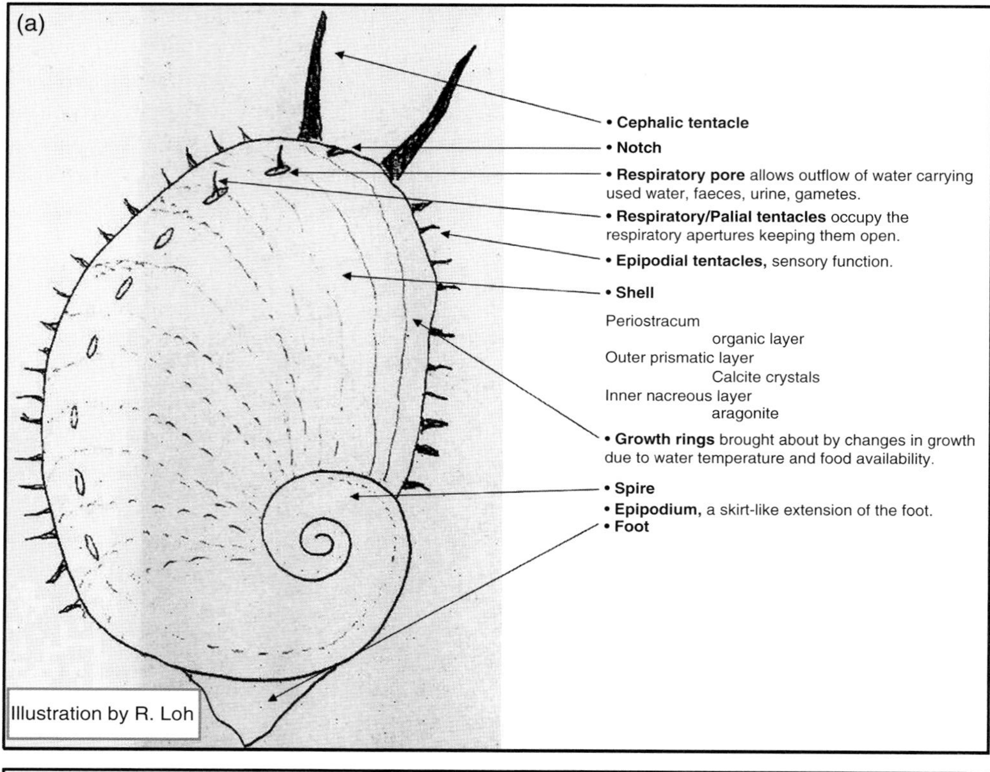

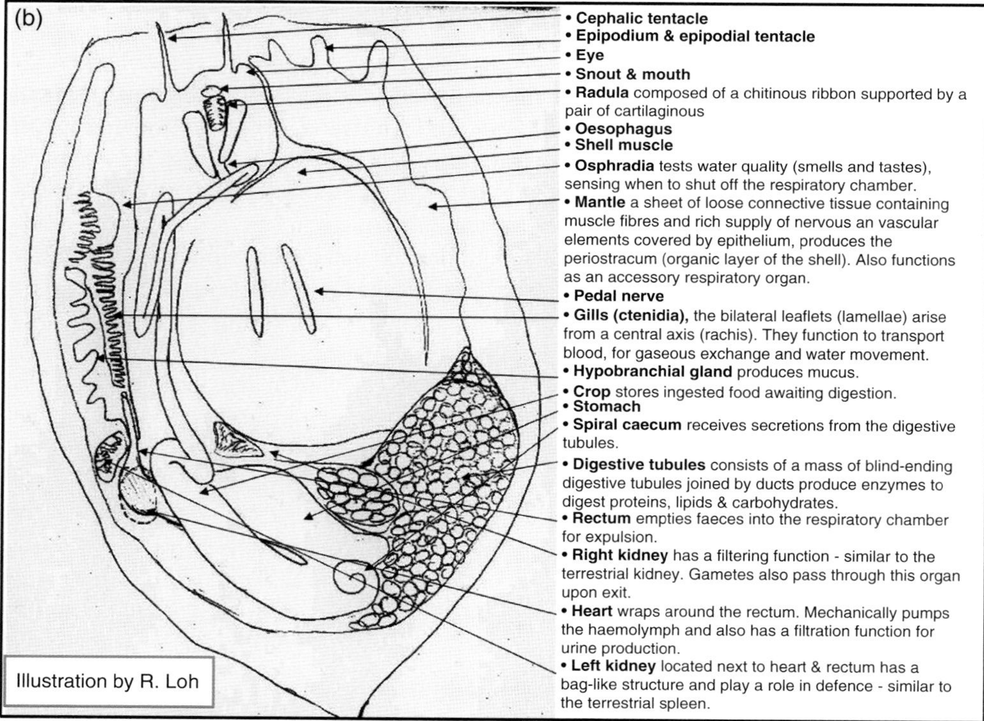

Figure 1.22 Anatomy and function of abalone. a) Dorsal view. b) Internal structure. (Illustrations by R. Loh).

Salinity:

- Optimal: 35 ppt
- Greenlip: 25–40 ppt
- Blacklip: 25–40 ppt
- Abalone do not tolerate freshwater and will develop skin blisters if exposed to raindrops.

Stocking density:

- No more than 40kg/m^3
- Average commercially 20kg/m^3

Ammonia:

- Chronic exposure is detrimental, and its effect depends on the interaction with dissolved oxygen.

Refuge:

- Abalone prefer dim to dark areas with increased activity, including feeding at night. Provide refuges and house in sheds or under thick shade cloth.

Infectious and Parasitic Diseases

Viral Abalone viral ganglioneuritis is a herpesvirus that causes intense hemocytic inflammation of the nervous tissue, causes weakness and paralysis with a rapid and high cumulative mortality of up to 90%. Radula may protrude, but usually, affected abalone are found dead. In wild populations, there may be large numbers of clean (empty) shells on the substrate due to predation or scavenging by other animals of moribund or dead abalone.

Bacterial Commonly *Vibrio* species cause "abscesses" or septicemia. Primary bacterial diseases are associated with *Vibrio splendidus*, *Vibrio alginolyticus*, *Vibrio parahaemolyticus* and *Vibrio harveyi*. Other bacterial infections tend to be secondary to stress, mainly due to heat stress, handling, and poor water quality.

Withering syndrome is a fatal disease caused by an intracellular *Rickettsia*-like bacterium *Xenohaliotis californiensis*, with upwards of 95% mortalities. It is a WOAH-listed disease. Other kinds of *Rickettsia*-like organisms are considered incidental. Superficial epithelial erosion is associated with *Flavobacterium*-like bacteria.

Fungal *Atkinsiella awabi* causes tubercle disease, with animals dying from rapidly progressing focal foot lesions with extensive inflammation. Histologically, fungal hyphae are poorly staining and are of variable thickness. Shell mycosis creates blisters of conchiolin and nacre on the interior rather than the shell's exterior. This results in loss of value of the shell and can be fatal if it affects the foot muscle attachment.

Protistans *Perkinsus olseni* is the most pathogenic. They are found systemically, incite intense hemocytic reaction and can cause vessel blockage (infarction) and gill necrosis. Other *Perkinsus* species are considered incidental. Detectable by histology, molecular tests, or incubating fresh gill tissues in Ray's thioglycollate broth for detecting Perkinsus infection.

The thraustochytrid *Labyrinthuloides haliotidis* only infects very young abalone when their cellular and humoral defenses are immature. Older animals (over one year) are refractory to becoming parasitized.

Incidental Findings

- Coccidian-like infection of the oesophageal pouch and intestinal mucosa.
- Cryptosporidian-like parasites have been observed in the intestinal epithelium.
- Holotrichous ciliates are found free in the lumen or adherent to the mucosa of the digestive gland, including the oesophageal pouch, in gills, and on the surface of the foot, with no associated host reaction.
- Mantoscyphidian-like ciliates (peritrichous ciliates) may be found attached to the gills, mantle cavity, and esophageal pouch epithelium, or attached to or cover without obvious host response or pathology.
- Intracellular parasites of the digestive gland.
- *Pseudoklossia*-type coccidia in the left kidney.
- *Nematopsis*-like gregarines are found in the interstitial tissue.

Helminths

Spionid Mudworms The polychetes *Boccardia knoxi*, *Boccardia chilensis*, *Polydora hoplura*, *Polydora*, *Polydora websterii*, and *Polydora armata* cause damage to the shells as they bore into the shell of abalone. The internal shell surfaces will have "mud blisters" covered by nacre. This diverts energy demand towards walling off the polychetes and potentially contaminates meat at processing or are unsightly for live trade. Small "chimneys" made by the worms may be observed on the external shell surfaces. The polychetes can be extracted for speciation from abalone shells by placing shells in a 50% alcohol and 50% seawater mix. This method causes the worms to either escape their burrows completely and then die where they can be easily collected, or at least expose themselves out of their burrows where they could be pulled out manually. An interactive key has been constructed (Wilson and McDiarmid 2004) and was used in conjunction with a review of the spionids present in Southern Australia by Blake and Kudenov (1978) to identify the key features of these taxa.

The sabellid polychete *Terebrasabella heterouncinata* causes poor productivity in abalone, and affected animals develop deformed capped-shaped shells. The sabellid larvae only settle on live gastropod shells as they rely on the host reaction to cover the parasite to form their burrows. Burrows appear as pinpoint lesions on the exterior surface from which the brachial crown of the worm protrudes during feeding.

Nematodes *Echinocephalus pseudouncinatus* causes foot muscle weakness and decreases the efficacy of this structure as a hold-fast organ making infected abalone easy to remove from the rock substrate. It is zoonotic, where consumption of live worms can lead to larval migrans. Abalone and sea urchins act as intermediate hosts, with adult worms maturing in elasmobranchs as definitive hosts. Other nematodes are found incidentally reported in the connective tissue near the mouth/esophagus.

Cestodes Plerocercids (the second intermediate host of the cestode) have been reported as incidental findings, with birds likely as the final host. They possibly belong to the genus *Polypocephalus* or *Tylocephalum* in the Family Lecanicephalidea.

Trematodes Metacercarial infections have been reported with little effect on survival. The abalone's gonad appeared to be the initial site of infection, and heavy infections in the gonad may occasionally cause castration. Imparts an orange discoloration if large numbers are encysted within the gills. Metacercariae may also be found in the right kidney and the esophagus's lamina propria.

Non-Infectious Diseases

Heat stress Abalone from temperate environments are prone to heat stress. The author's laboratory findings for heat-stressed greenlip abalone are summarized below:

- Intravascular glassy hypereosinophilic material (presumed fibrin) in the interstitium between digestive tubules.
- Left kidney fimbrial sinuses were expanded by moderate amounts of eosinophilic fluid (interpreted as hemolymph pooling), and others as hypereosinophilic glassy material (presumed fibrin).
- Gonads were consistent with the end of spawning or the beginning of a new cycle.
- Hemocytosis of the epipodium and mantle were seen in some.
- Reduced mucus cells at the gill tips (C. Hooper, personal communication, 2020).

Miscellaneous Findings

Wild-caught animals carry a range of fauna on their shells, including algae, sponges such as *Cliona* spp., cunjevoi (sea squirt), barnacles, oysters, other mollusks, and other harmless worms (spirorbids and *Pomatoceros* spp.). In the gills of wild abalone, there may be foreign-body type, hemocytic granulomatous reactions related to *Bacillariophyta* diatom algae or sponge spicules.

Sampling for Laboratory Testing

Necropsy A video detailing abalone anatomy and how to safely shuck (remove the abalone from its shell), draw hemolymph (abalone blood) for hemocyte analysis and bacteriology, and sampling organs for histopathology, *Perkinsus* testing and molecular analysis in a necropsy/autopsy by Dr. Loh the Fish Vet is available on YouTube (Biology lesson: Abalone autopsy/necropsy dissection of abalone, preparation for laboratory testing, 2016. https://youtu.be/vnms4gXOKik).

Hemocyte Counts A Neubauer hemocytometer is filled with undiluted hemolymph, and hemocyte counts are carried out immediately on five 0.2 mm squares. The average count is multiplied by a factor of 250 to derive the total chamber count for 1 cubic mm. The mean hemocyte count in greenlip abalone is 7317 cells/mm^3. Abalone infected with hemocyte parasites have lower counts, averaging 5680 cells/mm^3. The author has conducted hemocytes counts in heat-stressed sick animals, finding considerably lower counts at 450–2700 cells/mm^3.

Hemolymph Biochemistry It is thought that marine invertebrates are iso-osmotic with their environment. To investigate this preconception, the author has conducted some biochemistry testing by comparing heat-stressed ($n = 12$), recovered ($n = 15$) and healthy ($n = 10$) greenlip abalone. It is admittedly a small sample size; however, some patterns emerged. Healthy abalone appear able to achieve homeostasis for total protein ($\bar{x} = 4.7$ mmol/l), ammonia ($\bar{x} =$ 71–91 mmol/l), and creatinine ($\bar{x} =$ 108–126 mmol/l). The levels in sick abalone were unchanged for total protein ($\bar{x} = 5.0$ mmol/l) but were elevated for ammonia ($\bar{x}=130$ mmol/l), and reduced for creatinine ($\bar{x}=97$ mmol/l). All abalone appear to maintain above seawater levels for Ca ($\bar{x} =$ 12–13 mmol/l), Mg ($\bar{x} =$ 56–59 mmol/l), Na ($\bar{x} =$ 495–513 mmol/l), Cl ($\bar{x} =$

549–582 mmol/l), and K ($\bar{x}$ = 12.0–13.5 mmol/l). The results for these parameters in sick animals had a downward trend toward seawater levels. The iron level was higher in the recovering animals ($\bar{x}$ = 8.9 mmol/l) compared to the sick ($\bar{x}$ = 5.4 mmol/l) and healthy ($\bar{x}$ = 4.0 mmol/l) animals. Other biochemical parameters tested in the panel, with futile results, included creatine kinase, alanine transaminase, gamma-glutamyl transferase, glutamate dehydrogenase, total bilirubin, conjugated bilirubin, urea, phosphate, β-hydroxybutyric acid, cholesterol, albumin, and albumin/globulin.

Histology Assessment Examine for and quantify epithelial loss from foot, dilation of hemolymph channels, protein deposits in soft tissues or intravascular, pigmentation in the kidney or digestive gland, hemocytic response, necrosis, and infectious agents. A nutritional or general health assessment can be based on the digestive tubule spacing scoring system developed by Dr. Anna Mouton. Any separation of spaces between the digestive tubules is regarded as abnormal and indicates suboptimal conditions. Dilated right kidney tubules indicate poor water quality, overstocking, insufficient water flow, and poor tank hygiene, and also occur with returning abalone to water after handling and transport.

Cephalopods

A listing of clinical signs with differentials of cephalopods can be found in Appendix 1.1.

Gastropods

It is beyond the scope of this text to address all the current knowledge of this group. Some publications on gastropod diseases are included in the bibliography.

Crustacea

A listing of clinical signs with differentials of *Crustacea* is provided in Appendix 1.1.

Overview

The crustaceans are a group of invertebrate organisms containing many commercially important farmed and wild fisheries species. A great number of different aquaculture industries exist, but marine species Pacific white shrimp (*Penaeus vannamei*) and tiger shrimp (*Penaeus monodon*) are the most commonly farmed species, with the remainder of aquaculture crustaceans largely farmed in fresh water. The majority of this aquaculture occurs in Asia, but is also found in Central and South America. Crustacea of note in North America and Europe are largely obtained from fisheries, particularly focused on crabs and lobsters, although an industry for crayfish production does exist.

Each species and method of production has its own set of challenges and common disorders, some beyond the scope of this chapter to describe. Insight into the disease of both cultured and wild fisheries is, however, of importance to aquatic veterinary professionals, and an overview is provided here, with further reading recommended for greater detail. In addition to fisheries and aquaculture for food production, crustaceans are relatively popular in small aquaria, where multiple shrimp species, hermit crabs, and other small crabs are common ornamental additions.

Biology

Crustacea are a diverse subphylum within Arthropoda that includes copepods such as parasitic sea lice and even woodlice. The crustaceans identified as particularly of interest to aquatic veterinary specialists in this section are the decapods: crabs, lobsters, prawns, shrimp, and crayfish. The complex development, varied morphology, and divergent physiology of crustaceans must be appreciated to fully understand the approach to diagnosis and treatment of disease. This section provides a very brief overview of crustacean biology, with additional reading highly recommended. Not all diseases listed are documented as impacting all species within defined groups, so care must also be taken to avoid presumptive diagnosis without further reading.

A large amount of anatomical and physiological features separate crustaceans from fish (Figures 1.23, 1.24 and 1.25). Respiration is still achieved using gills, with similar important functions in osmoregulation and nitrogenous waste excretion. Unlike fish, however, a number of Crustacea species are able to breath atmospheric oxygen. Indeed, species such as hermit crabs are obligate air breathers and can drown. For many other crustaceans, though, provided that the gills are kept moist, respiration can be achieved both above and under water. Instead of blood, crustacean organs are bathed in oxygen-carrying fluid as part of an open circulatory system. The decapods addressed in this chapter use hemocyanin [KB(1)] as their oxygen-carrying pigment, a copper-based protein that is blue when oxygenated. Oxygen is supplied in this manner by the hemolymph plasma, rather than contained within erythrocyte cells. The hemocyanin gives a blue color appearance to the blood analog hemolymph, a color that can be seen externally in some thin-shelled species. When challenged by infectious agents, the repertoire of crustacean immune defenses is divergent from that of vertebrates. Crustaceans are not capable of building adaptive immunity and rely solely on innate responses. These responses are based mainly on the phagocytic

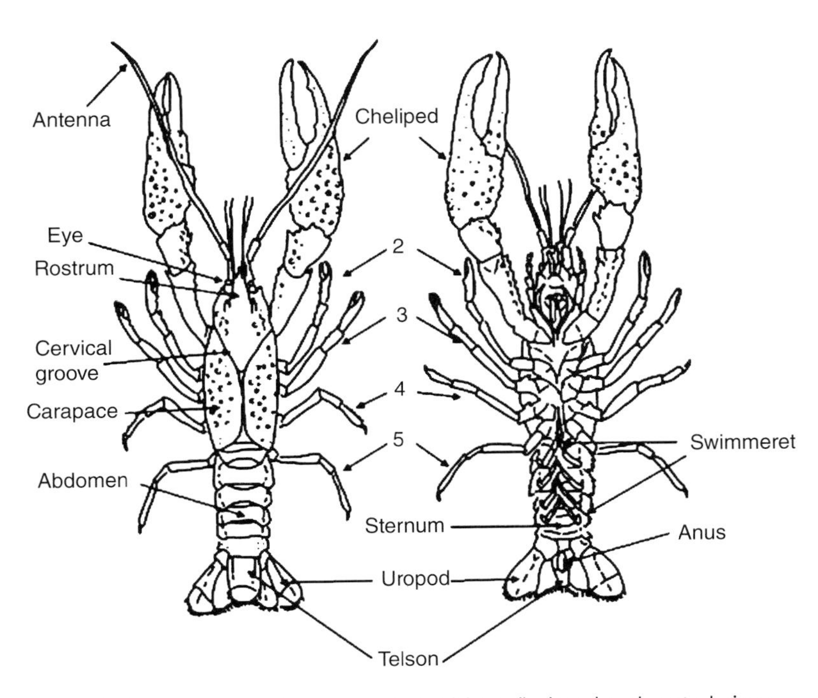

Figure 1.23 General anatomy of a lobster (clawed); dorsal and central views.

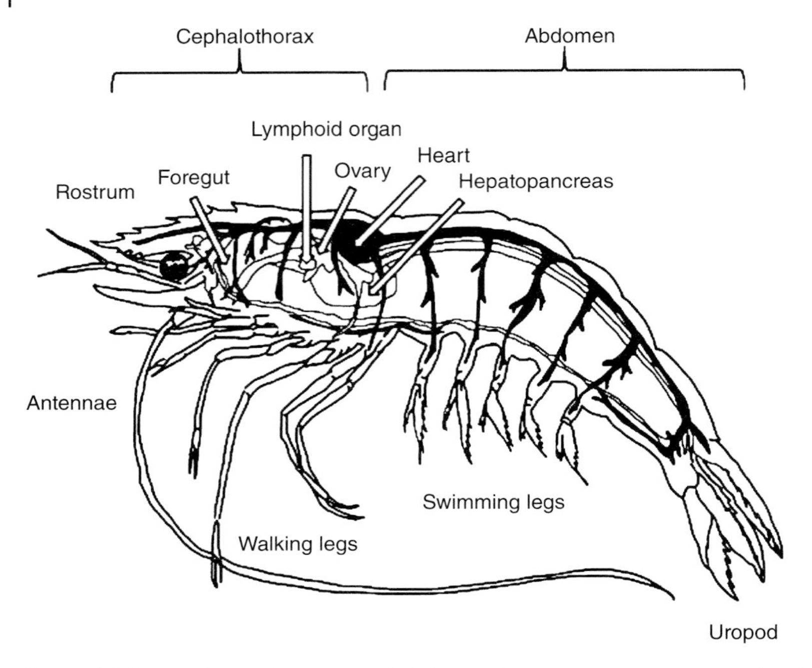

Figure 1.24 The internal anatomy of shrimp and prawns can, to an extent, be observed during the clinical examination. The majority of organs (anterior ganglion, brain, heart, gonads, foregut, and hepatopancreas) are located in the cephalothorax.

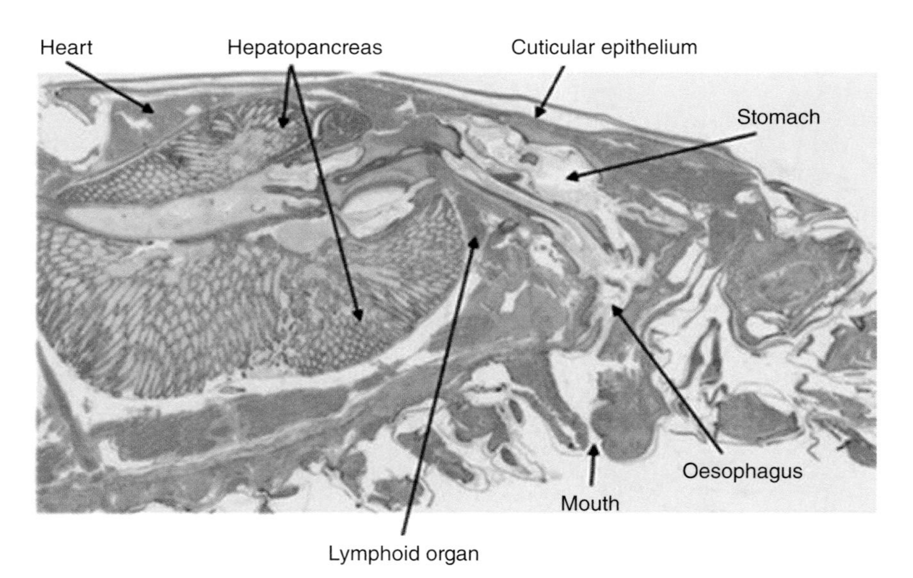

Figure 1.25 Penaeid shrimp cross-sectional anatomy.

and reactive oxygen species production capacity of immunologically active hemocytes as part of their alternative to blood, hemolymph, as well as antimicrobial peptides. Encapsulation and melanization of localized insults as "nodules" is considered an important aspect of host defense.

Individuals are usually of separate sexes, producing eggs that are either laid into the water column or remain attached to the female until they are ready to hatch. Larval development progresses through various stages of molting until adult morphology is achieved. Adult decapods are protected by an exoskeleton, which might include a carapace on the cranial aspect, the site of much externally observable pathology. The exoskeleton arrangement depends on the form and segmentation of the crustacean in question, with variation in antennae and appendage numbers.

Crustaceans shed their shells in a process called molting, which allows an increase in body size. This process occurs most frequently in larvae, but even adults molt [KB(2)], albeit less frequently. A new exoskeleton is laid down under the old, and regeneration of any lost limbs begins. The appearance and structure of various structures alters during this process, and this must be considered by clinicians when assessing animals for disease. The outer shell demineralizes and blood is withdrawn from appendages, which shrivel, grow soft, and take on a pale, almost blue appearance. Other color and externally apparent changes are documented and vary with the species in question. Many crustaceans cannot take on water for respiration during the metabolically expensive process of molting, and so if unnaturally prolonged, the individual can die. Immediately after molting, the flesh of crustacean is of lower quality and altered in appearance. Most fishery regulators do not allow the harvest of 'soft shelled' (post-molt) crustaceans such as crabs and lobsters. This is a stage of particular susceptibility to trauma and disease, and also easily confused with infectious pathology.

Reproduction occurs in crustaceans generally as an annual cycle. Crustaceans feed on a broad range of substrates, including small vertebrates, plankton, mollusks, other crustaceans, vegetation, and detritus. Females will, however, often not feed during the brooding period, depleting their body reserves. This impacts brown and white meat quality. Male and female individuals can be differentiated in different ways. For shrimp, males have two petasma on their first pleopods; small appendages for attaching onto females. Female shrimp do not have these. Differentiating using this method is similar in crayfish and lobsters, although species differences account for a lot of variation. There is a lot of information online regarding differentiating sex using other means, but this presence of a calcified appendage extension is the most reliable in these animals. Crab sex is differentiated by the shape of their apron (Figure 1.26).

Aquaculture and Economic Significance

Of the many varied aquacultured crustaceans, shrimp and prawns represent the largest combined industries. Although the major aquacultured shrimp and prawn species are tiger shrimp and Pacific white shrimp, also of note are other *Penaeus* species, such as the banana prawn

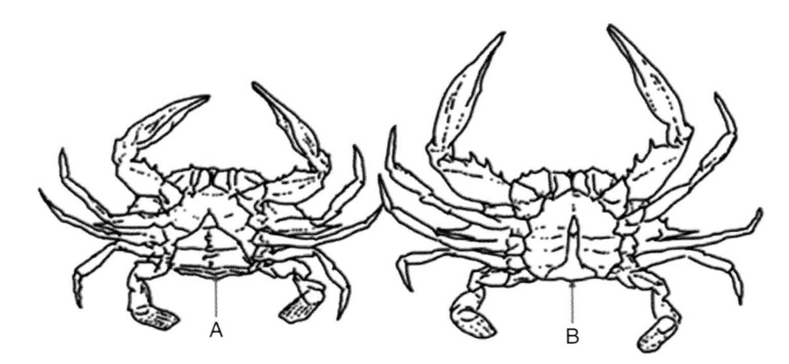

Figure 1.26 Male and female crabs can be differentiated by their external anatomy. In some species, the claws are a different color between males and females. Apron shape is also different between the sexes. Mature females (sooks) have a rounded apron (A) and males (jimmies) have a long, pointy apron (B). The apron of immature females can be more triangular.

(*Fenneropenaeus indicus*), kuruma prawn (*Marsupenaeus japonicus*) and fleshy shrimp (*Fenneropenaeus chinensis*). The majority of shrimp and prawn aquaculture occurs in Asia, with tiger shrimp and Pacific white shrimp being marine species. Aquaculture production of freshwater species is primarily of species such as the giant river prawn (*Macrobrachium rosenbergii*), crayfish, and freshwater crabs. The terms shrimp and prawn are often used interchangeably, despite taxonomic and morphological differences. A simple rule of thumb is that prawns have a "bend" to their body and release their eggs, whereas shrimp have a more linear form, and brood eggs on their underside.

Production of shrimp and prawns generally occurs in earthen pond systems, with a fresh or saline environmental water source depending on species adaptations. Although production times are short and profits can be very high, these organisms can be highly sensitive to environmental changes and stress. Infectious outbreaks can also be devastating, and a number of notifiable diseases with impact on production are detailed at the end of this section. Increasing use of recirculating aquaculture systems reduces the risk of disease outbreaks, although these come with their own suite of challenges. Large-scale wild fisheries of shrimp and prawns can have issues of sustainability owing to the focus on the use of trawling for capture, and although aquaculture removes some of the issues of seasonality in production and exploited fisheries, aquaculture has a number of issues too. Challenges such as sustainability, pollution and biosecurity all remain to the fully addressed.

The farming of a number of crab species such as *Eriochier sinensis* (Chinese mitten crab) and *Scylla* species occurs in Asia, but many others are harvested as part of fisheries. Commercially important crabs to Pacific fisheries include the horse crab (*Portunus trituberculatus*), flower crab (*Portunus pelagicus*), blue crab (*Callinectes sapidus*), mangrove mud crab (*Scylla serrata*) and *Charybdis* species. The edible or brown crab (*Cancer pagurus*) is an important catch species in the Atlantic, and several additional genera are important to northern fisheries, including genus *Chionoecetes* (snow crabs), *Metacarcinus magister* (Dungeness crab) and *Paralithodes camtschaticus* (king crab), [KB(3)].

Lobsters are a high value crustacean group, with varied taxonomy of members. Edible lobsters include the spiny lobster species (clawless species of genus *Panulirus* with robust antennae) and a group referred to as clawed lobsters that includes commercially important *Homarus* species. Spiny lobsters represent the only major aquacultured lobster species, farmed primarily in Vietnam, where wild-caught juveniles are raised to harvest. Culture efforts are currently being pursued, although a protracted larval phase limits entirely aquacultured individuals. European lobsters (*Homarus gammarus*) are generally dark blue in color (turning red only with cooking). American lobster (*Homarus americanus*) are generally brown/orange in color and can grow very large. Both species are found in the North Atlantic ocean. Closely related *Metanephrops*, also clawed, are commonly known as scampi.

Crayfish are an important aquacultured species in the Americas and Oceania and Asia. Red clawed crayfish (*Cherax quadricarinatus*) are farmed in Central America and Australia, whereas procambarid crayfishes, also known as 'crawdads', such as *Procambarus clarkia* (red swamp cray) and *Procambarus zonangulus* (white river crayfish), are commercially important to the Southern United States. Certain species of crayfish can be particularly invasive, and although desirable for harvest in their native regions, are considered pests elsewhere. Aquaculture production methodologies vary between species, but in general are less intensive than shrimp and prawn production [KB(4)]. *C. quadricarinatus* production can occur directly in ponds, without hatcheries, and omnivorous crayfish graze at night from the pond bottom without the requirement for high rate feeding of other aquaculture-farmed crustaceans. Important wild fisheries include those in Scandinavia and China.

Aquaria

Crustaceans such as shrimp make attractive editions to both freshwater and marine aquaria, and thus are popular amongst hobbyists. A huge variety of species are cultured for display, including *Neocaridina* and *Palaemonetes* commonly seen in freshwater tanks, Mantis shrimp (order Stomatopoda) in marine displays, and even microscopic daphnia. Different species have different environmental requirements that cannot be covered within the scope of this section. However, many clinical symptoms are shared across species, and similar principles can be applied in assessment of both aquacultured and home aquaria crustaceans. Further reading is required for specific species.

Disease and Diagnostics

Many infectious and environmental challenges exist to aquaculture production of crustaceans. Conditions impacting wild individuals are of importance to the aquatic health professional. For example, crustaceans obtained from fisheries are often transported live, and risk the spread of any pathogens they host not only to naïve wild populations, but also the geographical area of important aquacultured stock. Infections are potentially devastating in both commercially important wild populations and cultured stocks [KB(5)]. Many of the pathologies associated with high mortalities in aquaculture production require sophisticated diagnostics for definitive diagnosis. The clinical changes of crustaceans, although more varied than that of bivalves, are still fairly limited in their specificity to any given condition. Cageside diagnostic options include assessment of the clotting reaction of hemolymph, consistently delayed or even absent in many infections of shrimp, and non-destructive sampling for assessment of tissue squash preparations. Small sections of gill or pleopod connective tissue can allow observation of various indicators of disease, including presence of parasitic organisms, cellular changes such as hypertrophy of hemocytes or refractive aggregates of specific pathogens.

An appreciation of normal presentation for specific species is essential for performing accurate clinical assessments. For example, observation of reddening is a common feature of many pathological conditions. This color change occurs due to chromatophore expansion with carotenoid pigments (distributed throughout the body by hemolymph from the hepatopancreas) as part of necrosis. But reddening can also be a normal color change in lobsters due to seasonality, and in shrimp spawning, where broodstock can often be redder in color than expected (thought to be linked to a carotenoid-rich diet). Female lobsters can also take on a green coloration as part of reproductive cycling, where egg development gives the tail a green appearance. Diet can also give individuals a green appearance. This color can be striking, and easily mistaken for pathology.

Clinical assessment of crustaceans should proceed similarly to other aquatic organisms. An initial external assessment might include the notation of damage or loss to the eyes, antennae, pleopods (legs), and europod (tail), as well as appraisal of the gill tissue beneath the operculum. Identification of shell legions, testing for exoskeleton consistency and any discoloration can also be assessed. Owing to the more translucent nature of shrimp and prawn shells, the external examination of these animals can include assessment of internal body features. Stomach and intestinal fill, muscular coloration, and the appearance of the hepatopancreas can all be assessed. Noting deformities or deviation within a population provides essential initial information in building a clinical picture. Molt stage, sex, and carapace length can all be important information, and should be recorded.

Many of the pathologies associated with high mortalities in aquaculture production can be identified using sophisticated diagnostics. However, there is also a varied suite of initial investigations that can be explored. The clinical changes of crustaceans, although fairly limited in their specificity to any given condition, can be highly informative. Cageside diagnostic options include assessment of the clotting reaction of hemolymph, consistently delayed or even absent in many infections, and non-destructive sampling for assessment of tissue squash preparations. Appraisal of small sections of gill or pleopod connective tissue can allow observation of various indicators of disease, including presence of parasitic organisms, cellular changes such as hypertrophy of hemocytes, or refractive aggregates of specific pathogens. Microscopic assessment of pleopods involves removing a pleopod for examination with a compound microscope. This can be used to diagnose and even stage *Hematodinium* infections. Hemolymph smears stained with neutral red provides an easy method for observing pathogens and can always be photographed to share with colleagues if a clinician lacks experience in pathogen identification (Figure 1.27). Hemolymph smears, either fresh or stained, can demonstrate parasites and bacteria. If examination cannot be performed immediately, clinicians should avoid air drying smears to reduce artefacts. Even without microscopy however, assessment of the opacity or clotting ability of hemolymph can be informative.

The preferred method of euthanasia of lobsters and crabs [KB(6)] is through electrical stunning. Many other methods have been described (including boiling, freezing, and pithing), however electrical stunning is the only method that results in rapid loss of consciousness due to the decentralized nervous system of crustaceans. A number of water-soluble anesthetics have also been demonstrated as effective in multiple crustaceans, and might be used for sedation and euthanasia.

When performing disease diagnostics, moribund individuals should be selected for sampling, particularly for bacteriology and histopathology. In some suspected viral pathologies, however, hemolymph should be collected from clinically normal individuals cohabiting with moribund hosts, as hemocytes are depleted in later-stage infections. For the majority of conditions, juveniles and subadults provide the best samples for surveillance, although exceptions apply. Greater detail regarding sampling technique is available within WOAH disease guides.

Sampling should be performed as soon as possible following live transport of animals to avoid physiological stress. To avoid cannibalism for species such as crabs, holding individuals of varied size is not recommended. Small tissue sections of recently euthanized crustacean gill and hepatopancreas may be used in squash preparations and impression smears. The use of Davidson's fixative is recommended for routine histological studies of crustaceans. The formulation of the fixative should depend on the species to be studied, and the environment it resides in (freshwater or marine). A typical formulation of Davidson's fixative is 33% ethyl alcohol [95%], 22% formalin [approximately 37% formaldehyde], 11.5% glacial acetic acid and 33.5% distilled or tap water. Small individuals can be fixed whole following impregnation with fixative; approximately 5–10% of the body weight of the individual should be injected directly to the hepatopancreas and adjacent regions of the cephalothorax and abdomen. The cuticle should then be opened just lateral to the dorsal midline from the sixth

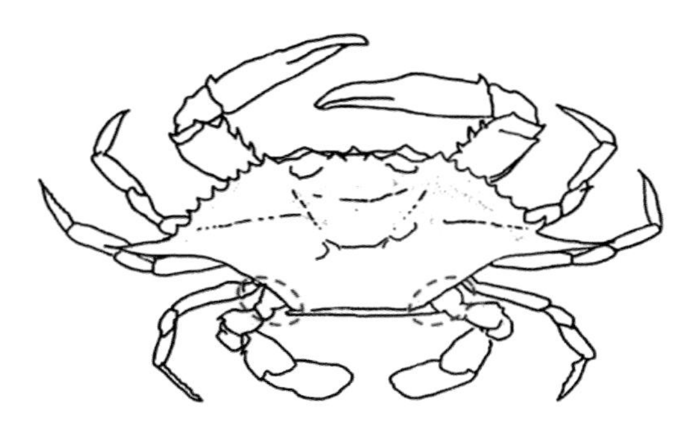

Figure 1.27 Hemolymph can be obtained via arthrodial membranes of the legs or the junction of the carapace and abdomen. Recommended sampling sites vary between species, but a common prebranchial site is from the base of the fifth leg. An appropriate gauge needle might be 27 gauge in crustaceans with a carapace greater than 15 mm, with small gauges for smaller individuals.

segment to rostrum base, to enhance penetration. Larger crustaceans such as lobsters, crabs and crayfish should be dissected, with tissues placed inside cassette(s) for fixation. Fixation should not exceed 48 hours, after which transfer to 70% ethyl alcohol for storage is necessary.

Clinical Signs

The research of pathogens of crustaceans is an emerging field, in which great progress has been made in recent years, particularly for those species of importance to aquaculture. There exists, however, a multitude of potentially pathogenic agents recently described, for which the gross clinical signs of infection are not yet fully understood.

Behavior Behavior can be assessed for animals within the pond, but by removing a subset of organisms to a bucket or bowl, observation becomes easier, particularly for smaller animals. Lethargy and altered feeding are particularly important clinical signs for most of the major diseases. Shrimp and prawns will also aggregate at the pond side in respiratory distress with many conditions, a behavioral change that might be first noticed due to the increased presence of predators that this attracts. Reduction or loss of the "tail flick" escape response can be an indication of continuing pathology and lethargy in some crustaceans. Poor coordination and collisions can also be helpful in diagnosis, often suggestive of blindness. Trying to escape, thrashing, spasms, and autotomy (limb shedding) can all be considered signs of distress in crabs and lobsters, sometimes due to as simple a reason as handling. Healthy lobsters can even be seen to avoid others within a cohort infected with disease (such as in the case of *Panulirus argus* virus 1, PaV1, in spiny lobsters).

Environmental Parameters Environmental changes can be an important cause of reported pathology within the *Crustacea*, and readings or assessment of the environment should be factored into any investigative approach. Algae, temperature, salinity, oxygen, turbidity, pH, and predator activity are just a few of the many changes that might be linked either directly or indirectly to apparent pathology in crustaceans. Recent run-off from nearby fields can be an important element of case history in pond-reared crustaceans, whereas fungal infections are considered more likely in recirculating systems, with high temperatures and high levels of nutrients within the water.

Shell Changes Shell changes are the most obvious clinical change that can be observed in crustaceans. Although the thin, semi-opaque shells of prawns and shrimp can allow visualization of organs within, shells are made of a very hard substance called chitin. As the exoskeleton is quite hard, many shell changes of thicker shelled crustaceans, such as lobsters and crabs, can be non-lethal. These changes can lead to rejection for sale of individuals on aesthetic grounds.

Environmental conditions are important factors in shell disease; ocean acidification, rough handling, high temperatures and poor water quality are considered predisposing to shell weakness across the decapod group. Crustacea are considered to be most vulnerable to shell lesions immediately after molting, when the new larger shell is potentially thinner and weaker due to relative mineral deficiency (calcium, phosphate and magnesium are all important dietary minerals for shell health). Shrimp and prawns have generally softer, thinner shells, and so many of the color changes observed in shrimp and prawns are not color changes to the carapace itself, rather internal changes visible through the shell.

Aggression and traumatic damage can induce shell lesions, but environmental stressors such as pollutants or temperature are also considered important factors in shell pathologies. Specific infectious agents of most shell disorders are not yet fully understood. Although bacteria are frequently isolated from lesions and researchers have seen limitation of lesion progression through experimental treatment with malachite green and formalin, these may represent secondary agents. Outcomes appear to depend on frequency of shell molts, meaning adults are most commonly observed as impacted due to their longer period between molts.

Incidental Findings Findings can at times be incidental, and of little significance to crustacean health. Some shell lesions are considered this way, determined to be merely melanized spots from previous trauma that do not extend full thickness through the carapace. Other findings without apparent clinical impact include intestinal parasites such as *Porospora nephropis* and *Stichocotyle nephropis* in lobsters, seen in squash or histological preparations of the gut as cyst like structures. *Histriobdella homari* worms can be found in the egg mass or gills of crustaceans, often without apparent ill effect, and documented findings of copepod and isopod infections, although rare within the literature, seem rarely of concern. Digenea infestations, often localized to the antennal gland in crayfish, are another incidental finding, and certain ciliates do not appear to be associated with direct pathology. Many apparently incidental pathogens can, however, cause disease given the correct set of circumstances. As with fish, the outcome of disease is predicated by a complex suite of contributory factors. Stress, nutritional status, age, stage of molt and a host of other factors influence disease outcome in crustaceans. Ultimately, lobster health status determines the outcome of survival in animals with disease such as shell lesions. General practice is to remove impacted individuals from an aquaculture population, whatever the causative agent. In many infectious outbreaks, destocking is required.

Specific Diseases

Similar to fish, crustaceans suffer a number of bacterial, viral, and parasitic infectious disorders, on top of non-infectious challenges such as water quality and temperature changes. Many clinical considerations are the same, such as the complexities of differentiating incidental findings from causative agents of observed clinical changes. Owing to the varied nature of host Crustacea and pathologies, only a limited number can be discussed in this chapter. The diseases presented here are majority WOAH notifiable conditions, of consequence not only to impacted farms, but regional production. Many of the listed diseases are associated with rapid high mortalities in shrimp and prawns. It is important to remember, however, that viral infections can be accompanied by secondary bacterial and epicommensal infestations, which may play a role in the ultimate cause of death. Many additional diseases can impact crustaceans beyond just those notifiable to the WOAH. Further reading is recommended from the expanding field of literature for a more complete overview of the topic.

Notifiable Diseases

White Spot Disease

Overview: White spot disease is highly infectious WOAH notifiable viral infection caused by white spot syndrome virus (WSSV), of which there are a number of genetic variants reported.

Etiology: WSSV has been assigned as the only member of the *Whispovirus* genus in the Nimaviridae family. It can be found in fresh, brackish, and marine environments and appears to be unrelated to other known viruses. Geographical isolates with genotypic variability have been identified, but they remain classified as a single species. The virus may remain viable in seawater for around 30 days at 30°C and 3–4 days in freshwater. Simulation of pond bottoms suggest sunlight will inactive it in a dried pond bed after 21 days or around 40 days in a pond with a still muddy bed. All life stages are susceptible, from eggs to broodstock.

Host range and distribution: WSSV infects crustaceans and all decapods (order Decapoda) including crabs and lobsters are considered susceptible. Indeed, to date, no decapod has shown any signs of being refractory to infection, although morbidity and mortality as a result of infection are variable and some species can carry high levels of virus without clinical signs. WSSV has been found in crustaceans in China, Japan, South Korea, South-East Asia, South Asia, the Indian Continent, the Mediterranean, the Middle East, and the Americas. Present within these regions are zones and compartments free from infection.

Signs/diagnosis: WSSV infections can be subclinical or clinical in nature. Affected shrimp are lethargic and exhibit abnormal swimming patterns such as swimming on their side, near the surface, or near pond edges. Feed consumption decreases or ceases. High morbidity and mortality are observed within days of the onset of signs, and some may die without showing any clinical signs. Non-penaeid species (e.g. crab, lobster) generally have subclinical infections under natural conditions.

WSSV is best detected following exposure to stressors such as eye-stalk ablation, spawning, molting, salinity fluctuation, temperature or pH changes, and during plankton blooms. The virus targets ectodermal and mesodermal tissues, especially the cuticular epithelium and subcuticular connective tissues and while it does infect connective tissues in the hepatopancreas and midgut, it does not infect the endodermis-derived tubular epithelial cells in either organ. Multifocal to coalescing white spots, seen within the exoskeleton, are the most commonly observed clinical sign and can range from barely discernible up to 3 mm in diameter. White spots are not a reliable diagnostic sign of infection, though, since environmental stress factors, such as high alkalinity or bacterial disease, can also cause white spots on the carapace of shrimp, and some WSSV-infected shrimp may have few, if any, white spots. Red to pink discoloration can also be seen in diseased populations.

The carapace can be loosely attached to underlying cuticular epithelium in clinically affected individuals and it can easily be removed (Figure 1.28); anorexia results in empty gastrointestinal tracts on inspection while debilitation results in excessive fouling of the gills and exoskeleton. Infected shrimp show delayed, or even absent clotting of hemolymph.

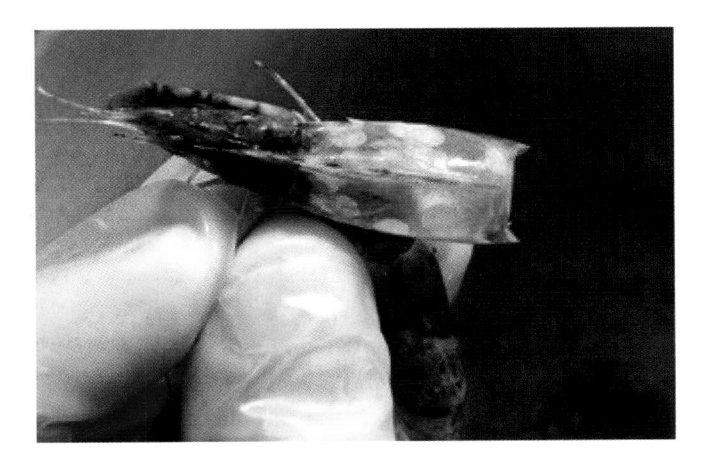

Figure 1.28 The carapace of a shrimp infected with white spot disease is loose and when removed, large smooth-edged white spots can be seen, often with smaller white spots also evident on the abdominal segments. Note that clinically affected shrimp may appear grossly normal. *Source:* Reproduced with permission B. Diggles/Department of Agriculture, Fisheries and Forestry/ CC BY 4.0.

Hypertrophied nuclei can be seen in squash preparations of the gills and cuticular epithelium, which can be stained or unstained (Figure 1.29). Otherwise, affected tissues can be identified in histopathology, where virus-infected cells exhibit hypertrophied nuclei with marginated chromatin, eosinophilic to pale basophilic (on hematoxylin and eosin, H&E) stained intranuclear viral inclusions within hypertrophied nuclei and multifocal necrosis associated with pyknotic and karyorrhectic nuclei in affected tissues of ectodermal and mesodermal origin. For details of polymerase chain reaction protocols, see the WOAH Manual of Diagnostic Tests for Aquatic Animals. Otherwise, diagnosis can be confirmed with in-situ hybridization, immunohistochemistry, and electron microscopy.

Differentials: Infection with infectious hypodermal and hematopoietic necrosis virus produce similar inclusions that need to be differentiated from those of WSSV as well as possibly white mottling of the shell. Environmental stress factors, such as high alkalinity, or bacterial disease can also cause white spots on the carapace of shrimp. Other viral conditions such as acute hepatopancreatic necrosis disease, infection with *Hepatobacter penaei*, infection with shrimp hemocyte iridescent virus, infection with Taura syndrome virus and infection with yellowhead virus genotype 1 (YHV1) should also be considered.

Treatment: There is no known treatment.

Management: Restocking with resistant species is not an option, although producers are attempting to breed improved resistant strains. Avoiding stocking in the cold season, use of specific pathogen-free or PCR-negative seed stocks, use of biosecure water and culture systems, and even polyculture of shrimp and fish have all apparently been attempted. Disinfecting eggs may help avoid trans-ovum transmission. Details on inactivation of the virus are available in the WOAH *Manual of Diagnostic Tests for Aquatic Animals.*

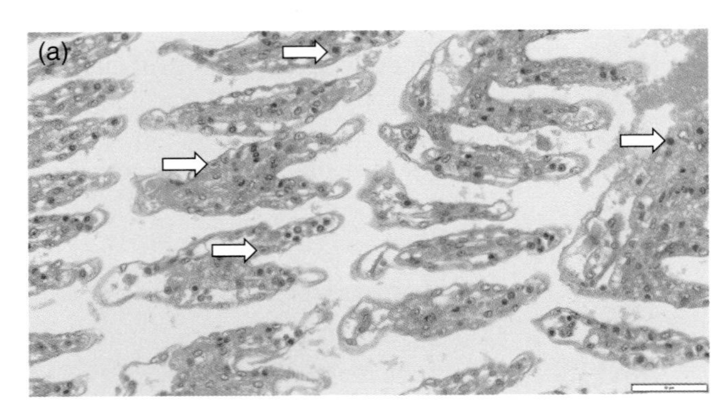

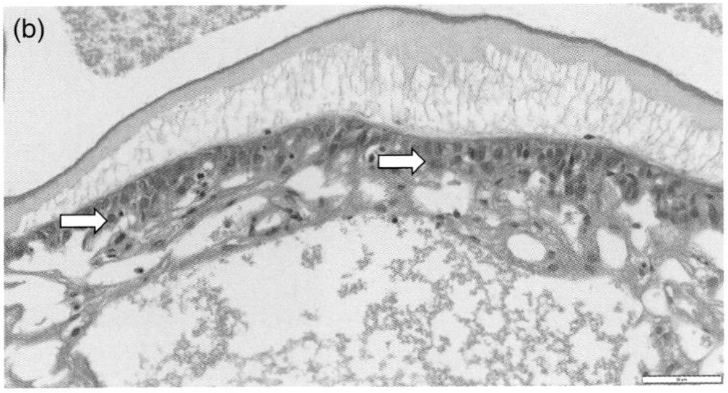

Figure 1.29 White spot syndrome virus infection in whiteleg shrimp (*Penaeus vannamei*). a) Virus infecting the nuclei of the circular epithelial cell lining in the gills. Infected nuclei appear hypertrophied with marginalized chromatin and containing an eosinophilic inclusion body (arrows). Hematoxylin and eosin stain. Scale bar = 50 µm. b) Virus infecting the nuclei of the cuticular epithelial cells lining the gut. Infected nuclei appear hypertrophied with marginalized chromatin and containing an eosinophilic inclusion body (arrows). Hematoxylin and eosin stain. Scale bar = 50 µm.

Taura Syndrome

Overview: Taura syndrome is a WOAH notifiable viral disease caused by infection with Taura syndrome virus (TSV), a small picorna-like RNA virus that belongs to the genus *Aparavirus* in the family Dicistroviridae. TSV replicates in the cytoplasm of host cells and has caused severe losses in shrimp farming regions of the Americas and Southeast Asia although impacts are declining due to improvements in good biosecurity practices and increasing use of tolerant stocks.

Etiology: TSV appears to remain infectious for up to 48 hours in the feces of sea gulls that have ingested infected shrimp carcasses, which may implicate birds as an important route of transmission of the virus within affected farms or farming regions. In addition, aquatic insects feeding on prawn carcasses, such as the water boatman (*Trichcorixa* spp.) may also act as vectors.

Host range and distribution: TSV causes disease in a wide range of penaeids and is known to be carried by a wide range of non-penaeids. *Penaeus monodon* and *Penaeus* (*Marsupenaeus*) *japonicus* susceptibility to TSV is unclear, but the whiteleg shrimp (*Litopenaeus vannamei*) and the western blue shrimp (*Litopenaeus stylirostris*) are probably the most susceptible species. The first known occurrence of a TSV outbreak was in 1992 when the virus impacted the shrimp population near the Taura river in Ecuador. The disease quickly spread to other countries in the Americas. By 1999, TSV was introduced into Southeast Asia through infected broodstock and post-larvae of *L. vannamei* intended for aquaculture and subsequently spread throughout much of the region.

Signs/diagnosis: Taura syndrome is seen mainly in the nursery phase of *Penaeus* (*Litopenaeus*) *vannamei*. It usually occurs within 14–40 days of stocking post-larvae into grow-out ponds or tanks. Mortalities are usually in the range of 40–90% in cultured populations of post-larval, juvenile, and subadult shrimp. Lesions usually appear during the acute phase of the disease and are present in specific target tissues, particularly the cuticular epithelium (hypodermis). Producers may notice lethargic prawns and cessation of feeding initially. Affected animals gather at the pond edge when moribund resulting in a sudden increase in seabird activity fishing in ponds. Producers will notice sudden onset of high mortalities in late post-larvae, juvenile, or subadult prawns.

The virus replicates mainly in the hypodermis but also in the gut, gills, and appendages. Gross pathology of the acute phase includes empty stomachs and pale red body surfaces and appendages, and notably, the uropods and pleopods may appear red due to the expansion of red chromatophores (Figure 1.30). The tail fan edges may also appear somewhat roughened by focal epithelial necrosis. Acutely affected shrimp may also exhibit soft shells and multiple, irregularly shaped, and randomly distributed melanized (dark) cuticular lesions in the transition phase. This will be accompanied by increased mortalities, usually at molting. There are few grossly obvious pathological signs of disease in the chronic phase.

Histopathology reveals necrosis of the cuticular epithelium of appendages, multiple melanized foci in the cuticular epithelium (transition phase), and abundant pyknotic and karyorrhectic nuclei, which have been described as giving Taura syndrome lesions a "peppered appearance" (Figure 1.31). In the chronic form of the disease, lymphoid organ spheroids may be apparent. Definitive diagnosis is based on consistent histopathology, positive in-situ hybridization in target tissues or reverse transcription PCR (rtPCR) followed by sequencing, or real-time PCR (Figures 1.32 and 1.33).

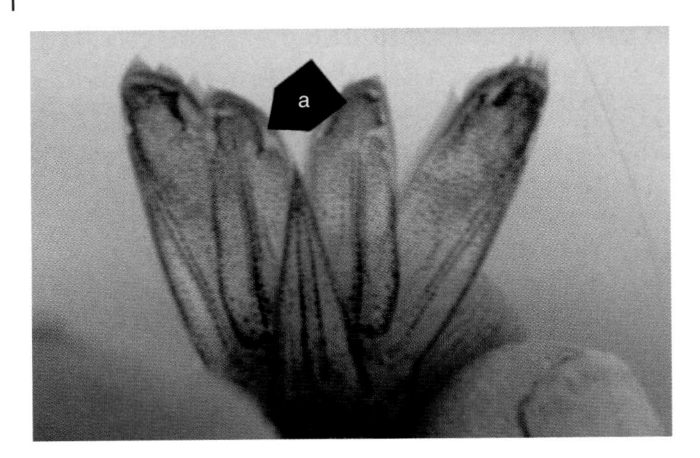

Figure 1.30 Reddened uropods with irregular edges suggesting focal necrosis caused by Taura syndrome virus. *Source:* Reproduced with permission from DV Lightner/Australia Department of Agriculture, Fisheries and Forestry/CC BY 4.0.

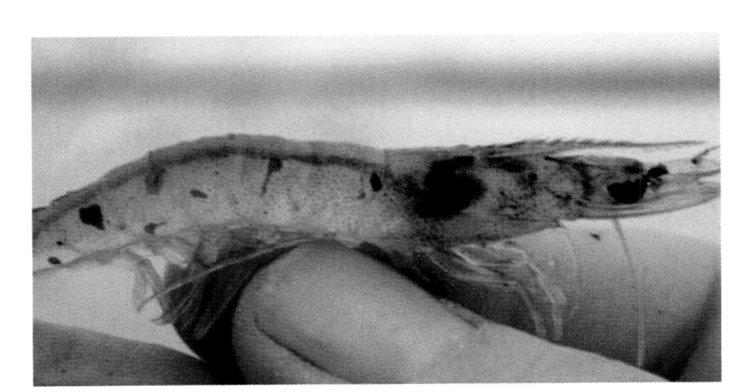

Figure 1.31 Multifocal melanization during a transitional phase infection with Taura syndrome virus. *Source:* Reproduced with permission from DV Lightner/Australia Department of Agriculture, Fisheries and Forestry/CC BY 4.0.

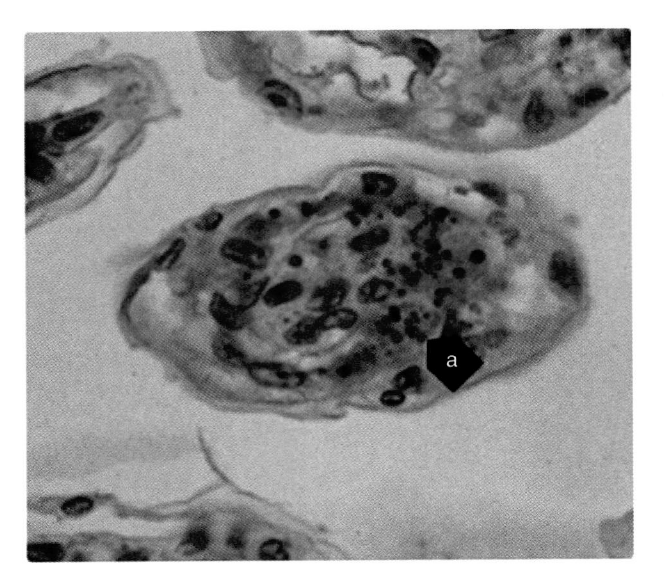

Figure 1.32 *Pennaeus vannamei* gill lesions exhibiting pyknosis, karyorrhexis, and a large number of cytoplasmic inclusion bodies (a). with Taura syndrome virus. *Source:* Reproduced with permission from DV Lightner/Australian Department of Agriculture, Fisheries and Forestry/CC BY 4.0.

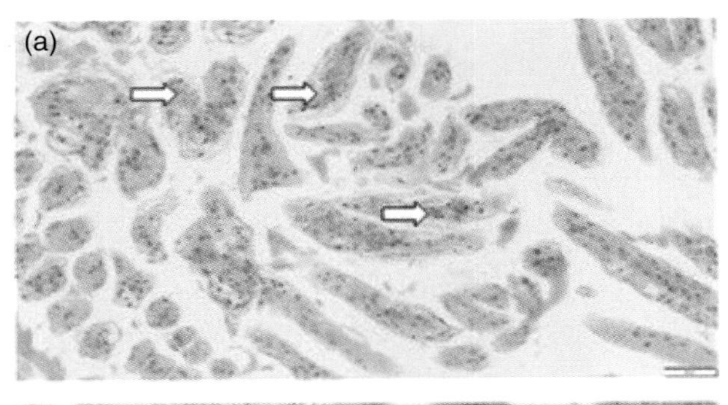

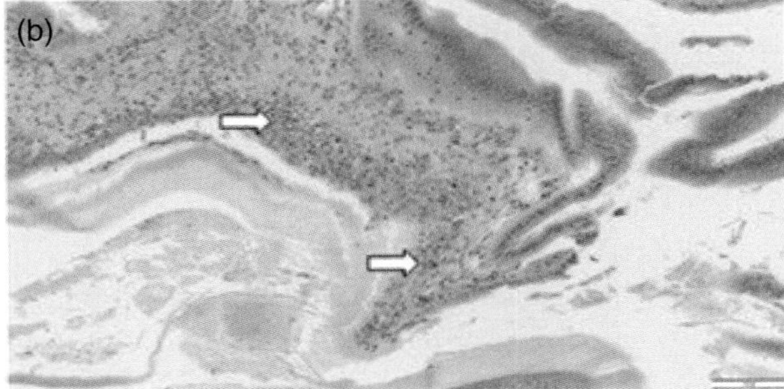

Figure 1.33 Taura syndrome virus and yellowhead virus 1 in whiteleg shrimp (*Pennaeus vannamei*). a) Infected cells within the cuticular epithelium of the gut are rounded with densely stained pyknotic nuclei (arrows). Hematoxylin and eosin stain. Scale bar = 100 μm. b) Infected cells within the cuticular epithelium of the gut are rounded with densely stained pyknotic nuclei (arrows). Hematoxylin and eosin stain. Scale bar = 100 μm.

Differentials: Affected prawn may show signs similar to yellowhead virus and WSSV.

Treatment: No confirmed effective treatments are in use, although blocking agents like injected short random double-stranded RNAi have been used with some improved resistance in trials. Some lines of TSV-resistant *P. vannamei* are available commercially.

Management: Outbreaks are reportedly more frequent when salinity falls below 30 ppt. Eradication methods for TSV depend on total depopulation of infected stocks, disinfection of the culture facility, avoiding the reintroduction of the virus from other nearby culture facilities, wild shrimp and fomites, and restocking with Taura syndrome-free post-larvae that have been produced from Taura syndrome-free broodstock. This approach has been successfully applied to certain aquaculture situations. It is good hygiene practice to disinfect eggs and larvae to reduce the potential of TSV contamination of spawned eggs and larvae produced from them.

Yellowhead Disease

Overview: Yellowhead disease is a WOAH notifiable concern in black tiger prawn aquaculture globally, with the majority of outbreaks reported in Southeast Asia. A number of viruses are included in the yellowhead complex: yellowhead virus genotype 1 (YHV1) is associated with yellowhead disease, while genotypes 2–6 are frequently isolated with apparently healthy individuals, and are rarely associated with disease, although genotype 2 is implicated with a gill-associated disease.

Host range and distribution: Yellowhead disease is infective in a wide array of prawn, shrimp, and krill species, both naturally and experimentally. Outbreaks have thus far been isolated however to *P. monodon* (black tiger prawn) and *P. vannamei* (white Pacific shrimp).

Transmission: Infective to post-larval organisms, this disease can be transmitted horizontally by cohabitation with live infected organisms, ingestion of infected material from deceased individuals, and through environmental water (where the virus can remain viable up to 72 hours). Infected organisms can remain lifelong carriers through viral persistence and chronic infections. Vertical transmission has been demonstrated for closely related genotype 2 yellowhead virus, but not yet for yellowhead disease.

Signs/diagnosis: Yellowhead disease is associated with rapid epidemics with high mortality, particularly in juvenile organisms. Behavioral changes common to many infectious pathologies are noted, including anorexia and congregation at pond edges. Producers report abnormally high feeding behavior prior to cessation and onset of clinical signs (two to four days). Total farm loss can occur within days of onset of clinical disease. The syndrome is named for the pallid, sometimes yellow, coloration of the dorsal cephalothorax area (due to enlargement and discoloration of the hepatopancreas). General appearance of an infected organism is a pallid/bleached presentation, with altered gill appearance, and a softened hepatopancreas. Presumptive diagnosis can be achieved using histopathology or Davidson-fixed, H&E-stained wet mounts with xylene alongside results of hemolymph smears (Figure 1.34).

Differentials: Cessation of feeding, congregation at pond edges, and lethargy of stock are shared features with many other pathologies in shrimp and prawns. In addition to infectious causes, yellow discoloration of individuals may occur due to stress or nutritional variation for altered metabolism and pigment deposition, as well as environmental toxicity (copper).

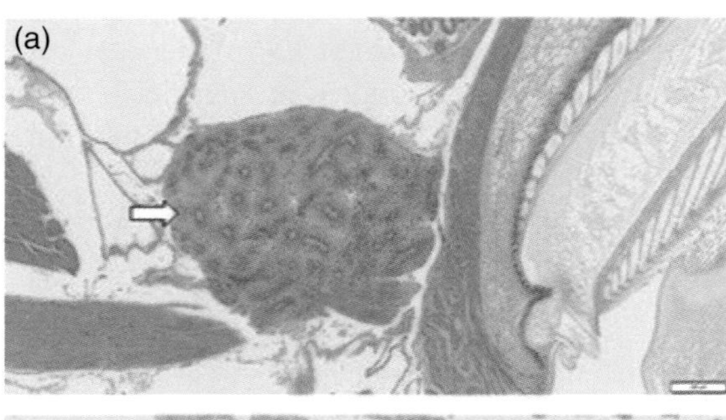

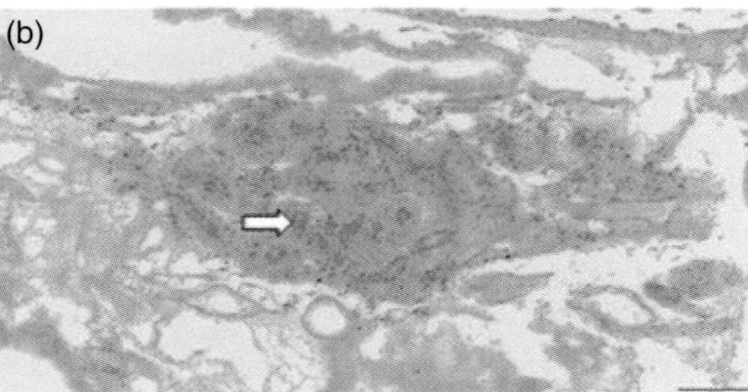

Figure 1.34 Taura syndrome virus (TSV) and yellowhead virus 1 in whiteleg shrimp (*Pennaeus vannamei*). a) TSV does not infect the lymphoid organ tissues; tubule structure is unaffected (arrow) and nuclei appear normal. Scale bar = 200 μm. b) Yellowhead virus infects the lymphoid organ tissues; loss of tubule structure is evident and nuclei rounded with densely stained pyknotic cells.

Treatment: No chemotherapy or preventative vaccinations are available for this pathogen. Specific disease-free animals are available for stocking. Following outbreaks, sites must be drained and treated to remove yellowhead virus particles. Yellowhead virus can be inactivated by heating and appears susceptible to chlorine treatment. Nested rtPCR is suggested as part of screening protocols for stock.

Infectious Hypodermal and Hematopoietic Necrosis Virus

Overview: The WOAH defines infection with infectious hypodermal and hematopoietic necrosis virus as infection with the non-enveloped and pathogenic DNA agent IHHNV of the Family Parvoviridae, an infection reportable to the WOAH and many state authorities. It is formally known as decapod Penstyldensovirus 1 but can also be known as *P. stylirostris* densovirus (PstDNV). In regions where the virus is endemic in wild stocks, the prevalence of IHHNV has been found in various surveys to range from 0% to 100%. Some reported mean values for IHHNV prevalence in wild stocks are 26% and 46%.

Host range and distribution: At least two distinct genotypes of IHHNV infectious to *P. vannamei* and *P. monodon* have been identified, with type 1 from the Americas and East Asia (principally the Philippines) and type 2 from South-East Asia (World Organisation for Animal Health, 2022a). Two sequences homologous to part of the IHHNV genome are found embedded in the genome of penaeids. These were initially described as type 3A from East Africa, India, and Australia, and type 3B from the western Indo-Pacific region including Madagascar, Mauritius, and Tanzania (World Organisation for Animal Health, 2022a; Tang and Lightner, 2006). In East Africa, Australia, and the western Indo-Pacific region, IHHNV-homologous sequences have been found in the *P. monodon* genome and are not infectious to the susceptible host species *P. vannamei* and *P. monodon*. Other susceptible species include yellowleg shrimp (*P. californiensis*), northern white shrimp (*Penaeus setiferus*), and blue shrimp (*P. stylirostris*). The northern brown shrimp (*Penaeus aztecus*) may be susceptible, and PCR positives (not active infection) have been reported from a number of other species: giant river prawn (*Macrobrachium rosenbergii*), kuruma prawn (*Penaeus japonicus*), green tiger prawn (*Penaeus semisulcatus*), Argentine stiletto shrimp (*Artemesia longinaruis*), Cuata swimcrab (*Callinectes arcuatus*), and some fish: Mazatlan sole (*Archirus mazatlanus*), yellowfin mojarra (*Gerres cinereus*), tilapias (*Oreochromis* sp.), Pacific piquitinga (*Lile stolifera*) and blackfin snook (*Centropomus medius*) (World Organisation for Animal Health, 2022a). IHHNV appears to be distributed worldwide in both wild and cultured penaeid shrimp (Owens et al., 1992). Infection has also been reported in farmed penaeids from Pacific islands including the Hawaiian Islands, French Polynesia, Guam, and New Caledonia. In the Indo-Pacific region, the virus has been reported from cultured and wild penaeid shrimp in East Asia, South-East Asia, and the Middle East (Bondad-Reantaso et al., 2001). An IHHN-like virus sequence was reported from Australia (Owens et al., 1992), and the presence of infection with IHHNV in farmed prawns in Australia was reported to the World Organisation for Animal Health in 2008.

Signs/diagnosis: IHHNV has been detected in all life stages (eggs, larvae, post-larvae, juveniles, and adults) of *P. vannamei*. When broodstocks are sourced from endemic areas, the hatching success of eggs is reduced, survival and culture performance of the larval and post-larval stages are lowered, and any nauplii produced from infected broodstock have a high prevalence of infection with IHHNV (Motte et al., 2003). Infection with IHHNV in this species is often acute, with very high mortalities occurring in the juvenile life stages of this species. Vertically infected larvae and early post-larvae do not become diseased, but in approximately 35-day-old or older juveniles, gross signs of the disease may be observed, followed by mass mortality. In horizontally infected juveniles, the incubation period and severity of the disease is somewhat size and/or age dependent, with young juveniles always being the most severely affected. Infected adults seldom show signs of the disease or mortalities. Gross signs are not specific, but juvenile *P. stylirostris* with acute infection with IHHNV refuse food, followed by changes in behavior and appearance. *P. stylirostris* have been observed in tanks to rise slowly to the surface, where they become motionless and then roll over and slowly sink (ventral side up) to the tank bottom. Shrimp exhibiting this behavior may repeat the process for several hours until they become too weak to continue, or until they are attacked and cannibalized by their healthier siblings. At this stage of infection, *P. stylirostris* often have white or buff-colored spots (which differ in appearance and location from the white spots that sometimes occur in shrimp with WSSV infections) in the cuticular epidermis, especially at the junction of the tergal plates of the abdomen, giving such shrimp a mottled appearance. This mottling later fades in moribund shrimp as such individuals become more bluish. In *P. stylirostris* and *P. monodon* with terminal-phase IHHNV infections, moribund shrimp are often distinctly bluish in color, with opaque abdominal musculature. Some surviving *P. stylirostris* and *P. vannamei* may carry the virus for life and may pass the virus to their progeny and other populations by vertical and horizontal transmission. Infections can be either acute or chronic depending on shrimp species and population. Some populations of *P. stylirostris* can suffer acute, usually catastrophic disease, with mortalities approaching 100% as described above. In contrast, infection in some populations of *P. vannamei*, *P. stylirostris*, and *P. monodon* results in a more subtle, chronic form of IHHVV disease, runt-deformity syndrome (RDS), in which high mortalities are unusual but where growth suppression and deformities of the cuticle are common (Kalagayan et al., 1991). The syndrome results in poor and highly disparate growth. RDS is a more commonly seen in *P. vannamei* where juvenile shrimp may display a bent (45–90-degree bend to left or right) or otherwise deformed rostrum, a deformed sixth abdominal segment, wrinkled antennal flagella, cuticular roughness, "bubble heads," and other cuticular deformities (Australia Department of Agriculture, Water and the Environment, 2020b). In *P. vannamei* and *P. stylirostris* with RDS, a deformed rostrum bent to the left or right, is said to be pathognomonic for infection with IHHNV. Affected shrimp show a wide distribution of sizes and the coefficient of variation, which should be between

10% and 30%, can approach 90% (World Organisation for Animal Health, 2022a). The principal target tissues for IHHNV include connective tissue cells, the gills, hematopoietic nodules and hemocytes, ventral nerve cord and ganglia, antennal gland tubule epithelial cells, and lymphoid organ parenchymal cells (World Organisation for Animal Health, 2022a). Hence, whole shrimp (e.g. larvae or post-larvae) or tissue samples containing the target tissues are suitable for most tests using molecular methods. In general, spawned eggs and larvae are not suitable samples for detection or certification (World Organisation for Animal Health, 2022a). Hemolymph or excised pleopods may be collected and used for testing (usually for PCR or dot-blot hybridization with specific probes) when non-lethal testing of valuable broodstock is necessary. IHHNV is a systemic virus, and it does not replicate in enteric tissues (e.g. the hepatopancreas, the midgut, or its caeca). Hence, enteric tissues are inappropriate samples for detection of IHHNV. Using Davidson's fixative, only live, moribund, or compromised shrimp should be selected for fixation and histological examination – dead shrimp should not be used. Selected shrimp are killed by injection of fixative directly into the hepatopancreas; the cuticle over the cephalothorax and abdomen just lateral to the dorsal midline is opened with fine-pointed surgical scissors to enhance fixative penetration (the abdomen may be removed and discarded), the whole shrimp (or cephalothorax less the abdomen) is immersed in fixative for 24–48 hours, and then transferred to 70% ethyl alcohol for storage. After transfer to 70% ethyl alcohol, fixed specimens may be transported (via post or courier to the diagnostic laboratory) by wrapping in cloth or a paper towel saturated with 70% ethyl alcohol and packed in leak-proof plastic bags. Acute (but not chronic) infections in *P. stylirostris* can be readily diagnosed using routine H&E-stained sections. For diagnosis of chronic infections, the use of molecular methods are recommended for IHHNV detection (e.g. by PCR or application of IHHNV-specific DNA probes to dot-blot hybridization tests or in-situ hybridization of histological sections). Histological demonstration of prominent intranuclear, Cowdry type A inclusion bodies provide a provisional diagnosis of infection with IHHNV (Australia Department of Agriculture, Water and the Environment, 2020b). These characteristic IHHNV inclusion bodies are eosinophilic and often haloed (with H&E stains of tissues preserved with fixatives that contain acetic acid, such as Davidson's AFA and Bouin's solution), intranuclear inclusion bodies within chromatin-marginated, hypertrophied nuclei of cells in tissues of ectodermal (epidermis, hypodermal epithelium of fore- and hindgut, nerve cord, and nerve ganglia) and mesodermal origin (hematopoietic organs, antennal gland, gonads, lymphoid organ, and connective tissue). Intranuclear inclusion bodies caused by and often haloed (with H&E stains of tissues preserved with fixatives that contain acetic acid, such as Davidson's AFA and Bouin's solution), intranuclear inclusion bodies within chromatin-marginated, hypertrophied nuclei of cells in tissues of ectodermal (epidermis, hypodermal epithelium of fore- and hindgut, nerve cord, and nerve ganglia) and mesodermal origin (hematopoietic organs, antennal gland, gonads, lymphoid organ, and connective tissue). Intranuclear inclusion bodies caused by infection with IHHNV may be easily confused with developing intranuclear inclusion bodies caused by WSSV infection. In-situ hybridization assay of such sections with a specific DNA probe to IHHNV provides a definitive diagnosis of infection with IHHNV. Direct detection methods using DNA probes specific for IHHNV are available in dot-blot and in-situ hybridization formats. PCR tests for IHHNV have been developed and a number of methods and commercial PCR detection kits are readily available (World Organisation for Animal Health, 2022a).

Infection with IHHNV is suspected if at least one of the following criteria are met: i) clinical signs indicative of infection with IHHNV; ii) histopathology indicative of infection with IHHNV; or iii) positive result by PCR. Infection is confirmed if two of the following criteria are met: i) positive result by in-situ hybridization; ii) positive result by PCR (always genotype specific); iii) and sequence analysis to confirm IHHNV nucleic acid sequence (World Organisation for Animal Health, 2022a).

Differentials: Clinical presentation and histological changes can be difficult to differentiate from white spot syndrome and abdominal segment deformity disease. In addition to infectious etiology, inappropriate nutrition or temperature for growth and development, as well as genetic defects, must be considered.

Treatment: No success with vaccination, chemotherapy, or immunostimulation has been described.

Management: The replication rate of IHHNV at high water temperatures appears to be significantly reduced. In one study with *P. vannamei*, after a suitable incubation period, shrimp held at 32°C had approximately 102 times lower viral load than shrimp held at 24°C (Montgomery-Brock et al., 2007). PCR prescreening of wild or pond-reared broodstock or their spawned eggs/nauplii and discarding those that test positive for the virus, as well as the development of specific pathogen-free shrimp stocks of *P. vannamei* and *P. stylirostris* have proven to help control the virus, with the latter being the most successful husbandry practice for the prevention and control of IHHN (Lightner, 2005). Selected stocks of *P. stylirostris* that are resistant to infection with IHHNV have been developed, and these have had some successful application in shrimp farms but they do not have increased resistance to other diseases, such as WSSV, so their use has been limited. A genetic basis for IHHN susceptibility in *P. vannamei* has been reported in some stocks. The relative resistance of these shrimp to infection with IHHNV is considered to be one of the main reasons that led to *P. vannamei* being the principal shrimp species farmed in the Western hemisphere, and since 2004, globally (Lightner, 2009).

Necrotising Hepatopancreatitis (Acute Hepatopancreatic Necrosis Disease)

Overview: Often observed as a protracted bacterial infection, this condition impacts post-larvae and juvenile giant tiger prawn (*Penaeus monodon*) and whiteleg shrimp (*Penaeus annamei*) following stocking.

Host range: Reported in susceptible organisms in China, Vietnam, Thailand, Malaysia, Mexico, and the Philippines. High salinity is considered a risk factor to infection, as is hot dry weather between April and July. It is unknown whether persistent carriers might transmit bacteria, but the causative agent *Vibrio parahaemolyticus* is common in environmental water; demonstrated as capable of surviving for more than two weeks. Vector species are suspected but not yet demonstrated.

Transmission: Transmission between infected individuals occurs via oral routes or cohabitation. Onset of infection often coincides with an external stressor such as poor water quality or algal blooms.

Signs/diagnosis: Onset of clinical signs and mortality occurs post-stocking. Changes include a pale, atrophied hepatopancreas, soft shells, and empty guts. Melanized spots and hardening can also occur within the hepatopancreas due to melanin deposition, hemocytes, and increase fibrous connective tissue content. Presumptive diagnosis by histopathology should be confirmed using PCR.

Differentials: General presentation is similar to numerous other viral and systemic bacterial infections.

Treatment: There are no recommended treatments for this infection, nor are there available resistant strains or disease-free strains.

Management: Strict feeding rate control and appropriate stocking density are considered important husbandry practices to reduce disease impact. Screening stock, sanitation, and strict biosecurity can reduce the likelihood of an outbreak. The bacterium is known to be sensitive to freezing, disinfection and heating, important considerations as it is associated with food poisoning in humans.

Acute Hepatopancreatic Necrosis Disease, Vibrio parahaemolyticus

Overview: Acute hepatopancreatic necrosis disease (AHPND) was formally known as early mortality syndrome and refers to infection with strains of *Vibrio parahaemolyticus* (Vp AHPND), a Gram-negative rod-shaped bacterium that contains an approximate 70-kbp plasmid with genes that encode homologues of the *Photorhabdus* insect-related (Pir) binary toxins, PirA and PirB (World Organisation for Animal Health, 2022b) and is capable of causing rapid death of infected shrimp. *Photorhabdus* is a genus of bioluminescent, gram-negative bacilli known to be pathogenic to a wide range of insects and has been used as biopesticide in agriculture. Although other *Vibrio* species have been isolated from clinical cases of AHPND, only Vp AHPND has been demonstrated to cause AHPND. Removal (or "curing") of the plasmid pVA1 abolishes the AHPND-causing ability of Vp AHPND strains. It is important to recognise from a diagnostic perspective that the Pirvp operon may be deleted naturally due to the instability of repeat sequences that flank the Pir toxin operon. Any affected Vp AHPND strain will lose its ability to cause AHPND. If the Pir toxin sequence is used as a target for detection, a false negative may occur if the colony isolated has this deletion even though the colony was derived from an isolate of AHPND-causing Vp AHPND. The pVA1 plasmid also carries genes related to conjugation, meaning this plasmid is potentially transferable to other bacteria.

Host range and distribution: The giant tiger prawn (*Penaeus monodon*) and whiteleg shrimp (*Penaeus vannamei*, also known as king prawn or Pacific white shrimp) are currently listed by the WOAH as fulfilling all the criteria for susceptible species; there are possibly more, including the fleshy prawn (*Penaeus chinensis*) that partially fulfils the criteria, or the kuruma prawn (*Penaeus japonicus*) that has demonstrated a PCR-positive product in the absence of clinical signs. The disease has been reported from China, Vietnam, Malaysia, Thailand, Mexico, and the Philippines.

Signs/diagnosis: In regions where the bacterium is endemic in farmed shrimp, evidence suggests a prevalence approaching 100% (Tran et al., 2013a). AHPND is characterised by sudden, mass mortalities (up to 100%) usually within 30–35 days of stocking grow-out ponds with post-larvae or juveniles (Food and Agriculture Organization, 2013), although older juveniles may also be affected (de la Peña et al., 2015). The onset of clinical signs and mortality can start as early as 10 days post-stocking, with moribund prawns sinking to the bottom of the pond.

Clinical signs include hepatopancreatic pallor and atrophy, soft shells, intestines with discontinuous or no contents, black foci or linear streaks visible within the hepatopancreas (due to melanized tubules). In addition, the hepatopancreas does not squash easily between the thumb and forefinger (possibly due to increased fibrous connective tissue and hemocytes) (Network of Aquaculture Centres in Asia-Pacific, 2014). The disease has been described as having two distinct phases: an acute phase characterized by a massive and progressive degeneration of the hepatopancreatic tubules from proximal to distal, with significant rounding and sloughing of tubule epithelial cells into the tubules, collecting ducts and posterior stomach in the absence of bacterial cells, and a terminal phase characterised by marked intratubular hemocytic inflammation and development of massive secondary bacterial infections that occur in association with the necrotic and sloughed HP tubule cells (Food and Agriculture Organization, 2013; Tran et al., 2013a).

Wet mounts and smears are not appropriate, nor are fixed sections for in-situ hybridization or electron microscopy. Vp AHPND can be isolated on standard media used for isolation of bacteria from diseased shrimp and species identification may be carried out using 16S rRNA PCR or toxR-targeted PCR and sequencing. AHPND-specific PCR methods, protocols and primers that target the Vp AHPND toxin genes are described in the *Manual of Diagnostic Tests for Aquatic Animals* (World Organisation for Animal Health, 2017b).

Differentials: Infection with *Enterocytozoon hepatopenaei*, *Hepatobacter penaei* or shrimp hemocyte iridescent virus (Australia Department of Agriculture, Water and the Environment. 2020a).

Treatment: There are no known treatments, vaccinations, immunostimulants or resistance-breeding successes to-date (Food and Agriculture Organization, 2013).

Management: *Vibrio* spp. are ubiquitous in the marine environment, and the possibility that there are vector species, particularly various genera of polychete worms that are thought to be naturally susceptible (World Organisation for Animal Health, 2022a), can be expected, although to date none has been conclusively identified. The bacteria are thought to be naturally transmitted through horizontal oral transmission and cohabitation. Low salinity (< 20 ppt) seems to reduce the incidence of the disease and peak occurrence appears during the hot and dry season from April to July. Overfeeding, poor seed, water, and feed quality, algal blooms or crashes are also factors that may lead to occurrences of AHPND in endemic areas (Food and Agriculture Organization, 2013). As with other infectious diseases of shrimp, establishing good sanitary and biosecurity practices, such as improvement of hatchery sanitary conditions and post-larval screening are likely to be beneficial; good broodstock management, use of high-quality post-larvae and good shrimp farm management (strict feeding rate control, appropriate stocking density) are all well-established practices that reduce the impact of disease, including AHPND (Network of Aquaculture Centres in Asia-Pacific, 2012).

Vp AHPND is expected to possess similar properties to other strains of *V. parahaemolyticus* found in seafood that have been shown to survive up to 9 days in filtered estuarine water and 18 days in filtered seawater at an ambient temperature of 28°C ± 2°C (Karunasagar et al., 1987). Experimental studies have shown that Vp AHPND could not be transmitted via frozen infected shrimp (Tran et al., 2013a). Other strains of *V. parahaemolyticus* are known to be sensitive to freezing, refrigeration, heating, and common disinfectants.

Shrimp White Tail Disease The clinical disease based on appearance of "white tail" has been associated with several etiological agents in both shrimp and freshwater prawns. These are:

- infectious myonecrosis virus (IMNV)
- *Macrobrachium rosenbergii* nodavirus (MrNV)
- extra-small virus-like particle (XSV).

Infectious Myonecrosis Virus

Overview: IMNV is similar to the Totiviridae and is related to the *Giardia lamblia* virus. IMNV infects penaeid shrimp, including the most commonly farmed species, causing mortalities that can reach to 70% in farmed *Penaeus vannamei*. Losses due to IMNV from 2002 through 2011 were estimated to be more than US $ 1 billion (Lightner, 2012). In regions where the infection is endemic in farmed stocks of *P. vannamei*, its prevalence may reach 100%.

Host range and distribution: Anecdotal information on the introduction of *P. vannamei* stocks from Brazil to Indonesia in 2006 was confirmed when investigations of stock in both countries revealed a shared 99.6% similar genome sequence identity. The virus appeared to be contained in Indonesia until 2008, when it subsequently spread to multiple provinces including East Java, Bali, Lampung, Central Java, West Kalimantan, and West Nusa Tenggara. Susceptible species include the brown tiger prawn (*Penaeus esculentus*), banana prawn (*Penaeus merguiensis*), and whiteleg shrimp (*P. vannamei*) (World Organisation for Animal Health, 2022a), while it is thought that the giant tiger prawn (*Penaeus monodon*) and blue shrimp (*Penaeus stylirostris*) may be susceptible, and the southern brown shrimp (*Penaeus subtilis*) has yielded a PCR-positive only.

Transmission: IMNV has been demonstrated to be transmitted horizontally by cannibalism, and although vertical transmission is suspected from anecdotal evidence, it is not known whether this occurs transovarially or by surface contamination of newly spawned eggs. Transmission via water probably occurs. Real Time PCR for screening pond-reared broodstock and/or their spawned eggs/nauplii and discarding those that test PCR-positive, fallowing and restocking of affected farms or entire culture regions with IMNV-free stocks of *P. vannamei*, and the development of specific pathogen-free shrimp stocks of *P. vannamei* most suited to local culture conditions have proven to be the most successful husbandry practice for preventing and controlling other virus diseases of shrimp, and should be applicable to control and prevent infection with IMNV (Tang et al., 2019).

Signs/diagnosis: Juveniles and subadults of *P. vannamei*, farmed in marine, brackish, and low salinity brackish water, appear to be most severely affected by infection with IMNV (Lightner, 2011). The virus targets the striated muscles (skeletal and less often cardiac), connective tissues, hemocytes, and the lymphoid organ parenchymal cells (Figure 1.35). Simple dissection will allow the hypertrophied (three to four times their normal size) paired lymphoid organs to be seen. On histopathology, lesions in striated muscles and lymphoid organs are not pathognomonic for infection with IMNV since white tail disease of penaeid shrimp caused by *P. vannamei* nodavirus (PvNV) can mimic infection with IMNV. Hence, diagnostic information from other sources (e.g. history, gross signs, morbidity, mortality, or rtPCR findings) may be required to confirm a diagnosis of infection with IMNV (Tang et al., 2019). Routine H&E-stained paraffin sections of acute-phase infections with IMNV show myonecrosis with characteristic coagulative necrosis of striated (skeletal) muscle fibers, often with marked edema among affected muscle fibers. Some shrimp may present a mix of acute and older lesions. In this shrimp, affected muscle fibers appear to progress from coagulative necrosis to liquefactive necrosis, accompanied by moderate infiltration and accumulation of hemocytes (Tang et al., 2019). In the most advanced lesions, hemocytes and inflamed muscle fibers are replaced by a loose matrix of fibrocytes and connective tissue fibers that are interspersed with hemocytes and presumed foci of regenerating

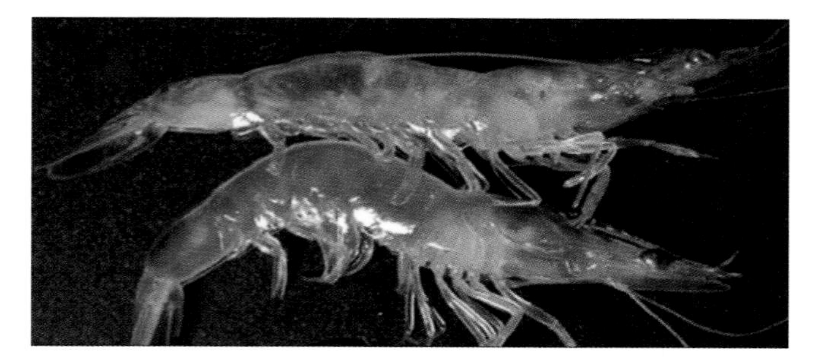

Figure 1.35 Opaque muscle in the abdominal sections and an erythematous tail caused by infectious myonecrosis virus. *Source:* Reproduced with permission from DV Lightner/Australia Department of Agriculture, Fisheries and Forestry/CC BY 4.0.

muscle fibers (Poulos et al., 2006). Significant hypertrophy of the lymphoid organ caused by accumulations of lymphoid organ spheroids (LOS) is a highly consistent lesion in shrimp with acute or chronic-phase infection with IMNV lesions. Often, many ectopic LOS are found in other tissues not near the main body of the lymphoid organ. Common locations for ectopic LOS include the hemocoelom in the gills, heart, near the antennal gland tubules, and ventral nerve cord (Poulos et al., 2006). Stained or unstained tissue squashes of skeletal muscle when examined with phase or reduced light microscopy may show loss of the normal striations. Fragmentation of muscle fibers may also be apparent. Squashes of the lymphoid organ may show the presence of significant accumulations of spherical masses of cells (LOS) among normal lymphoid organ tubules. See the *Manual of Diagnostic Tests for Aquatic Animals* for further details on sampling and diagnosis based on antibody and molecular techniques (Tang-Nelson F-J. 2017a).

In endemic areas, following stressful events such as capture by cast netting, feeding, and sudden changes in water salinity or temperature, there may be outbreaks of infection associated with sudden high mortalities in early juvenile, juvenile, or adult *P. vannamei*. In the acute phase, IMNV presents as focally extensive areas of white necrosis in striated (skeletal) muscles, especially in the distal abdominal segments, uropods and telson, which can become reddened and necrotic in some shrimp. Severely affected shrimp become moribund with high mortalities following a "stress" event that may continue for several days. Only shrimp with the acute phase of disease exhibit behavioral changes. Typically, severely affected shrimp become lethargic during or soon after stressful events. Feed conversion ratios of affected populations can increase from a normal value of approximately 1.5 up towards 4.0 or higher. Some *P. vannamei* that survive IMNV infections or epidemics may carry the virus.

Differentials: Whitish, necrotic tail muscle is observed in dead and moribund shrimp, especially in samples from Brazil, Indonesia, India, and Malaysia. IMNV should be included in the list of diseases for diagnosis. However, this clinical sign can also be caused by a number of factors other than IMNV infection (e.g. hypoxia, crowding, sudden changes in temperature or salinity, PvNV, and MrNV; Tang, 2019).

Management: The virus is non-enveloped and it is likely that IMNV will remain infectious in the gut and feces of birds that feed on dead or moribund shrimp at farms with continuing infection, and spread within and among farms by feces or regurgitated shrimp carcasses. Anecdotally, IMNV appears to be more difficult to inactivate with typical pond disinfection procedures (e.g. sun drying, chlorination, etc.) than other penaeid shrimp viruses like WSSV, YHV1, TSV, and IHHNV; however, disinfection of eggs and larvae is a good management practice recommended to reduce the transmission potential of a number of penaeid shrimp diseases from female spawners to their eggs or larvae, and the practice may reduce IMNV contamination of spawned eggs and larvae produced from them. Reservoir hosts are suspected, but none have been documented consistently. There are no specific data on vectors.

Macrobrachium rosenbergii Nodavirus

Overview: The MrNV virus is infective to brown tiger prawn (*Penaeus esculentus*), banana prawn (*Penaeus merguiensis*), and whiteleg shrimp (*Penaeus vannamei*) and is identified with no clinical signs in southern brown shrimp (*Penaeus subtilis*). Juveniles and subadults appear most severely impacted.

Transmission: Transmission occurs from infected tissue, including possibly within the gastrointestinal tract of predatory birds, through feces or regurgitate. Horizontal transmission is demonstrated, and vertical suspected, however this might be through contamination of eggs after laying.

Signs/diagnosis: High mortalities following stressful events such as handling or sudden alterations to environmental conditions. This disease impacts the striated muscles (skeletal and cardiac) and lymphoid organ parenchymal cells, causing white necrotic areas within the musculature. Reddening is seen in some shrimp in the distal abdominal segments and tail fan. Animals become moribund and high mortalities (40–70%) can be seen for a number of days. Confirmatory diagnosis can be achieved through histopathology and a careful clinical history, or molecular techniques such as PCR or in-situ hybridization.

Differentials: Differential diagnoses include other white tail disease agents. Necrotic muscle tissue can also occur due to stresses such as low dissolved oxygen or altered temperature.

Management: There is currently no treatment or verified prevention strategy for this disease, although research does support the existence of more resistant lines of *P. vannamei* (a species that, in general, appears more susceptible to this disease than others). Screening broodstock is recommended to prevent outbreaks, and specific pathogen-free lines of *P. vannamei* seem the most successful prevention strategy. This virus appears particularly resistant to traditional disinfection protocols.

Enterocytozoon hepatopenaei

Overview: *Enterocytozoon hepatopenaei* (EHP) is a microsporidian parasite of emerging concern in aquaculture production. Although infection does not appear to be associated with mortalities, it has been linked to notable reduction in growth performance.

Host range and transmission: EHP is known to infect *Penaeus monodon*, *Penaeus vannamei* and *Penaeus stylirostris* and is potentially endemic to the Australasian Pacific region. The full life cycle remains to be characterized, although infection is known to occur via infective spores, considered to be acquired through excretion in the feces or through cannibalism of infected tissue.

Signs/diagnosis: Clinical signs appear to be exclusively in a retardation of growth of infected individuals. Diagnosis is best achieved via molecular means due to the small spore size of this organisms.

Differentials: A general lack of clinical signs typifies this infection. Generalized poor growth can occur due to a multitude of different conditions in shrimp (poor nutrition, altered temperature as well as viral and bacterial pathologies) and is therefore not pathognomonic.

Treatment: No treatment is currently available for this condition.

Management: PCR screening can be used to detect infection within a population and screen juveniles prior to stocking. Various trials have been aimed at killing spores, including temperature and chemical water treatments.

Freshwater Infections

Prawn "White Tail" Disease

Overview: White tail disease is a viral infection of brackish and freshwater environments that can present entirely without clinical signs for variable mortality in non-adult freshwater prawns.

Transmission: Infects giant freshwater prawn (*Macrobrachium rosenbergii*) by both vertical from broodstock and horizontal (via infected individuals and contaminated water) transmission. Larvae, post-larvae, and early juveniles are impacted, with variable mortality up to 95%.

Signs/diagnosis: Infection impacts striated muscle tissue and intratubular connective tissue of the hepatopancreas. Externally visible discoloration begins at the tail and extends cranially to cephalothorax, with extensive necrosis of muscle fibers, followed by death. Presumptive diagnosis can be reached by observation of post-larval stock with milky, opaque tails, and high mortality. Confirmatory diagnosis of MrNV and/or XSV is via rtPCR and loop-mediated isothermal amplification.

Treatment: No vaccination protocols or treatments are currently available for this infection.

Management: Broodstock screening with rtPCR is highly recommended.

Necrotizing Hepatopancreatitis

Overview: The WOAH defines infection with *Hepatobacter penaei* as infection with the pathogenic agent *Candidatus Hepatobacter penaei*, an obligate intracellular bacterium of the Order α-Proteobacteria that targets all hepatopancreatic cell types. The disease is commonly known as necrotizing hepatopancreatitis (World Organisation for Animal Health, 2022a). In *Penaeus vannamei*, it can result in an acute, usually catastrophic disease, with mortalities approaching 100%. Infection with *H. penaei* has been demonstrated in juveniles, adults, and broodstock of *P. vannamei* but other penaeids are susceptible.

Host range and distribution: Prevalence of *H. penaei* in wild stocks has been estimated between 5% and 17% in *Penaeus duorarum* and *Penaeus aztecus* in Mexico. Reported values for *H. penaei* prevalence in shrimp farms are between 0.6% and 1.3% in *P. vannamei* from shrimp farms in Belize, Brazil, Guatemala, Honduras, Mexico, Nicaragua, and Venezuela. *H. penaei* appears to have a Western hemisphere distribution in both wild and cultured penaeid shrimp and in addition to those territories above, is also found in Colombia, Costa Rica, Ecuador, El Salvador, Honduras, Panama, Peru, and the United States. On-farm infection may increase during long periods of high temperatures (> 29°C) and high salinity (20–38 ppt). In Mexico, the bacterium has a prevalence of less than 7% in shrimp farms between April and August; however, in September and October when temperatures are high during the day and low at night, a high prevalence and mortality (> 20%) are observed (Morales-Covarrubias, 2010).

Signs/diagnosis: No clinical signs are pathognomonic. Infection with *H. penaei* often causes an acute disease with very high mortalities in young juveniles, adult, and broodstock. In horizontally infected young juveniles, adult, and broodstock, the incubation period and severity of the disease is often size and/or age dependent. Gross signs are not specific, but acute infection with *H. penaei* shows a marked reduction in food consumption, followed by changes in behavior and appearance. These include lethargy, reduced food intake, atrophied hepatopancreas, anorexia, and empty guts, noticeably reduced growth and poor length to weight ratios ("thin tails"), soft shells and flaccid bodies, black or darkened gills, heavy surface fouling by epicommensal organisms, bacterial shell disease, including ulcerative cuticle lesions or melanized appendage erosion, and expanded chromatophores resulting in the appearance of darkened edges in uropods and pleopods. The principal target tissue for *H. penaei* is hepatopancreas but it infects most enteric tissues meaning feces may be collected and used for testing (usually by PCR, or dot-blot hybridization with specific probes) when non-lethal testing of valuable broodstock is necessary (Morales-Covarrubias et al., 2012). *H. penaei* do not replicate in the midgut, caeca, connective tissue cells, the gills, hematopoietic nodules, and hemocytes, ventral nerve cord and ganglia, antennal gland tubule epithelial cells, and lymphoid organ parenchymal cells, and these tissues are not appropriate for sampling (World Organisation for Animal Health, 2022a, chapter 2.2.3).

Differentials: Infection with EHP, infection with Vp AHPND and infection with (SHIV) (World Organisation for Animal Health, 2022a).

Transmission: Surviving prawns may be able to carry the intracellular bacterium for life and act as a source of infection by horizontal transmission, which is typically via cannibalism or contaminated water (Aranguren et al., 2006; Morales-Covarrubias, 2010). Feces shed into water has also been suggested as a source of transmission.

Management: Prevention includes early detection of the initial phase of clinical infection because of the potential for cannibalism to amplify and transmit the disease; sufficient feeding since starvation and cannibalism of infected shrimps with positive conditions for *H. penaei* multiplication are important factors for spread of the bacterium; using hydrated lime to treat pond bottoms during pond preparation before stocking can help reduce infection with *H. penaei*; preventive measures including raking, tilling, and removing sediments from the bottom of the ponds, fallowing ponds with prolonged drying (through exposure to sunlight) of ponds and water distribution canals for several weeks, disinfection of fishing gear and other farm equipment using calcium hypochlorite, and extensive liming of ponds between batches; employing best practice and using specific pathogen-free broodstock where possible (World Organisation for Animal Health, 2022a).

In the face of an outbreak, the best treatment currently available is antibiotic treatment with oxytetracycline and florfenicol in medicated feeds every 8 hours for 10 days, particularly if infection with *H. penaei* is detected in the initial phase (Morales-Covarrubias et al., 2012). There are no vaccinations or confirmed successes with immunostimulants, breeding for resistance, restocking with resistant strains or blocking agents. Disinfection of eggs and larvae is good management practice (Lee & O'Bryen, 2003) and is recommended for its potential to reduce *H. penaei* contamination of spawned eggs and larvae (and is good hygiene practice to prevent contamination by other infectious agents). The prevalence and severity of infection with *H. penaei* may be increased by rearing shrimp in relatively crowded or stressful conditions. Some husbandry practices have been successfully applied to the prevention of infection with *H. penaei* including the application of PCR to prescreen wild or pond-reared broodstock.

Non-Notifiable Diseases

Epizootic Shell Disease

Overview: A number of shell conditions are described in lobster, *Homarus americanus*, including impoundment shell disease (ISD), burn-spot or rust-spot shell disease, epizootic shell disease (ESD), and the enzootic form of ESD. ESD is a form of shell disease that presents differently to "classical" shell pathologies in that it develops rapidly with high prevalence in a population.

Host range and transmission: ESD impacts clawed lobsters. Important factors in onset appear to be water temperature, as well as environmental contaminants. Shell pathologies are considered to be predisposed by conditions that reduce the integrity of the carapace, including altered environmental pH or direct trauma, but the full causality of epizootic shell disease appears complex, involving multiple anthropogenic factors. Various bacteria can be cultured from lesions, including *Aquimarina homari* and *Thalassobius* species (also observed in ISD). These mixed bacterial communities appear to be associated with subsequent necrosis of tissues.

Signs/diagnosis: Shell erosions (moderate to deep) occur in the carapace along the dorsum of the cephalothorax and abdomen. Lesions are generally thin and deep, with pillars of unpigmented tissue seen deeper within the erosion. Diagnosis is based on clinical presentation and a case history of high prevalence of shell disease within a population.

Differentials: Several forms of shell disease can present clinically similarly, and most shell disease syndromes linked to bacterial infection are documented as presenting with irregular "cigarette burn marks" that progress and overlap. They can be distinguished by their characteristic clinical signs and prevalence. Chitinolytic bacterial infections can impact all lobster species, as can diet-induced shell disease. Additional shell diseases, including traumatic damage from substrate or aggression and "rust spot" disease (linked to aquatic pollution) cause brown necrotic pits across the shell surface, both often localized to claws and appendages. Impoundment shell disease, linked with overcrowding, poor water quality or inadequate diets, is seen bilaterally on the dorsal carapace, centered on setal pores, but also progresses to coalescing lesions. Fusarium fungal infection can also cause black discoloration to the carapace. Blackspot (auto-oxidation and polymerization of polyphenol oxidase oxidizing diphenols to form dark pigments during traumatic events such as molting and rough handling) is cosmetic only.

Treatment: As causation appears to be multifactorial, prevention must also be multifactorial. At this stage, treatments are only used in the study of this condition.

Gaffkemia

Overview: Gaffkemia (also known as red-tail) is an extremely virulent infectious disease of lobsters caused by the bacterium *Aerococcus viridans*.

Host range and distribution: Gaffkemia is thought to be a risk in all species of lobster but appears particularly virulent in European lobsters.

Signs/diagnosis: Dark orange to pink discoloration to the ventral surface of infected individuals occurs due to stress-associated pigmentation of hemolymph with astaxanthin, seen through thin ventral membranes. Lethargy and anorexia are also common findings, with infection progressing to moribund individuals that may lie on their sides or lose appendages. Rate of progression is impacted by temperature but can occur within a few days of infection in warm conditions. Diagnosis can be achieved by culture, PCR or fluorescent antibody techniques.

Differentials: Lethargy and inappetence are common findings as with most diseases. Reddening of the tail is a finding also seen in generalized stress syndromes, as well as with *Hematodinium* (parasitic) and *Haliphthoros* (fungal) infections.

Treatment: Antibiotics can be successful in the treatment of this condition, although legislation varies globally on their use.

Management: Good hygiene and low stress environments are key to prevention. Low stocking density and prevention of traumatic injury that might allow bacterial ingress are thought to be key.

Hematodinium

Overview: *Hematodinium* are parasitic dinoflagellates documented in a number of crustacean species globally and one of the most economically significant pathogens of decapod crustaceans (Figure 1.36).

Host range and distribution: *Haematodinium* infections are documented in many crustacean hosts, including the Atlantic blue crab (*Callinectes sapidus*), Norwegian lobster (*Nephrops norvegicus*), mud crabs (*Scylla serrata*), snow crab (*Chionoecetes opilio*), tanner crab (*Chionoecetes bairdi*), velvet swimming crab (*Necora puber*) and ridgetail white prawns (*Exopalaemon carinicauda*). European lobsters do not appear to be susceptible. The currently described species are *Haematodinium perezi* and *Haematodinium australis*, and they appear to have varied host prevalence.

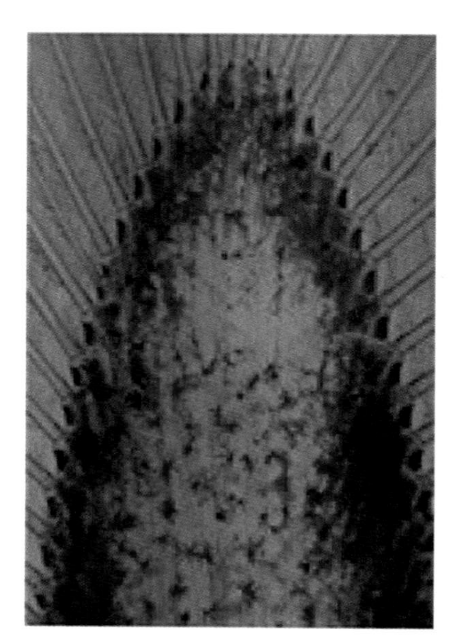

Figure 1.36 *Hematodinium* infection of *Nephrops norvegicus* pleopod. Pleopod assessment is used for diagnosis and staging severity. Cells similar in size to the hemocytes are seen as darkened areas due to dense aggregations using compound light microscopy. Intensely red pigmentation is due to carotenoid pigment released from the hepatopancreas during disease. This reddening can be observed macroscopically but is considered a less reliable indicator of disease. *Source:* Image kindly provided by Irene Molto-Martin, Institute of Aquaculture, Stirling and Cefas, Weymouth.

Transmission: Transmission is thought to occur horizontally through release of spores from infected animals.

Signs/diagnosis: Sometimes described as "bitter crab disease" due to the impact infection imparts on the taste of these animals, this disease causes high mortalities, with seasonal mortalities or even near eradication of stock occurring in wild crustaceans. Other clinical signs include altered carapace coloration, as well as paling and necrosis of muscle tissues. Hemolymph is cloudy, and animals can display altered swimming behavior and lethargy.

Dead animals sink to the bottom and are not observed unless washed upon the shoreline in wild populations. Infections can therefore go unnoticed in juveniles and females not targeted by fisheries. Diagnosis can be achieved using wet smears, histology, and molecular detection techniques. Neutral red stains *Hematodinium* well for wet mounts, although histology can allow observation of parasites in multiple tissue types.

Differentials: Pallid muscle due to glycogen depletion can occur in many chronic conditions, as well as naturally with seasonal variation. Pallid shell appears similar to recently molted individuals. Clouded hemolymph in crabs can be due to a number of systemic diseases, including *Paramoeba* and bacterial infections.

Treatment: Currently, there are no practical treatments or means of prevention.

Paramoeba perniciosa

Overview: *Paramoeba perniciosa* causes paramoebiasis (also known as "gray crab disease") in multiple *Crustacea* and is of concern to fisheries globally.

Host range and distribution: Infection occurs in crabs (*Callinectes sapidus* and *Cancer irroratus*) and lobsters (*Homarus americanus*).

Transmisison: Transmission appears to be horizontal through contact.

Signs/diagnosis: Infection causes pallid or a grayish discoloration of the shell, often accompanied by altered behavior ranging from reduced activity to flaccid paralysis. Reduced or absent clotting of the hemolymph can be indicative of disease presence, and high mortalities can be observed following stressful events. Parasites can be observed in squash preparations, hemolymph smears, and histology, as well as being diagnosed by PCR.

Differentials: Diseased species may provide an indication of which condition to expect; however, cloudy hemolymph and altered shell coloration are both symptoms seen in paramoebiasis and *Hematodinium* infections in crabs. Systemic infections of bacteria or viral diseases can also cause mass mortalities such as can be seen with paramoebiasis.

Treatment: There are currently no methods of treatment or control for this organism.

Zoonoses

Handling shellfish often leads to cuts or mild abrasions of the skin because of their tough shells and ability to pinch. Similar to mycobacterial infection from tropical fish, care must be taken to avoid infection of the skin with *Erysipelothrix rhusiopathiae*, particularly from lobsters. If infection does occur, a red-purple circular lesion will develop, progressing to a blister. Systemic infection leading to sepsis is rare but possible.

Like many aquatic organisms, crustaceans can also pose a risk to human health if improperly cooked or prepared. Bacterial infections such as *Vibrio* can be transmitted from crustaceans to human hosts to cause gastritis, and digenea of the *Paragonimus* species are considered zoonotic from uncooked crayfish. Crayfish-related rhabdomyolysis (Haff disease) is a condition reported in humans following consumption of crayfish but the toxicity is currently unclear. Similarly, to bivalves, toxic algae may be a concern (although less so than in filter-feeding mollusks) and *Paragonimiasis* (lung fluke) can also be contracted by eating uncooked crayfish or crabs.

References

Abrams MJ, Basinger T, William Y, et al. 2015. Self-repairing symmetry in jellyfish through mechanically driven reorganization. *PNAS* 112(26) E3365–E3373.

Adams A, Thompson KD. 2012. Advances in diagnostic methods for mollusc, crustacean and finfish diseases. In: Austin B, eds. *Infectious Disease in Aquaculture: Prevention and Control*. Woodhead Publishing Series in Food Science, Technology and Nutrition. Amsterdam: Elsevier, pp. 129–146.

Aeby GS, Ushijima B, Campbell JE, et al. 2019. Pathogenesis of a tissue loss disease affecting multiple species of corals along the Florida Reef tract. *Front Marine Sci 6*: https://doi.org/10.3389/fmars.2019.00678.

American Fisheries Society. 2020. *Fish Health Section Blue Book*. Corvallis, OR: AFS. https://units.fisheries.org/fhs/fish-health-section-blue-book-2020 (accessed 24 August 2022).

Andrews JD. 1996. History of *Perkinsus marinus*, a pathogen of oysters in Chesapeake Bay 1950–1984. *J Shellfish Res* 15:13–16.

Aranguren LF, Briñez B, Aragon L, et al. 2006. Necrotizing hepatopancreatitis (NHP) infected *Penaeus vannamei* female broodstock: effect on reproductive parameters nauplii and larvae quality. *Aquaculture* 258:337–343.

Australia Department of Agriculture, Water and the Environment. 2020a. *Aquatic Animal Diseases Significant to Australia: Identification Field Guide*, 5th ed. Canberra: Australia Department of Agriculture, Water and the Environment.

Australia Department of Agriculture, Water and the Environment. 2020b. *Infection with Infectious Hypodermal and Haematopoietic Necrosis Virus (IHHNV)*. Canberra: Department of Agriculture, Water and the Environment.

Bakus GJ, Schulte B, Jhu S, et al. 1990. Antibiosis and antifouling in marine sponges: Laboratory versus field studies. In: Rützler K, ed. *New Perspectives in Sponge Biology*. Washington, DC: Smithsonian Institution Press; pp. 102–108.

Barnes DB, Harrison FW. 1994. Introduction to the Mollusca. In: Harrison FW, Kohn AJ, eds. *Microscopic Anatomy of Invertebrates, Mollusca One*, Volume 5 New York, NY: Wiley, pp. 1–13.

Batista FM, Arzul I, Pepin JF, et al. 2007. Detection of ostreid herpesvirus-1 DNA in bivalve molluscs: a critical review. *J Virol Methods* 139(1):1–11.

Bell TA, Lightner DV. 1984. IHHN virus: infectivity and pathogenicity studies in Penaeus stylirostris and Penaeus vannamei. *Aquaculture* 38:185–194.

Bell TA, Lightner DV. 1988. *A Handbook of Normal Penaeid Shrimp Histology*. Special Publication No. 1. Baton Rouge, LA: World Aquaculture Society.

Berthe FCJ, Le Roux F, Adlard RD, Figueras A. 2004. Marteiliosis in molluscs: a review. *Aquat Living Resources* 17:433–448.

Bevelander G. 1988. *Abalone Gross and Fine Structure*. Monterey Bay, CA: Boxwood Press.

Bielmyer-Fraser GK, Patel P, Capo T, Grosell M. 2018. Physiological responses of corals to ocean acidification and copper exposure. *Mar Poll Bull* 133:781–790.

Bondad-Reantaso MG, McGladdery SE, East I, Subasinghe RP. 2001. *Asia Diagnostic Guide to Aquatic Animal Diseases*. FAO Fisheries Technical Paper 402, Supplement 2. Rome, Italy: Food and Agriculture Organization.

Boonstra JL, Koneval ME, Clark JD, et al. 2015. Milbemycin oxime (Interceptor) treatment of amphipod parasites (*Hyperiidae*) from several host jellyfish species. *J Zoo Wildl Med* 46:158–160.

Borneman E. (2007). Two potential molluscicides useful against pest aeolid nudibranchs common on species of montipora in aquariums. *Reefkeeping Magazine* http://reefkeeping.com/issues/2007-09/eb (accessed 24 August 2022).

Bower SM. 2010. *Synopsis of Infectious Diseases and Parasites of Commercially Exploited Shellfish*. Nanaimo, BC: Fisheries and Oceans Canada. https://www.dfo-mpo.gc.ca/science/aah-saa/diseases-maladies/index-eng.html (accessed 28 August 2022).

Bower SM. 2001a. Hazards and risk management of Mikrocytos mackini in oysters. In: Rodgers CJ, ed. Proceedings of the OIE International Conference on Risk Analysis in Aquatic Animal Health. Paris, France: World Organisation for Animal Health, 164–166.

Bower SM. 2001b. Synopsis of infectious diseases and parasites of commercially exploited shellfish: nematode parasitism of abalone. Nematode parasitism of abalone. Government of Canada. https://www.dfo-mpo.gc.ca/science/aah-saa/diseases-maladies/nemparab-eng.html (accessed 25 August 2022).

Bower SM, McGladdery SE, Price IM. 1994. Synopsis of infectious diseases and parasites of commercially exploited shellfish. *Ann Rev Fish Dis* 4:1–199.

Bradbury PC. 1994. Parasitic protozoa of molluscs and crustacea. In: Kreier JP, eds. *Parasitic Protozoa*, 2nd ed. San Fransisco, CO: Elsevier, pp. 139–263.

Brown HH, Galtsoff PS, Smith CL, Smith FWG. 1939. Sponge mortality in the Bahamas. *Nature (Lond)* 143:807–808.

Burke CM, Harris JO, Hindrum SM, et al. 2001. *Environmental Requirements of Abalone*. Project No. 97/323. Launceston: University of Tasmania.

Butler IV, MJ, Hunt JH, et al. 1995. Cascading disturbances in Florida Bay, USA: Cyanobacteria blooms, sponge mortality, and implications for juvenile spiny lobsters Panulirus argus. *Mar Ecol Prog Ser* 129:119–125.

Carballo JL, Naranjo SA, Garcia-Gomez JC. 1996. Use of marine sponges as stress indicators in marine ecosystems at Algeciras Bay (southern Iberian Peninsula). *Mar Ecol Prog Ser* 135:109–122.

Carnegie RB, Burreson EM, Hine PM, et al. 2006. *Bonamia persporan*. Sp. (Haplosporidia), a parasite of the oyster *Ostreaola equestris*, is the first Bonamia species known to produce spores. *J Eukaryot Microbiol* 53:232–245.

Castro-Longoria R, Quintero-Arredondo N, Grijalva-Chon JM, Ramos-Paredes J. 2008. Detection of the yellow-head virus (YHV) in wild blue shrimp, Penaeus stylirostris, from the Gulf of California and its experimental transmission to the Pacific white shrimp, Penaeus vannamei. *J Fish Dis* 31:953–956.

Cawthorn RJ. 2011. Diseases of American lobsters (*Homarus americanus*): a review. *J Invert Pathol* 106(1):71–78.

Chaijarasphonga T, Munkongwongsiri N, Stentiford GD, et al. 2020. The shrimp microsporidian Enterocytozoon hepatopenaei (EHP): biology, pathology, diagnostics and control. *J Invert Pathol* 186:107458.

Chen SN, Chang PS, Kou GH. 1992. Infection route and eradication of monodon baculovirus (MBV) in larval giant tiger prawn, *Penaeus monodon*. In: Fulks W, and Main KL, eds. *Diseases of Cultured Penaeid Shrimp in Asia and the United States*. Honolulu, HI: Oceanic Institute, pp. 177–184.

Cheng TC, Rifkin E, Yee HWF. 1968a. Studies on the internal defense mechanisms of sponges. II. Phagocytosis and elimination of India ink and carmine particles by certain parenchymal cells of *Terpios zeteki*. *J Invertebr Pathol* 11:302–309.

Cheng TC, Yee HWF, Rifkin E, Kramer MD. 1968b. Studies on the internal defense mechanisms of sponges. III. Cellular reactions in Terpios zeteki to implanted heterologous biological materials. *J Invertebr Pathol* 11:29–35.

Chistoserdov AY, Quinn RA, Gubbala SL, Smolowitz R. 2012. Bacterial communities associated with lesions of shell disease in the American lobster. *Homarus americanus Milne-Edwards. J Shellfish Res* 31(2):449–462.

Chistoserdov AY, Smolowitz R, Mirasol F, Hsu A. 2005. Culture-Dependent Characterization of the Microbial Community Associated with Epizootic Shell Disease Lesions in American Lobster, *Homarus americanus*. Journal of Shellfish Research 24(3):741–747.

Christie BL, Raines JA. 2016. Effect of an otic milbemycin oxime formulation on *Tegastes Acroporanus* infesting corals. *J Aquatic Anim Health 28*(4):235–239.

Cobb J, Phillips B. 1980. *The Biology and Management of Lobsters*, Volume I Physiology and Behaviour. New York, NY: Academic Press.

Couch JA. 1983. Diseases caused by protozoa. In: AJ. Provenzano, Jr., ed. *The Biology of the Crustacea, Volume 6, Pathobiology*. New York, NY: Academic Press, pp. 79–111.

Crane M. 2018. Acute hepatopancreatic necrosis disease. In: Manual of Diagnostic Tests for Aquatic Animals. Paris, France: World Organisation for Animal Health, chapter 2.2.1. https://www.woah.org/en/what-we-do/standards/codes-and-manuals/aquatic-manual-online-access (accessed 25 August 2022).

Crane M, Corbeil S. 2022. Infection with abalone herpesvirus. In: World Organisation for Animal Health. *Manual of Diagnostic Tests for Aquatic Animals*. Paris, France: WOAH, chapter 2.4.1. https://www.woah.org/en/what-we-do/standards/codes-and-manuals/aquatic-manual-online-access (accessed 25 August 2022).

Crossley SMGS, George AL, Keller CJ. 2009. A method for eradicating amphipod parasites (hyperiidae) from host jellyfish, *Chrysaora fuscescens* (Brandt, 1835), in a closed recirculating system. *J Zoo Wildl Med* 40:174–180.

Cuellar-Anjel J, Corteel M, Galli L, et al. 2010. Principal Shrimp Infectious Diseases, Diagnoses, and Management. In: Alday-Sanz V, ed. *The Shrimp Book*. Nottingham, UK: Nottingham University Press, pp. 517–621.

Davis AR, Roberts DE, Cummins SP. 1997. Rapid invasion of a sponge-dominated deep-reef by Caulerpa scalpelliformis (Chlorophyta) in Botany Bay, New South Wales. *Aust J Ecol* 22:146– 150.

De La Peña LD, Cabillon NA, Catedral DD, et al. 2015. Acute hepatopancreatic necrosis disease (AHPND) outbreaks in *Penaeus vannameiand P. monodon* cultured in the Philippines. *Dis Aquat Organ* 116:251–254.

De Vos L, Rützler K, Boury-Esnault N, et al. 1991. *Atlas of Sponge Morphology*. Washington, DC: Smithsonian Institution Press.

Deschaseaux E, Hardefeldt J, Graham J, Reichelt-Brushett A. 2018. High zinc leads to reduced dimethylfulfoniopropionate (DMSP) levels in both the host and endosymbionts of the reef-building coral Acropora aspera. *Mar Poll Bull.* 126:93–100.

Diggles BK, Cochennec-Laureau N, Hine PM. 2003. Comparison of diagnostic techniques for *Bonamia exitiosus* from flat oysters *Ostrea chilensis* in New Zealand. *Aquaculture* 220:145–156.

Dodge RE, Aller RC, Thomson J. 1974. Coral growth related to resuspension of bottom sediments. *Nature (Lond)* 247:574–577.

Doerr M, Stoskopf MK. 2019. Evaluation of euthanasia of moon jellyfish (Aurelia aurita) using simple salt solutions. *J Zoo Wildl Med* 50(1):123–126.

Doores S, Cook TM. 1976. Occurrence of*Vibrio* and other bacteria on the sea nettle,*Chrysaora quinquecirrha*. *Microb Ecol* 3:31–40.

Dungan C, Reece K. 2020. 5.2.1 *Perkinsus* sp. infections of marine molluscs. In: *American Fisheries Society. Fish Health Section Blue Book*. Corvallis, OR: AFS. https://units.fisheries.org/fhs/fish-health-section-blue-book-2020 (accessed 24 August 2022).

Ein-Gil N, Ilan M, Carmeli S, et al. 2009. Presence of *Aspergillus sydowii*, a pathogen of gorgonian sea fans in the marine sponge *Spongia obscura*. *ISME J* 3(6):752–755.

Elson R. 1993. Infectious diseases of the Pacific oyster, *Crassostrea gigas*. *Ann Rev Fish Dis* 3:259–276.

Fleming NEC, Harrod C, Griffin DC, et al. 2014. Scyphozoan jellyfish provide short-term reproductive habitat for hyperiid amphipods in a temperate near-shore environment. *Mar Ecol Prog Ser* 510:229–240.

Florida Department of Environmental Protection. Stony coral tissue loss disease (SCTLD) case definition. 2018. https://floridadep.gov/rcp/coral/documents/stony-coral-tissue-loss-disease-sctld-case-definition (accessed 24 August 2022).

Food and Agriculture Organization 2013. *Report of the FAO/MARD Technical Workshop on Early Mortality Syndrome (EMS) or Acute Hepatopancreatic Necrosis Syndrome (AHPNS) of Cultured Shrimp (under TCP/VIE/3304), Hanoi, Viet Nam, 25–27 June 2013*. Rome. Italy: FAO.

Fossa SE, Nilsen AJ. 2002. Mollusca. In: Brockman D, Schmettkamp W, eds. *The Modern Coral Reef Aquarium*, Volume 4. Bornheim, Germany: Birgit Schmettkamp, 29–208.

Francis JC, Harrison FW. 1988. Copper and zinc toxicity in *Ephydatia fluviatilis* (Porifera: Spongillidae). *Trans Am Microsc Soc* 107:67–78.

Freeman KA. 2001. *Aquaculture and related biological attributes of abalone species in Australia – A Review*. Fisheries Research Report, No. 128. North Beach, WA: Western Australia Marine Research Laboratories Department of Fisheries.

Freeman KS, Lewbart GA, Robarge WP, et al. 2009. Characterization of eversion syndrome in captive Scyphomedusa jellyfish. *Am J Vet Res* 70:1087–1093.

Gaino E, Pronzato R. 1989. Ultrastructural evidence of bacterial damage to Spongia officinalis fibres (Porifera, Demospongiae). *Dis Aquat Organ* 6:67–74.

Gaino E, Pronzato R, Corriero G, Buffa P. 1992. Mortality of commercial sponges: Incidence in two Mediterranean areas. *Boll Zool* 59:79–85.

Gao Z, Li B, Zheng C, Wang G. 2008. Molecular detection of fungal communities in the Hawaiian marine sponges Suberites zeteki and Mycale armata. *Appl Environ Microbiol* 74(19):6091–6101.

Gerrodette T, Flechsig AO. 1979. Sediment -induced reduction in the pumping rate of the tropical sponge Verongia lacunosa. *Mar Biol* 55:103–110.

Gestal C, Pascual S, Guerra Á, et al. 2019. *Handbook of Pathogens and Diseases of Cephalopods*. Cham, Switzerland: Springer Open.

Gomez-Chiarri M, Cobb JS. 2012. Shell disease in the American lobster, *Homarus americanus*: a synthesis of research from the New England Lobster Research Initiative: lobster shell disease. *J Shellfish Res* 31(2):583–590.

Gosling E. 2015. *Marine Bivalve Molluscs*, 2nd ed. Ames, IA: Wiley.

Guzman EA, Johnson JD, Carrier MK, et al. 2009. Selective cytotoxic activity of the marine-derived batzelline compounds against pancreatic cancer cell lines. *Anticancer Drugs* 20(2):149–155.

Handlinger J, Bastianello S, Callinan R, et al. 2006. *Abalone Aquaculture Subprogram: A National Survey of Commercially Exploited Abalone Species to Support Trade and Translocation Issues and the*

Development of Health Surveillance Programs. Final Report May 2006. FRDC Project No. 2002/201. Canberra: Fisheries Research and Developmewnt Corporation.

Hansen IV, Weeks JW, Depledge MH. 1995. Accumulation of copper, zinc, cadmium and chromium by the marine sponge *Halichondra panicea* Pallas and the implications for biomonitoring. *Mar Pollut Bull* 31:133–138.

Hasson KW, Lightner DV, Mohney LL, et al. 1999. Taura syndrome virus (TSV) lesion development and the disease cycle in the Pacific white shrimp *Penaeus vannamei*. *Dis Aquat Organ* 36:81–93.

Hatch Accelerator Holding. 2022. Taura syndrome. *The Fish Site*. https://thefishsite.com/disease-guide/taura-syndrome (accessed 26 August 2022).

Hill M, Stabile C, Steffen LK, Hill A. 2002. Toxic effects of endocrine disrupters on freshwater sponges: Common developmental abnormalities. *Environ Pollut* 117:295–300.

Hine PM. 1991a. The annual pattern of infection by *Bonamia* sp. In New Zealand flat oysters *Tiostrea chilensis*. *Aquaculture* 93:241–251.

Hine PM. 1991b. Ultrastructural observations on the annual infection pattern of *Bonamia* sp. In flat oysters *Tiostrea chilensis*. *Dis Aquat Org* 11:163–171.

Hine PM, Jones JB. 1994. *Bonamia* and other aquatic parasites of importance to New Zealand. *N Z J Zool* 21:49–56.

Hine PM, Diggles BK, Parsons MJD, et al. 2002. The effects of stressors on the dynamics of *Bonamia exitiosus* Hine, Cochennec-Laureau and Berthe, infections in flat oysters *Ostrea chilensis* (Philippi). *J Fish Dis* 25:545–554.

Hirose E, Kumagai A, Nawata A, Kitamura S-I. 2014. *Azumiobodo hoyamushi*, the kinetoplastid causing soft tunic syndrome in ascidians, may invade through the siphon wall. *Dis Aquat Organ* 109:251–256.

Hirose E, Nozawa A, Kumagai A, Kitamura S-I. 2012. *Azumiobodod hoyamushi* gen. nov. et sp. Nov. {Euglenoza, Kinetoplastea, Neobodonida}: a pathogenic kinetoplastid causing the soft tunic syndrome in ascidian aquaculture. *Dis Aquat Organ* 97:227–235.

Hooper JNA, Van Soest RWM. 2002. *Systema Porifera: A Guide to the Classification of Sponges*, Volumes 1 and 2. New York, NY: Kluwer Academic/Plenum.

Howard DW, Lewis EJ, Keller BJ, Smith CS. 2004. *Histological Techniques for Marine Bivalve Mollusks and Crustaceans*. NOAA Technical Memorandum NOS NCCOS 5. Oxford, MD: National Oceanic and Atmospheric Administration.

Jackson JBC, Goreau TF, Hartman WD. 1971. Recent brachiopod–coralline sponge communities and their paleoecological significance. *Science* 173:623–625.

Jaenike F, Gregg K, Hamper L. 1992. Shrimp production in Texas using specific pathogen-free stocks. In: Fulks W, and Main K, eds. *Diseases of Cultured Penaeid Shrimp in Asia and the United States*. Honolulu, HI: Oceanic Institute, pp. 295–302.

Jafarabadi AR, Bakhtiari AR, Spanó N, Capello T. 2018. First report of geochemical fractionation distribution, bioavailability and risk assessment of potentially toxic inorganic elements in sediments of coral reef islands of the Persian Gulf, *Iran. Mar Poll Bull* 137:185–197.

Jithendran KP, Poornima M, Balasubramanian CP, Kulasekarapandian S. 2010. Diseases of mud crabs (*Scylla* spp.): an overview. *Indian J Fisheries* 57(3):55–63.

Joshi J, Srisala J, Sakaew W, et al. 2014. Identification of bacterial agent(s) for acute hepatopancreatic necrosis syndrome, a new emerging shrimp disease. *Suranaree J Sci Technol* 21:315–320.

Kalagayan G, Godin D, Kanna R, et al. 1991. IHHN virus as an etiological factor in runt-deformity syndrome of juvenile Penaeus vannamei cultured in Hawaii. *J World Aquacult Soc* 22:235–243.

Karunsagar I, Venugopal MN, Nagesha CN. 1987. Survival of *Vibrio parahaemolyticus* in estuarine and sea water and in association with clams. *Syst Appl Microbiol* 9:316–319.

Keyzers RA, Davies-Coleman MT. 2005. Anti-inflammatory metabolites from marine sponges. *Chem Soc Rev* 34(4):355–365.

Kitamura SI, Ohtake SI, Song JY, et al. 2010. Tunic morphology and viral surveillance in diseased Korean ascidinas: soft tunic syndrome in the edible ascidian, *Halocynthia roretzi* (Drasche), in aquaculture. *J Fish Dis* 33:153–160.

Kochanowska AJ, Rao KV, Childress S, et al. 2008. Secondary metabolites from three Florida sponges with antidepressant activity. *J Nat Prod* 71(2):186–189.

Kogovšek TT, Klun K, Malej A, et al. 2019. Jellyfish-associated microbiome in the marine environment: exploring its biotechnological potential. *Mar Drugs* 17(2):94.

Krediet CJ, Meyer JL, Gimbrone N, et al. 2014. Interactions between the tropical sea anemone *Aiptasia pallida* and *Serratia marcescens*, an opportunistic pathogen of corals. *Environ Microbiol Rep* 6(3):287–292.

Kuhns WJ, Ho M, Burger MM, Smolowitz R. 1997. Apoptosis and tissue regression in the marine sponge *Microciona prolifera*. *Biol Bull* 193:239–241.

Kumagai A, Suto A, Ito H, et al. 2011. Soft tunic syndrome in the edible ascidian *Halocynthia roretzi* is caused by a kinetoplastid protist. *Dis Aquat Organ* 95:153–161.

Kumagai A, Suto A, Ito H, et al. 2010. Mass mortality of cultured ascidians *Halocynthia roretzi* associated with softening of the tunic and flagellate-like cells. *Dis Aquat Organ* 90:223–234.

Kuris AM, Lafferty KD. 1992. Modelling crustacean fisheries: effects of parasites on management strategies. *Can J Fish Aquat Sci* 49:327–336.

LaDouceur EEB, Garner MM, Wynne J, et al. 2013. Ulcerative umbrellar lesions in captive moon jelly (*Aurelia aurita*) medusae. *Vet Pathol* 50(3):434–442.

Lauckner G. 1980. Diseases of Porifera. In: Kinne O, ed. *Diseases of Marine Animals*, Vol. 1. New York, NY: Wiley, pp. 139–165.

Levine JF, Law M, Corsin F. 2012. Bivalves. In: Lewbart GA. ed. *Invertebrate Medicine*, 2nd ed. Chichester, UK: Wiley-Blackwell, pp. 127–152.

Levine JF, Law M, Corsin F. 2012. Crustaceans. In: Lewbart GA, ed. *Invertebrate Medicine*, 2nd ed. Chichester, UK: Wiley-Blackwell.

Lightner DV. 2011. Virus diseases of farmed shrimp in the Western Hemisphere (the Americas): a review. *J Invertebr Pathol* 106:110–130.

Lightner DV. 2005. Biosecurity in shrimp farming: pathogen exclusion through use of SPF stock and routine surveillance. J World Aquaculture Soc 36:229–248.

Lightner DV, ed. 1996. *A Handbook of Shrimp Pathology and Diagnostic Procedures for Diseases of Cultured Penaeid Shrimp*. Baton Rouge, LA: World Aquaculture Society.

Lightner DV, Redman RM. 1998. Shrimp diseases and current diagnostic methods. *Aquaculture* 164:201–220.

Lightner DV, Redman RM, Pantoja CR, et al. 2012. Historic emergence, impact and current status of shrimp pathogens in the Americas. J. *Invert Pathol* 110:174–183.

Lightner DV, Redman RM, Arce S, Moss SM. 2009. Specific pathogen-free (SPF) shrimp stocks in shrimp farming facilities as a novel method for disease control in Crustaceans. In: Shumway S. and Rodrick G, eds. *Shellfish Safety and Quality*. London, UK: Woodhead, pp. 384–424.

Lightner DV, Pantoja CR, Poulos BT, et al. 2004. Infectious myonecrosis: new disease in Pacific white shrimp. *Global Aquaculture Advocate* 7:85.

Lightner DV, Bell TA, Redman RM, Perez LA. 1992. A collection of case histories documenting the introduction and spread of the virus disease IHHN in penaeid shrimp culture facilities in Northwestern Mexico. *ICES Marine Sci Symp* 194: 97–105.

Lo GC-F. 2018. Infection with white spot syndrome virus. In: Manual of Diagnostic Tests for Aquatic Animals. Paris, France: World Organisation for Animal Health, 2.2.8. https://www.woah.org/en/what-we-do/standards/codes-and-manuals/aquatic-manual-online-access (accessed 26 August 2022).

Longshaw, M. Diseases of crayfish: a review. *J Invert Pathol* 106:54–70.

Longshaw M, Feist SW, Matthews A, Figueras A. 2001. Ultrastructural characterisation of *Marteilia* species (Paramyxea) from *Ostrea edulis*, *Mytilus edulis* and *Mytilus galloprovincialis*. *Dis Aquat Org* 44:137–142.

López-Flores I, De La Herran R, Garrido-Ramos MA, et al. 2004. The molecular diagnosis of *Marteilia refringens* and differentiation between *Marteilia* strains infecting oysters and mussels based on the rDNA IGS sequence. *Parasitology* 129:411–419.

Luter HM, Whalan S, Webster NS. 2010. Prevalence of tissue necrosis and brown spot lesions in a common marine sponge. *Mar Freshw Res* 61(4):484–489.

Lynch SA, Villalba A, Abollo E, et al. 2013. The occurrence of haplosporidian parasites, *Haplosporidium davi* and *Haplosporidium* sp., in oysters in Ireland. *J Invert Pathol* 112(3):208–112.

Madri PP, Hermel M, Claus G. 1971. The microbial flora of the sponge Microciona porifera Verrill and its ecological implications. *Bot Mar* 14:1–5.

Madri PP, Claus G, Kunen SM, Moss EE. 1967. Preliminary studies on the *Escherichia coli* uptake of the redbeard sponge (*Microciona prolifera* Verill). *Life Sci* 6:889–894.

Marine Scotland Directorate. 2020. Diseases of finfish, molluscs and crustaceans. https://www.gov.scot/collections/diseases-of-finfish-molluscs-and-crustaceans (accessed 25 August 2022).

McDiarmid H, Day RW. 2004. The ecology of polychaetes that infest abalone shells in Victoria, Australia. *J Shellfish Res* 23:1179–1188.

McGladdery SE, Drinnan RE, Stephenson MF. 1933. *A Manual of Parasites, Pest and Diseases of Canadian Atlantic Bivalves. Canadian technical report of fisheries and aquatic sciences*. Ottawa, Canada: Department of Fisheries and Oceans.

Meiling S, Muller EM, Smith TB, Brandt ME. 2020. 3D photogrammetry reveals dynamics of Stony Coral Tissue Loss Disease (SCTLD) lesion progression across a thermal stress event. *Front Mar Sci* 7:597643.

Meyer GR, Bower SM, Lowe G, Davies S. 2008. Resistance of the Manila clam (*Venerupis philippinarum*) to infection with *Mikrocytos mackini*. *J Invert Pathol* 98:54–57.

Meyer GR, Bower SM, Carnegie RB. 2005. Sensitivity of a digoxigenin-labelled DNA probe in detecting Mikrocytos mackini, causative agent of Denman Island disease (mikrocytosis) in oysters. *J Invert Pathol* 88:89–94.

Mizoguchi H, Watanabe Y. 1990. Collagen synthesis in *Ephydatia fluviatilis*. In: Rützler K, ed. *New Perspectives in Sponge Biology*. Washington, DC: Smithsonian Institution Press, pp. 188–192.

Mohamed AR, Sweet M. 2019. Current knowledge of coral diseases present within the Red Sea. In: Rasul NMA and Stewart ICF eds. *Oceanographic and Biological Aspects of the Red Sea*. Geneva: Springer Oceanography, pp. 387–400.

Moiseeva E, Rabinowitz C, Yankelelvich I, Rinkervich B. 2004. "Cup cell disease" in the colonial tunicate Botryllus schlosseri. *Dis Aquat Organ* 60:77–84.

Monniot C. 1990. Diseases of urochordata. In: Kinne O, ed. *Diseases of Marine Animals*, Volume 3. Hamburg, Germany: Biologische Anstalt, pp. 569–636.

Montgomery-Brock D, Tacon AGJ, Poulos B, Lightner DV. 2007. Reduced replication of infectious hypodermal and hematopoietic necrosis virus (IHHNV) in Litopenaeus vannamei held in warm water. *Aquaculture* 265:41–48.

Morado J. 2011. Protistan diseases of commercially important crabs: a review. *J Invert Pathol* 106(1):27–53.

Morals-Covarrubias MS, Tlahuel-Vargas L, Martínez-Rodríguez IE, et al. 2012. Necrotising hepatobacterium (NHPB) infection in *Penaeus vannamei* with florfenicol and oxytetracycline: a comparative experimental study. *Rev Cient Vet* 22:72–80.

Morals-Covarrubias MS, Lozano-Olvera RY, Hernández-Silva AJ. 2010. Necrotizing hepatopancreatitis in cultured shrimp caused by extracellular and intracellular bacteria. *Tilapia Camarones* 5:33–39.

Morales-Covarrubias MS, Nunan LM, Lightner DV, et al. 1999. Prevalence of IHHNV in wild broodstock of Penaeus stylirostris from the upper Gulf of California, *Mexico. J Aqua. Anim Health* 11:296–301.

Moss JA, Burreson EM, Cordes JF, et al. 2007. Pathogens in *Crassostrea ariakensis* and other Asian oyster species: implications for non-native oyster introduction to Chesapeake Bay. *Dis Aquat Org* 77:207–223.

Motte E, Yugcha E, Luzardo J, et al. 2003. Prevention of IHHNV vertical transmission in the white shrimp Litopenaeus vannamei. *Aquaculture* 219:57–70.

Mouton A. 2003. Histological changes associated with stress in intensively cultured South African abalone, *Haliotis midae*. In: Fleming AE, *ed. Proceedings of the 10th Annual Abalone Aquaculture Workshop, 19–21st November 2003, Port Lincoln, Australia*. Canberra, Australia: Abalone Aquaculture Subprogram, Fisheries Research and Development Corporation, pp. 123–128.

Müller WEG, ed. 2003. *Sponges (Porifera): Progress in Molecular and Subcellular Biology*. Springer, Berlin.

Neely KL, Macaulay KA, Hower EK, Dobler MA. 2020. Effectiveness of topical antibiotics in treating corals affected by stony coral tissue loss disease. *PeerJ* 8: e9289.

Negri AP, Smith LD, Webster NS, Heyward AJ. 2002. Understanding ship-grounding impacts on a coral reef: Potential effects of antifoulant paint contamination on coral recruitment. *Mar Pollut Bull* 44:111–117.

Network of Aquaculture Centres in Asia-Pacific. 2014. *Diseases of Crustaceans: Acute hepatopancreatic necrosis disease*. Bangkok, Thailand: NACA.

Newton AL, Smolowitz R. 2020. Invertebrates. In: Terio KA, McAloose D, St. Leger J, eds. *Pathology of Wildlife and Zoo Animals*. London, UK: Academic Press, pp. 1011–1043.

Nigrelli RF, Jakowska S, Calventi J. 1959. Ectyonin, an antimicrobial agent from the sponge *Microciona prolifera* Verrill. *Zoologica (NY)* 44:173–176.

Norton JH, Jones GW. 1992. *The Giant Clam: An Anatomical and Histological Atlas*. Townsville, Queensland, Australia: Queensland Department of Primary Industries.

Olson JB, Gochfeld DJ, Slattery M. 2006. Aplysina red band syndrome: a new threat to Caribbean sponges. *Dis Aquat Organ* 71(2):163–168.

Owens L, La Fauce K, Juntunen K, et al. 2009. *Macrobrachium rosenbergii* nodavirus disease (white tail disease) in Australia. *Dis Aquat Organ* 85:175–180.

Owens L, Anderson IG, Kenway M, et al. 1992. Infectious hypodermal and hematopoietic necrosis virus (IHHNV) in a hybrid penaeid prawn from tropical Australia. *Dis Aquat Org* 14:219–228.

Park KH, Zeon S-R, Lee J-G, et al. 2014. in vitro and in vivo efficacy of drugs against the protozoan parasite *Azumiobodo hoyamushi* that causes sotunic syndrome in edible ascidian *Halocynthia roretzi* (Drasche). *J Fish Dis* 37: 308–317.

Patel PP, Bielmyer-Fraser GK. 2014. Influence of salinity and copper exposure on copper accumulation and physiological impairment in the sea anemone, *Exaiptasia pallida*. *Comp Biochem Physiol C* 168:39–47.

Pepin JF, Roiu A, Renault T. 2008. Rapid and sensitive detection of ostreid herpesvirus 1 in oyster samples by real-time PCR. *J Virol Methods* 149:269–276.

Poulos BT, Lightner DV. 2006. Detection of infectious myonecrosis virus (IMNV) of penaeid shrimp by reverse-transcriptase polymerase chain reaction (rt-PCR). *Dis Aquat Org* 73:69–72.

Poulos BT, Tang KFJ, Pantoja CR, et al. 2006. Purification and characterization of infectious myonecrosis virus of penaeid shrimp. *J Gen Virol* 87:987–996.

Proctor HC, Pritchard G. 1989. Variability in the life history of Unionciola crassipes, sponge-associated water mite (Acari: Unionicolidae). *Can J Zool* 68:1227–1232.

Ravi M, Nazeer Basha A, Taju G, et al. 2010. Clearance of *Macrobrachium rosenbergii* nodavirus (MrNV) and extra small virus (XSV) and immunological changes in experimentally injected *Macrobrachium rosenbergii*. *Fish Shellfish Immunol* 28:428–433.

Reece KS, Duncan CF, Burreson EM. 2008. Molecular epizootiology of *Perkinsus marinus* and *P. chesapeaki* infections among wild oysters and clams in Chesapeake Bay, USA. *Dis Aquat Org* 82:237–248.

Reitzel AM, Sullivan JC, Brown BK, et al. 2007. Ecological and developmental dynamics of a host-parasite system involving a sea anemone and two ctenophores. *J Parasitol* 93:1392–1402.

Robledo JAF, Santarem MM, Gonzalez P, Figueras A. 1995. Seasonal variations in the biochemical composition of the serum of *Mytilus galloprovincialis* Lmk. and its relationship to the reproductive cycle and parasitic loads. *Aquaculture* 133:311–322.

Ruppert EE, Fox RS, Barnes RD. 2004. *Invertebrate Zoology: A Functional Evolutionary Approach*, 7th ed. Belmont, CA: Brooks/Cole Thomson Learning.

Rützler K. 1988. Mangrove sponge disease induced by cyanobacterial symbionts: Failure of a primitive immune system? *Dis Aquat Organ* 5:143–149.

Rützler K. 1970. Spatial competition among Porifera: Solution by epizoism. *Oecologia (Berl)* 5:85–95.

Scimeca JM. 2012. Cephalopods. In: Lewbart GA, ed. *Invertebrate Medicine*. Ames, IA: Wiley-Blackwell, pp. 113–125.

Shields JD. 2011a. Collection techniques for the analyses of pathogens in crustaceans. *J Crust Biol* 37(6):753–763.

Shields JD. 2011b. Diseases of spiny lobsters: a review. *J Invert Pathol* 106:79–91.

Smith FGW. 1941. Sponge disease in British Honduras, and its transmission by water currents. *Ecology* 22:415–421.

Smith FGW. 1939. Sponge mortality at British Honduras. *Nature (Lond)* 144:785.

Smith IM, Oliver DR. 1986. Review of parasitic associations of larval water mites (Acari: Parasitengona: Hydrachnida) with insect hosts. *Can Entomol* 118: 407–472.

Smolowitz AQR. 2012. Gastropods. In: Lewbart G, ed. *Invertebrate Medicine*, 2nd ed. Ames, IA: Wiley Blackwell.

Spaulding JG. 1972. The life cycle of *Peachia quinquecapitata*, an anemone parasitic on medusae during its larval development. *Biol Bull* 143:440–453.

Sprung J. 2001. Mollusks. In: Sprung J. ed. Invertebrates: A quick reference guide. Oceanographic Series. Miami, FL: Ricordea, pp. 86–133.

Sprung J, Delbeek JC. 1997. *The Reef Aquarium: A Comprehensive Guide to the Identification and Care of Tropical Marine Invertebrates*, Volume 2. Coconut Grove, FL: Ricordia.

Srivastava M, Simakov O, Chapman J, et al. 2010. The *Amphimedon queenslandica* genome and the evolution of animal complexity. *Nature* 466:720–726.

Stegeman N, Allender M, Arnold J, Bonar C. 2020. Aquatic invertebrates. In: Heatley J, Russell KE, eds. *Exotic Animal Laboratory Diagnosis*. John Ames, IA: Wiley, 383–408.

Stentiford GD, Shields GD. 2005. A review of the parasitic dinoflagellates *Hematodinium* species and *Hematodinium*-like infections in marine crustaceans. *Dis Aquat Organ* 66:47–79.

Stewart JE, Arie B, Zwicker BM, Dingle JR. 1969. Gaffkemia, a bacterial disease of the lobster, Homarus americanus: effects of the pathogen, *Gaffkya homari*, on the physiology of the host. *Can J Microbiol* 15(8):925–932.

Stewart ZK, Pavasovic A, Hock DH, Prentis PJ. 2017. Transcriptomic investigation of wound healing and regeneration in the cnidarian *Callictis polypus*. *Sci Rep* 7:41458.

Su YC, Liu C. 2007. *Vibrio parahaemolyticus*: a concern of seafood safety. *Food Microbiol* 24:549–558.

Sweet MJ, Croquer A, Bythell AC. 2014. Experimental antibiotic treatment identifies potential pathogens of white band disease in the endangered Caribbean coral *Acropora cervicornis*. *Proc R Soc B* 281(1788): 20140094.

Tang KFJ, Lightner DV. 2006. Infectious hypodermal and hematopoietic necrosis virus (IHHNV)-related sequences in the genome of the black tiger prawn Penaeus monodon from Africa and Australia. *Virus Res* 118:185–191.

Tang KFJ, Lightner DV. 2001. Detection and quantification of infectious hypodermal and hematopoietic necrosis virus in penaeid shrimp by real-time PCR. *Dis Aquat Organ* 44:79–85.

Tang KFJ, Bondad-Reantaso MG, Arthur JR. 2019. *Shrimp Infectious Myonecrosis Strategy Manual*. FAO Fisheries and Aquaculture Circular No. 1187. Rome: Food and Agriculture Organisation.

Tang-Nelson F-J. 2018. Infection with infectious hypodermal and haematopoietic necrosis virus. In: *Manual of Diagnostic Tests for Aquatic Animals*. Paris, France: World Organisation for Animal Health, chapter 2.2.4. https://www.woah.org/en/what-we-do/standards/codes-and-manuals/aquatic-manual-online-access/ https://www.woah.org/en/what-we-do/standards/codes-and-manuals/aquatic-manual-online-access (accessed 25 August 2022).

Tang-Nelson F-J. 2017a. Infection with infectious myonecrosis virus. In: *Manual of Diagnostic Tests for Aquatic Animals*. Paris, France: World Organisation for Animal Health, chapter 2.2.5. https://www.woah.org/en/what-we-do/standards/codes-and-manuals/aquatic-manual-online-access (accessed 26 August 2022).

Tang-Nelson F-J. 2017b. Infection with Taura syndrome virus. In: *Manual of Diagnostic Tests for Aquatic Animals*. Paris, France: World Organisation for Animal Health, chapter 2.2.7. https://www.woah.org/en/what-we-do/standards/codes-and-manuals/aquatic-manual-online-access (accessed 26 August 2022).

Taylor MW, Radax R, Steger D, Wagner M. 2007. Sponge-associated microorganisms: Evolution, ecology, and biotechnological potential. *Microbiol Mol Biol Rev* 71(2):295–347.

Thakur NL, Hentschel U, Krasko A, et al. 2003. Antibacterial activity of the sponge Suberites domuncula and its primmorphs: Potential basis for epibacterial chemical defense. *Aquat Microb Ecol* 31:77–83.

Thébault A, Bergmann S, Pouillot S, et al. 2005. Validation of in situ hybridization and histology assays for the detection of the oyster parasite *Marteilia refringens*. *Dis Aquat Organ* 65(1):9–16.

Tran L, Nunan L, Redman RM, et al. 2013a. EMS/AHPNS: Infectious disease caused by bacteria. *Global Aquaculture Advocate* July/August:18–20.

Tran L, Nunan L, Redman RM, et al. 2013b. Determination of the infectious nature of the agent of acute hepatopancreatic necrosis syndrome affecting penaeid shrimp. *Dis Aquat Organ* 105:45–55.

Vacelet J. 1994. *Control of the Severe Sponge Epidemic: Near East and Europe: Algeria, Cyprus, Egypt, Lebanon, Malta, Morocco, Syria, Tunisia, Turkey, Yugoslavia. Technical Report: The struggle against the epidemic which is decimating Mediterranean sponges*. FI:TCP/RAB/8853. Rome: Food and Agriculture Organization, pp 1–39.

Vacelet J, Donadey C. 1977. Electron microscope study of the association between some sponges and bacteria. *J Exp Mar Biol Ecol* 30:301–314.

Vacelet J, Vacelet E, Gaino E, Gallissian MF. 1994. Bacterial attack of spongin skeleton during the 1986–1990 Mediterranean sponge disease. In: Van Soest RWM, van Kempen TMG, and Braekman JC, eds. *Sponges in Time and Space*. Rotterdam: AA Balkema, pp. 355–362.

Van de Vyver G, Buscema M. 1990. Diversity of immune reactions in the sponge Axinella polypoides. In: Rützler K, ed. *New Perspectives in Sponge Biology*. Washington, DC: Smithsonian Institution Press, pp. 96–101.

Van Etten, JL, Meints RH, Kuczmarski D, et al. 1982. Hydra virus. *Proc Natl Acad Sci U S A* 79:3867–3871.

Van Soest RWM, Boury-Esnault N, Hooper JNA, et al. 2008. World Porifera database. http://www.marinespecies.org/porifera/index.php (accessed 24 August 2022).

Vasque-Yeomans R, Garcia-Ortega M, Caceres-Martinez J. 2010. Gill erosion and herpesvirus in *Crassostrea gigas* cultured in Baja California, Mexico. *Dis Aquat Org* 89:137–144.

Vigneron V, Solliec G, Montanie H, Renault T. 2004. Detection of ostreid herpes virus 1 (OsHV-1) DNA in seawater by PCR: influence of water parameters in bioassays. *Dis Aquat Org* 62:35–44.

Villalba A, Mourelle SG, Carballal MJ, Lopez MC. 1993a. Effects of infection by the protistan parasite Marteilia refringens on the reproduction of cultured mussels *Mytilus galloprovincialis* in Galicia (NW Spain). *Dis Aquat Org* 17:205–213.

Walker PJ, Cowley JA, Spann KM, et al. 2001. Yellow head complex viruses: Transmission cycles and topographical distribution in the Asia-Pacific Region. In: Browdy CL, and Jory DE, eds. *The New Wave, Proceedings of the Special Session on Sustainable Shrimp Culture, Aquaculture 2001*. Baton Rouge, LA: World Aquaculture Society, pp. 292–302.

Wallis C, Melnick J. 1965. Thermostabilization and thermosensitization of herpesvirus. *J Bacteriol* 90:1632–1637.

Webster NS. 2007. Sponge disease: A global threat? *Environ Microbiol* 9(6):1363–1375.

Webster NS, Xavier JR, Freckelton M, et al. 2008. Shifts in microbial and chemical patterns within the marine sponge *Aplysina aerophoba* during a disease outbreak. *Environ Microbiol* 10(12):3366–3376.

Webster NS, Negri AP, Webb RI, Hill RT. 2002. A spongin-boring proteobacterium is the etiological agent of disease in the Great Barrier Reef sponge *Rhopaloeides odorabile*. *Mar Ecol Prog Ser* 232:305–309.

White BL, Schofield PJ, Poulos BT, Lightner DV. 2002. A laboratory challenge method for estimating Taura syndrome virus resistance in selected lines of Pacific white shrimp *Penaeus vannamei*. *J World Aquacult Soc* 33:341–348.

Wongteerasupaya C, Boonsaeng V, Panyim S, et al. 1997. Detection of yellow-head virus (YHV) of *Penaeus monodon* by RT-PCR amplification. *Dis Aquat Organ* 31:181–186.

World Organisation for Animal Health. 2022a. *Manual of Diagnostic Tests for Aquatic Animals*. Paris, France: WOAH. https://www.woah.org/en/what-we-do/standards/codes-and-manuals/aquatic-manual-online-access (accessed 25 August 2022).

World Organisation for Animal Health. 2022b. Animal Diseases. https://www.woah.org/en/what-we-do/animal-health-and-welfare/animal-diseases (accessed 25 August 2022).

Yusa Y, Yamato S, Kawamura M, Kubota S. 2015. Dwarf males in the barnacle *Alepas pacifica* Pilsbry, 1907 (*Thoracica, Lepadidae*), a symbiont of jellyfish. *Crustaceana* 88(3):273–282.

Zahn RK, Zahn G, Müller WEG, et al. 1983. DNA damage by PAH and repair in a marine sponge. *Sci Total Environ* 26:137–142.

Zannella C, Mosca F, Mariani F, et al. 2006. Microbial diseases of bivalve mollusks: infections, immunology and antimicrobial defense. *Marine Drugs* 15(6):182.

Zaragosa WJ, Krediet CJ, Meyer JL, et al. 2014. Outcomes of infections of sea anemone Aiptasia pallida with Vibrio spp. pathogenic to corals. *Microb Ecol* 68:388–396.

Appendix 1.1

Etiology and clinical signs: coelenterates

Condition/body part affected	Etiology/clinical signs
Cnidarians	
Scyphozoa (jellyfish)	
Sudden death	Toxicity, trauma, extreme water quality parameters
Poor growth	Inadequate nutritional quality, inadequate food supply, loss of symbiotic bacteria, water pollution
Major diseases:	
Trauma	Nearly any species is susceptible. Healing and even regeneration is possible. The term "symmetrization" has been used to describe injured jellyfish healing and regaining their radial symmetry
Toxicity	Heavy metals like copper are known to be toxic to medusae and polyps
Aging	In some cases, it is possible that animals are merely undergoing senescence, although, it is very easy to make this "diagnosis" despite the fact that husbandry-related problems could be in play
Infectious diseases	Numerous species of bacteria have been cultured from jellyfishes, but in many cases these may represent normal flora. *Bacillus* spp. have been associated with moribund sea nettles (Doores and Cook, 1976). No viral or fungal diseases have been reported in jellyfish
Parasitic diseases:	
Nematodes	Larval nematodes of the genus *Thynnascaris* have been found associated with several species of jellyfish but successful treatment has not been reported
Digenean trematodes	Jellyfish can serve as an intermediate host for digenean trematodes, with the first host being a mollusk. In most cases the definitive host is a vertebrate such as a fish. It is not clear what clinical affect these infections have on the jellyfish
Cestodes	Cestode plerocercoids have been widely reported in jellyfish but their clinical impact is not well understood. It is likely that fish are the definitive hosts for many of these infections
Amphipods	The parasite of most concern in captive situations are the hyperiid amphipods. It appears the amphipods use the jellyfish as a haven for seasonal reproductive efforts (Crossley et al., 2009; Boonstra et al., 2015; Newton and Smolowitz, 2020). Treatment includes manual removal and chitin synthesis inhibitors like diflubenzuron (Crossley et al., 2009). Milbemycin oxime (0.66 mg/l) has been used to successfully treat *Hyperia medusarum* in the crystal jellyfish (*Aequorea victoria*) (Boonstra, 2015)
Isopods	Isopods have been reported in jellyfish and include the infestation of *Catostylus mosaicus* with *Cymodoce gaimardii* (Browne, 2017)
Crustaceans	Barnacles and decapod crustaceans are commonly found "hitch-hiking" in medusae of many jellyfish species. While some of these relationships may be deleterious to the host, others may be neutral, or even symbiotic (Yusa et al., 2015)

Condition/body part affected	Etiology/clinical signs
Anthozoa (sea anemones)	
Sudden death	Toxicity, trauma, extreme water quality parameters
Poor growth	Inadequate nutrition, inadequate lighting, inadequate water flow/motion, water pollution, loss of symbiotic bacteria
Trauma	All species are susceptible. Healing and regeneration occurs in many species
Major diseases:	
Toxicity	Heavy metals like copper are known to be toxic to anemones (Patel et al., 2014)
Aging	In some cases, it is possible that animals are merely undergoing senescence, although, its very easy to make this "diagnosis," despite the fact that husbandry-related problems could be in play
Inadequate environment	Anemones require at least some water current to respire, feed, and expel waste
Infectious diseases	No viral or fungal diseases have been reported in true anemones. Hydra adenovirus causes disease in the form of decreased growth in the hydrozoan *Hydra vulgaris* (Van Etten et al., 1982). There is no known treatment. It appears that anemones are not susceptible to at least some of the bacteria (*Vibrio* sp.) that affect their coral cousins based on in vivo studies (Zargoza et al., 2014). However, one laboratory study found that *Serratia marcescens* results in clinical disease in *Aiptasia pallida* (Krediet et al., 2014)
Parasitic diseases	Protozoal parasites have the potential to impact anemones. *Helicostoma nonatum*, a marine ciliate, has been implicated in "brown jelly infection" of corallimorph anemones (Sprung and Delbeek, 1997). It is possible, if not likely, that this is an opportunistic infection secondary to trauma
Anthozoa (corals)	
Sudden death	Toxicity, trauma, predation, extreme water quality parameters
Poor growth	Inadequate nutritional quality, inadequate food supply, loss of symbiotic bacteria, water pollution, interspecific competition
Brown jelly presence	A brown gelatinous material appears suddenly on the surface of a coral or soft coral. The material is the product of necrosing polyp tissues, and bare skeletal material will become visible as the condition progresses
Coral bleaching (loss of symbiotic zooxanthellae)	Increased temperature, pH, carbon dioxide; decreased light, wave action/water current; other water quality aberrations, bacterial infection, fungal infections
Goniopora slow wasting	The lower marginal polyps stop expanding and then die. The condition can progress vertically until all polyps are gone
Gorgonian sloughing	This spontaneous condition starts at the base, the tissue becomes soft and spongy, and then separates from the dark core
Large polyp recession	Apparently healthy large polyp corals begin to lose tissue at the polyp margins. Algal growth or brown jelly reactions may follow
Leather coral collapse	Distinct from normal shedding of leather corals. The polyps stop expanding, darken, after several weeks the tissue loses integrity, and degenerates. Rotting tissue ulcers appear on the capitulum or stalks and increase in size

(*Continued*)

Condition/body part affected	Etiology/clinical signs
Mushroom shrink	Corallimorphs shrink, cannot fully expand, and appear mottled
Polyp coagulative necrosis	Polyps becomes soft, display an external white friable deposit, and usually progress to death
Polyp extrusion	This is similar to bleaching, but small spherical structures (intact polyps) float out from the coral's skeleton. This is common and normal for pocillioprids but can also be a response to disease or stress
Polyp shutdown	Colonial polyps do not open for prolonged periods even after water changes
Soft coral collapse	Loss of turgor; the coral may wilt or even collapse
Stony coral tissue loss	Known as stony coral tissue loss disease, this disease syndrome has caused major stony coral mortality in Florida since 2014 (Aeby et al., 2019). To date, an etiological agent(s) has not been identified
White film	Excessive mucus, when draped over the coral, appears like a white film. White film can be a response to chemical irritation, rough handling, or areas of anaerobic decay
White paste	More extreme than white film. This aggressive response to irritants results in a thick white pasty substance engulfing stony corals
Xeniid melt	Healthy soft corals, particularly in the family Xeniidae, melt into a pile of small fragments and stumps within 24 hours
Trauma	Nearly all species are susceptible. Healing and regeneration is possible and probably common if the environmental conditions are good
Toxicity	Heavy metals like copper and zinc are known to be toxic to coral polyps of many species (Bilemyer-Fraser et al., 2018; Deschaseaux et al., 2018). Other heavy metals, such as iron, nickel, and vanadium are also toxic to at least some reef-building corals (Jafarabadi et al., 2018)
Infectious diseases	This is a very complicated area but one of much active research. Rarely have Koch's postulates been fulfilled for any soft or hard coral infectious disease. Mohamed and Sweet (2019) provide a comprehensive review that includes a very helpful and fully referenced table. Bacterial organisms that have been associated with specific disease are *Aurantimonas* spp. and *Sphingomonas* spp. (white plague types II and III), *Geitlerinema* spp., *Leptolyngbya* spp., *Oscillatoria* spp., *Pseudoscillatoria* spp. (black band disease), Serratia marcescens. (white pox disease), *Vibrio* sp. (yellow band disease), *Vibrio harveyi* and *Vibrio alginolyticus* (rapid tissue necrosis), *Vibrio coralliilyticus* and *Vibrio shiloi* (bacterial bleaching), *Oscillatoria* spp. (red band disease), *Vibrio* spp. (ulcerative white spot disease), *Vibrio charcharia* (white band disease type II), *Vibrio* spp. (porites white patch syndrome). A number of fungal organisms have been associated with coral disease. These include *Aspergillus sidowii* (aspergillosis), *Rhystisma* spp., (dark spots syndrome), *Curvularia* lunata (pink line syndrome – also includes *Phormidium valderianum*, a cyanobacterium)
Parasitic diseases	Protozoans are known to cause disease in corals. *Philaster* sp., a ciliate, has been implicated in brown band disease and brown jelly syndrome. *Halofolliculina* spp. has been linked to Caribbean ciliate infection. *Halofolliculina corallasia* is the causative agent for skeleton eroding band of *Acropora* and *Pocillopora* spp. *Amakusaplana acroporae*, *Acropora*-eating flatworm. *Tegastes acropranus*, red bug. *Heterotrich* spp. (ciliate). *Phestilla* sp., *Montipora*-eating nudibranch, *Dendrophilia*-eating nudibranch. *Polyclad* spp., *Euphyilla* flatworms. Zoanthid-eating nudibranch. *Pycnogonida* sp., zoanthid sea spider. *Convolutriloba retrogemma*, red planaria. *Vermetidae* spp. vermentid snail

Condition/body part affected	Etiology/clinical signs
Hydrozoa	
Hydras, colonial hydroids, colonial pelagic jellies (Portuguese Man-o-War)	Little is known about the pathology and diseases of this phylum
Ctenophora	
Comb jellies	Little is known about the pathology and diseases of this phylum
Urochordata	
Sea squirts, salps	
Infectious diseases	Secondary invasion of bacteria from injury or decomposition of dead epibiota
Cup cell diseases	Parasitic disease caused by a haplosporidian. Affects Botryllus schlosseri
Soft tunic syndrome	Thinning, softening of the body wall (tunic) of cultured *Halocynthia roretzi*. Causative agent is the kinetoplastid *Azumiobodo hoyamushi*
Mollusca	
Bivalves (oysters, mussels, clams, abalone)	
Sudden death	Parasites (*Haplosporidia/Minchinia*, *Bonamia*, *Hexamita*), transmissible hemocytic neoplasia, *Vibrio*, *Oyster herpesvirus*, acute viral necrosis of scallops, iridoviruses, malacoherpesvirus
Poor growth	*Perkinsus*, insufficient food
Larval death	Velar virus disease (iridovirus), vibriosis
Biofouling	Generalized sign of disease
Ulcers/pustules	Mikrocytos, *Nocardia*, *Bonamia*, foreign-body haemocytic granulomas (metacercariae, nematodes, *Crustacea*, algae)
Emaciation/gaping	*Perkinsus*, *Haplosporidia/Minchinia*, *Marteilia*, hinge erosion (bacteria), Oyster herpes virus, *Mikrocytos*
Gills:	
Ulcers	*Bonamia* (parasite)
Nodules	*Marteila* (parasite)
Inflammation	*Trubellaria*, *Trichodina*
Brown discoloration	*Haplosporidia*
Shell:	
Deformity/poor growth	Juvenile oyster disease, shell disease (mudworm, boring mussels – *Lithophaga*, boring sponges – clina, pine, possibly fungus), *Haplosporidia*, *Mikrocytos*, thickening or marked extension of shells in oysters caused by disturbance of calcium metabolism
Mantle:	Rickettsia-like organisms (aka prokaryote inclusion bodies, *Chlamydia*-like organisms, intracellular microcolonies of bacteria)
Brown/yellow digestive gland	Necrosis (*Marteila*)
Gametes	Viral gametocytic hypertrophy, *Marteilioides chungmuensis*, metacercariae, nematodes, transmissible hemocytic neoplasia, hermaphrodites

(*Continued*)

Condition/body part affected	Etiology/clinical signs
Digestive gland	*Ancistrocoma* (incidental)
Unknown etiology	Akoya oyster disease, oyster edema disease
Cephalopods	
Sudden death	Bacterial septicemia (*Vibrio*), water quality issues (ammonia, oxygen, hydrogen sulfide), toxicosis (heavy metal-copper, herbicide, pesticide), parasites, trauma, gas supersaturation, handling stress
Poor growth, emaciation	Anorexia, insufficient caloric intake, nutritional deficiency, stress/water quality issues, heavy parasitism
Uncoordinated swimming/ nervousness	Generalized infectious disease (bacteria,fungal, protist infection), electrocution, copper toxicosis, central nervous system disease, water quality issues, gas bubble disease, parasitism, low strontium
Asphyxia	Gill disease (parasites), anemia (parasites), low dissolved oxygen, toxin exposure/ammonia, organic/inorganic contaminants
Skin/mantle:	
Petechiae	Bacterial septicemia
Increased mucus	Water quality issues, parasitism
Hemorrhage/ulcers/ necrosis	Trauma (handling, tankmate aggression/contact), improper pH, bacterial infection (*Vibrio*, *Lactococcus*, *Photobacterium*, *Pseudomonas*, *Aeromonas*, *Staphylococcus*), labyrinthulomycetes (thraustochytrid) infection, fungus (*Cladosporidium*, *Fusarium*) infection, irritant exposure, cuttlebone fracture
Parasites	Isopods, copepods, branchiurans
Nodules/lumps	Granulomatous disease (bacteria, fungi), parasites (coccidians – Aggregata), virus (iridovirus-like), foreign body
Pale spots	Acute skin injury, neurologic injury, scarring, deep infection
Edema	Trauma, skin ulcers, fatal idiopathic condition
Gills:	
Hemorrhage/ulcers	Bacterial infection (*Vibrio*), parasites, toxins
Pallor	Anemia, mild hyperplasia
Parasites	Copepods, cestodes, trematodes, coccidians
Hyperplasia/fusion	Water quality issues, chronic inflammation, parasitism (ciliates – Ancistromidae)
Gas bubbles	Supersaturation
Necrosis	High/low pH, chlorine, toxins
Nodules	Encysted trematodes, coccidians, cysts, neoplasia, bacteria (*Vibrio*, *Rickettsia*-like organisms) fungus, labyrinthulomycetes (thraustochytrid) infection, fibrosis, spermatophores (other cephalopods)
Hemorrhage/ulcers	Bacterial infection (*Vibrio*), parasites, toxins
Pallor	Anemia, mild hyperplasia
Increased mucus	Water quality issues, bacterial infection, parasites
Eyes:	
Exophthalmia/ buphthalmia	Bacterial septicemia, trauma, gas bubble disease/supersaturation, idiopathic

Condition/body part affected	Etiology/clinical signs
Ulcers/hemorrhage	Fungus, bacterial septicemia, viral infection, trauma
Corneal edema	Poor water quality, sepsis, fungus, labyrinthulomycetes (thraustochytrid) infection
Ophthalmitis	Trauma, bacteria (*Lactococcus*, *Photobacterium*), hematogenous spread of pathogens
Cataract	Rapid osmolar fluctuations, gas bubble disease
Gas bubbles	Supersaturation, bacterial infection, corneal perforation
Nodules	Granulomas (bacteria, fungi, parasite
Enucleation	Trauma, severe ophthalmitis
Heart:	
Inflammation/pericarditis	Bacterial sepsis (*Vibrio*)
Nodules	Granulomas (bacteria, fungus)
Skeleton:	
Cuttlebone fracture	Trauma
Deformity	Trauma, hereditary, nutritional deficiency, adverse environment conditions, toxicant exposure, healing cuttlebone fracture
Loss of limb	Autophagy (self-destruction)
Small cuttlebone	Hypercapnia
Stomach	Ulcers
Digestive tract:	
Nodules	Coccidians, encysted trematodes, encysted cestodes
Connective tissues	Coccidians, encysted cestodes, encysted nematodes, fibrosis, neoplasia
Crustacea (shrimps, lobsters, crabs, crayfish)	
Sudden death/ lethargy	Viruses (many), bacteria (*Vibrio*, *Micrococcus*, *Aerococcus*, *Rickettsia*), water quality, *Aphanomyces*, aflatoxin, pesticides, herbicides, ultraviolet light
Floating	Gas supersaturation
Milky hemolymph	Bacteria (*Rickettsia*), microsporidians, dinoflagellates, scuticociliates, amoeba
Dwarfism/deformity/poor growth	Viruses (IHHNV, hepatopancreatic parvovirus, monodon slow growth syndrome), vibriosis, diet
Cramped tail	Nutritional imbalance
Muscle opacity	Viruses (iridovirus, totivirus, nodavirus), microsporidians (Ameson), muscle necrosis (exertion/stress), vibriosis, trematodes, asbestos fibers, selenium deficiency, *Aphanomyces*
Cuticle:	
Black spots	Melanin production (inflammation: bacterial sepsis – *Vibrio*, especially secondary to viral disease), fungus, *Lagenidium*, virus (Taura syndrome), parasite (microsporidians), Aphanomyces, water quality); ultraviolet light
Yellow spots	Viruses, bacteria

(*Continued*)

Condition/body part affected	Etiology/clinical signs
White spots	white spot virus, mineral deficiency (water quality), bacteria (Bacillus), phosphatidylcholine deficiency
Pink coloration	Chromatophore expansion, especially of telson, due to stress, sepsis
Mucus	Bacteria
Ulcers	Bacteria (*Vibrio*, *Mycobacterium*), fungi, neoplasia, ultraviolet light, *Aphanomyces*
Biofouling of gills, cuticle	Poor water quality, generalized debility from disease
Dysecdysis	Multiple causes, especially viruses, phosphatidylcholine deficiency
Nodules	Granulomas, neoplasia (rare)
Soft shell	Nutritional imbalance, rancid feeds, pesticides
Luminescence	Luminescent vibriosis
Gills:	
Biofouling	Poor water quality, generalized debility from disease
Black spots	Inflammation (bacteria, fungi, protozoans), sediment, heavy metals (iron, cadmium, chromium, copper), oxidants (chlorine, potassium permanganate), ultraviolet light, gas supersaturation, ammonia, acids, crude oil, ascorbic acid imbalances
Parasites	Isopods
Hepatopancreas:	
Nodules	Granulomas (bacterial, parasite – cestode, trematode, fungus)
Yellow/pale	Can be normal, necrosis (yellowhead virus), microsporidians
Atrophy	Emaciation, viral infection, bacterial infection (*Vibrio*, spirochetes)
Dark	Emaciation/atrophy, lack of lipid
Speckles (various colors)	Granulomas – bacteria, microsporidians, fungus
Gut:	
Darkened	Vibriosis, parasites
Red feces	Virus (suspected parvovirus)
Parasites	Gregarines, cestodes, nematodes
Antennal gland nodules	Granulomas (melamine)
Gonads: black spermatophore (penaeids)	Unknown etiology
Eye: Corneal plaques	Unknown etiology

2

Teleost Fish

Laura Urdes and Marius Hangan

The etiology and clinical signs of the diseases of salmonids and coldwater food fish, warm water food fish, and elasmobranchs are shown in Appendix 2.1, Appendix 2.2, and Appendix 2.3, respectively, at the end of this chapter.

Parasitic Diseases

Ectoparasites

Flukes (Monogenean Parasites)

Overview/Etiology The Monogenea group comprises 6000–7000 species, many being parasites of gill and skin of fish. Some monogeneans have also been found in amphibians and reptiles (Hutson et al., 2018; Kohn et al., 2006; Aisien et al., 2004). To complete their lifecycle, monogeneans require one host. Four genera commonly affect freshwater fish: *Ancyrocephalus*, *Dactylogyrus*, *Gyrodactylus*, and *Paradiplozoon*, with *Dactylogyrus* and *Gyrodactylus* being most dominant. *Dactylogyrus* is more commonly found on the gills, whereas *Gyrodactylus* prefers fish skin. Both genera are hermaphroditic. Monogeneans pathogenic to marine fish include monopisthocotyleans in the Capsalidae family, parasitizing the skin, fins, and gills of marine fish. In cultured marine fish, capsalids can sometime cause epizootic events. The most common genera of pathogenic capsalids are *Benedenia*, *Capsala*, *Entobdella* and *Neobenedenia*. The representatives of these genera parasitize many elasmobranch and teleost species, including sturgeons (Whittington, 2004). Flukes have a spoliatory, toxic, and irritative effect on their hosts, feeding on mucus, detritus, and epithelial tissue and blood.

- *Dactylogyrus* are hermaphroditic flukes with an elongated, dorsoventrally flattened body, of 1–2 mm length and 0.1–0.4 mm width. The head has four contractile papillae and four eye (pigmentary) spots. At the posterior end of the body there is a haptor, a fixation disk with two hooks placed in the disk's center and an additional 14 marginal, smaller, paired hooks (Figure 2.1). The parasite uses the haptor to attach to the gill lamellae of the fish host.
- *Gyrodactylus* spp. have a flattened body. Depending on the species involved, the body length varies between 0.2 mm (*Gyrodactylus salmonis*) and 1.3 mm (*Gyrodactylus katharineri,* Malmberg,

Pathology and Epidemiology of Aquatic Animal Diseases for Practitioners, First Edition.
Edited by Laura Urdes, Chris Walster, and Julius Tepper.

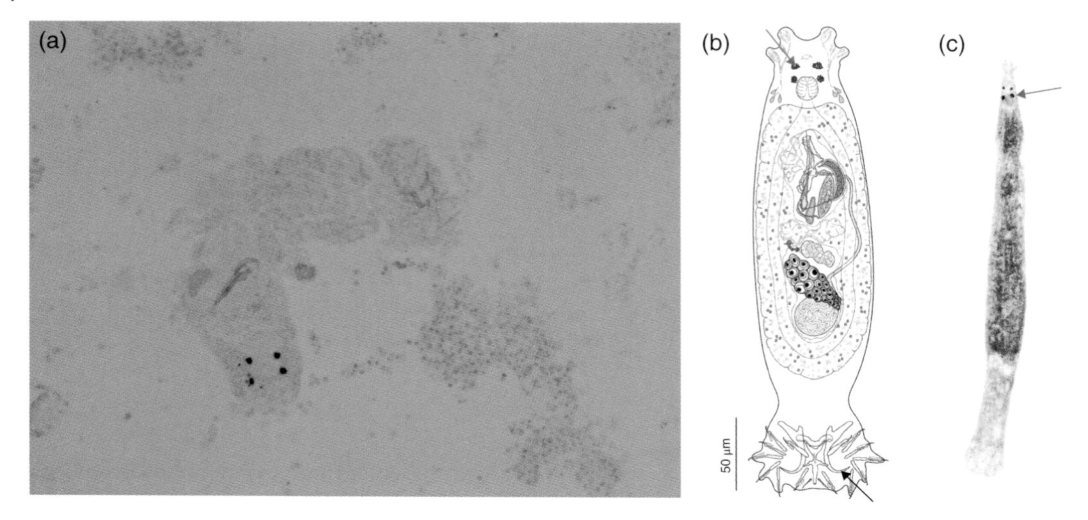

Figure 2.1 *Dactylogyrus* species, showing two pairs of pigmentary eye spots (red arrows) and the haptor (black arrow); skin scrape from a koi carp (a–c). *Source:* Yuriy Kvach/Wikimedia Commons; Eva Řehulková, Michal Benovics and Andrea Šimková/Wikimedia Commons; sinhyu/Adobe Stock.

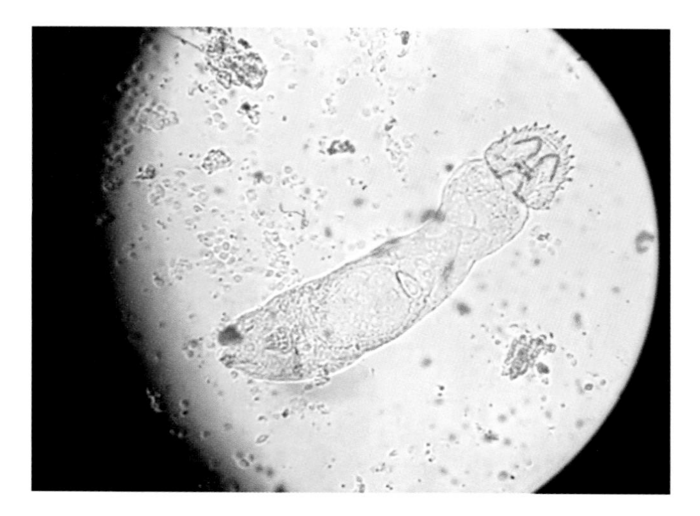

Figure 2.2 *Gyrodactylus* species; skin scrape from a koi carp. *Source:* Flickr/KoiQuestion.

1964). The anterior end has two contractile papillae. Compared with *Dactylogyrus*, these flukes lack the pigmentary spots. The fixation organ, placed at the posterior end of the body, is equipped with two large, centered hooks and an additional 16 smaller, marginal hooks (Figure 2.2).

Host Range and Transmission The genus *Dactylogyrus* is found worldwide, commonly affecting cyprinid species of freshwater fish. Many *Gyrodactylus* species are found in North America, Europe, and Asia, parasitizing both marine and freshwater fish. *Gyrodactylus* flukes are commonly observed in wild and farmed salmonids, in Alaska (Meyers at al., 2019). Flukes are transmitted horizontally, by physical contact of susceptible fish with infested individuals, high-density

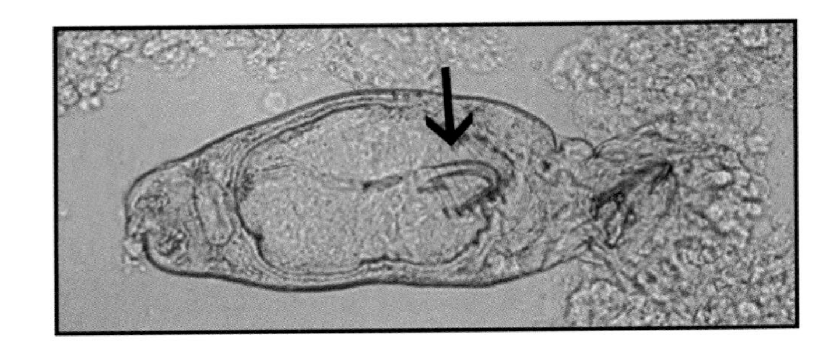

Figure 2.3 *Gyrodactylus* showing visible internal embryos with hooks (arrow), 200× magnification. *Source:* Meyers et al., 2019/Alaska Department of Fish and Game.

populations being among the favoring factors, thus increasing the risk of transmission within receptive fish populations. *Dactylogyrus* produces fertilized eggs that hatch into the water. The juveniles usually attach to a different host, while *Gyrodactylus* is viviparous, releasing juveniles, which often attach to the same host as their adult parent.

Signs and Diagnosis *Dactylogyrus* parasitizes the gills of the host fish, causing lamellar hyperplasia, excessive mucus production, and signs of asphyxia, shown by rapid respiratory movements. *Gyrodactylus* attach to skin causing excess mucus production and hyperpigmentation of the skin, fin erosions, flashing behavior, and lethargy. Gill localizations of *Gyrodactylus* flukes cause similar signs as in the case of *Dactylogyrus*. In trout, *Gyrodactylus* may also cause physical damage to the olfactory system leading to olfactory impairment (Lari and Pyle, 2017). Wet mounts of skin scrapes or gill samples are sufficient to establish a fluke infestation diagnosis. The dactylogyrid fluke has four pigmentary eye spots. In the "uterus," there are present pedunculate eggs that can be viewed by light microscopy. Gyrodactylus has no pigmentary spots at their anterior end, but contain embryos (with well-developed hooks) inside their body (Figure 2.3).

Treatment/Management Formalin treatments are used to eliminate these external flukes from affected hatcheries. Fluke infestations are problematic because of the associated risks of secondary infections and immunosuppression, which are common to chronic parasitic infestations. The prognosis is good for fish with low to mild infestations. However, fins, skin, and/or gill lesions produced by attached flukes often become entry points for opportunistic pathogens and spoilage of fish. Recently, praziquantel has become the treatment of choice in ornamentals and koi ponds. Effective levels must be maintained for complete elimination of flukes. This can be a problem in systems where biological deactivation occurs. Regular assays of the levels when in use can mitigate this problem.

Digenean Black Spot Disease

Overview/etiology Black spot disease is caused by digenean trematodes (flukes) in the family Diplostomidae (*Posthodiplostomum cuticola* – sin. *Diplostomum cuticola*, *Diplostomum spathaceum*, *Posthodiplostomum minimum*, *Neascus cuticola*, *Neascus nolfi*, *Austrodiplostomum mordax*, etc.) and family Heterophyidae (*Apophalus*/*Rossicotrema*/*donicum*, *Apophalus muehlingi* (Jägerskiöld, 1899), *Cryptocotyle concavum*, *Cryptocotyle jejunum*, *Cryptocotyle lingua*, *Metagonimus yokogawai*, etc.). These parasites have a complex life cycle, with up to three intermediary hosts, fish being either intermediary or definitive hosts. In fish, metacercaria are found in skin, muscle, fins, eye (lens), and/or operculum. Sometimes, gills and visceral organs are also affected (e.g. *Austrodiplostomum mordax* in brain; *Posthodiplostomum*/*Neascus minimum* in kidney, liver, spleen and heart).

Host range and transmission Aquaculture, wild freshwater and marine fish species of all ages are affected. Most fluke species have gastropods and fish as intermediary hosts. Aquatic birds and mammals, including humans, act as definitive hosts for the adult parasite, releasing the fluke's eggs through feces into the water. *P. cuticula* (Nordmann, 1832) has aquatic birds as definitive host, affecting most often farmed cyprinids.

Signs and Diagnosis In most cases, evolution is subclinical. Pinpoint-sized black spots, multifocal and slightly raised on the skin and/or fin epithelium, gills, operculi, or in the muscle (hypermelanosis; Figure 2.4) indicate the location of metacercariae within the tissue, aiding in establishing a presumptive diagnosis. Sometimes, difficulty in swimming, as well as necrosis and hemorrhage, accompany the black spots. Massive infestations can cause subnutrition of affected fish. Ocular sites (often involving *D. spathaceum* or *A. mordax*) may lead to clouding of the lens (cataracts) followed by partial or total blindness.

Diagnostics Sampling of black spots and observations of the samples in light microscopy on wet mount preparations and histological sections allow for identification of the metacercariae in the cysts. Genus and species identification is based on marine or freshwater habitat, location of the parasitic cyst, and a more detailed morphological description of the encysted metacercariae. Most metacercariae have an oval body of a length ranging from 0.1 mm to 0.5 mm encysted in cysts of elliptical or spherical shape. The encysted metacercariae are found within a fibrinous capsule surrounded with numerous melanocytes.

Differentials Hypermelanosis of genetic or other causes.

Treatment and Management The disease is usually self-limiting and fish may recover on their own with time. If cysts are accessible, metacercariae can be removed surgically. Praziquantel added to the system is efficient in eliminating metacercariae from the water. Removal of any dead fish will prevent the parasitic larvae from multiplying. Eliminating the source of infection for fish in the aqua system (e.g. aquatic gastropods) will help break the chain of transmission, as will regular and efficient water treatments.

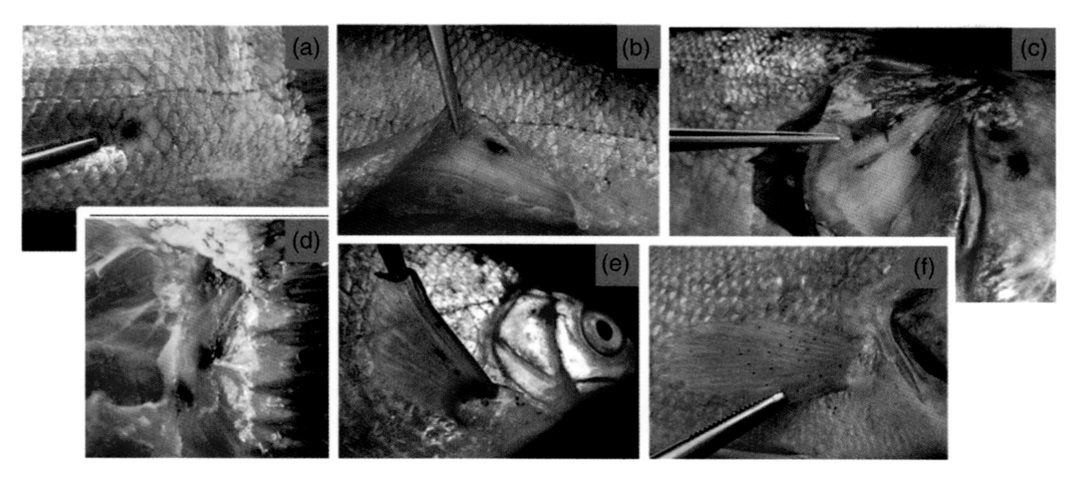

Figure 2.4 *Posthodiplostomum cuticola* metacercariae, in (a) skin, (b) connective tissue, (c) operculum, (d) muscle of the caudal peduncle, (e and f) pectoral fin epithelium. Silver carp (*Hypophtalmichthys molitrix*).

Turbellarian Black Spot Disease (Tang Disease, Black Itch)

Overview/Etiology Most *Turbellaria* are free-living organisms. Parasitic *Turbellaria* are pathogenic to several marine fish species (Jean-Lou et al., 2009) and some invertebrates, such as mollusks. In tropical fish, species from the genus *Paravortex* and genus *Piscinquilinus* (formerly named *Ichthyophaga*) are known to cause black spot disease.

Host Range and Transmission Parasitic turbellarian flukes are pathogenic to a wide variety of fish species, including yellow tang (*Zebrasoma flavescens*), clown fish (*Amphiprion ocellaris*), and unicorn tang or bluespine unicornfish (*Naso unicornis*) (Figure 2.5), the cottid *Bero elegans*, the greenling *Hexagrammos decagrammus*, and the tropical serranid *Cephalopholis pachycentron*. *Piscinquilinus* species may be more host specific (Jean-Lou et al., 2009). *Paravortex* spp. and *Piscinquilinus* spp. are believed to have a single-host life cycle.

The reproductive cycle takes place in the aquatic substrate. After hatching, the juvenile, measuring around 200 μm in length and 50 μm width, swim freely seeking a host fish, where it burrows into the epithelium of the skin or gills and start to feed on tissue and cell fluids for around six days. It remains attached to feed and grow for a few days until it becomes an adult turbellaria. The parasite may reach adulthood in 6–10 days, when they reach 2500 μm length and 750 μm width. Once matured, *Turbellaria* leave the fish, descend into the substrate and form a reproduction cyst. Five days later, the encysted worm ruptures and releases a new population of over 100 young juveniles, which immediately swim to find and feed on a new host. *Piscinquilinus* species may have a longer life cycle (Jean-Lou et al., 2009).

Signs and Diagnosis The primary symptom is the presence of small black swellings, about 2–4 mm in diameter, in the skin and fin epithelia. Black spots are easier to see on light-colored fish. On dark-colored fish the lesions may go unnoticed until other more visible symptoms appear. As the worms have the ability to move about freely on fish, black spots may disappear from one place and appear in other locations of the body surface. The infested fish scratches against objects or the substrate in an attempt to remove the parasites. As infestations progress, infested fish can become lethargic, anorexic, and lose skin color. In gill infestations, asphyxia may also occur, complicating disease evolution. Secondary opportunistic pathogens often enter through damaged tissue sites. Diagnosis is made following parasite examination. The parasite is obtained from the host by pressing black spots. This usually will cause the release of a whitish or yellowish fluke of 2–4 mm in length (Figure 2.5d). Microscopic examination of the parasites between a slide and a cover slip, as well as preserved preparations (hematoxylin and eosin), aid in identifying the species involved.

Differentials *Turbellaria* can be distinguished from metacercariae causing black spots identical to turbellarian black spots during the examination of the black lesions by cutting the cyst and releasing the parasite. *Turbellaria* move by gliding using its cilia, which are present on the body surface, whereas metacercariae move by peristalsis, as they lack cilia. *Paravortex* spp. have both the eyes and pharynx located at the anterior end of the body, whereas *Piscinquilinus* spp. have the eyes placed anteriorly and the pharynx, posteriorly (Cannon & Lester 1988).

Treatment and Management The most effective treatments are praziquantel and formalin. Praziquantel treatment is 2 mg/l in a single dose for seven days in the quarantine tank. Treatment with formalin consists of a 45–60-minute treatment bath, followed by transfer into a sterile quarantine tank. Osmotic shock (freshwater dips) is an alternative treatment option but is not always effective as it may not result in complete eradication. Another option is to treat at 1.009 SG

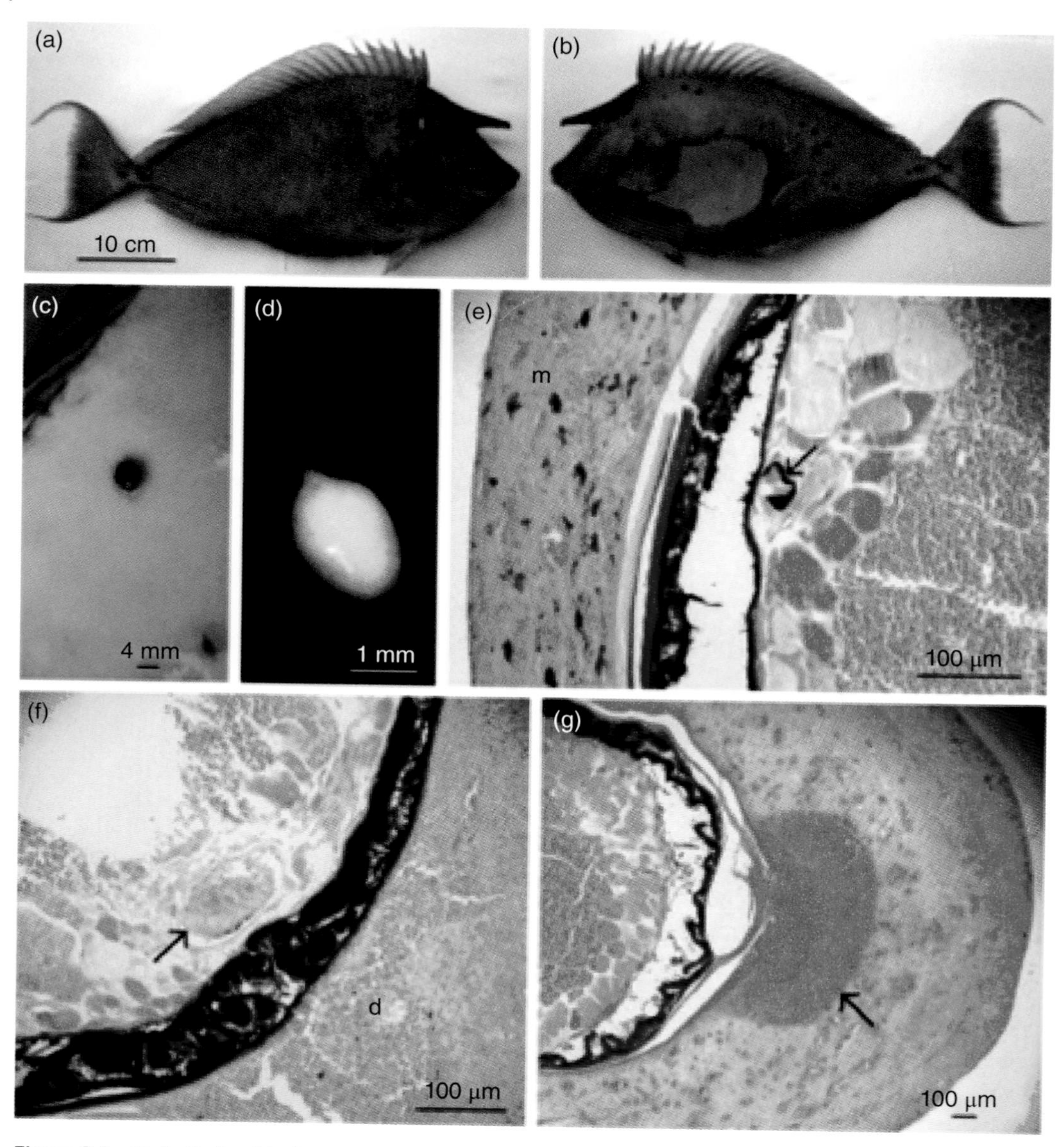

Figure 2.5 Turbellarian black spot disease in bluespine unicornfish. (a, b) Bluespine unicornfish (*Naso unicornis*) infected with black spot disease. Photographs of both sides of the dead fish; the discoloured area in the centre of the fish in b is an artifact due to wet skin. (c) Black spot on the skin. (d) Live turbellarian, *Piscinquilinus* sp., extracted from a cyst and swimming in sea water. (e–g) *Piscinquilinus* sp. in the skin of *Naso unicornis*, hematoxylin and eosin section. (e) Arrow, eye spot; m melanophore. (f) Arrow, pharynx; d, developing granuloma with free erythrocytes and leucocytes. (g) Margin of cyst showing region of dying host cells (arrow). Scale bars in (c) and (d) are approximate. *Source:* Jean-Lou et al. 2009/Inter-Research.

for at least 10 days. The resulted hyposalinity (decreased salt concentration) kills the infective and free-living stages of the parasite. Hyposalinity can be applied only in fish-only tanks, or marine aquariums containing no freshwater-sensitive invertebrates. Vacuuming the aquarium gravel may help remove encysted worms from the substrate during the outbreak.

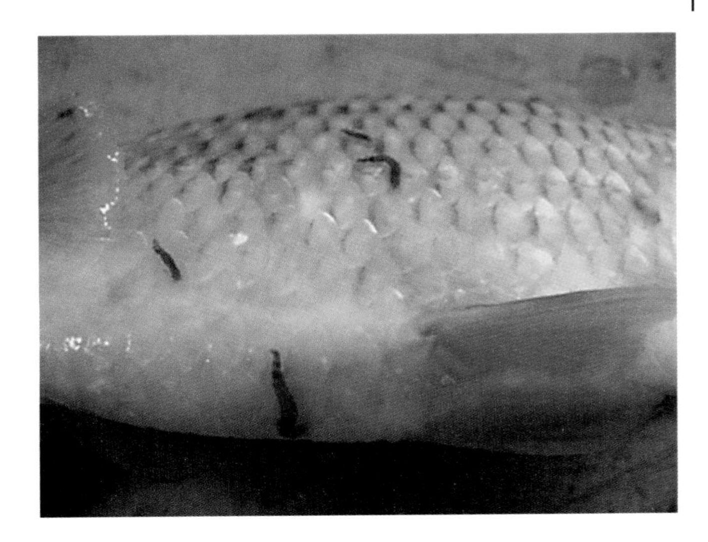

Figure 2.6 *Piscicola* spp. attached to skin of *Rutilus rutilus*.

Piscicolosis

Overview/Etiology *Piscicola* is a freshwater segmented worm (leech) in the phylum Annelida, which can be abundantly found on the bottom of lakes, ponds and streams. The parasite is found in many species of freshwater fish, in Europe and North America.

Piscicola has a subcylindrical and elongate body (Figure 2.6), 2.5 cm in length. Adult leeches are hermaphroditic and produce eggs. There is one juvenile stage. Eggs are encased in cocoons attached to the substrate at the bottom of lakes, ponds, and streams. Juvenile leeches begin looking for a fish host when they hatch from the eggs. They usually require several blood meals before becoming adults. The leech attaches for several days to the fish skin to feed on blood and other tissue fluids. Apart from being a nuisance for the host, serving as vectors for infectious agents, such as infectious hematopoietic necrosis virus, and causing portals of entry for secondary pathogens, leeches do not cause direct harm to their hosts, as the tissue damage is localized at the sites of attachment. However, when present in large numbers, leeches can cause extensive skin damage, such as hemorrhage and necrosis, and anemia.

Signs and Diagnosis Leeches are easily identified by visual examination of the parasitized fish. Under a dissecting microscope, the morphological characteristics help identify the genus *Piscicola*.

Treatment and Management Leeches should be removed from the fish's skin. The best way to remove a leech from fish directly is by bathing them in a 2.5% aquarium salt solution for 10–15 minutes. This causes the leech to either drop away from the fish or facilitate manual removal of the leech. The skin erosions should also be treated with topical antimicrobial ointment. In addition, the aquarium, tank or pond should be treated or sanitized (e.g. trichlorfon solution) to kill any adult parasites, larvae or eggs (Urdeş, 2007).

Fish Henneguya (Henneguyosis)

Overview and Etiology *Henneguya* is a histozoic parasite, a metazoan in the class Myxosporea, phylum Cnidaria. There are over 120 species, with only a few being pathogenic to fish. Of these, some species are host and tissue specific. The parasite affects both freshwater and marine, wild and cultured fish worldwide. *Henneguya* causes sporadic mortality to fish populations, parasitizing in

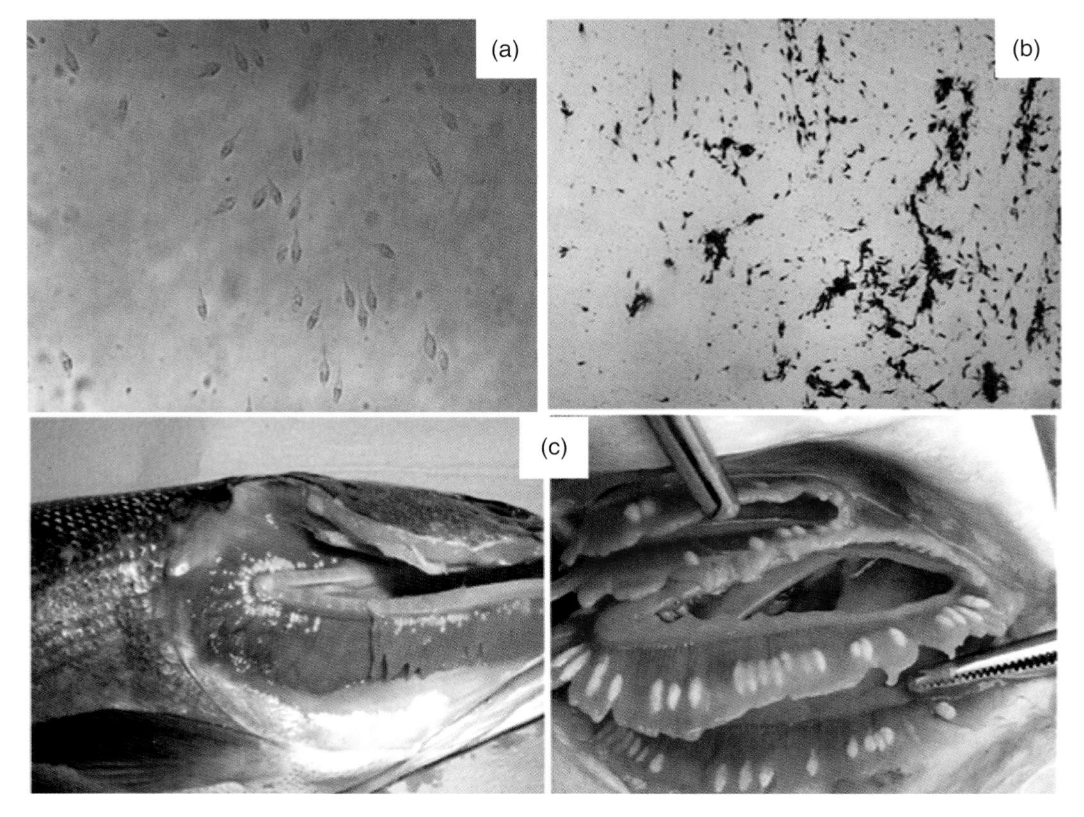

Figure 2.7 Spores of *Henneguya psorospermica* in Sander lucioperca, 400× magnification. (a) Wet smears. (b) Malachite green. (c) Cysts of *Henneguya psorospermica* on gill lamellae, hyperplastic branchiitis, and necrosis in *Esox lucius*.

the muscle, gills, skin, and fins of fish hosts. The parasite is an ovoid spore of 11 × 9 μm with two polar capsules and two long caudal appendages of 26–40 μm.

H. psorospermica commonly affects pike perch (*Esox lucius*), perch (*Sander lucioperca*), and bass (*Perca fluviatilis*). It parasitizes in the gills, where it forms spindle-like, white, 7-mm long cysts (pansporoblast), (Figure 2.7c). *H. psorospermica* spores are oval, with two piriform apical polar capsules. At their basal pole, the spores are provided with a pair of symmetrical caudal appendages (Figure 2.7a,b).

H. salminicola is found in Pacific salmon, in the muscle and under the skin, causing a condition known as "milky flesh disease" (also known as "tapioca disease"). The name comes from the creamy white fluid that oozes from the cysts during filleting of the infested fish (Figure 2.8).

Signs and Diagnosis The white pansporoblasts (cysts) containing thousands of spores are present in gills, fins, muscle, or skin. White cysts are examined microscopically for the typical 2-tailed spores. Histological examination of tissues can also reveal the presence of the parasite. Species differentiation is determined by further spore morphology.

Treatment and Management To prevent infection in cultured salmon use sources of water free from *Henneguya* spores. There are no treatment or control measures available.

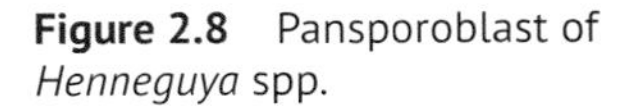

Figure 2.8 Pansporoblast of *Henneguya* spp.

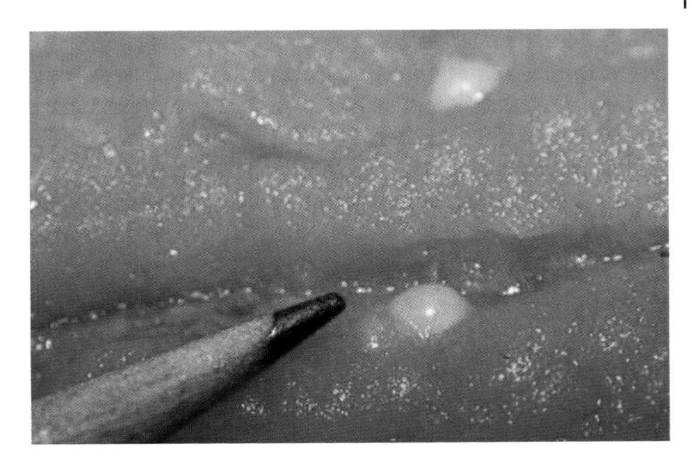

Parasitic Crustacean Infestations

Overview and Etiology Most commonly, ectoparasites in the Order Copepoda (*Ergasilus* spp., *Lernaea* spp. or "anchor worm," and *Caligus* spp.), subclass Branchiura (*Argulus* spp. or "fish lice"), Order Isopoda (*Gnathia* spp.) and Order Siphonostomatoida (*Lepeophtheirus salmonis salmonis*, Krøyer, 1837, or "sea lice"). Most of these crustaceans live a parasitic life, affecting both marine and freshwater fish, and generally showing a low species specificity. Most commonly, these infestations occur in lakes and ponds. Crustaceans are generally found on the gills, skin, fins, and external mucous membranes of susceptible fish, feeding on the host's mucus, skin epithelial cells, or blood. At the site of attachment, these parasites damage the epithelium possibly causing bleeding, inflammation, or ulcer. Secondarily, they create gateways for opportunistic agents and cause stress in the infested fish.

Parasitic copepods are ectoparasites of the skin, gills, and fins. They live either fixed to the tissue (through their anterior extremity, which is provided with fixing apparatus), or move freely to the surface of the host's body (these forms lack a fixing apparatus). Both female and male copepods attach to the host to mate, but after mating the male dies. Subsequently, the female (oviparous) moves deeper into the host's skin to lay embryonated eggs into the water. From the eggs the young, free forms hatch, undergoing up to 16 developmental stages before they reach the infectious stage for fish, and two more stages as an ectoparasite, until they become adults (Longshaw and Feist, 2001). Water temperature plays an important role in the life cycle of these copepods. Below 15 degrees C, mating no longer takes place.

Ergasilus spp. lives in freshwater systems, is up to 3 mm in length and resembles the free form of the copepod (Vulpe, 2007), with an additional fixing device. After mating, the female attaches to the host's gills and skin. As with *Ergasilus*, the female of *Lernaea* spp. has a parasitic life. In fish, it is found on the skin, at the base of the scales, on the gills, around the eyes, in the oral cavity and on the fins. *Lernaea cyprinacea* parasitizes the gills of carp, Gibel carp, and other cyprinids. Infestations with *Lernaea cyprinacea* are also documented in trout. The female's body is vermiform, with a length of approximately 2 cm.

Signs and Diagnosis In severe copepod infestations, death occurs due to osmoregulation disorders. *Ergasilus* spp., through its localization on the gills, causes epithelial necrosis and destruction of the secondary lamellae, which leads to hypoxia, reduced growth, and death. Low infestations with *Lernaea* spp. can cause serious problems in the affected fish stocks. Fish become listless, dashing

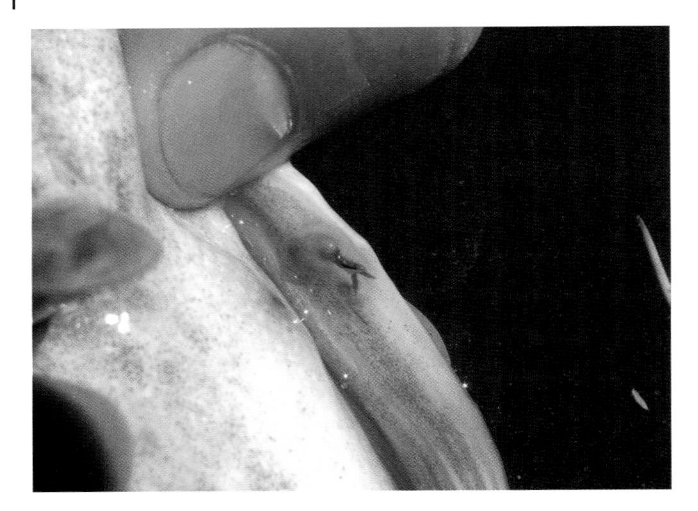

Figure 2.9 Female of *Lernea spp.* attached (arrows). *Source:* Dnatheist/ Wikimedia Commons.

quickly, lethargic, and off feed. The fish are susceptible to secondary infections through wounds caused by the parasite when it attaches to the body. Infested fish may be seen gasping and rubbing their body against the pond's wall. Agitation, ulcers, and redness at the base of the fins are also often present in infested fish. The parasites are visible with the naked eye (Figure 2.9).

Treatment and Management Infested fish should be isolated to prevent the spread of the copepods. Copepod infestations at all stages of their development can be controlled with organophosphates. It should be noted that dryness affects all copepods, regardless of the biological stage. The system should therefore be completely drained of water and disinfected to interrupt the transmission cycle of the parasite (especially in the infestations involving *Ergasilus* spp.). Localized inflammation and bleeding caused by parasite attachment, are treated directly with disinfectants and antimicrobial to prevent secondary infections.

Branchiurids affect freshwater fish. The most important branchiurid is *Argulus* spp. (fish lice). The parasite has an oval, dorsoventrally flattened body (Figure 2.10). There are two eye-shaped spots on the carapace. The body is up to one cm long. *Argulus* lives an ectoparasitic life, feeding on the host's blood. *A. foliaceus* is commonly found in wild fish, inhabiting natural aquatic systems, while *A. japonicus* affects fishponds, affecting koi carp and goldfish. Both sexes have a parasitic life. After mating, the female lays eggs on various substrates into the water. The young stages which emerge from the eggs require the fish host to reach the adult stage.

Signs and Diagnosis Depending on the intensity of the infestation, fish may exhibit some distress. Excessive mucus may also be present on the surface of the skin. Skin inflammation and hemorrhage indicate the spots where the parasite is attached to the epithelium. *Argulus* can act as a vector for infectious agents (e.g., spring viremia of carp), which it can transmit while feeding.

Diagnosis is established by examining the fish and parasite. When an infested fish is taken out of the water, the parasite can be seen dropping off the fish to enter back into the water, where it swims to find another host. Fish lice (*Argulus* spp.) are highly irritative, causing the fish to move rapidly and jump out of the water.

Treatment and Management The parasite must be mechanically removed from the fish's skin and the wounds should be treated topically with disinfectants and antimicrobial to prevent secondary

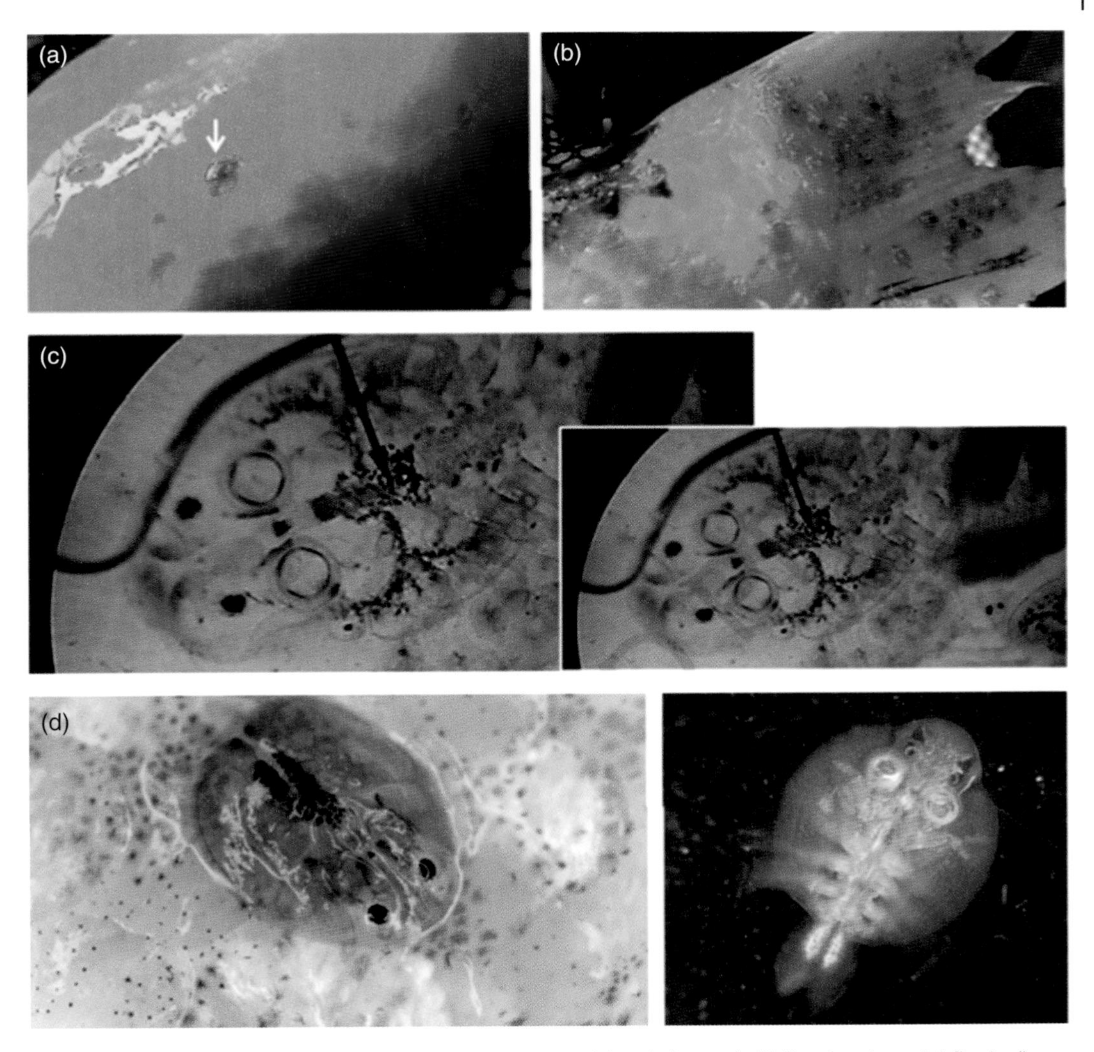

Figure 2.10 Heavy infestation with fish lice (Argulus spp.) in a koi carp. (a, b) Head and caudal fin. (c, d) Argulus spp. from a gill skin scrape. *Source:* Henrik Larsson/Adobe Stock; Keisotyo/Wikimedia Commons.

infections from occurring. Water can be treated with organophosphorus, formalin, or potassium permanganate, which are effective on adult stages only. Salt destroys the young forms, so the fish can be placed in a 2% salt bath to accomplish this. Drainage and drying of ponds are effective in eradicating the disease. Alternatively, various egg-laying surfaces may be placed into the water, and then removed and left to dry every three days. Currently, in closed systems and where regulations allow, chitin inhibitors, such as lufenuron and diflubenzuron, have shown to be safe and effective.

Parasitic isopods are found in marine waters. These copepods have a very low species specificity. Two groups of isopods are known: *Flabellifera* and *Gnathiidae*. *Flabellifera* spp. has an elongated body, up to 6 cm in length. Gnatids are less than 1 cm. The life cycle of isopods involves one host. Only the larval stages need a host, living on the skin, gills, and oral mucosa of fish. Adult isopods are free-living stages, inhabiting the mud at the bottom of ponds.

Signs and Diagnosis Flabellifera causes problems even when the infestation is low, due to the parasite's large size. In the case of oral localizations, Flabellifera often obstructs the host's mouth, so the fish can no longer feed. Gnathia infestations can lead to death in small fish as it often causes bleeding and anemia in the affected fish. Isopods are easily identified by external clinical examination.

Treatment and Management Manual removal of the isopod, followed by local treatment of existing wounds with disinfectants and antimicrobials to prevent secondary infections. The interruption of the biological cycle of the parasite should be aimed at removal of the fish from the affected pond and eliminating adult isopods from the system. The latter can be achieved by removing the water and mud followed by treating the basin with organophosphates. If this is not possible, prediluted organophosphates can be applied into the fish water by using a can so as it is evenly distributed.

Sea lice (*Lepeophtheirus salmonis salmonis*, Krøyer, 1837) occur naturally in salmon and sea trout, presenting a major economic challenge for farmed salmonids. In these populations, they cause severe infestations, chronic stress, anemia, reduced osmoregulation, and death (Coates et al., 2021; Bui et al., 2016). Aquaculture practices create favorable conditions for the farmed salmon to become heavily parasitized by sea lice. Wild juvenile salmon start becoming infected by sea lice when salmon return from spawning grounds, as they travel migratory routes in close proximity to salmon farms (Levin, 2013). These copepods feed on blood, skin tissue and mucus, impacting salmon survival, productivity, and migration, creating welfare concerns, and causing significant economic costs (Liu & Bjelland, 2014; Krkošek et al. 2013, cited by Coates et al., 2021).

The female salmon louse lay eggs the number of which may vary with time of year, louse size, louse age and host species (Whelan, 2010). One female can produce 6–11 broods during her lifetime. To complete its lifecycle, *L. salmonis* requires only the salmonid host. It has two initial larval stages, termed nauplii, both of which are non-feeding and planktonic. Following release, the eggs float within the surface plankton. At 5–15 days, the larvae turn into infective free-living copepodids, locate a host to which they attach by means of their antenna. The copepodid molts, then a further four successive sessile chalimus stages feed on the host skin around their point of attachment. Two additional preadult stages follow, during which the lice move freely at the surface of the host body to feed on its skin. Adults can overwinter on wild salmon (Whelan, 2010).

Signs and Diagnosis Sea lice can occur anywhere on the skin, but often congregate on the head and behind the fins. They grasp tightly to their host with their second pair of antennae and maxillipeds, causing the epithelium to bleed and to produce increased mucus discharge. Tissue necrosis and loss of physical and microbial protective function by chemical changes of the skin mucus also occur, exposing fish to secondary infections. Infested fish have reduced appetite, growth and food conversion efficiency, manifesting stress and discomfort. Changes to the host blood include anemia, reduced lymphocytes, ion imbalance and elevated cortisol (Whelan, 2010). The adult stages are highly visible on infested fish. Examination of the sea lice under a microscope, aids in identification of the parasite.

Treatment and Management As sea lice are ubiquitous in the marine environment, prevention of these infestations in farmed salmonids is difficult. The disease control consists in using licensed veterinary medicines and cleaner fish, such as wrasse and lumpfish that feed on sea lice. Veterinary medicines are either applied as a bath or via feed. There is the potential for salmon lice to adapt to current prevention and control methods, by its ability to evolve resistance to chemical therapeutants.

The industry has shifted to alternative non-chemical approaches. Other measures include the coordination of fallowing and stocking within agreed management areas (Powell et al., 2018). Vaccination has been proposed to control salmon lice, but there are no licensed vaccine available.

Endoparasites

Fish Eustrongylides (Eustrongylidosis)

Overview and Etiology Disease caused by the third and fourth larval stages of the nematode *Eustrongylides* spp., Jägerskiöld, 1909 (Phylum Nematoda, Family Dioctophymidae). Eustrongylidosis occurs worldwide, in marine, brackish, and freshwater fish species. Although a total of 19 Eustrongylides species have been described based on the morphology of the adult and larval stages, three species are commonly being referred to in the literature: *Eustrongylides tubifex*, *Eustrongylides ignotus* and *Eustrongylides excisus*. The nematode has a complex life cycle, requiring a definitive host (wading birds) and intermediate hosts; that is, oligochaetes or annelid worms (for earlier larval stages – to ensure development from L1 to L2 stages, or only for L2) and finfish (for both L3 and L4 stages, or just for L4). *Eustrongylides ignotus* may be able to complete its lifecycle without a tubifex worm, whereas some fish species may act as definitive hosts of the nematode. Amphibians (frogs), reptiles (alligators, caimans, grass and dice snakes) and humans are occasional hosts of the nematode. Most studies would recognize the larvae at the genus level, as there are no sufficient discriminant morphological characteristics to identify them to the species level.

Host Range and Transmission Adult nematodes live in the proventriculus of wading birds. These birds excrete the parasite's unhatched eggs into the water, where L1 hatches to find an oligochaete (e.g. *Tubifex tubifex*, *Limnodrilus hoffmeisten*). In infested oligochaetes, the parasite moves to L2 stage, which is the stage of the parasite where it is transmissible to fish. When fish feed on infested oligochaetes, the parasite is able to continue the lifecycle, by passing through two successive larval stages, to L3 and then to L4. In fish, these two stages coexist in the same host, moving freely or being trapped into parasitic cysts. When infected fish are consumed by predatory fish, the parasite disseminates within the predator, as well. Aquatic birds are definitive hosts of the adult nematode, infestations in these occurring when they feed on infested fish. In humans, sporadic infestations ("larva migrans") are reported, with a predominantly digestive localization, caused by the consumption of raw, infested fish. Many species of wild and farmed fish are susceptible (e.g. perch, pike, catfish, avat, pikeperch, redfish, slug, crucian carp, oblate, eel). Larvae situate in the viscera and muscles of the host, compromising reproduction and depreciating the value of the muscle meat. The incidence of parasitism (measured at the population level) and the intensity of the parasitism (measured at the individual level) vary according to the species and the individual resistance to infestation, and depending on the season.

Signs and Diagnosis Larval eustrongylidosis in fish is mostly subclinical. The debilitated, severely infested, and young fish may become anorexic and emaciated. They may also show abdominal dilation, dyspnea, and swimming abnormalities. Necropsy reveals pallor of gills and internal organs, ascites, necrosis, and liver degeneration, petechiae and hyperemia in the digestive tract and peritoneum. Free and encysted larvae are present in the peritoneal cavity on the peritoneal serosa, in the body muscles, and on the visceral serosae (Figure 2.11a,b). A leukocytic infiltrate surrounding the parasitic cysts is formed in the affected tissues (Figure 2.11c,d).

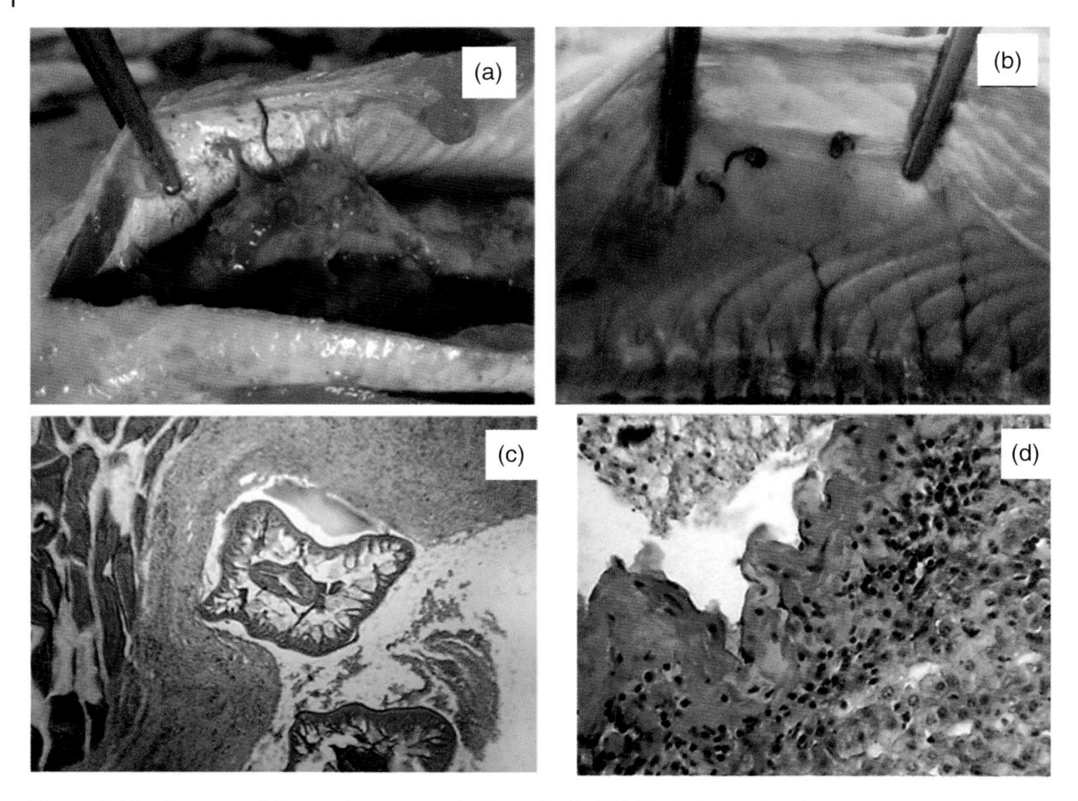

Figure 2.11 *Eustrongylides* spp. larvae, perch (*Perca fluviatilis*). (a) Peritoneal and visceral adhesion. (b) Hemorrhage and encysted larvae in the peritoneum. (c) Leukocytic infiltrate surrounding cysts with *Eustrongylides* spp. in muscle of *Perca fluviatilis*. (hematoxylin and eosin stain, 40× magnification, 5.6 zoom), (d) Liver, *Sander lucioperca* (hematoxylin and eosin stain, 100× magnification, 7.1 zoom).

The larvae have a wire-like appearance, are reddish in color, and vary in size up to a few tenths of centimeters. Necropsy and parasitological examinations of the larvae allow for genus-level identification. Molecular tools, such as polymerase chain reaction (PCR), loop-mediated isothermal amplification, recombinase polymerase amplification, PCR plus sequencing or real-time PCR (qPCR), are required to identify the species involved for monitoring and control purposes.

Treatment and Management Treatment of fish is not possible. Disease prevention and control measures are difficult to implement in aquaculture and wild fish populations for several reasons. The parasite's eggs remain viable in the water for up to 2.5 years. Eustrongylides larvae (including encysted larvae) are infectious throughout the life of the host. The nematode may continue to remain alive even after the fish host dies. From personal observations, shortly after fish death a number of larvae actively migrate to exit the fish body (Figure 2.12). Once freed into the water, they may remain viable some time, being able to infest other susceptible hosts. Eutrophication and heating of the water temperature (at 20–30°C) provide optimal conditions for the development of the parasite. Environmental pollution (including heavy metal contaminants) appears to play an important role in the epizootiology of larval eustrongylidosis, enhancing the resistance of the parasite and increasing the susceptibility of fish to infestation (Urdeş and Warren, 2022). Improving water quality and rigorous control of fish feed are currently the only means available to prevent infestation.

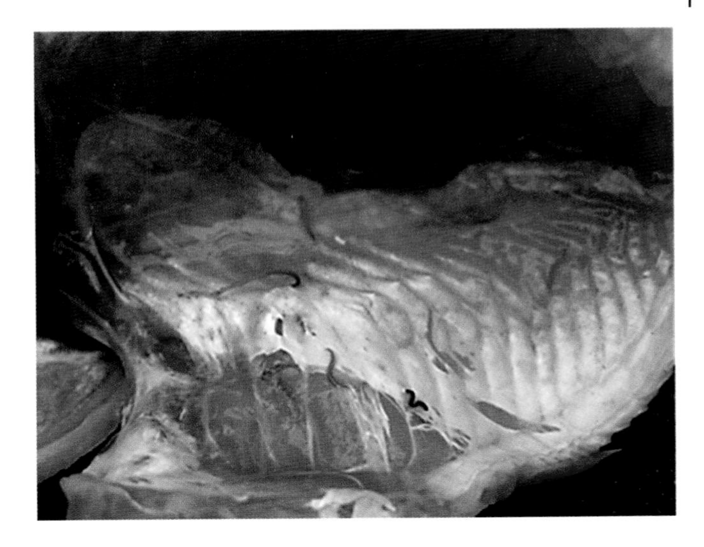

Figure 2.12 *Eustrongylides* species postmortem larval migration from muscle, *Perca fluviatilis*.

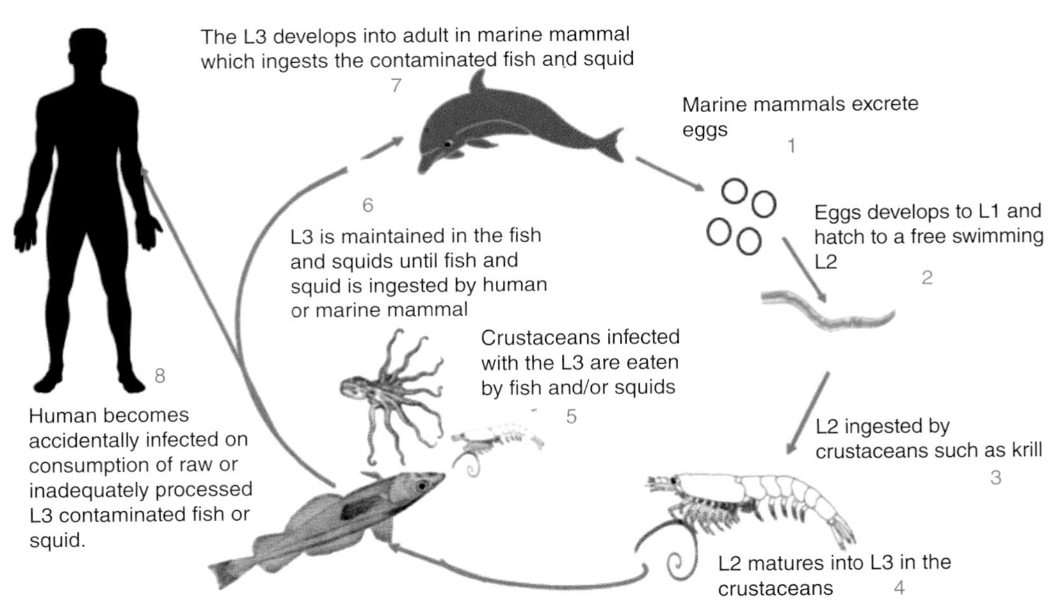

Figure 2.13 Lifecycle of the anisakids. *Source:* Aibinu, et al. 2019/with permission of Elsevier.

Fish *Anisakis* (Anisakidosis)

Overview and Etiology A widespread nematodosis affecting a large variety of aquatic hosts, including marine mammals and aquatic birds (e.g. pelicans). Marine mammals, especially cetaceans (such as whales, dolphins, and seals) and aquatic birds are the definitive hosts of anisakids. Aquatic invertebrates such as cephalopods, shrimps, crustaceans (especially crustaceans of the order Euphausiacea, krills) and fish act as intermediate or paratenic hosts (Figure 2.13). Freshwater fish (cyprinids and silurids) and a wider variety of marine fish species such as herring (*Clupea harengus*), mackerel (*Scomber scombrus*), cod (*Gadus morhua*), hake (*Merluccius merluccius*), sardines (*Sardina pilchardus*), and anchovy (*Engraulis encrasicolus*), are the most commonly affected fish. Marine fish are the major causes of anisakid infections in humans. Humans are incidental hosts of the parasite, anisakidosis occurring by consumption of seafood, particularly fish, undercooked or raw, contaminated with the infective stage (L3) of the nematode (Audicana et al., 2002; Guardone et al., 2018, Cipriani et al., 2018; Mladineo et al., 2016). Atlantic salmon (Salmo salar) and sea trout (*Salmo trutta*) have also been found infected with anisakid larvae (Buchmann and Mehrdana, 2016).

Anisakidosis is caused by members of the family Anisakidae (Skrjabin and Karokhin, 1945). The anisakid genera includes *Anisakis, Pseudoterranova, Hysterothylacium* and *Contracaecum*. Nematodes from *Anisakis* (particularly, *A. simplex* and *A. pegreffii)* and the *Pseudoterranova* genera have been involved in human anisakiasis globally, causing gastrointestinal and ectopic infections, accompanied by allergic reactions and immunological cross-reactivity with invertebrate proteins (Pampiglione et al., 2002; Aibinu et al., 2019).

Signs and Diagnosis Symptomatology may vary, depending on the intensity of the parasitism and the age of the fish. Fish with chronic and heavy infestations lose weight and become hypodynamic and anorexic. The growth rate of affected fish slows. Necropsy reveals organ atrophy, fibrosis with visceral adhesions, muscle hemorrhage and ulcers of the intestinal mucosa.

The morphology of *Anisakis* varies with the different stages of the nematode. In fish, the coiled larvae (L3 stage) form cysts of 2–3 mm diameter, on the peritoneum, musculature, liver, intestines, gonads, and other visceral organs. Uncoiled larvae are about 2 cm length. The larvae are a grayish or yellowish color (Figure 2.14a). Morphology of the larvae is part of the diagnosis protocol. However, molecular tools such as sequencing of the internal transcribed spacer region of ribosomal DNA and PCR coupled with restriction fragment length polymorphism are the most commonly employed methods to identify species involved (Iglesias et al., 2008; Shamsi et al., 2009; Umehara et al., 2006).

Treatment and Management As in the case of eustrongylidosis, anisakidosis occurs in the natural environment. The parasite has a complex lifecycle involving a wide variety of host species. Consequently, efficient control measures are not applicable.

Fish Tapeworm Infection (Diphyllobothriasis)

Overview and Etiology Plerocercoids of the tapeworm in the genus *Diphyllobothrium* are found worldwide. Common species are *Diphyllobothrium latum*, *Diphyllobothrium nihonkaiense* (Japan, Korea, eastern Russia, and North America), *Diphyllobothrium dendriticum* (in the northern part

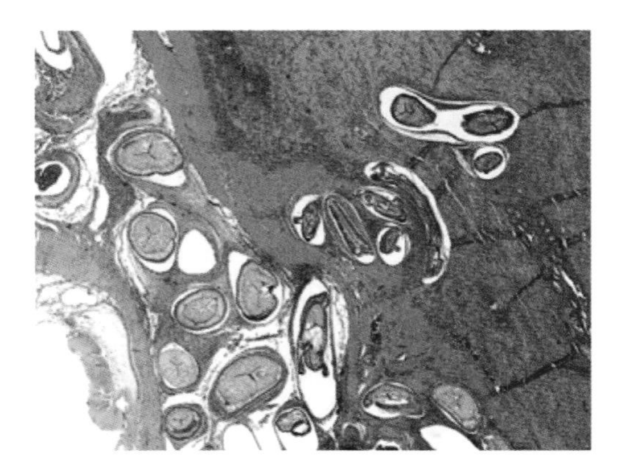

Figure 2.14 Histological section through the anus and hind gut of salmon infected with *A. simplex*. Localized inflammatory response surrounds the parasitic cysts. *Source:* Longshaw (2012).

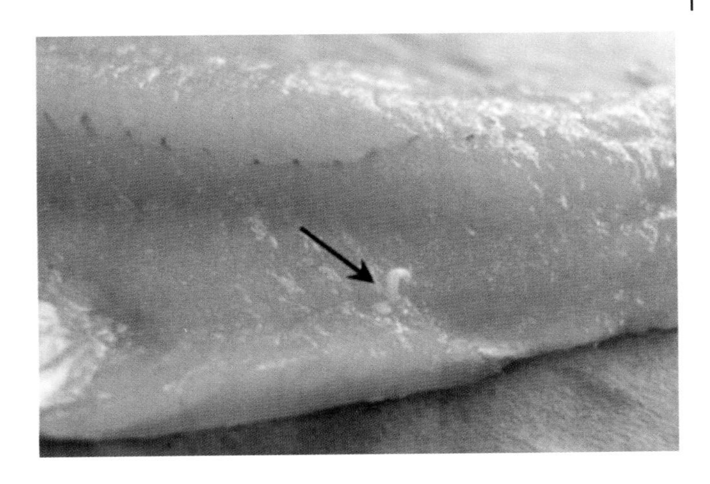

Figure 2.15 Plerocercoid of *Diphyllobothrium latum* in a perch fillet (*Perca fluviatilis*) from Lake Maggiore, Switzerland. *Source:* Lake Maggiore/Elsevier.

of the northern hemisphere) and *Diphyllobothrium pacificum* (in Argentina, Chile, Peru), (Dupouy-Camet & Peduzzi, 2014). Fish diphyllobotriasis occurs in predatory fish, with pike, perch, and salmonids being among the most affected fish. The plerocercoid larva morphology is white-gray or yellowish, elongated, unsegmented, rounded in section, of 2 mm to a few cm in length (Figure 2.15). In parasitized fish, the worm moves freely in the body or becomes encysted in the muscles and internal organs. Copepod crustaceans are the first intermediate host, and fish are the second. Mammals (including humans) and piscivorous birds are definitive hosts of the parasite. Fish infestations occur through the consumption of crustaceans infested with procercoids. Once into the fish digestive system, the procercoid larvae are released. They pass through the wall of the digestive tract and migrate into the body cavity, establishing in the muscle or in gonads, liver, and other organs. Here, they develop into the plerocercoid stage. Predatory fish become infested by consumption of small fish that do not normally participate in the biological cycle of the parasite, but which accumulate the worm by eating procercoid-infested copepod crustaceans. Humans and carnivorous mammals become infested by consuming raw fish infested with plerocercoid. In the intestines of these hosts, the plerocercoid larvae become adults, initiating the egg production.

Signs and Diagnosis There are no obvious clinical signs of the disease in acute infestations in fish. In chronic infestations, a reduced growth rate may be noticed in some infested fish. Externally, small nodules of less than one centimeter in diameter are observed protruding through the skin, giving the skin an uneven appearance. In the peritoneal cavity, free larvae and nodular proliferations (with trapped larvae), necrosis and hemorrhage are present. Mortality is rare, occurring only in the young and debilitated fish. Direct examination (including microscopically) is used to confirm the presumptive diagnosis.

Treatment and Management No treatment is available. Prevention aims at interrupting the biological cycle of the parasite, rigorous checks of fish destined for human consumption, and eliminating those fish infested with plerocercoids.

Fish Triaenophorus (Triaenophorosis)

Overview and Etiology Cestods in the genus *Triaenophorus*, order Pseudophyllidea (*Triaenophorus nodulosus* and *Triaenophorus crassus*) are affected.

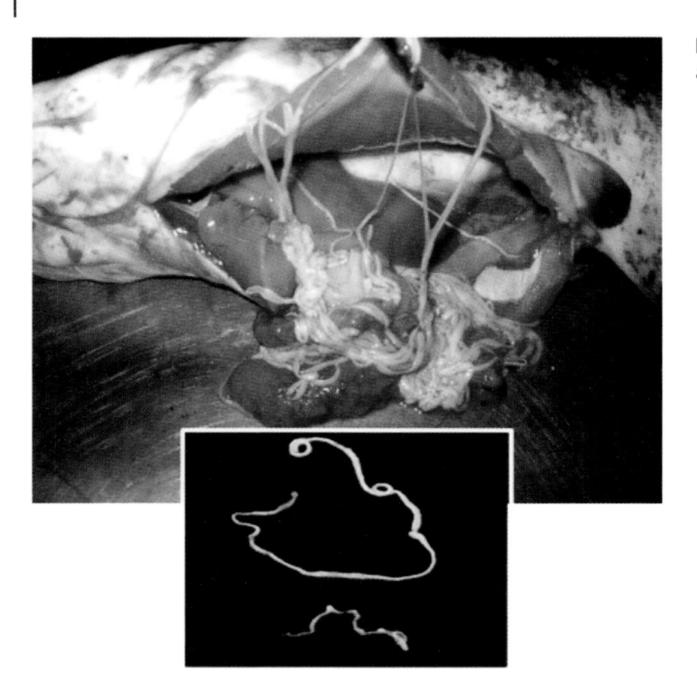

Figure 2.16 *Triaenophorus* species in a catfish (*Silurus glanis*).

Fish trienophorosis is found in freshwater fish in Europe, North America, and Asia. Receptive fish species include pike, perch, native trout, rainbow trout, catfish, salmon, and eel. *T. nodulosus* is considered more pathogenic and invasive than *T. crassus*. The biological cycle of the worm involves three larval stages (trienophorosis, procercoid, and plerocercoid), two intermediate hosts (copepod crustaceans and phytophagous fish species), and one definitive host (predatory fish). Adults are oviparous.

The body of *T. nodulosus* has the appearance of a white ribbon, being 300 mm long and 2-4 mm wide (Figure 2.16). Adult worms are found in the intestine of piscivorous fish, such as European catfish, pike, perch, pike, perch, or trout. *T. crassus* is 250–400 mm long and 4–5 mm wide. Adults of *T. crassus* are found in the gut of pike.

Signs and Diagnosis The infestation is often subclinical. In massive infestations, abdominal distension can be observed due to the size and number of parasites in the viscera and muscles. Fish can show discomfort and reduced growth due to intestinal obstruction and inflammation of the intestinal epithelium (Urdeș, 2015) (Figure 2.17). The migration of the parasite through the body cavity and viscera can cause localized tissue damage. Multiparasitism with *Triaenophorus* is not an uncommon finding in natural aquasystems (Figure 2.18). Macroscopic and histologic exams lead to identification of the parasite to the genus level.

Treatment and Management There is no treatment for larval infestations. Praziquantel or other anthelmintics are used to treat the disease in the definitive host, aiming at adult stages of the cestode. To avoid reinfestation, during the treatment, the fish subjected to dehelminthization should be maintained in quarantine throughout treatment duration. The water in these quarantine systems must not come into contact with the source of water intended for growing fishponds. Avoid introducing infested fish and live food into healthy ponds.

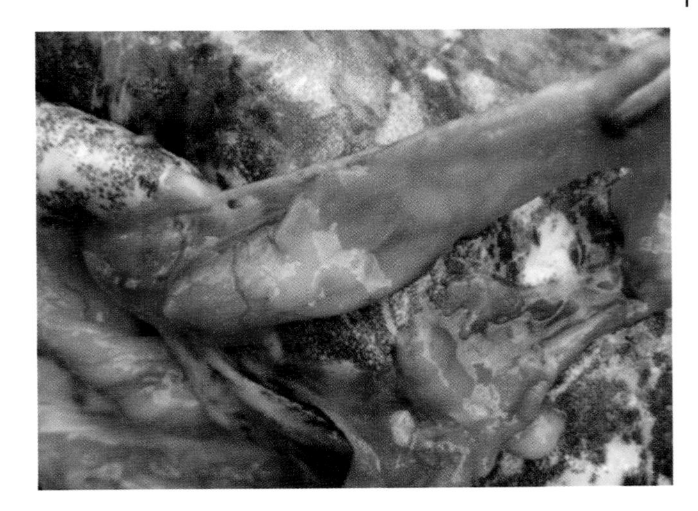

Figure 2.17 Catarrhal enteritis, triaenophorosis in catfish (*Silurus glanis*).

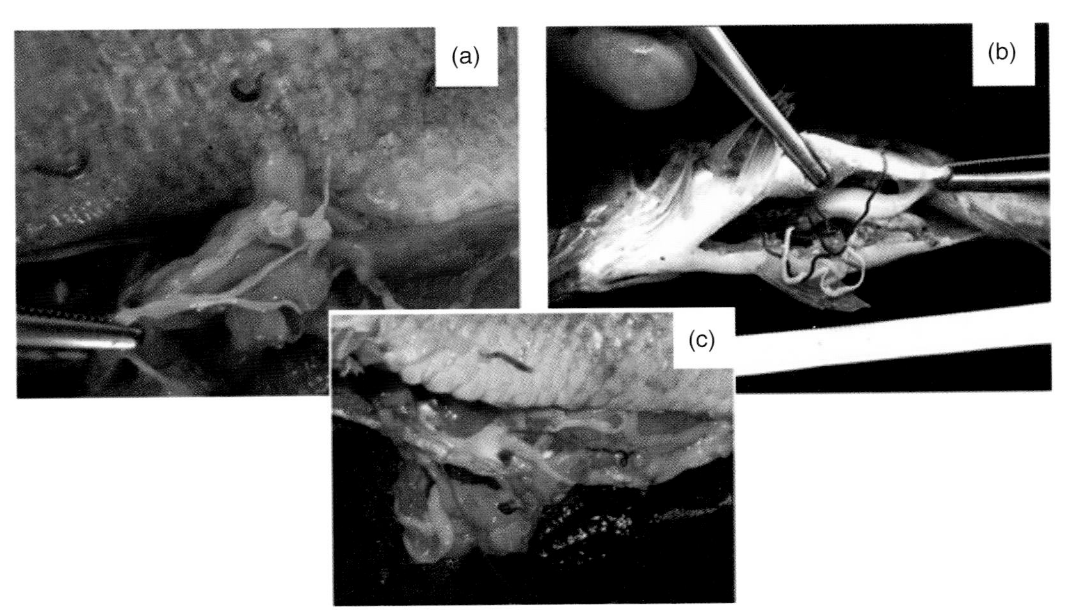

Figure 2.18 *Triaenophorus* spp. in perch *(Perca fluviatilis)*, with (a) *Piscicola* spp., (b) *Eustrongylides spp.*, and (c) *Eustrongylides* and *Piscicola* spp.

Intestinal Ligulosis

Overview and Etiology The genus *Ligula* includes three species: *Ligula intestinalis* (in Cyprinidae and Catostomidae), *Ligula colymbi* (in Cobitidae) and *Ligula Pavlovskii* (in Gobiidae). These parasitic species have aquatic crustaceans (family Cyclopidae) as an intermediate host of the first order. The adult parasitizes the intestine in ichthyophagous birds from the families Lariidae, Podicipedidae, and Ardeidae. Second-order intermediate hosts are freshwater fish. In these hosts, the plerocercoid larva parasitizes the abdominal cavity.

Signs and Diagnosis The parasite is 20–100 cm in length and 0.5–1.8 cm wide *(L. intestinalis)* (Figure 2.19). Affected fish swim at the surface or on their sides or back, have a swollen belly, and

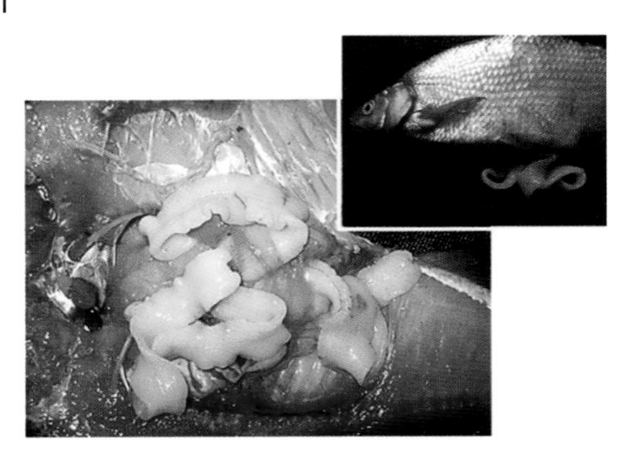

Figure 2.19 Plerocercoid of *Ligula intestinalis* in *Abramis brama*.

stop feeding. Pathological changes consist of fibrosis, inflammation, and atrophy of the abdominal viscera by displacement and compression, with an accompanying accumulation of blood stained ascitic fluid.

Treatment and Management Praziquantel is directly applied or mixed into pellets and fed to infested fish. The treatment requires the control of copepods for more effectiveness. Remove infested fish and disinfect the water. Discourage the presence of fish-eating birds.

References

Aibinu IE, Smooker PM, Lopata AL. 2019. *Anisakis* nematodes in fish and shellfish: from infection to allergies. *Int J Parasitol* 9:384–393.

Aisien SO, Salami LA, Obaro FE, Erakpoweri SO. 2004. The influence of climate on the distribution of monogeneans of anurans in Nigeria. *J Helminthol* 78(2):101–104.

Amlacher E, Conroy, DA, Herman RL. 1970. *Textbook of Fish Diseases*. Jersey City, NJ: Crown Publishers.

Audicana MT, Ansotegui IJ, de Corres LF, Kennedy MW. 2002. *Anisakis simplex*: dangerous-dead and alive? *Trends Parasitol* 18:20–25.

Benz GW, Bullard SA. 2004. Metazoan Parasites and associates of chondrichthyans with emphasis on taxa harmful to captive hosts. In: Smith M, Warmolts D, Thoney D, Hueter R, eds. *The Elasmobranch Husbandry Manual: Captive care of sharks, rays, and their relatives*. Columbus, OH: Ohio Biological Survey, pp. 325–416.

Bruno DW, Noguera PA, Poppe TT. 2013. *A Colour Atlas of Salmonid Diseases*, 2nd ed. Dordrecht, Germany: Springer.

Buchmann K, Mehrdana F. 2016. Effects of anisakid nematodes *Anisakis simplex* (s.l.), *Pseudoterranova decipiens* (s.l.) and *Contracaecum osculatum* (s.l.) on fish and consumer Health. *Food Waterborn Parasitol.* 4:13–22.

Bui S, Oppedal F, Stien L, Dempster T. 2016. Sea lice infestation level alters salmon swimming depth in sea-cages. *Aquaculture Environ Interact* 8: 429–435, 2016. DOI:10.3354/aei00188.

Cain KD, Polinkski MP. 2014. Infectious diseases of coldwater fish in fresh water. In: Woo PTK, and Bruno D, eds. *Diseases and Disorders of Finfish in Cage Culture*. Wallingford, UK: CABI International, pp. 60–113.

Cannon LRG, Lester RJG. 1988 Two turbellarians parasitic in fish. *Dis Aquat Org* 5:15–22.

Cheung P. 1993. Parasitic diseases of elasmobranchs. In: Stoskopf MK, ed. *Fish Medicine*. Philadelphia, PA: Saunders, pp. 782–807.

Cipriani P, Sbaraglia GL, Palomba, M, et al. 2018. *Anisakis pegreffii* (Nematoda: *Anisakidae*) in European anchovy, *Engraulis encrasicolus*, from the Mediterranean sea: fishing ground as a predictor of parasite distribution. *Fish Res* 202:59–68.

Coates A, Phillips B, Bui S, et al. 2021. Evolution of salmon lice in response to management strategies: a review. *Rev Aquacult* 13:1397–1422.

Colorni A, Diamant A. 2014. Infectious diseases of warmwater fish in marine and brackish waters. In: Woo PTK, and Bruno D, eds. *Diseases and Disorders of Finfish in Cage Culture*. Wallingford, UK: CABI International, pp. 155–192.

Dove DM, Clauss TM, Marancik DP, Camus AC. 2017. Emerging diseases of elasmobranchs in aquaria. In: Smith M, Warmolts D, Thoney D, et al., eds. *Elasmobranch Husbandry Manual II: recent advances in the care of sharks, rays and their relatives*. Columbus, OH: Ohio Biological Survey, pp. 263–275.

Dupouy-Camet J, Peduzzi R. 2014. *Encyclopedia of Food Safety Volume 2: Hazards and Diseases*. San Diego, CA: Academic Press.

Guardone L, Armani A, Nucera D, et al. 2018. Human anisakiasis in Italy: a retrospective epidemiological study over two decades. *Parasite*. 25:41.

Harris P, Shinn A, Cable J, Bakke T. 2004. Nominal species of the genus *Gyrodactylus* von Nordmann 1832 (Monogenea: *Gyrodactylidae*), with a list of principal host species. *Syst Parasitol* 59(1):1–27.

Hutson KS, Brazenor AK, Vaughan DB, Trujillo-González A. 2018. monogenean parasite cultures: current techniques and recent advances. *Adv Parasitol* 99:61–91.

Iglesias R, D'Amelio S, Ingrosso S, et al. 2008). Molecular and morphological evidence for the occurrence of *Anisakis* sp. (Nematoda, *Anisakidae*) in the Blainville's beaked whale *Mesoplodon densirostris*. *J. Helminthol.* 82:305–308.

Jansson E, Vennerström P. 2014. Infectious diseases of coldwater fish in marine and brackish waters. In: *Diseases and Disorders of Finfish in Cage Culture*, 2nd ed. Woo PTK, and Bruno D, eds. Wallingford, UK: CABI International, pp. 15–59.

Jean-Lou J, Leblanc P, Florent K, Robert L. 2009. Turbellarian black spot disease in bluespine unicornfish, *Naso unicornis*, in New Caledonia, due to the parasitic turbellarian *Piscinquilinus* sp. *Dis Aquat Organ* 85:245–249.

Jones SRM, Smith PA. 2014. Sporadic emerging diseases and disorders. In: Woo PTK, and Bruno D, eds. *Diseases and Disorders of Finfish in Cage Culture*. Wallingford, UK: CABI International, pp. 287–312.

Kohn A, Cohen SC, Salgado-Maldonado G. 2006. Checklist of *Monogenea* parasites of freshwater and marine fishes, amphibians and reptiles from Mexico, *Central America and Caribbean. Zootaxa* 1289(1): https://doi.org/10.11646/zootaxa.1289.1.1.

Lari E, Pyle GG. 2017. *Gyrodactylus salmonis* infection impairs the olfactory system of rainbow trout. *J Fish Dis.* 40(10):1279–1284.

Levin SA. 2013. *Encyclopedia of Biodiversity*. 2nd ed. San Diego, CA: Academic Press.

Lewbart GA. 2017. *Ornamental Fishes and Aquatic Invertebrates: Self-assessment color review*, 2nd ed. Philadelphia, PA: Routledge.

Lio-Pio GD, Lim LHS. 2014. Infectious diseases of warmwater fish in fresh water. In: Woo PTK, and Bruno D, eds. *Diseases and Disorders of Finfish in Cage Culture*. Wallingford, UK: CABI International, pp. 193–253.

Loh R. 2014. *Fish vetting techiques and practical tips. The Fish Vet's Blog 8 September*. Perth, Australia: Richmond Loh Publishing. https://thefishvet.com/2015/09/08/fish-vetting-techniques-practical-tips (accessed 29 August 2022).

Longshaw M. 2012. *Anisakis Larvae ("Herringworm"; Nematoda) in Fish*. ICES Leaflet No. 8. Copenhagen, Denmark: International Council for the Exploration of the Sea.

Longshaw M, Feist SW. 2001. Parasitic diseases. In: Wildgoose WH, ed. *BSAVA Manual of Ornamental Fish*, 2nd ed. Gloucester, UK: British Small Animal Veterinary Association, pp. 167–184.

Lumsden JS. 2006. Gastrointestinal tract, swimbladder, pancreas and peritoneum. In: Ferguson HW, ed. *Systemic Pathology of Fish*. London: Scotian, pp. 169–199.

McAllister PE. 1993. Cold-water marine fish viruses. In: Stoskopf MK, ed. *Fish Medicine*. Philadelphia, PA: Saunders, pp. 697–711.

McAllister PE, Stoskopf MK. 1993. Shark viruses. In: Stoskopf MK, ed. *Fish Medicine*. Philadelphia, PA: Saunders, pp. 780–782.

Meyers T, Burton T, Bentz C, et al. 2019. *Diseases of Wild and Cultured Fishes in Alaska*. Anchorage, AK: Alaska Department of Fish and Game Fish, Pathology Laboratories.

Mladineo I, Popovic M, Drmic-Hofman I Poljak V. 2016. A case report of *Anisakis pegreffii* (Nematoda, *Anisakidae*) identified from archival paraffin sections of a Croatian patient. *BMC Infect Dis* 16:42.

Pampiglione S, Rivasi F, Criscuolo M, et al. 2002. Human anisakiasis in Italy: a report of eleven new cases. *Pathol Res Pract.* 198:429–434.

Pike CS, Manire CA, Gruber SH. 1993. Nutrition and nutritional diseases in sharks. In: Stoskopf MK, ed. *Fish Medicine*. Philadelphia, PA: Saunders, pp. 763–769.

Powell A, Treasurer JW, Pooley CL, et al. 2018. Use of lumpfish for sea-lice control in salmon farming: challenges and opportunities. *Rev Aquacult* 10: 683–702.

Schmidt-Posthaus H, Marcos-López M. 2014. Non-infectious disorders of coldwater fish. In: Woo PTK, and Bruno D, eds. *Diseases and Disorders of Finfish in Cage Culture*. Wallingford, UK: CABI International, pp. 114–154.

Shamsi S, Eisenbarth A, Saptarshi S, et al. 2011. Occurrence and abundance of anisakid nematode larvae in five species of fish from southern Australian waters. *Parasitol Res* 108:927–934.

Stedman NL, Garner MM. 2018. Chondrichthyes. In: Terio KA, McAloose D, St. Leger J. *Pathology of Wildlife and Zoo Animals*. San Diego, CA: Academic Press, pp. 1003–1018.

Stoskopf MK. 1993. Bacterial diseases of sharks. In: Stoskopf MK, ed. *Fish Medicine*. Philadelphia, PA: Saunders, pp. 774–776.

Stoskopf MK. 1993. Fungal and algal diseases of sharks. In: Stoskopf MK, ed. *Fish Medicine*. Philadelphia, PA: Saunders, pp. 776–780.

Terrell SP. 2004. An introduction to viral, bacterial, and fungal diseases of elasmobranchs. In: *Elasmobranch Husbandry Manual: Captive care of sharks, rays, and their relatives*. Smith M, Warmolts D, Thoney D, Hueter R, eds. Columbus, OH: Ohio Biological Survey, pp. 427–431.

Umehara A, Kawakami Y, Matsui T, et al. 2006. Molecular identification of *Anisakis simplex* sensu stricto and *Anisakis pegreffii* (Nematoda: Anisakidae) from fish and cetacean in Japanese waters. *Parasitol Int* 55:267–271.

Urdeş L, Alcivar-Warren A. 2022. *A comparative study on metals and parasites in shellfish J Shellfish Research* 40(3):565–588.

Urdeş LD. 2015. *Ihtiopatologie*. Bucharest, Romania: Editura Granada.

Urdeş LD. 2007. *Ihtiopatologie şi elemente de tehnică sanitar-veterinară în acvacultură*. [*Ichthyopathology and Elements of Sanitary Veterinary Technique in Aquaculture*] Bucharest: Romania: Printech.

Vulpe V. 2007. *Paraziţi şi parazitoze ale peştilor dulcicoli [Parasites and Parasitosis of Freshwater Fish]*. Iaşi, Romania: Ed. Stef.

Whelan K. 2010. *A Review of the Impacts of the Salmon Louse, Lepeophtheirus salmonis (Krøyer, 1837) on Wild Salmonids*. Perth, Scotland: Atlantic Salmon Trust.

Whittington ID. 2004. The capsalidae (Monogenea: Monopisthocotylea): a review of diversity, classification and phylogeny with a note about species complexes. *Folia Parasitol (Praha)* 51(2–3):109–122.

Appendix 2.1

Etiology and clinical signs: salmonids and coldwater food fish

Clinical signs	Etiology
Sudden death	Bacterial septicemia (*Aeromonas*, *Bacillus*, *Pseudomonas*, *Proteus*), water quality issues (ammonia, oxygen, hydrogen sulfide), toxicosis (heavy metal, herbicide, pesticide), trauma, electrocution, botulism, methemoglobinemia/ brown blood disease, gas supersaturation, salmonid alphavirus (sleeping disease)
Poor growth	nutritional deficiency, stress/water quality issues, insufficient caloric intake, heavy parasitism (*Chilodonella*, *Ichthyophthirius*), salmonid alphavirus, *Mycobacterium*
Uncoordinated swimming/ nervousness/buoyancy	generalized infectious disease (virus, fungi, bacteria, myxozoans, microsporidians), electrocution, spinal trauma, toxicosis, central nervous system disease, water quality issues, gas bubble disease, thiamine/ riboflavin/pyridoxine deficiency, botulism, Ichthyophonus hoferi, algal blooms, jellyfish
Gasping/asphyxia:	Low dissolved oxygen, high water temperature, high carbon dioxide, toxin exposure/ammonia, organic/inorganic contaminants, suspended sediments, physical impediment/obstruction to gas exchange
Gill disease	Branchiomycosis, Flavobacterium, Epitheliocystis, parasites
Anemia	Piscirickettsia, salmon leukemia virus, infectious hematopoietic necrosis, hemorrhagic smolt syndrome, zinc toxicosis, lipoid liver disease (rancid feed)
Skin/fins:	
Petechiae	Virus, bacterial septicemia, low pH
Increased mucus	Water quality issues, parasitism
Hemorrhage, necrosis, ulcers	Overcrowding (fin nipping, soreback), improper pH, trauma, sunburn, bacterial infection (*Aeromonas*, *Pseudomonas*, *Moritella*, *Flavobacterium*, *Aliivibrio – Vibrio*, *Tenacibaculum*, *Piscirickettsia*, *Mycobacterium*), *Saprolegnia*, *Phialophora*, *Aphanomyces*, infectious hematopoietic necrosis (especially young fish), spring viremia of carp, rhabdoviruses (including viral hemorrhagic septicemia), herpesvirus, cardiomyopathy syndrome, red mark syndrome (coldwater strawberry disease), gas bubble disease
Parasites	*Monogenes*, ciliates, flagellates, amoeba, copepods, branchiurans, bivalves, leeches, hydroids
Yellow/white flat lesions	*Flavobacterium* infection, necrosis, epidermal hyperplasia, dermal edema, *Saprolegnia*
Depigmentation	Epidermal/dermal injury of any type, toxicosis/environmental
Nodules/lumps	Papillomatosis, neoplasia, granulomatous disease (Mycobacterium, other bacteria, fungi), virus (lymphocystis, adenovirus, herpesvirus), *Ichthyophthirius*, foreign body, *Dermocystidium*, furunculosis, encysted trematodes
Segmental darkening	Neurologic disease/infection (*Myxobolus*, *Mycobacterium*, betanodavirus)
Edema/lepidorthosis	Hypoalbuminemia, renal disease, severe skin disease

(*Continued*)

Clinical signs	Etiology
Red vent	Red vent – internal disease (bacterial, viral), *Anisakis* larvae, *Ceratomyxa*
Black spots/nodules	Melanocyte hyperplasia, melanoma, encysted trematodes, microsporidian infection, pigmented fungal granulomas
Gills:	
Hemorrhage/ulcers	Bacterial septicemia, toxins, virus, *Flavobacterium*, *Sanguinicola*, diatoms, jellyfish, protozoan parasites
Hyperplasia	Gill necrosis virus, water quality issues, dietary imbalance (vitamin B5), chronic inflammation, parasitism (amoeba, flagellates, ciliates)
Necrosis	High/low pH, chlorine, *Flavobacterium*, *Branchiomycosis*, *Saprolegnia*, jellyfish, protozoan parasites
Nodules	Encysted trematodes, myxozoan cysts, neoplasia, bacteria (*Nocardia*, *Mycobacterium*), amoebic gill disease, *Dermocystidium*, microsporidian (*Loma*), *Ichthyophthirius*
Pallor	Anemia, salmon leukemia virus, infectious hematopoietic necrosis (especially in young fish.), spring viremia of carp, amoebic gill disease
Gas bubbles	Supersaturation of water by gas
Increased mucus	Water quality issues, bacterial infection, parasites
Parasites	*Monogenes*, ciliates, flagellates, copepods, branchiurans, bivalves, amoeba
Yellow/white lesions	*Flavobacterium* infection, necrosis, *Saprolegnia*
Pseudobranch:	
Necrosis	*Parvicapsula*, *Flavobacterium*, toxins (herbicides, metals, pesticides)
Swelling	*Xcellia* (X cell disease), *Parvicapsula*
Calcification	Vitamin E deficiency, lipoid liver disease, nephrocalcinosis
Mouth:	
Gasping/asphyxia	See general comment above; screamer disease (mouth locked open)
Hemorrhage/ulcers	Bacterial septicemia (*Yersinia*, *Flavobacterium*, *Tenacibaculum*, *Vibrio*), parasites (metacercariae, isopods), trauma
Increased mucus/ exudate	Bacterial infection (*Flavobacterium*), parasitism
Gas bubbles	Gas supersaturation
Malocclusion	Inappropriate food sources, trauma
Nodules	Granulomas, papilloma (*Oncorhynchus masou* virus), dental neoplasia, parasitic cyst, thyroid hyperplasia, thyroid neoplasia, goiter, thymic neoplasia
Eye:	
Exophthalmia	Bacterial septicemia, multiple viral infections (spring viremia of carp), *Mycobacteria*, vitamin A/E/pantothenic acid deficiency, nephrocalcinosis, gas bubble disease/supersaturation, white-eye syndrome (salmon)
Ulcers	Fungus, bacterial septicemia, trauma, blindness
Corneal edema/ cloudiness	Poor water quality, conspecific aggression, bacterial, viral, fungal, parasitic disease, white-eye syndrome (salmon)
Ophthalmitis	Trauma, hematogenous spread of pathogens, thermal damage, *Piscirickettsia*, *Tenacibaculum*, zinc deficiency, *Diplostomum*, *Tylodelphys*

Clinical signs	Etiology
Cataract	*Diplostomum*, deficiencies (zinc, vitamin A, thiamine, riboflavin, methionine, tryptophan, histidine), rapid osmolar fluctuations, ultraviolet exposure, temperature fluctuations, gas bubble disease
Gas bubbles	Supersaturation, bacterial infection, corneal perforation
Lens luxation	Trauma
Enucleation	Trauma (predator, stocking density too high, jellyfish), severe ophthalmitis (*Tenacibaculum*)
Muscle:	
Atrophy	Emaciation, denervation, riboflavin deficiency
Liquefaction/ necrosis	Microsporidians, myxozoans, bacterial infection
Nodules/swelling	Encysted trematodes, granulomas, microsporidians, myxozoans, emphysematous bacterial infection, Ichthyophonus hoferi, neoplasia
Hemorrhage	Viral hemorrhagic septicemia, bacterial sepsis, trauma, vascular disease, myonecrosis
White foci	Magnesium deficiency, other dietary imbalances, necrosis, microsporidians, white-eye syndrome (salmon)
Skeletal deformity	Vitamin A/C/E deficiency, *Myxobolus*, *Mycobacterium*, abnormal egg incubation temperatures, trauma, hereditary, adverse environment conditions, toxicant exposure
Abdomen/Coelom:	
Enlarged (general)	Neoplasia, overweight, egg binding/dystocia, gastrointestinal impaction, peritonitis, cardiovascular/hepatic disease leading to ascites, renal disease, other causes of hypoproteinemia, gastrointestinal impaction, parasites
Ascites	Bacterial septicemia, piscine reovirus, cardiomyopathy syndrome, viral hemorrhagic septicemia, vegetative valvular endocarditis
Peritonitis, nodular/ granulomatous	Mycobacteriosis, streptococcosis, *Francisella*, parasites, (including encysted cestodes), fungus, egg binding, *Dermocystidium*, vaccination, steatitis (sequela to pancreatitis, antioxidant deficiency), neoplasia
Petechiae	Infectious pancreatic necrosis, salmon leukemia virus, viral hemorrhagic septicemia, infectious hematopoietic necrosis (especially in young fish), salmonid alphavirus, *Listonella*
Cysts	Polycystic renal disease, blocker ureter
Gas	Swimbladder or gut rupture, body wall perforation, inflammation with gas-producing microbes or fungi
Kidney:	
Diffuse swelling	Virus (salmon leukemia virus), bacterial septicemia, *Sphaerothecum*, immune stimulation, neoplasia
Cystic change	*Hoferellus carassii*, polycystic kidney disease (genetic/environmental), chronic renal disease
Necrosis	Virus, bacterial sepsis, parasite/protozoa (*Spironucleus*), riboflavin deficiency, heavy metals
Granulomas/nodules	Granulomas: bacterial (*Renibacterium*, *Mycobacterium*, *Nocardia*, *Francisella*), fungi, *Ichthyophonus hoferi*, proliferative kidney disease, nephrocalcinosis, neoplasia
Urinary bladder stones	Salinity/cation imbalances, renal/gill disease, genetic

(*Continued*)

Clinical signs	Etiology
Spleen:	
Diffuse swelling	Bacterial septicemia, reovirus, salmon leukemia virus, *Sphaerothecum*, proliferative kidney disease
Nodules	granulomas (bacterial, fungal, parasitic (*Spironucleus*), *Ichthyophonus*, neoplasia hoferi), *Dermocystidium*, hematoma, cysts (polycystic syndrome)
Liver:	
Necrosis	Virus (infectious pancreatic necrosis, reovirus, others), bacterial sepsis, heavy metals, algal toxin, rancid food, carbohydrates fed to carnivores
Hemorrhage	Infectious pancreatic necrosis, *Listonella*, *Aliivibrio* (*Vibrio*), *Carnobacterium*, infectious salmon anemia (diffuse hemorrhage)
Tan/yellow liver	Fat accumulation – excessive nutrition, toxicosis, choline deficiency, inadequate antioxidants, vitamin E deficiency, lipoid liver disease (rancid feed), seasonal accumulation (especially gadoids); fibrosis/iron accumulation; necrosis (see above)
Nodules	*Piscirickettsia*, *Spironucleus*, *Yersinia*, *Renibacterium*, *Mycobacterium*, *Nocardia*, myxozoan infection, encysted parasites (*Anisakis*), fungi, *Ichthyophonus hoferi*, *Dermocystidium*, neoplasia, mineral (biliary lithiasis)
Cysts	Polycystic liver, cestode larvae
Jaundice	Hemolysis, toxins, genetic abnormalities, erythrocytic inclusion body syndrome, infectious hemolytic anemia, erythromycin toxicosis
Stomach:	
Nodules	Granulomas (fungi, mycobacteria), microsporidians, myxozoans, nematodes
Dilation	Gastric dilation and airsacculitis syndrome, foreign bodies
Intestines:	
Hyperemia/ hemorrhage	Rainbow trout gastroenteritis, bacterial enteritis (*Clostridium*), infectious pancreatic necrosis, acanthocephalans
Mucoid feces/casts	Rainbow trout gastroenteritis, infectious pancreatic necrosis, infectious hematopoietic necrosis, parasites (*Spironucleus*), spring viremia of carp, coccidian infection, bacterial enteritis (*Vibrio*), dietary
Nodules	Foreign bodies, granulomas, coccidian cysts, myxozoan cysts, neoplasia, encysted worms
Diffuse thickening	*Piscirickettsia*, *Ceratomyxa*
Swimbladder:	
Enlarged	Hyperinflation: gas supersaturation, torsion, physostome blockage, betanodavirus, acid/base imbalance; fluid: exudate (bacteria), protozoa (*Spironucleus*), viral hemorrhagic septicemia; fungi: *Isaria farinosa* (*Paecilomyces*), *Phialophora*, *Phoma*, microsporidians, myxozoans; thickened wall: nematodes, chronic inflammation;
Atrophy	Rupture
Hemorrhage	Virus, bacteria
Reproductive nodules/ enlarged	*Mycobacterium*, *Ichthyophonus*, egg binding, microsporidians, myxozoans, neoplasia
Heart:	
Pallor	Necrosis, sanguinicola, fat deposition
Fibrosis	Reovirus

Clinical signs	Etiology
Inflammation/ pericarditis	bacterial sepsis (*Pseudomonas*, *Renibacterium*, *Piscirickettsia*, *Francisella*, *Lactobacillus*), cardiomyopathy syndrome, Spironucleus, metacercariae (*Apatemon*, *Cotylurus*, *Ichthyocotylurus*, *Stephanostomum*)
Hemopericardium	Cardiomyopathy syndrome, heart rupture
Nodules	Granulomas (bacteria, fungus, Ichthyophonus hoferi), metacercariae, ventricular aneurysms
Brown/bronze	Lipoid liver disease (rancid feed)

Appendix 2.2

Etiology and clinical signs: warm water food fish

Clinical signs	Etiology
Sudden death	Bacterial septicemia (*Aeromonas*), water quality issues (ammonia, oxygen, hydrogen sulfide), toxicosis (heavy metal, herbicide, pesticide), trauma, electrocution, botulism, methemoglobinemia/brown blood disease, gas supersaturation
Poor growth	Nutritional deficiency, stress/water quality issues, insufficient caloric intake, heavy parasitism (*Chilodonella*, *Ichthyophthirius*, *Enteromyxum*, cestodes), *Mycobacterium*
Uncoordinated swimming/ nervousness/buoyancy	Generalized infectious disease (virus – betanodavirus), bacteria (*Eubacterium tarantellus*), myxozoans, microsporidians, electrocution, spinal trauma, toxicosis, central nervous system disease, water quality issues, gas bubble disease, thiamine/riboflavin/pyridoxine deficiency, botulism, *Ichthyophonus hoferi*, fungal infection, algal blooms, parasitism
Gasping/asphyxia:	Low dissolved oxygen, high water temperature, high carbon dioxide, toxin/ ammonia exposure, organic and inorganic contaminants, suspended sediments, physical impediment/obstruction to gas exchange
Gill disease	Branchiomycosis, *Flavobacterium*, epitheliocystis, parasites
Anemia	Red sea bream iridovirus, zinc toxicosis
Skin/fins:	
Petechiae	Virus, bacterial septicemia (*Aeromonas*, *Photobacterium*, *Streptococcus*, *Lactococcus*), low pH
Increased mucus	Water quality issues, parasitism (*Cryptobia*, *Ichthyophthirius*, *Amyloodinium* and other dinoflagellates)
Hemorrhage, necrosis, ulcers	Overcrowding (fin nipping, soreback), trauma, improper pH, sunburn, bacterial infection (*Aeromonas*, *Flavobacterium*, *Pseudomonas*, *Mycobacterium*, *Vibrio*, *Edwardsiella*, *Tenacibaculum*, *Epitheliocystis*), *Saprolegnia*, *Aphanomyces*, virus infection (koi herpesvirus, grass carp reovirus, channel catfish virus), gas bubble disease, head and lateral line erosion syndrome

(Continued)

Clinical signs	Etiology
Parasites	*Monogenea*, ciliates, flagellates, amoeba, copepods, branchiurans, bivalves, leeches, hydroids
Yellow/white flat lesions	*Flavobacterium* infection, necrosis, epidermal hyperplasia, dermal edema, *Saprolegnia*
Depigmentation	Epidermal/dermal injury of any type, toxicosis/environmental
Nodules/lumps	Papillomatosis, carp pox, neoplasia, granulomatous disease (*Mycobacterium*, other bacteria, fungi), *Ichthyophthirius*, *Dermocystidium*, encysted trematodes, lymphocystis, foreign body, furuncles (Gram-negative bacteria)
Segmental darkening	Neurologic disease/infection (*Mycobacterium*, betanodavirus)
Edema/lepidorthosis	Hypoalbuminemia, renal disease, severe skin disease
Red vent	Red vent – internal disease (bacterial, viral, parasites)
Black spots/nodules	Melanocyte hyperplasia, melanoma, encysted trematodes, microsporidian infection, pigmented fungal granulomas
Gills:	
Hemorrhage/ulcers	Bacterial septicemia, *Flavobacterium*, viral infection (red sea bream iridovirus, koi herpesvirus, channel catfish virus), toxins, diatoms, protozoan parasites
Hyperplasia	Water quality issues, dietary imbalance (vitamin B5), chronic inflammation, parasitism (myxozoans, amoeba, flagellates, ciliates)
Necrosis	High/low pH, chlorine, *Flavobacterium*, *Branchiomycosis*, *Streptococcus*, koi herpesvirus, protozoan parasites
Nodules	Encysted trematodes, myxozoan cysts, neoplasia, bacteria (*Nocardia*, *Mycobacterium*), amoebic gill disease, *Dermocystidium*, microsporidians, *Ichthyophthirius*
Pallor	Anemia, viral infection (spring viremia of carp), mild hyperplasia
Gas bubbles	Supersaturation of water by gas
Increased mucus	Water quality issues, bacterial infection, parasites
Parasites	*Monogenea*, ciliates, flagellates, copepods, branchiurans
Yellow/white lesions	*Flavobacterium* infection, necrosis, *Saprolegnia*
Pseudobranch:	
Necrosis	*Flavobacterium*, toxins (herbicides, metals, pesticides)
Swelling	*Xcellia* (X cell disease)
Calcification	Vitamin E deficiency
Mouth:	
Gasping/asphyxia	See general comment above, screamer disease (mouth locked open)
Hemorrhage/ulcers	Bacterial septicemia (*Yersinia*, *Flavobacterium*), trauma
Increased mucus/ exudate	Bacterial infection (*Flavobacterium*), parasitism
Gas bubbles	Gas supersaturation
Malocclusion	Inappropriate food sources, trauma
Nodules	Granulomas, papilloma, dental neoplasia, parasitic cyst, thyroid hyperplasia, thyroid neoplasia, thymic neoplasia

Clinical signs	Etiology
Eye:	
Exophthalmia	Bacterial septicemia, multiple viral infections (grass carp reovirus, channel catfish virus, golden shiner virus), *Mycobacteria*, vitamin A/E/pantothenic acid deficiency, nephrocalcinosis, gas bubble disease/supersaturation
Ulcers	Fungus, bacterial septicemia, trauma, blindness
Corneal edema/ cloudiness	Poor water quality, conspecific aggression, bacterial, viral, fungal, parasitic disease
Ophthalmitis	Trauma, hematogenous spread of pathogens, thermal damage, zinc deficiency, *Diplostomum*
Cataract	*Diplostomum*, deficiencies (zinc, vitamin A, thiamine, riboflavin, methionine, tryptophan, histidine), rapid osmolar fluctuations, ultraviolet exposure, temperature fluctuations, gas bubble disease
Gas bubbles	Supersaturation, bacterial infection, corneal perforation
Lens luxation	Trauma
Enucleation	Trauma (predator, stocking density too high, jellyfish), severe ophthalmitis (*Streptococcus*, *Aeromonas*)
Muscle:	
Atrophy	Emaciation, denervation, riboflavin deficiency
Liquefaction/ necrosis	Microsporidians, myxozoans, bacterial infection (Gram-negative and anaerobe bacteria)
Nodules/swelling	Encysted trematodes, microsporidians, myxozoans, granulomas, emphysematous bacterial infection, *Ichthyophonus hoferi*, neoplasia
Hemorrhage	Trauma, vascular disease, myonecrosis, viral hemorrhagic septicemia, grass carp reovirus, bacterial sepsis
White foci	Magnesium deficiency, other dietary imbalances, necrosis (winter disease of Mediterranean fishes)
Skeletal deformity	Vitamin A/C/E deficiency, *Myxobolus*, *Mycobacterium*, abnormal egg incubation temperatures, trauma, hereditary, adverse environment conditions, toxicant exposure
Abdomen/coelom:	
Enlarged (general)	Neoplasia, overweight, egg binding/dystocia, gastrointestinal impaction, peritonitis, cardiovascular/hepatic disease leading to ascites, renal disease, other causes of hypoproteinemia, gastrointestinal impaction, parasites
Ascites	Bacterial septicemia (*Aeromonas*, *Vibrio*, *Edwardsiella*, *Streptococcus*, *Lactococcus*, *Pseudomonas*), viral infection (channel catfish virus, viral hemorrhagic septicemia, spring viremia of carp)
Peritonitis, nodular/ granulomatous	Mycobacteriosis, streptococcosis, *Francisella*, parasites, (including encysted cestodes), virus, fungus, egg binding, vaccination, steatitis (sequela to pancreatitis, antioxidant deficiency), neoplasia
Petechiae	Bacterial septicemia (*Aeromonas*, *Vibrio*, *Edwardsiella*), viral infection (spring viremia of carp)
Cysts	Polycystic renal disease, blocker ureter
Gas	Swimbladder or gut rupture, body wall perforation, inflammation with gas-producing microbes or fungi

(*Continued*)

Clinical signs	Etiology
Kidney:	
Diffuse swelling	Virus, bacterial septicemia, immune stimulation, neoplasia
Cystic change	*Hoferellus carassii*, polycystic kidney disease (genetic/environmental), chronic renal disease
Necrosis/ hemorrhage	Virus, bacterial sepsis, parasite/protozoa (*Spironucleus*), riboflavin deficiency, heavy metals
Granulomas/nodules	Granulomas: bacterial (*Mycobacterium*, *Nocardia*, *Edwardsiella*, *Francisella*), fungi, Ichthyophonus hoferi, nephrocalcinosis, neoplasia, trematode (*Acolpenteron* in bass)
White ureters	Nephrocalcinosis
Urinary bladder stones	Salinity/cation imbalances, renal/gill disease, genetic
Spleen:	
Diffuse swelling	Bacterial septicemia, viral infections (red sea bream iridovirus, grass carp reovirus)
Nodules	Granulomas (bacterial, fungal, parasitic, *Ichthyophonus*, neoplasia, *Dermocystidium*, hematoma
Liver:	
Necrosis	Virus, bacterial sepsis, heavy metals, algal toxin, rancid food, carbohydrates fed to carnivores
Hemorrhage	Virus, bacterial sepsis
Tan/yellow liver	Fat accumulation – excessive nutrition, toxicosis, choline deficiency, inadequate antioxidants, vitamin E deficiency, winter disease of Mediterranean fishes; fibrosis/iron accumulation; necrosis (see above)
Nodules	Bacteria (*Mycobacterium*, *Nocardia*, *Francisella*, *Pseudomonas*, *Edwardsiella*, among others), myxozoan infection, encysted parasites (*Anisakis*), fungi, *Ichthyophonus hoferi*, *Dermocystidium*, neoplasia, mineral (biliary lithiasis)
Cysts	Polycystic liver, cestode larvae
Jaundice	Hemolysis, toxins, genetic abnormalities, *Staphylococcus aureus*, rancid feeds
White liver	Necrosis with inflammation (carbohydrate consumption in carnivorous fish)
Stomach:	
Nodules	Granulomas (fungi, mycobacteria), microsporidians, myxozoans, nematodes
Dilation	Ileus, foreign bodies
Intestines:	
Hyperemia/ hemorrhage	Bacterial septicemia (*Aeromonas*, *Vibrio*, *Edwardsiella*), viral infections (grass carp reovirus), cestodes, acanthocephalans
Mucoid feces/casts	Parasites, hypothermia, dietary, winter disease of Mediterranean fishes, spring viremia of carp
Nodules	Foreign bodies, granulomas, myxozoan cysts, neoplasia, encysted worms
Swimbladder	
Enlarged	Hyperinflation: gas supersaturation, torsion, physostome blockage, betanodavirus, acid/base imbalance; fluid: exudate (bacteria), protozoa (*Sphaerospora*), viral hemorrhagic septicemia; fungi, microsporidians, myxozoans; thickened wall – nematodes, chronic inflammation
Atrophy	Rupture
Hemorrhage	Virus (iridovirus), bacteria

Clinical signs	Etiology
Reproductive enlarged nodules	*Mycobacterium*, *Ichthyophonus*, egg binding, microsporidians, myxozoans, neoplasia
Heart:	
Pallor	Amyloid
Inflammation/ pericarditis	Bacterial sepsis (*Vagococcus*)
Hemopericardium	Heart rupture, virus
Nodules	Granulomas (bacteria, fungus, *Ichthyophonus hoferi*), metacercariae, ventricular aneurysms

Appendix 2.3

Etiology and clinical signs: elasmobranchs

Clinical signs	Etiology
Sudden death	Bacterial septicemia (*Vibrio*), water quality issues (ammonia, oxygen, hydrogen sulfide), toxicosis (heavy metal-copper, herbicide, pesticide), parasites, trauma, electrocution, gas supersaturation, handling stress
Poor growth	Nutritional deficiency, stress/water quality issues, insufficient caloric intake, heavy parasitism (*Eimeria southwelli*)
Uncoordinated swimming/ nervousness/buoyancy	generalized infectious disease (virus, bacteria – *Vibrio*, *Flavobacterium*), fungal infection, electrocution, spinal trauma, toxicosis, central nervous system disease, water quality issues, gas bubble disease, algal blooms, parasitism (skin/gill, central nervous system, viscera), otitis/ endolymphatic duct inflammation
Gasping/asphyxia:	Low dissolved oxygen, high water temperature, high carbon dioxide, toxin exposure/ammonia, organic/inorganic contaminants, suspended sediments, physical impediment/obstruction to gas exchange
Gill disease	Epitheliocystis, *Monogene* parasites
Anemia	Viral erythrocytic necrosis, iridovirus, parasites, heavy metals
Skin/fins:	
Petechiae	Virus, bacterial septicemia, algae, low pH
Increased mucus	Water quality issues, parasitism
Hemorrhage, necrosis, ulcers	trauma, improper pH, bacterial infection (Vibrio), algae, virus infection (adenovirus, herpesvirus), fungus infection (*Aspergillus*, *Fusarium*, *Exophiala*, *Saprolegnia*), monogenes, scuticociliates, copepods, gas bubble disease, tumoral calcinosis, fenbendazole, irritant exposure to (ventrum)
Parasites	Monogenes, scuticociliates, Dinoflagellates (Amyloodinium), leeches, nematodes, arthropods (fish lice, copepods, isopods, barnacles)
Yellow/white flat lesions	necrosis, gas bubble disease, herpesvirus, Fusarium

(*Continued*)

Clinical signs	Etiology
Serpigenous tattoo	Huffmanela nematodes
Nodules/lumps	Papillomas, granulomatous disease (bacteria, fungi), parasites (copepods, monogenes), tumoral calcinosis, viral hyperplasia (herpesvirus), foreign body
Prominent lymphatics	*Eimeria southwelli*
Black spots/nodules	Melanocyte hyperplasia, melanoma, pigmented fungal granulomas
Gills:	
Hemorrhage/ulcers	Bacterial infection (*Vibrio*), parasites (monogenes), toxins
Hyperplasia	Qater quality issues, chronic inflammation, parasitism (*Monogenes*)
Necrosis	High/low pH, chlorine, toxins
Nodules	Encysted trematodes, cysts, neoplasia, bacteria, epitheliocystis
Pallor	Anemia, viral infection (viral erythrocytic necrosis), mild hyperplasia
Gas bubbles	Supersaturation of water by gas
Increased mucus	Water quality issues, bacterial infection, parasites
Parasites	*Monogenea*, copepods
Yellow/white lesions	*Flavobacterium* infection, necrosis, *Saprolegnia*
Mouth:	
Hemorrhage/ulcers	Bacterial septicemia, trauma
Increased mucus/exudate	Bacterial infection, parasitism
Gas bubbles	Gas supersaturation
Nodules	Granulomas, gingival hyperplasia, dental neoplasia, goiter, parasitic cyst, thyroid hyperplasia, thyroid neoplasia, thymic neoplasia, tumoral calcinosis
Parasites	Copepods, leeches
Everted stomach	Complication of gastric eversion reflex
Eye:	
Exophthalmia	Bacterial septicemia, multiple viral infections, gas bubble disease/ supersaturation
Ulcers/hemorrhage	Fungus, bacterial septicemia, viral infection, trauma, blindness
Corneal edema/ cloudiness	Poor water quality, conspecific aggression, bacterial, viral, fungal, parasitic disease
Ophthalmitis	Trauma, hematogenous spread of pathogens, thermal damage
Cataract	Rapid osmolar fluctuations, gas bubble disease
Gas bubbles	Supersaturation, bacterial infection, corneal perforation
Lens luxation	Trauma
Enucleation	Trauma (predator, stocking density too high), severe ophthalmitis
Nodules	Granulomas (bacteria, fungi, parasite), tumoral calcinosis
Muscle:	
Atrophy	Emaciation, denervation
Liquefaction/necrosis	Bacterial infection, barnacles
Nodules/swelling	Encysted trematodes, microsporidians, granulomas, neoplasia
Hemorrhage	Exertional rhabdomyolysis

Clinical signs	Etiology
White foci	Necrosis
Skeletal deformity	Trauma, hereditary, deficiency (zinc, potassium, vitamins C and E, inadequate space to swim), adverse environment conditions, toxicant exposure
Abdomen/coelom	
Enlarged (general)	Neoplasia, overweight, egg binding/dystocia/mucometra, gastrointestinal impaction, peritonitis, cardiovascular/hepatic disease leading to ascites, renal disease, other causes of hypoproteinemia, parasites
Ascites	Bacterial septicemia, coccidians (*Eimeria southwelli*)
Peritonitis, nodular/ granulomatous	Bacteria, parasites (coccidians, encysted cestodes, scuticociliate), virus, fungus, neoplasia
Petechiae	Bacterial septicemia
Gas	Gut rupture, body wall perforation, inflammation with gas-producing microbes or fungi
Kidney:	
Diffuse swelling	Virus, bacterial septicemia, immune stimulation, neoplasia
Necrosis/hemorrhage	Virus, bacterial sepsis (*Vibrio*), parasite/protozoa, riboflavin deficiency, heavy metals
Granulomas/nodules	Granulomas: bacterial, fungi, neoplasia, tumoral calcinosis
Spleen:	
Diffuse swelling	Bacterial septicemia (*Vibrio*), viral infections
Nodules	Granulomas (bacterial, fungal, parasitic), neoplasia, hematoma
Liver:	
Necrosis	Bacterial sepsis (*Carnobacterium*, *Vibrio*), fungal infection, heavy metals, algal toxin, scuticociliate infection, rancid food
Hemorrhage	Viral infections, fungal infection, scuticociliate infection
Tan/yellow liver (sharks normally contain abundant lipid in their livers)	Fat accumulation – excessive nutrition, toxicosis, linolenic/linoleic acid deficiency, inadequate antioxidants, vitamin E deficiency; fibrosis/iron accumulation; necrosis (see above)
Nodules	Bacteria, myxozoan infection (biliary), encysted parasites, fungi, neoplasia
Stomach:	
Nodules	Granulomas (fungi, bacteria, parasites), neoplasia
Dilation	Ileus, foreign bodies
Intestines:	
Hyperemia/hemorrhage	Bacterial septicemia (*Vibrio*)
Necrosis	Bacteria, parasites (coccidians), fenbendazole
Everted spiral valve	Complication of eversion reflex
Nodules	Granulomas (fungi, bacteria, parasites), tumoral calcinosis
Reproductive:	
Nodules	Egg binding, tumoral calcinosis, neoplasia, egg case impaction, cystic ovaries
Mucus/exudate	Parasites (coccidians, ciliates), mucometra, pyometra

(*Continued*)

Clinical signs	Etiology
Enlarged ovary/uterus	cysts, mucometra, pregnancy
Fetal Demise	*Fusarium*
Brain (meningitis)	*Vibrio*, *Carnobacterium*
Heart:	
Pallor	Necrosis, exertional rhabdomyolysis, fibrosis
Inflammation/pericarditis	Bacterial sepsis
Hemopericardium	Heart rupture
Nodules	Granulomas (bacteria, fungus), tumoral calcinosis
Parasites	Isopods, nematodes

3

Amphibians

María J. Forzán

The etiology of amphibian diseases is presented in Appendix 3.1 at the end of this chapter.

Ranavirosis

Overview

Ranavirosis can affect all cold-blooded vertebrates: amphibians, reptiles, and fish. Although no amphibian extinctions have been linked to ranavirosis, outbreaks in the wild and in captive collections can result in mortality rates of up to 100% of individuals, particularly at the tadpole stage. Ranaviruses are one of three pathogens reportable to the World Animal Health Organisation (WOAH).

Etiology

Viruses are in the *Ranavirus* genus, part of the Iridoviridae family. The most commonly reported amphibian outbreaks are the frog virus 3 (Figure 3.1), *Ambystoma tigrinum* virus, common midwife toad virus and Bohle iridovirus (BIV).

Host Range and Transmission

Among amphibians, ranavirosis causes severe disease and mortality in anurans (frogs and toads) and *Caudata* (salamanders and newts); little to nothing is known about infection in caecilians. In North America, ranavirosis is particularly fatal to tadpoles, whereas in the United Kingdom, deaths are often reported in adults. Transmission is achieved through consumption of infected material (particularly important in tadpoles, given their cannibalistic habits) and direct contact with infected individuals, particularly if it involves abraded skin. The possibility of transmission through vectors (mosquitoes) has been hypothesized but remains unconfirmed.

Signs and Diagnosis

Lethargy, regurgitation, increased shedding with decreased consumption of shed skin, petechiae to frank hemorrhage in the oral cavity, ventral skin, particularly in the digits and legs, eventually leading to severe depression, loss of withdrawal or righting reflexes, and death. Severely ill amphibians will likely

Pathology and Epidemiology of Aquatic Animal Diseases for Practitioners, First Edition.
Edited by Laura Urdes, Chris Walster, and Julius Tepper.

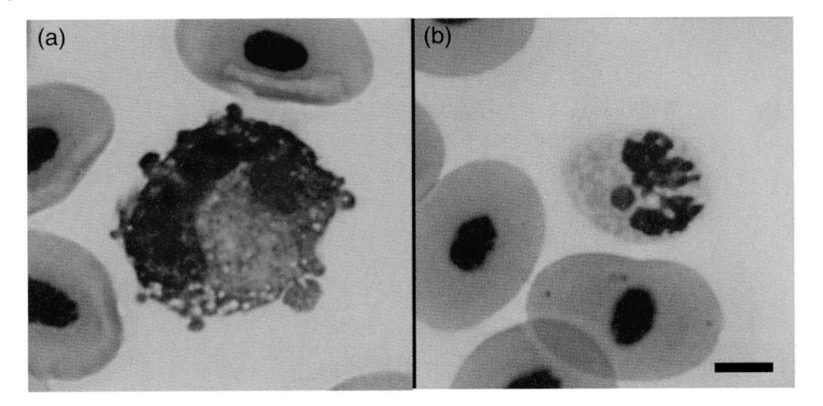

Figure 3.1 Frog virus 3 (*Ranavirus* sp.) intracytoplasmic inclusions in a monocyte (a) and neutrophil (b) from an infected wood frog, *Rana sylvatica*. Scale bar = 10 microns.

display lymphopenia and intracytoplasmic viral inclusion bodies in the various leukocytes. At necropsy, external lesions are striking hemorrhage and bruising in the skin, sometimes with frank blood in the oral cavity; internally, there are hemorrhages in the wall of the gastrointestinal tract, liver, spleen, kidney, and fat bodies, the spleen is often enlarged (splenomegaly) and the stomach filled with air.

Diagnosis relies on histologic lesions consistent with ranavirosis (widespread epithelial, hematopoietic and endothelial necrosis, and hemorrhage, often with intracytoplasmic inclusion bodies in affected tissues), identification of the virus via polymerase chain reaction (PCR) performed on postmortem tissues or, in severely ill individuals, antemortem samples including skin sheds and fecal swabs; skin swabs or other samples from clinically healthy individuals are unlikely to yield positive results even in infected individuals.

Differential Diagnosis

Severe skin hemorrhages and some internal lesions may be also present in bacterial dermatosepticemia, gas bubble disease, and other causes of systemic intravascular coagulation. See also the differential diagnoses for sudden death, buoyancy problems, skin erythema/petechia, skin hemorrhage and necrosis, skin edema, gill erythema/hemorrhage and necrosis, oral cavity hemorrhage, spleen enlargement, liver necrosis, kidney edema and pallor, stomach and intestinal hemorrhage.

Prevention, Treatment, and Control

Antemortem detection of infection is mostly unreliable, so investigation of mortalities, including full postmortem examination and PCR testing, is crucial in preventing and controlling ranavirosis in wild or captive populations through movement restriction and/or quarantine. No treatment for ranavirosis exists.

Bacterial Dermatosepticemia (Red Leg Syndrome)

Overview

Until the latter half of the 20th century "red leg syndrome" was considered a disease in its own right, caused by Gram-negative bacteria. Currently, we know that it is most commonly caused by secondary bacterial sepsis that either develops opportunistically in poor habitat conditions (such as overcrowding, poor water quality, malnutrition), or is secondary to other infections (e.g. chytridiomycosis and ranavirosis) or neoplastic diseases.

Etiology

Gram-negative bacteria are normally found in the aquatic or riparian habitats, particularly *Aeromonas hydrophila*, *Enterobacter* and *Citrobacter* species.

Host Range and Transmission

All amphibian species are susceptible; in early tadpole stages, before the legs are developed, lesions manifest in the ventral skin, mouth parts and tail. As secondary invaders, Gram-negative bacteria may be acquired from the environment or, in overcrowded captive environments, from direct contact with affected individuals.

Signs and Diagnosis

Erythema of the legs and ventral skin of other body parts may progress to frank hemorrhage, skin necrosis, and subcutaneous or generalized edema. Bacterial culture of liver, spleen, or kidney can be used to determine the species of bacterium involved in the secondary sepsis, but emphasis must be placed on determining the underlying disease process. Cultures of skin or gastrointestinal tract are not indicated as the bacteria often associated with red leg syndrome are common inhabitants of both tissues.

Differential Diagnosis

Differential diagnosis is focused on the underlying problem, particularly on determining whether chytridiomycosis or ranavirosis are involved. See also the differential diagnoses for sudden death, skin erythema/petechia, skin hemorrhage and necrosis, skin edema, coelom ascites, liver necrosis, kidney edema and pallor, stomach and intestinal hemorrhage.

Prevention, Treatment, and Control

Good husbandry practices will avoid opportunistic bacterial invasions, while preventive measures for diseases such as chytridiomycosis or ranavirosis will also prevent development of secondary bacterial sepsis. Treatment of the bacterial infection (usually parenteral broad-spectrum antibiotics) will need to be performed in parallel with the measures to treat the underlying cause (for specific recommendations on treatment of sepsis in amphibians, see Wright and Whitaker, 2001, pages 314–315).

Ammonia Toxicity

Overview

Ammonia concentrations in water tanks above tolerable levels are toxic to the aquatic stages of captive amphibians, sometimes causing sudden death to entire collections.

Etiology

Ammonia is excreted in the urine of larval amphibians (tadpoles) and adult aquatic species as the end result of protein metabolism. Toxic ammonia concentrations are caused by poor water quality from lack of filtration, either mechanical (filters) or organic (plants and bacteria).

Host Range

Ammonia toxicity is mostly a problem in tadpoles, and possibly problematic to adults of species with entirely aquatic life cycles (e.g. newts).

Signs and Diagnosis

Sudden death of large numbers of individuals within a tank, buoyancy problems (tadpoles swimming upside down), occasionally with ascites and/or ventral skin erythema will be seen. Diagnosis is based on measurements of water ammonia above acceptable levels (most commercially available aquaria water quality kits are useful).

Differential Diagnosis

Differential diagnoses include other water quality problems, such as inappropriate temperature, or pH. Mortalities are sudden (hyperacute) and involve numerous individuals. See also differential diagnoses for sudden death.

Prevention, Treatment, and Control

Establish an organic ammonia balance prior to introduction of tadpoles in the tank (plants and bacteria) or use a mechanical water filtration system. No effective treatment exists for tadpoles. Once ammonia reaches lethal levels, even rapid water changes are unlikely to avoid the death of all individuals in the tank. Less severely affected adults may benefit from supportive treatment, mainly the provision of fresh, well-oxygenated water, but prognosis in all cases is poor. Control is based on prevention – monitoring water parameters and providing mechanical or biological filtration systems to ensure that ammonia levels are kept within acceptable limits.

Gas Bubble Disease

Overview and Etiology

Gas bubble disease is caused by supersaturation of gases in the water environment, mostly nitrogen. Municipal (tap) water rich in air bubbles is used directly in water tanks, often accompanied by a sudden drop in water temperature followed by a quick increase, which results in gas supersaturation. Similar to the 'bends' in divers, lesions and death are due to tissue damage secondary to gas emboli formation.

Host Range

Gas bubble disease is most common in African clawed frog adults (*Xenopus laevis*) (Figure 3.2), but potentially affects any aquatic amphibian species, adults or tadpoles.

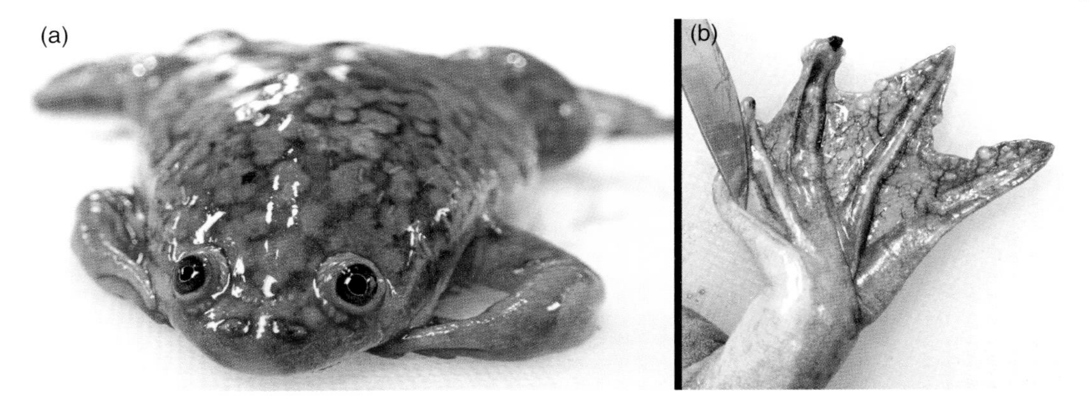

Figure 3.2 Gas bubble disease in a female adult African clawed frog, *Xenopus laevis*. Note the multifocal dermal hemorrhages (a) and characteristic bubbling of the skin in the interdigital webbing (b).
Source: Diagnostic case provided by Dr. Erica Feldman, Cornell University.

Signs and Diagnosis

Signs include severe erythema and bruising (intradermal hemorrhage) of the ventral skin, ascites, buoyancy problems (frogs or tadpoles find it difficult to submerge, often swimming upside down); if frogs survive for a few days, they may develop dermatosepticemia or other chronic poorly defined illnesses that result in their death or euthanasia.

Diagnosis is based on characteristic bubbling of the skin, easily visible in the digits and interdigital web, together with gas saturation measurements or a history of sudden water temperature change (hours/days), together with the appearance of clinical signs.

Differential Diagnosis

Dermatosepticemia can be a differential diagnosis in some cases, but bubbles in the skin are practically pathognomonic. See also the differential diagnoses for sudden death, buoyancy problems, skin hemorrhage and necrosis, and coelom gas.

Prevention, Treatment, and Control

Prevention consists of air stones in tank water and temperature control. No practical treatment exists, so control is based on prevention by maintaining gas saturation under acceptable limits.

Frog Chytridiomycosis

Overview

Chytridiomycosis due to *Batrachochytrium dendrobatidis* has caused extinctions and severe population declines of amphibians worldwide. It affects primarily frogs and toads (anurans). Deaths are most common in recently metamorphosed individuals (froglets), and in some very susceptible species, adults. Once the disease appears in a collection or in a wild habitat, it is difficult or impossible to eradicate as the etiologic agent can survive outside the host (facultative fungus).

Etiology

Batrachochytrium dendrobatidis is a chytrid fungus, and until recently was the only pathogenic species in its order. The fungus reproduces through motile zoospores produced inside a characteristic flask-shaped sporangium. When infecting an amphibian, the fungus restricts its growth to the epidermis, never invading any deeper tissues or internal organs. Infections usually result in hyperkeratosis (thickening of the corneal layer of the epidermis).

Host Range and Transmission

Most frogs and toads are susceptible, although pathogenicity varies greatly among species. For instance, African clawed frogs (*Xenopus laevis*) usually act as carriers, suffering no ill effects from infection, while chytridiomycosis is often fatal to species like the yellow-legged frog of the Sierra Nevada, United States (*Rana muscosa* and *Rana sierrae*), and to many species of Central American and Australian frogs. Transmission occurs through direct contact with infected substrate (water or organic matter), infected individuals, or through fomites.

Signs and Diagnosis

Erythema of skin in ventral patch, legs, and palmar/plantar surfaces, followed by increased shedding are seen. During the agonal stage, muscular tremors are sometimes observed. Diagnosis is achieved through PCR testing of skin swabs (live amphibians) or histologic detection (biopsy or necropsy examination) of characteristic lesions with fungal structures aided by PCR or specific in-situ hybridization to confirm fungal species.

Differential Diagnosis

Differential diagnoses include bacterial dermatosepticemia and other systemic diseases, such as ranavirosis. See also the differential diagnoses for sudden death, neurologic signs, skin erythema/petechia.

Prevention, Treatment, and Control

Quarantine of new animals and testing prior to translocations in the wild are crucial in preventing the introduction of *Batrachochytrium dendrobatidis* into a collection or wild habitat. Treatment is effective for captive collections, but is impractical in wild populations. Itraconazole baths are most commonly used, but alternatives such as topical (sprayed) voriconazole or increase environmental temperature can also be used. Disinfection of the habitat and removal of all organic matter is necessary to prevent treated animals from becoming reinfected after treatment.

Salamander Chytridiomycosis

Overview

A significant threat to wild and captive salamanders and newts (caudata), *Batrachochytrium salamandrivorans* was discovered less than a decade ago as the cause of massive mortalities in a wild population of fire salamanders (*Salamandra salamandra*) in the Netherlands. Since then, the disease has been found in wild populations in Germany, Belgium, and Spain, and in captive collections in several European countries. Mortalities occur in recent metamorphs (efts) as well as in adults. As of the time of writing, *B. salamandrivorans* has not been detected in wild amphibians outside its native South-East Asia and invasive range in continental Europe, but concerns exist regarding is possible introduction into North America, a hotspot of salamander biodiversity.

Etiology

B. salamandrivorans, like the better known *B. dendrobatidis*, is a chytrid fungus, and as such reproduces through motile zoospores that are produced in sporangia. Also like *B. dendrobatidis*, *B. salamandrivorans* is restricted to the epidermal layers of the skin, but it is more likely to cause ulceration than hyperkeratosis (thickening of the corneal layer).

Host Range and Transmission

Fire salamanders (*S. salamandra*) were the index case and have suffered significant population declines in the areas where *B. salamandrivorans* was first discovered and described. Most salamanders and newts are susceptible to infection, but development of disease varies depending on the family or species. Asian salamanders are thought to act as carriers, being infected without clinical signs, and yet are capable of transmitting the disease to naïve individuals, particularly European and North American salamanders and newts. Frogs and toads may become infected, but are usually subclinical, developing no ill effects from infection. Transmission occurs through direct contact with infected substrate (water or organic matter), infected individuals, or through fomites.

Signs and Diagnosis

Ulcers, sometimes described as "crater-like," are randomly scattered on the skin of lethargic salamanders and newts; sometimes dark pigmentation of irregular areas of the skin occur. Diagnosis is achieved through PCR testing of skin swabs (live amphibians) or histologic detection (biopsy or necropsy examination) of characteristic lesions with fungal structures aided by PCR or specific in-situ hybridization to confirm fungal species.

Differential Diagnosis

Differential diagnoses include environmental or traumatic lesions to skin, other bacterial and fungal dermatitis. See also the differential diagnoses for sudden death, skin hemorrhage, and necrosis.

Prevention, Treatment, and Control

Quarantine of new animals and testing prior to translocations in the wild are crucial in preventing the introduction of *B. salamandrivorans* into a collection or wild habitat. Treatment is possible in captive collections, but impractical in wild populations. Treatment requires a mixture of polymyxin E (bath) and voriconazole (topical spray), ideally at ambient temperature around 20 degrees C. Disinfection of the habitat and removal of all organic matter is necessary to prevent treated animals from becoming reinfected after treatment.

Renal Calculi (Oxalate Toxicity or Nephrocalcinosis)

Overview

Oxalate calculi in renal tubules is associated with disease or death in captive amphibians. Feeding of oxalate-rich vegetables during the tadpole stage has been linked to acute mortality in froglets. Similarly, providing insect prey that have fed on oxalate-rich vegetation to adults has been suggested to cause disease in adult frogs.

Etiology

Oxalate calculi accumulate in the lumen of renal tubules and causes tubular necrosis.

Host Range

Reported mostly in ranid (true) frogs, mortalities are not noted during the tadpole stage when the oxalate-rich vegetables are consumed. Instead, acute mortalities are observed in froglets, approximately two weeks after completing metamorphosis.

Signs and Diagnosis

Acute death of froglets, sometimes together with ascites, lethargy, and loss of righting reflex are seen. A history of oxalate-rich feeding during the tadpole stage, deaths at two weeks past metamorphosis, and histopathology of kidneys revealing characteristic birefringent crystals in the lumen of renal tubules with varying degrees of epithelial necrosis confirm the diagnosis.

Differential Diagnosis

Other husbandry problems (poor temperature control, improper feeding, etc.), and infectious diseases such as chytridiomycosis are differential diagnoses. See also the differential diagnoses for sudden death.

Prevention, Treatment, and Control

Avoid feeding oxalate-rich vegetables, such as spinach or rhubarb leaves, to tadpoles. No treatment exists.

Mycobacteriosis

Overview

Rarely encountered in the wild, mycobacteriosis is a significant problem in captive amphibians, whether aquatic or terrestrial (Figure 3.3). A zoonotic disease, mycobacteriosis can be transmitted to humans through abraded skin, usually causing local nodular lesions (granulomas) in hands and feet, and known sometimes as “fish tank” or “swimming pool” granulomas. Subclinical infection may smolder for months or years, controlled by a competent immune response. Disease may develop after a stressor weakens the immune system, and cause mortality within a few weeks.

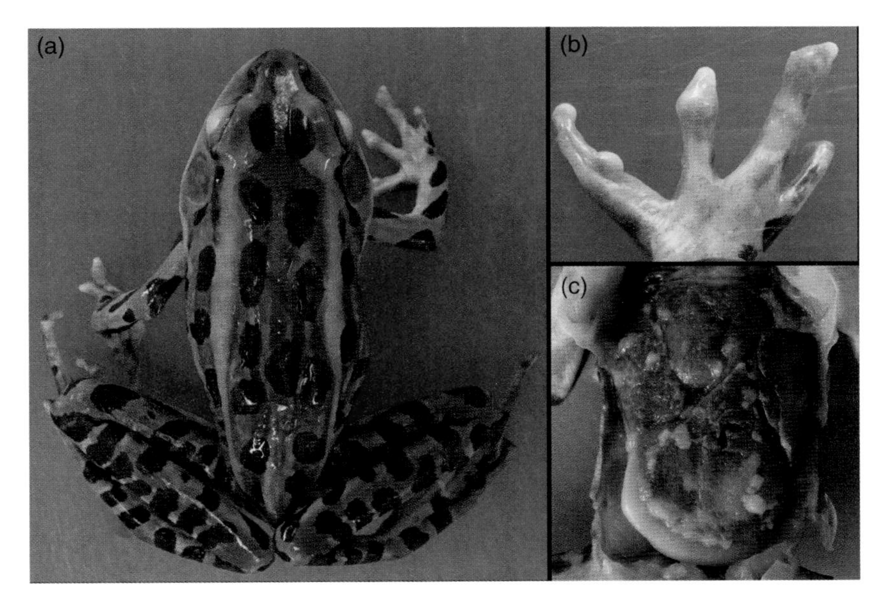

Figure 3.3 Mycobacteriosis and emaciation in a male adult northern leopard frog (*Rana pipiens*). Note the thinness of the legs (a), and muscle atrophy nodules in the digits (a and b); caseous exudate covers the visceral surfaces of the heart and liver (c).

Etiology

Most commonly caused by *Mycobacterium marinum*, and less commonly by *Mycobacterium chelonae*, *Mycobacterium xenopi*, and other species. *M. marinum* is a saprophytic bacterium, normally inhabiting water environments in the wild or captivity. At least one report documented infection of a captive frog (American bullfrog, *Rana catesbeiana*) with *Mycobacterium bovis*, a species usually associated with mycobacteriosis in mammals, including humans.

Host Range and Transmission

All amphibians at every stage are susceptible, although aquatic stages and species are more frequently affected. Bacterial infections are acquired through ingestion or contact between contaminated water and abraded skin; transmission can also be achieved through contact between infected and naïve individuals, or via fomites (such as aquarium tools). The chronicity of the disease means that by the time clinical signs are noted or mortalities recorded, transmission to all individual housed together is almost inevitable.

Signs and Diagnosis

Prolonged weight loss and ill thrift before lesions become evident. Externally, firm nodules (granulomas) are found on the skin and joints, particularly of the digits. Internally, dull to pearl-white, firm nodules may be present in viscera and/or coelomic cavity; sometimes caseous exudate fills the coelom, thickening the pericardial sac and sometimes causing adhesions between viscera.

Diagnosis is based on identification of acid-fast bacteria in nodular lesions (granulomas) via impression smears, biopsies, or necropsy samples; amphibian mycobacteriosis is usually a paucibacillary infection, requiring perseverance in the search for acid-fast bacilli. Determination of the species involved requires either culture in specialized labs (zoonotic and slow-growing organisms) or PCR testing of tissues either frozen or fixed in 70% ethanol, or less ideally, 10% formalin.

Differential Diagnosis

Differentials incude other systemic granulomatous bacterial and fungal infections. In aquatic stages, particularly tadpoles, small nodules may be confused with infection with *Ichthyophonus* species; a rule of thumb to distinguish between the two is that 'Ich' nodules are evenly small, whereas mycobacterial granulomas are usually larger and will vary in size and shape. See also the differential diagnoses for emaciation, skin edema, skin nodule, skin rostral abrasions, coelom granulomas/caseous exudate, muscle nodules, skeletal deformities, spleen/liver/kidney nodules.

Prevention, Treatment, and Control

Treatment is not recommended, in part at least because of the zoonotic potential of the disease. Euthanasia of infected animals and disinfection of housing materials are needed to control mycobacteriosis in a captive population.

Pulmonary Nematodiasis

Overview

Rhabdiasis (pulmonary nematodiasis) is not uncommon in wild amphibians, who manage to maintain a host–pathogen balance that rarely results in disease. Captivity, however, presents the perfect opportunity for superinfection and, as parasitism increases beyond tolerable levels, clinical signs and mortality may ensue.

Etiology

Rhabdias species are nematodes with a facultative life cycle, capable of reproducing in the environment, independent of the amphibian host (free-living stage), as well as in the lungs or coelomic cavity of amphibians. Within the pulmonary lumen or coelomic cavity, infective larvae (L3) develop into hermaphroditic adults. Larvated eggs (L1) produced in the lungs are expelled into the trachea, swallowed, and released into the environment, to mature into sexually dimorphic adults or infect an amphibian host.

Host Range and Transmission

Adult stages of terrestrial anurans (frogs and toads) and *Caudata* (salamanders and newts) species are affected. Experimentally, recent metamorphs (froglets or efts) may become infected and develop severe disease from an overwhelming visceral larva migrans syndrome. Transmission occurs when L3 larvae, produced by either parasitic or free-living adults, penetrate intact skin.

Signs and Diagnosis

Signs are non-specific, usually progressive weakness, possible weight loss, and if infections are severe enough or secondary complications ensue, death. Antemortem diagnosis consists of fecal examination for larval nematodes (i.e. Baerman's technique). At necropsy, numerous hair-thin, pale nematodes, approximately 1 cm long, will be found in the lumen of the lungs and, sometimes, free in the coelomic cavity.

Differential Diagnosis

Differentials include progressive debilitating disease, such as mycobacteriosis, malnutrition, poor habitat conditions (improper temperature or humidity). See also differential diagnosis for emaciation, lung parasitism.

Prevention, Treatment, and Control

Prevention and control are only necessary for captive amphibians, or wild-caught amphibians who will spend some time in captivity. Identification of infected animals (via Baerman's examination of feces), followed by deworming and isolation of infected animals in enclosures lacking organic substrate (to eliminate the possibility of free-living larval development), will prevent and/or control infections in captive collections. Topical ivermectin, applied weekly until Baerman's fecal examination is clear of larvae, must be followed with placing of amphibians in parasite-free substrate.

Hypovitaminosis A (Short-Tongue Syndrome)

Overview

Although little is known about amphibian vitamin A metabolism, studies on amphibian subjects have demonstrated its importance in embryonic development, vision, and limb regeneration. Amphibians cannot produce vitamin A, and thus must acquire it through their diet. Unfortunately, it seems that minimal requirements of vitamin A vary greatly among species.

Etiology

Captive diets deficient in vitamin A, meaning diets consisting of insects fed on low vitamin A foods, can cause chronic disease in amphibians.

Host Range

Most frequently reported in anurans, adult frogs and toads.

Signs and Diagnosis

Difficulty in capturing prey results in lethargy, weight loss and, if untreated, death. Diagnosis is based on histopathological detection of lingual squamous metaplasia and may be supported by vitamin A level determination in affected animals compared with healthy species-specific controls.

Differential Diagnosis

Other infectious diseases or poor management responsible for lethargy; inappropriate prey offerings (resulting in difficulty in capturing them) may be seen. See also the differential diagnoses for emaciation, oral cavity short-tongue, esophageal mucosal thickening.

Prevention, Treatment, and Control

Flakes (tadpoles) or prey (adults) supplemented with vitamin A should be fed. "Dusting" of insects with vitamin powder supplements is common practice in feeding adult amphibians. Care should be taken to avoid too much vitamin A (hypervitaminosis), which may result in skin ulceration, excess shedding, liver fibrosis or, in tadpoles, developmental anomalies.

Corneal Lipidosis

Overview

Corneal lipidosis causes severe eye lesions and death from starvation in captive tree frogs.

Etiology

The etiology is high cholesterol and triglyceride levels in the blood, with subsequent deposition of cholesterol in corneal tissues. It is hypothesized to be associated with inadequate diet (insect prey fed on high fat food items, such as dog kibble) and lack of normal "basking" behavior.

Host Range

Tree frog adults are affected; the disease is reported mostly in White's tree frog (*Litoria caerulea*) and Cuban tree frogs (*Osteopilus septentrionalis*) (Figure 3.4).

Signs and Diagnosis

Signs are opacity or whitening of the cornea, worsening with time, and eventually forming a raised, pitted surface that impedes blinking. Corneal lesions impede prey capture and result in progressive weight loss and starvation. Lesions may begin in one eye, but eventually they will become bilateral. Ocular examination revealing corneal infiltration in a horizontal striate pattern, together with high cholesterol levels in serum or plasma (8 mmol/l or above).

Differential Diagnosis

Traumatic corneal ulceration may be suspected at the onset, but the gross appearance and progressive course of the disease are almost unmistakable. See also the differential diagnoses for emaciation and corneal opacity.

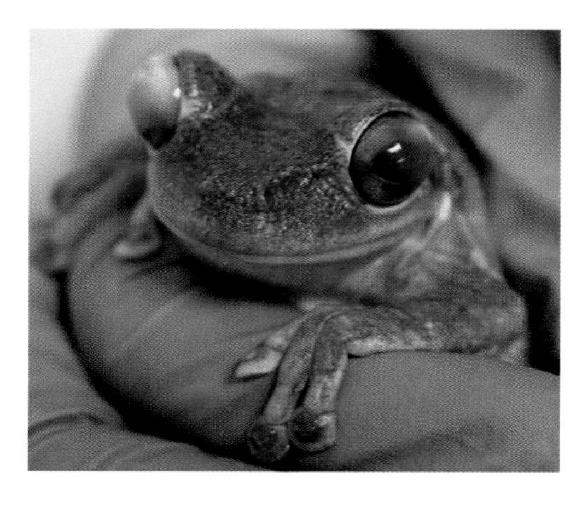

Figure 3.4 Cuban tree frog (*Osteopilus septentrionalis*) with corneal lipidosis in late (right eye) and early stages (left eye).

Prevention, Treatment, and Control

Reduce cholesterol in diet fed to insect prey, provide areas of high temperature (43 degrees C or above) to promote basking. Treatment is unrewarding, and based on published reports and experience, once lesions appear the disease progression is unrelenting.

Renal (Lucké's) Adenocarcinoma

Overview

Frogs developing transmissible tumors in the kidneys were described in the early 20th century by Lucké, which were subsequently proved to be caused by a virus.

Etiology

Renal adenocarcinoma is caused by ranid herpesvirus 1 (RHV1), of the genus *Batrachovirus*.

Host Range and Transmission

Northern leopard frogs (*Rana pipiens*) are the only amphibian species known to be naturally susceptible to developing renal adenocarcinoma from infection with RHV1. Metastasis is uncommon except when frogs are maintained in warm temperatures. Transmission from infected adults to eggs or larvae occurs in the spring, during breeding season; frogs exposed to the virus as adults are refractile to infection.

Signs and Diagnosis

Renal failure signs such as ascites or generalized edema are seen. Diagnosis is based on postmortem observation of large firm tan to red masses that may present in one or both kidneys, often obliterating the kidney almost entirely (Figure 3.5). Histopathology will reveal cords of epithelial neoplastic cells with little stroma and, if detected soon after overwintering (hibernation), with Cowdry type A intranuclear inclusion bodies.

Differential Diagnosis

Differential diagnoses include other causes of renal failure, and spontaneous (non-infectious) neoplasms. See also the differential diagnoses for emaciation, coelom neoplasia, and kidney neoplasia.

Prevention, Treatment, and Control

Prevalence in the wild varies greatly, both temporarily and geographically, but has not been associated with population declines, so that prevention and control are likely unnecessary in the wild. If animals are to be brought into captivity, it may be wise to avoid known areas with high prevalence, remove eggs soon after oviposition to raise tadpoles in a virus-free environment. No treatment exists.

Herpesvirus Skin Disease

Overview

After nearly a century of thinking that the only herpesvirus causing disease in amphibians was RHV1 associated with Lucké's renal adenocarcinoma, other strains have been found in wild anurans in Europe.

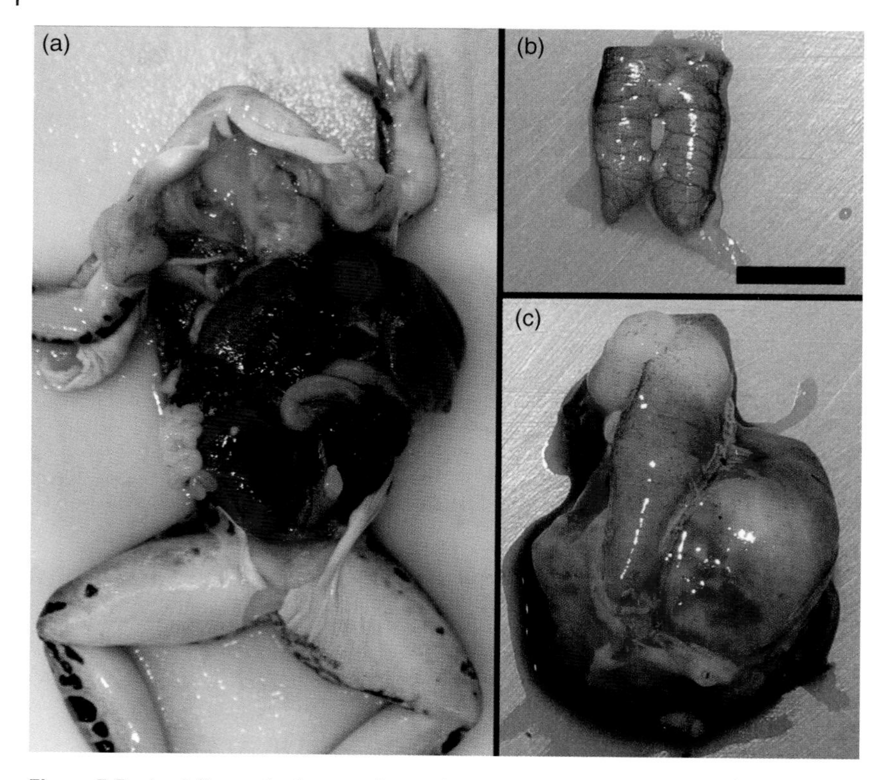

Figure 3.5 Lucké's renal adenocarcinoma in the kidney of a female adult northern leopard frog (*Rana pipiens*), displaces other viscera and ovary (a). Healthy kidneys of an age-matched frog (b) compared with large adenocarcinoma replacing most of the right kidney (c). Scale bar = 1 cm

Etiology

Causes are the ranid herpesvirus 3 (RHV3) and bufonid herpesvirus 1 (BfHV1), which are strains (or species) of the genus *Batrachovirus*.

Host Range and Transmission

RHV1 infects the common frog (*Rana temporaria*) while BfHV1 infects common toads (*Bufo bufo*). Mode of transmission is unknown.

Signs and Diagnosis

Firm raised nodules or plaques, usually paler than the surrounding skin, are present mostly on the dorsum and ventrum of the body, and only occasionally in the limbs. A consensus PCR test is used to detect various strains of amphibian herpesviruses.

Differential Diagnosis

Differential diagnosis is mycobacteriosis. See also the differential diagnoses for skin edema, and skin proliferative patches.

Prevention, Treatment, and Control

No recommendations specific to herpesviral skin disease are yet available. Quarantining of new amphibians in a collection and testing prior to transportation of amphibians between wild habitats are indicated for this and any other infectious diseases.

Hemoparasites

Overview

Hemoparasites (*Hepatozoon* and *Trypanosoma* spp.) are usually found only in wild amphibians or captive collections maintained at least partly outdoors, as infection depends on exposure to insect vectors. Hemoparasites are not generally thought to cause disease in amphibians, but it is important for the veterinary clinician to recognize them. As they are often prominent findings in blood smears, they run the risk of being blamed for an amphibian's poor health when they are, in the majority of cases, not associated with disease.

Etiology

Hemoparasites most commonly found in blood smear examination are protozoans of the genera *Hepatozoon* (apicomplexa) and *Trypanosoma* (flagellate) (Figure 3.6). Small merozoites and banana-shaped gamonts of *Hepatozoon* species are found within the cytoplasm of erythrocytes, where they replicate through binary fission. Trypanosoma species are large extracellular protozoans, round to comma-shaped, depending on the life stage present, deeply basophilic and identifiable from the presence of a distinct undulating membrane.

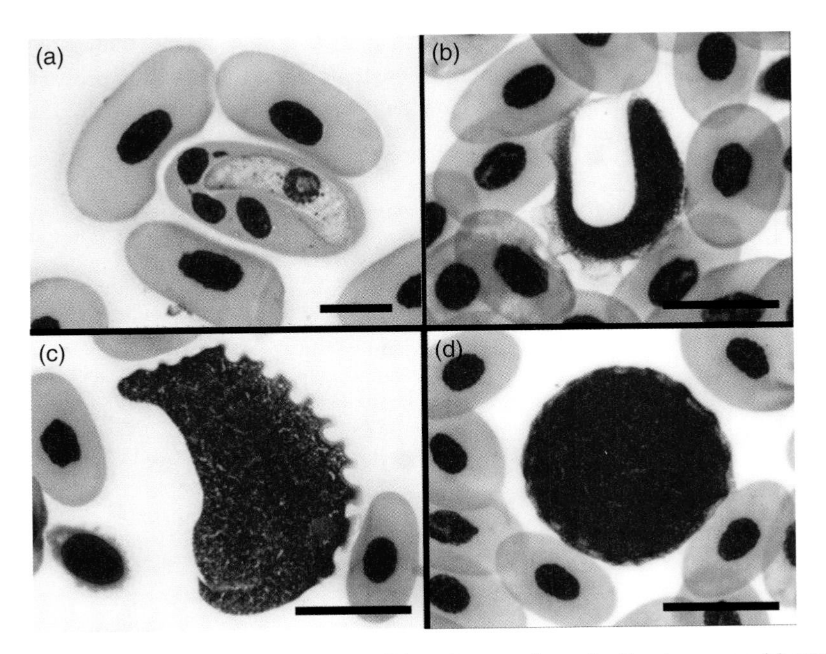

Figure 3.6 Hemoparasites of amphibians. Intraerythrocytic *Hepatozoon* sp. (a), and various stages of extracellular *Trypanosoma* sp. (b, c and d). Scale bars = 10 microns.

Host Range and Transmission

Hepatozoon and *Trypanosoma* are ubiquitous parasites, most often reported in ranid (true) frogs and tree frogs, and occasionally in some *Caudata* species, namely eastern hellbenders (*Cryptobranchus alleganiensis alleganiensis*). Transmission is accomplished through vectors: mosquitoes for *Hepatozoon* species, and both mosquitoes and leeches for *Trypanosoma* species.

Signs and Diagnosis

Increased immature erythrocyte counts have been reported in the Australian white-lipped tree frog (*Litoria infrafrenata*) infected with *Hepatozoon* and other hemogregarines, but no clinical signs were reported in this or any other amphibian species, even in individuals carrying a high infection load.

Differential Diagnosis

Differential diagnoses include other hemogregarines, artifacts, or contaminants during sample collection.

Prevention, Treatment, and Control

Isolating individuals from the vectors will prevent infection. No treatment is recommended, as infections usually run their course without causing disease.

Ascites/Lymphedema

Overview

More a clinical sign than a disease entity, ascites or generalized edema (anasarca) is often present in amphibians suffering from metabolic, infectious, or neoplastic disease (Figure 3.7). Tadpoles

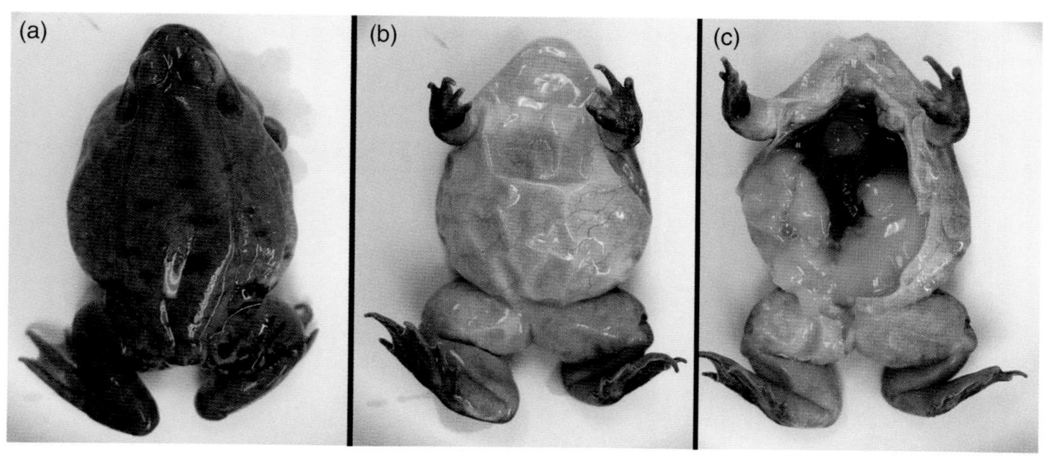

Figure 3.7 Green frog adult (*Rana clamitans*) with severe subcutaneous and coelomic edema (anasarca), due to renal failure (a, b). Material in the coelom is high in protein and has formed a white coagulum postmortem (c).

usually develop ascites, while more generalized edema is more frequently found in adults. As the skin of amphibians, particularly adult frogs, is attached to the underlying musculature by discontinuous thin fibrous tags, subcutaneous fluid accumulation is often spectacular.

Etiology

Electrolyte imbalance, endothelial damage, impaired lymphatic drainage, and deficient fluid excretion through urine are some possible underlying causes resulting in generalized edema.

Host Range

All life stages and species may develop generalized edema; high or low susceptibility depends on species susceptibility to the underlying cause.

Signs and Diagnosis

Expansion of the coelomic cavity due to fluid accumulation (ascites), accompanied in adults with fluid accumulation and expansion of subcutaneous spaces. Diagnosis should aim at determining the underlying cause. Begin with fluid examination to determine whether it is an exudate (leading toward a bacterial or systemic fungal etiology), a transudate, or a modified transudate (due to either infectious or non-infectious causes, sometimes found in cases of underlying neoplasia such as Lucké's renal adenocarcinoma).

Differential Diagnosis

Multiple causes result in generalized edema, including poor water quality (aquatic stages), systemic inflammation (e.g. mycobacteriosis), renal disease (e.g. nephritis, renal adenocarcinoma), liver disease (e.g. mycobacteriosis, *Perkinus*-like infections), and alterations in electrolyte balance (e.g. chytridiomycosis).

Prevention, Treatment, and Control

Prevention, treatment, and control are dependent on determining the underlying cause.

Other Fungal Diseases

For other fungal diseases, see oomycete infection in fish.

Bibliography

Brunner JL, Schock DM, Davidson EW, Collins JP. 2004. Intraspecific reservoirs: complex life history and the persistence of a lethal ranavirus. *Ecology* 85(2):560–566.

Miller DL, Pessier AP, Hick P, Whittington RJ. 2015. Comparative pathology of ranaviruses and diagnostic techniques. In: Gray M, Chinchar V., eds. Ranaviruses Cham, Switzerland: Springer, pp. 171–208.

Berger L, Roberts AA, Voyles J, et al. 2016. History and recent progress on chytridiomycosis in amphibians. *Fungal Ecol* 19:89–99.

Blooi M, Martel A, Haesebrouck F, et al., 2015. Treatment of urodelans based on temperature dependent infection dynamics ofBatrachochytrium salamandrivorans. *Sci Rep* 5(1):1–4.

Blooi M, Pasmans F, Rouffaer L, et al. 2015. Successful treatment of Batrachochytrium salamandrivorans infections in salamanders requires synergy between voriconazole, polymyxin E and temperature. *Sci Rep* 5:11788.

Chatfield MW, Richards-Zawacki CL. 2011. Elevated temperature as a treatment for Batrachochytrium dendrobatidis infection in captive frogs. *Dis Aquat Organ* 94(3):235–238.

Clugston RD, Blaner WS. 2014. Vitamin A (retinoid) metabolism and actions: What we know and what we need to know about amphibians. *Zoo Biol* 33(6):527–535.

Col, J, Orwicz K, Brooks D. 1984. Gas bubble disease in the African clawed frog, *Xenopus laevis*. *J Herpetol* 18:131–137.

Forzán MJ, Horney BS. 2020. Amphibians. In: Heatley JJ, Russell KE, eds. *Exotic Animal Laboratory Diagnosis*. Ames, IA: Wiley, pp. 347–368.

Forzán MJ, Jones KM, Ariel E, et al. 2017. Pathogenesis of frog virus 3 (*Ranavirus*, *Iridoviridae*) infection in wood frogs (*Rana sylvatica*). *Vet Pathol* 54(3):531–548.

Forzán MJ, Ferguson LV, Smith TG. 2015a. Calcium oxalate nephrolithiasis and tubular necrosis in recent metamorphs of Rana sylvatica (*Lithobates sylvaticus*) fed spinach during the premetamorphic (tadpole) stage. *Vet Pathol* 52(2):384–387.

Forzán MJ, Jones KM, Vanderstichel RV, et al. 2015. Clinical signs, pathology and dose-dependent survival of adult wood frogs, Rana sylvatica, inoculated orally with frog virus 3 *Ranavirus* sp., *Iridoviridae*. *J Gen Virol* 96(5):1138–1149.

Hopkins WA, Fallon JA, Beck ML, et al. 2016. Haematological and immunological characteristics of eastern hellbenders (*Cryptobranchus alleganiensis alleganiensis*) infected and co-infected with endo-and ectoparasites. *Conserv Physiol* 4(1):cow002.

Ikuta CY, Reisfeld L, Silvatti B, et al. 2018. Tuberculosis caused by Mycobacterium bovis infection in a captive-bred American bullfrog (*Lithobates catesbeiana*). *BMC Vet Res* 14(1):1–4.

Jones ME, Paddock D, Bender L, et al. 2012. Treatment of chytridiomycosis with reduced-dose itraconazole. *Dis Aquat Organ* 99(3):243–249.

Laking AE, Ngo HN, Pasmans F, et al. 2017. Batrachochytrium salamandrivorans is the predominant chytrid fungus in Vietnamese salamanders. *Sci Rep* 7:44443.

Licheri M, Origgi FC, 2020. Consensus PCR protocols for the detection of amphibian herpesviruses (*Batrachovirus*). *J Vet Diagn Invest* 32(6):864–872.

Lucké B. 1952. Kidney carcinoma in the leopard frog: a virus tumor. *Ann N Y Acad Sci* 54(6):1093–1109.

Martel A, Spitzen-van der Sluijs A, Blooi M, et al. 2013. Batrachochytrium salamandrivorans sp. nov. causes lethal chytridiomycosis in amphibians. *Proc Natl Acad Sci* 110(38):15325–15329.

Martel A, Van Rooij P, Vercauteren G, et al. 2011. Developing a safe antifungal treatment protocol to eliminate Batrachochytrium dendrobatidis from amphibians. *Med Mycol* 49(2):143–149.

Martinho F, Heatley JJ, 2012. Amphibian mycobacteriosis. *Vet Clin North Am Exot Anim Pract* 15(1):113–119.

McKinnell RG. 1973. The Lucké frog kidney tumor and its herpesvirus. *Am Zool* 13(1):97–114.

Origgi FC, Schmidt BR, Lohmann P, et al. 2017. Ranid herpesvirus 3 and proliferative dermatitis in free-ranging wild common frogs (*Rana temporaria*). *Vet Pathol* 54(4):686–694.

Origgi FC, Schmidt BR, Lohmann P, et al. 2018. Bufonid herpesvirus 1 (BfHV1) associated dermatitis and mortality in free ranging common toads (*Bufo bufo*) in Switzerland. *Sci Rep* 8(1):1–12.

Pessier AP. 2018. Amphibia. In: Terio K, Mcaloose D, St. Leger J. *Pathology of Wildlife and Zoo Animals*. Philadelphia, PA: Academic Press, pp. 921–951.

Poole VA, Grow S. 2012. *Amphibian Husbandry Resource Guide*. Silver Spring, MD: Association of Zoos and Aquariums.

Reavill DR, Schmidt RE. 2012. Mycobacterial lesions in fish, amphibians, reptiles, rodents, lagomorphs, and ferrets with reference to animal models. *Vet Clin North Am Exot Anim Pract* 15(1):25–40.

Shilton CM, Smith DA, Crawshaw GJ, et al. 2001. Corneal lipid deposition in Cuban tree frogs (*Osteopilus septentrionalis*) and its relationship to serum lipids: an experimental study. *J Zoo Wildlife Med* 32(3):305–319.

Smith TG, Kim B, Hong H, Desser SS. 2000. Intraerythrocytic development of species of Hepatozoon infecting ranid frogs: evidence for convergence of life cycle characteristics among apicomplexans. *J Parasitol* 86(3):451–458.

Spitzen-van der Sluijs A, Martel A, Asselberghs J, et al. 2016. Expanding distribution of lethal amphibian fungus Batrachochytrium salamandrivorans in Europe. *Emerg Infect Dis* 22(7):1286–1288.

Wright K. 2003. Cholesterol, corneal lipidosis, and xanthomatosis in amphibians. The Veterinary Clinics of North America. *Exot Anim Pract* 6(1):155–167.

Wright KM, Whitaker BR. 2001. *Amphibian Medicine and Captive Husbandry*. Malabar, FL: Krieger.

Yap TA, Nguyen NT, Serr M, et al. 2017. Batrachochytrium salamandrivorans and the risk of a second amphibian pandemic. *Ecohealth* 14(4):851–864.

Young S, Warner J, Speare R, et al. 2012. Hematologic and plasma biochemical reference intervals for health monitoring of wild Australian tree frogs. *Vet Clin Pathol* 41(4):478–492.

Appendix 3.1

Etiology of amphibian diseases

Amphibians	Life stage	Etiology (most likely)
Sudden death	All	Bacterial sepsis, ranavirosis, toxicosis (various chemicals, including DEET, herbicides, pesticides), trauma, stress from handling
	Tadpoles[1] and Aquatic adults[2]	Water quality (increased ammonia, gas supersaturation/gas bubble disease)[1,2], ranavirosis[1], Perkinsus-like infection[1]
	Froglets and adults	Chytridiomycosis, oxalate toxicity (froglets at 2 weeks)
Emaciation (e.g., atrophied fat bodies, muscle atrophy), poor growth	All	Nutritional deficiency, stress, poor habitat (water quality, temperature, humidity, etc.), inadequate diet (e.g. insufficient caloric intake, wrong prey item for the species, insufficient feeding frequency), parasitism (e.g. pulmonary nematodiasis superinfection with *Rhabdias* sp.), oral trauma, mycobacteriosis
	Froglets[1] and adults[2]	Hypovitaminosis A (short tongue syndrome),[1,2] corneal ipidosis[1,2], renal (Lucké's) adenocarcinoma[2]
Neurologic signs (e.g., ataxia, torticollis, seizures)	Froglets[1] and adults[2]	Chytridiomycosis,[1,2] otitis/panophthalmitis (bacterial) [2], toxicosis (various chemicals, including DEET, herbicides, pesticides)[1,2], Other CNS disease[1,2]
Buoyancy problems	Tadpoles[1] and aquatic adults[2]	Ranavirosis[1], gas supersaturation/gas bubble disease)[1,2], other CNS disease[1,2]
Skin: erythema, petechia	All (except tadpoles[1])	Chytridiomycosis (*Batrachochytrium dendrobatidis*)[1], early ranavirosis, bacterial sepsis (including *Chlamydia* sp.), topical irritation (handling, contact with irritants such as detergents, bleach, etc.)
Skin: severe hemorrhage, necrosis, ulceration	All (except tadpoles[1])	Chytridiomycosis (*Batrachochytrium salamandrivorans*)[1], advanced ranavirosis, bacterial sepsis (including *Chlamydia* sp.), severe topical irritation (handling, contact with irritants such as detergents, bleach, etc.), gas supersaturation/gas bubble disease[1]
Skin: edema (cutaneous, subcutaneous)	All (except tadpoles[1])	Ranavirosis (dermal edema most common around the mouth), bacterial sepsis (including *Chlamydia* sp.), *Perkinsus*-like infection, mycobacteriosis,[1] ranid herpesvirus 3,[1] bufonid herpesvirus 1,[1] hepatic or renal disease, poor water quality
Skin: nodules	All (except tadpoles[1])	*Ichthyophonus*-like infection, mycobacteriosis, neoplasia[1], encysted parasites (nematodes)
Skin: proliferative patches or discoloration	Froglets and adults	Ranid herpesvirus 3, bufonid herpesvirus 1, idiopathic discoloration
Skin: rostral abrasions	Froglets and adults	Trauma, mycobacteriosis
Gills: erythema, hemorrhage, necrosis	Tadpoles and aquatic adults	Ranavirosis, poor water quality, bacterial/fungal infections

Amphibians	Life stage	Etiology (most likely)
Blood: hemoparasites	Froglets and adults	Hepatozoon and *Trypanosoma* spp.
Lung: parasitism	Adults	*Rhabdias* sp. (nematodes)
Coelom: ascites	Froglets and adults	Renal (Lucké's) adenocarcinoma, renal disease, bacterial sepsis
Coelom: ascites	Tadpoles and aquatic adults	Low osmolality in water, renal/cardiac/hepatic or systemic disease
Coelom: Granulomas/ caseous exudate	Adults	Mycobacteriosis, neoplasia, encysted parasites
Coelom: gas	Tadpoles and aquatic adults	Gas supersaturation/gas bubble disease
Oral cavity: hemorrhage	Froglets and adults	Ranavirosis, trauma
Oral cavity: 'short-tongue', keratin cysts	Froglets and adults	Hypovitaminosis A
Eye: cornel ulcer	All	Trauma, bacterial infection
Eye: corneal opacity	Adults	Corneal lipidosis (tree frogs), edema, ophthalmitis
Muscle nodules	All	Mycobacteriosis, *Ichthyophonus*-like infection, encysted parasites
Skeletal deformities	All	Mycobacteriosis, malnutrition, excessive or lack of ultraviolet B light (froglets), vitamin b deficiency (theorized for scoliosis in tadpoles), metabolic bone disease (calcium: potassium imbalance), metacercaria of *Ribeiroia odantrae* (polymelia, amelia, hypomelia), toxins
Esophageal, mucosal thickening	Adults	Hypovitaminosis A, cryptosporidiosis (esophagus and stomach)
Spleen, enlargement and necrosis	All	Ranavirosis, bacterial sepsis, other infectious diseases
Liver: necrosis	All	Ranavirosis, bacterial sepsis, *Perkinsus*-like Infection
Liver: fibrosis	Unknown	Biliary disease (myxozoan cyst)
Kidney: neoplasia	Adults	Ranid herpesvirus 1 (Lucké's adenocarcinoma, northern leopard frogs)
Kidney: edema and pallor	All	Ranavirosis, *Perkinsus*-like infection, bacterial sepsis, toxins (aminoglycosides, metals, polyvinyl chloride glue)
Spleen, liver, kidney: nodules	All	Mycobacteriosis, encysted parasites
Stomach and intestine: hemorrhage	All	Ranavirosis, bacterial sepsis, intussusception

[1,2] Life stage relating to etiology seen.
CNS, central nervous system; DEET, N, N-Diethyl-meta-toluamide.

4

Reptiles

Karina Jones and Ellen Ariel

Introduction to the Manifestation of Disease and Major Pathogens of Aquatic Reptiles

There are currently over 11500 recognized species within the class Reptilia (Uetz, 2021). All animals in this class are ectothermic and covered in scales or scutes. Oviparity is common to most animals in this class, although some species are viviparous or ovoviviparous (Doneley, 2018). Living animals in this class can be divided into the orders Testudines (turtles and tortoises), Crocodilia (crocodiles, alligators, gharials, and caimans), Squamata (snakes, lizards, and amphibians) and Rhynchocephalia (tuataras). Ecology and habitat use varies greatly, even within orders. This chapter focuses on reptiles with primarily aquatic lifestyles, namely marine and freshwater turtles (Testudines), crocodiles, alligators, gharials, and caimans (Crocodilia), sea snakes, and marine iguanas (Squamata).

Although generally thought of in the context of the wild, some of the species considered in this chapter can be encountered in animal production systems (e.g. crocodiles) or kept as pets (e.g. some freshwater turtle species). Such species have benefited from being more closely studied and the knowledge surrounding diseases of these animals tends to be more substantial than that of wild aquatic reptiles. When the biology of the captive species is considered in husbandry and enclosure design, an environment can be created that will allow these reptiles to thrive in captivity. Conversely, suboptimal temperatures, feeding, and/or overcrowding can lead to the development of clinical signs and otherwise harmless microorganisms turning pathogenic.

Because of their longevity and close association with the aquatic environment, some wild aquatic reptile species are considered indicators of aquatic environmental health. In addition to being sentinel species for long-term pollution exposure, they are also at risk of habitat loss or degradation, invasive species, and diseases, among other threats (Doupe et al., 2009; Flint et al., 2011; Gibbons et al., 2000; Rowe, 2008; Aguirre and Lutz, 2004). Another calamity of their long life cycle and low reproductive output is that they are exceptionally slow to recover from population declines, even after the cause has been removed (Doupe et al., 2009; Rowe, 2008). Add to this the endangered status of many aquatic reptile species and the above mentioned threats become very real and an urgent conservation issue.

Wildlife diseases are difficult to study and characterize. Unlike farmed aquatic animals, there is often no direct financial return in understanding or mitigating disease in wild aquatic species. Moreover, wild aquatic reptiles are typically dispersed in relatively remote locations that are

Pathology and Epidemiology of Aquatic Animal Diseases for Practitioners, First Edition.
Edited by Laura Urdes, Chris Walster, and Julius Tepper.

difficult for researchers and managers to access; in comparison with animals in aquaculture, wild aquatic reptiles cannot be easily observed and monitored. As a result, relatively few diseases of wild aquatic reptiles have been well characterized and these diseases are often challenged by knowledge gaps. The literature is interspersed with case descriptions reporting clinical signs but in many instances these cases are not linked to a major, well-defined disease. While it is likely that knowledge in this area will expand in the future, this chapter reports only on well-characterized major diseases of aquatic reptiles. The chapter highlights major, more well-defined diseases in aquatic reptiles with an indication (where possible) of disease etiology, transmission pathways, clinical signs, diagnosis, treatment, prevention, and control. Appendix 4.1 lists the etiologies of amphibian diseases.

Marine Turtles

Of the seven species of marine turtle, the hawksbill (*Eretmochelys imbricata*) and the Kemp's ridley (*Lepidochelys kempii*) turtles are globally recognized as critically endangered (Mortimer and Donnelly, 2008; Wibbels and Bevan, 2019); the green turtle *(Chelonia mydas)* is listed as endangered (Seminoff, 2004); and the loggerhead *(Caretta caretta)*, olive ridley (*Lepidochelys olivacea*), and leatherback (*Dermochelys coriacea*) turtles are considered vulnerable (Casale and Tucker, 2017; Abreu-Grobois and Plotkin, 2008; Wallace et al., 2013). The remaining species, the flatback turtle *(Natator depressus)*, is formally listed as data deficient, which makes it impossible to assign a status to it (Red List Standards and Petitions Subcommittee, 1996). The threatened population status of marine turtle species, coupled with their iconic and charismatic nature, has led them to be considered a key flagship species for conservation. Although many aspects of marine turtle health are yet to be fully understood, their unique status has led them to be one of the more well-studied wild aquatic reptiles afflicted by several well-defined major diseases. While there are several case reports of smaller-scale disease outbreaks in marine turtles, there is not enough evidence to suggest that these diseases are of major risk to turtles. However, this could be a misinterpretation because of the challenges associated with studying wild animals. The diseases outlined in this chapter are those that have been ranked by an international panel of experts to be of major risk to marine turtle health (Mashkour et al., 2020).

All species of marine turtles share the same key life stages and have a primarily aquatic lifecycle. While there are some differences in diet and distribution between species, there is significant overlap in these key habitat determinants, and as such, several marine turtle species can often be found cohabiting the same locations. As a consequence of these shared life histories, reported diseases are typically marine turtle specific but not species specific; sympatric species of marine turtle will often be afflicted by the same conditions (e.g. cold stunning).

Determining whether a marine turtle is unwell can often be challenging. Gross clinical signs which indicate that further investigation is needed include lesions, listlessness/lethargy, inappetence, floating (inability to dive below the surface), and stranding (washing ashore on the beach). Differential diagnoses are challenged by these signs of general health, which are likely to be observed in almost all major marine turtle diseases. Basking is a natural behavior employed by marine turtles to rest and regulate their body temperature and/or metabolism. This behavior may initially be difficult to distinguish from a potential stranding or floating case. Further diagnostic tools, including hematology and x-ray, can be invaluable for establishing pathology in such cases.

Prevention and Control of Marine Turtle Diseases

The knowledge gaps surrounding marine turtle health, in addition to their global distribution across a range of jurisdictions, has led to considerable challenges in preventing and controlling disease in these species. Captive turtles will likely benefit from proper husbandry, quarantine procedures, veterinary care, and preventive medicine. However, the management of disease in wild marine turtles is markedly more difficult. The transmission pathways are not yet described for any of the infectious marine turtle diseases outlined in this chapter and although they are likely waterborne and ubiquitous, they only cause disease under some conditions. Similarly, the life cycles of many of the known disease-causing pathogens discussed here are still being investigated. Until these knowledge gaps are resolved, effective prevention and control protocols cannot be established.

Viral Disease

Fibropapillomatosis

Overview Fibropapillomatosis is a globally distributed neoplastic condition. The growth of fibropapillomatosis lesions may inhibit a turtle's ability to see, feed, breathe, or locomote. Prevalence varies both spatially and temporally, with the higher prevalence reported in juvenile turtles (Figure 4.1). Contribution to mortality varies by region (Jones et al., 2016; Hargrove et al., 2016). Multiple cases of lesion regression and turtle recovery have been documented but the rate at which this occurs is yet to be determined.

Etiology Chelonid alphaherpesvirus 5 (ChHV5) is the leading etiological candidate for fibropapillomatosis, as it has been consistently detected in fibropapillomatosis tumors. This virus is a herpesvirus, belonging to the subfamily Alphaherpesvirinae. However, Koch's postulates for ChHV5 have yet to be fulfilled. Recently, *Chelonia mydas* papillomavirus 1 (CmPV1) was also reported in fibropapillomatosis lesions. In some cases, both ChHV5 and CmPV1 were both detected in the same lesions. However, the role of CmPV1 in fibropapillomatosis is not yet understood.

Host Range and Transmission Fibropapillomatosis can affect all marine turtle species but is most prevalent in the green turtle. Transmission of ChHV5 is thought to occur horizontally upon recruitment to neritic zones but the mechanism for this has not been confirmed. Spirorchiid trematodes, coral reef cleaner fish, saddleback wrasse, and a range of epibiota including marine leeches (*Ozobranchus* spp.) have all been proposed as potential vectors of ChHV5, with marine leeches currently considered the leading candidates for a mechanical vector. However, the exact role of marine leeches has not been confirmed. Studies have noted that the latent nature of herpesviruses and the indication of other cofactors in expression of fibropapillomatosis have hampered the understanding of transmission.

Gross and Clinical Signs The disease is characterized by the growth of benign lesions which may be smooth or verrucous and range in pigmentation and size (0.1–30 cm), (Figure 4.1). These lesions predominantly grow on the soft tissue but may also be present on the carapace, plastron, or viscera. Turtles afflicted are also often immunosuppressed and chronically stressed. Chronic inflammation such as anemia, lymphocytopenia, neutrophilia, monocytosis, hypoproteinemia, and hyperglobulinemia may be observed. Body condition in afflicted turtles can vary from emaciated to good. Fibropapillomatosis can be diagnosed through a combination of histological

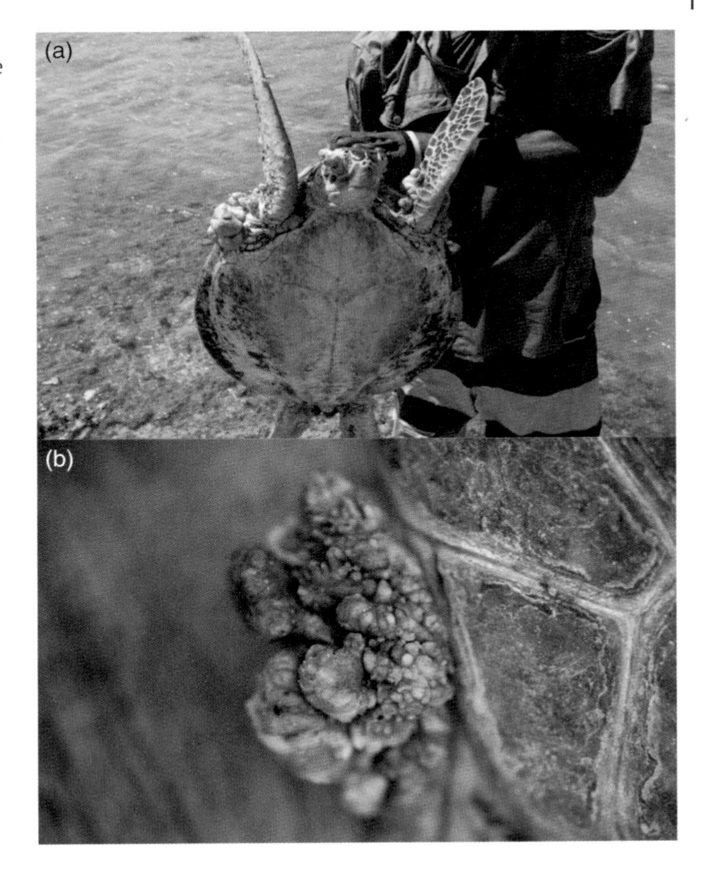

Figure 4.1 (a) A Saibai Mura Buway ranger holding a juvenile green turtle (*Chelonia mydas*) with fibropapillomatosis tumors. Photo taken on Warul Kawa, Torres Strait, by Mr Tristan Simpson. (b) A close-up image of a verrucous fibropapillomatosis tumor on a sub-adult green turtle, captured in Cleveland Bay, Townsville, Australia.

and molecular methods. Key histologic features observed in lesions include orthokeratosis hyperkeratosis, varying degrees of epidermal hyperplasia, cytoplasmic vacuolation, and ballooning degeneration of superficial epidermal cells.

Diagnosis and Differential Diagnosis Molecular detection of ChHV5 through polymerase chain reaction (PCR) or qualitative PCR is currently the most widely used diagnostic tool for ChHV5. There is no standardized test for this virus but several published assays are available in the literature. Viral detection is most successful in tissues sourced from lesions but some assays have been successful in detecting virus in clinically healthy tissues. Established enzyme-linked immunosorbent assay (ELISA) tests are also available and have demonstrated success in identifying both past exposure and subclinical infections.

Proliferative dermatitis, characteristic of papillomaviral infection, has been reported in green and loggerhead turtles (Manire et al., 2008). Although initially not considered to be linked with fibropapillomatosis infection, results of some studies suggest that this link requires further investigation (Mashkour et al., 2021; Mashkour et al., 2018). Thus, *Chelonia mydas* papillomavirus (CmPV1) and *Caretta caretta* papillomavirus infection should also be investigated in the diagnosis of fibropapillomatosis.

Prevention, Treatment, and Control High prevalence has consistently been linked with regions of poor water quality; this includes areas of high anthropogenic activity such as urbanization, industrialization, and agricultural runoff. This relationship is complex and is still being investigated; however, it has been suggested that improving the water quality of these inshore areas could reduce the prevalence of fibropapillomatosis. Individual tumors can be removed successfully using laser surgery; however, it is important to consider the initial cost and long recovery time in captivity, which may not be realistic in all scenarios.

Lung–Eye–Trachea Disease

Overview Lung–eye–trachea disease (LETD) as the name indicates, is characterized by lesions on the lung, eye and/or trachea of affected turtles.

Etiology This disease is believed to be caused by a herpesvirus known as LETD–associated virus or Chelonid alphaherpesvirus 6 (ChHV6). Serological studies suggest that this virus is distinct from ChHV5. However, the virus has not been genetically sequenced and is not recognized by the International Committee on Taxonomy of Viruses.

Host Range and Transmission LETD has been reported in captive green turtles and wild populations of both green and loggerhead turtles.

Gross and Clinical Signs Case reports of LETD describe gross clinical signs consistent with respiratory tract disease, including periglottal necrosis, tracheitis with intraluminal caseous and laminated necrotic debris, and severe pneumonia.

Diagnosis and Differential Diagnosis At present, observation of these lesions and detection of ChHV6 would be sufficient for a diagnosis of LETD. However, future cases would benefit from more in–depth investigation and reporting to better characterize this disease and the etiological agent.

Treatment Data are deficient.

Gray Patch Disease

Overview One case of gray patch disease has been reported in captive reared post–hatchling green turtles. Although considered by experts as a major viral disease of concern in marine turtles due to its potential impact on captive turtles (Mashkour et al., 2020), there have been no published reports on this disease since 1978 (Haines, 1978).

Etiology Electron microscopy studies linked this disease to a herpesviral infection (Chelonid alphaherpesvirus 1). However, this virus has not been molecularly characterized and is not recognized by the International Committee on Taxonomy of Viruses.

Host Range and Transmission Experimental transmission was successful in 100% of turtles through scratch inoculating bacteria–free preparations of gray patch skin lesion scrapings into the epidermis of immature turtles. Non–experimental transmission is data deficient.

Gross and Clinical Signs Skin lesions are most commonly obvious gray patches, which may spread over large areas of the epidermal surface. In some cases, this disease may present as pustular–like skin lesions.

Diagnosis and Differential Diagnosis Observation of these lesions and evidence of herpesviral infection under electron microscopy are presently the only means of diagnosis. Future cases would benefit from more in–depth investigation and reporting to better characterize this disease and the etiological agent. Gray skin lesions may occasionally be observed on turtles afflicted with fibropapillomatosis, but fibropapillomatosis lesions are typically pedunculated, raised masses while gray patch lesions present as flat discolorations of the skin. Diagnosis can be resolved with molecular analyses of lesions.

Prevention, Treatment, and Control Reports suggest that both higher water temperatures and overcrowding of hatcheries can worsen the symptoms. Strict hygiene and quarantine procedures for a minimum of three months can be effective in reducing impact of this disease in a hatchery. Although, if it is a herpesvirus as expected, this could just be a reduction in impact rather than eradication.

Parasitic Disease

Parasites are to be expected in wild animals but the relationship should be balanced and should not compromise the host. If other factors are at play, such as starvation and other immunosuppressive factors, low level parasitemia may suddenly increase opportunistically and reach levels that are of pathogenic impact.

Spirorchiidiasis

Overview Spirorchiidiasis is often considered to be one of the most significant diseases of marine turtles as a result of its widespread occurrence and the perceived associated high mortality rates in afflicted turtles. However, *Spirorchiid* spp. have also been reported in turtles where no associated clinical signs were elicited (Stacy et al., 2010, Chapman et al., 2019).

Etiology This disease is caused by trematodes belonging to the Spirorchiidae family, a form of blood fluke. While it is common for these flukes to be reported with no ill effects on the host, there are an extensive range of pathologies associated with these blood flukes which can be observed in an array of organs and tissues (Chapman et al., 2019).

Host Range and Transmission Most commonly described in greens and loggerhead turtles, there have also been reports of *Spirorchiid* species in hawksbill, olive ridley, and Kemp's ridley turtles. There are presently no reports of these blood flukes in leatherback or flatback turtles (Chapman et al., 2019). The exact mode of transmission is not yet understood. However, Cribb et al. (2017) reported a *Spirorchiid* infection in a vermetid gastropod, which could well be the intermediate host.

Gross and Clinical Signs Antemortem signs of spirorchiidiasis are non–specific. Poor body condition (emaciation, plastron concavity, muscle wastage, sunken eyes; Figure 4.2), as well as lethargy, may be associated with *Spirorchiid* infection. Neurological signs can also be indicative of neurospirorchiidiasis, linked to *Neospirorchis* spp. (Stacy et al., 2010). Vascular occlusions may lead turtles to develop limb edema (Walden et al., 2020).

Diagnosis and Differential Diagnosis Although antemortem diagnosis is possible through ELISA and/or identification of eggs under microscopic examination of feces, these methods have limitations; currently available ELISA assays cannot yet distinguish between past exposure and current infections (Chapman et al., 2019) while fecal collection and species identification based on

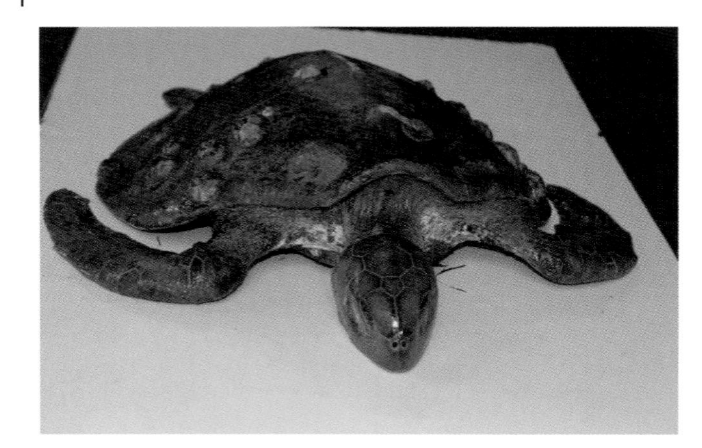

Figure 4.2 An emaciated juvenile green turtle (*Chelonia mydas*). Not pictured, concave plastron and sunken eyes. *Source:* Courtesy of Stephen Menzies, Reef HQ Aquarium, Great Barrier Reef Marine Park Authority, Australia.

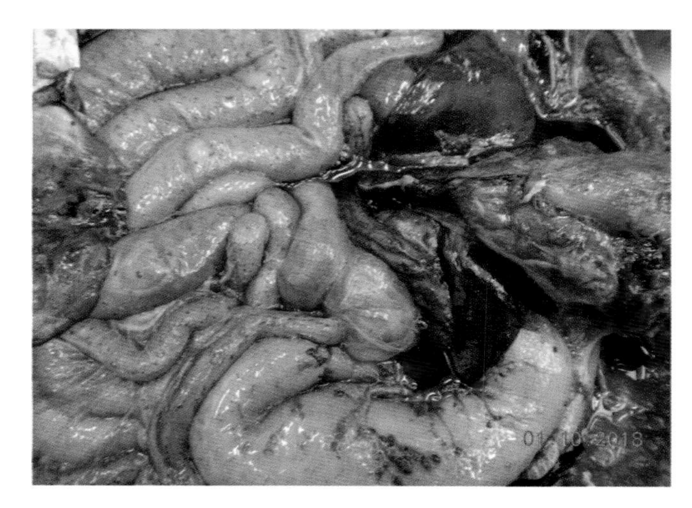

Figure 4.3 Widespread distribution of small, dark, raised lesions throughout the serosal surfaces of the gastrointestinal tract of a juvenile green turtle (*Chelonia mydas*). These lesions, observed during necropsy, are characteristic of Spirorchiid eggs. *Source:* courtesy of Erina Young, Murdoch University, Australia.

egg morphology is unlikely (Stacy et al., 2010).Visual observation of these flukes and/or their eggs during gross necropsy is the most common approach for diagnosing this disease. Eggs and granulomatous inflammation associated with these eggs can be observed as small, black, or white raised lesions (Figure 4.3). Protruding nodules on serosal surfaces have been reported to contain substantial numbers of *Spirorchiid* spp. eggs (Walden et al., 2020). Such lesions can be observed on nearly all organs, but are commonly seen in the gastrointestinal tract, lungs, spleen, and thyroid (Chapman et al., 2019; Stacy et al., 2010). Endocarditis, arteritis, thrombosis, aneurysm, and granulomatous inflammation are associated with adult flukes, which are most commonly reported in the heart and great vessels (Chapman et al., 2019). Flukes or eggs observed in the central nervous system are most likely to be *Neospirorchis* spp. and so are unlikely to be associated with granulomatous inflammation (Stacy et al., 2010). Further microscopic investigation of the parasites or their eggs is recommended for species identification, regardless of the location of detection. Antemortem clinical signs are synonymous with general ill health and are therefore unreliable for diagnosis. Flukes, eggs, and their associated lesions are characteristic to spirorchiidiasis.

Treatment Praziquantel has demonstrated success in controlling adult flukes, although its effects may be delayed in cases involving egg embolization. Appropriate dosage has been debated;

however, oral administration of 25 mg/kg^{-1} three times daily at three–hourly intervals (Jacobson et al 2003) is generally considered the most suitable according to a review by Chapman et al. (2019). A greater understanding of the lifecycle of *Spirorchiid* spp. is critical to effective control strategies. While a range of other anthelminthics may also be effective in treating parasitic infections in turtles, ivermectin is not recommended owing to its linkage to acute toxicity and death in chelonian species (Teare and Bush, 1983).

Coccidiosis

Overview Originally reported from farmed turtles on Grand Cayman island, coccidiosis in marine turtles has now been reported in wild turtles in several regions globally. This disease has also been linked to multiple mass mortality events in both Australia and Florida (Chapman et al., 2016; Gordon et al., 1993; Stacy et al., 2019).

Etiology Coccidiosis is induced by the presence of protozoans belonging to the subclass Coccidia. Several novel Coccidia species have been reported in marine turtles, of which only two have been formally described: *Caryospora cheloniae* and *Eimeria carrettae* (Stacy et al., 2017). It should be noted that there have been no reports of *E. carrettae* since the initial report in 1990 (Upton et al., 1990).

Host Range and Transmission *C. cheloniae* is considered a significant pathogen of green turtles but has also been reported in loggerheads. To date, *E. carrettae* has only been reported to infect loggerhead turtles. Other novel Coccidia species have also been reported in both green and leatherback turtles (Stacy et al., 2017). Mode of transmission is unknown.

Gross and Clinical Signs Live turtles affected by coccidiosis can appear to be emaciated, lethargic and/or weak. They may also display neurological signs such as circling, nystagmus, and head tilts. Gross lesions may include severe fibrinous or necrotizing enteritis, nephritis, thyroiditis, or meningoencephalitis (Walden et al., 2020; Stacy et al., 2017).

Diagnosis and Differential Diagnosis Diagnosis of coccidial infection in live turtles can be achieved through detection of Coccidia oocysts in fecal floats. In deceased turtles, a combination of gross necropsy and histopathology methods is effective; gross lesion identification consistent with the clinical signs outlined above and identification of Coccidia in sampled tissues through histopathology allows for a definitive diagnosis. Molecular methods can also be used to isolate coccidial DNA and formally characterize the detected species.

Treatment Ponazuril, sulfonamides, and metronidazole may be effective antiprotozoals for marine turtles, with varying degrees of success (Stacy et al., 2017; Innis et al., 2017). Manire and Montgomery (2014) suggest that oral administration of metronidazole (50 mg/kg daily for four or five doses) is an effective treatment for coccidiosis in marine turtles, although appetite suppression may occur during treatment; a reduced dosage may be equally effective while avoiding inappetence. Treatment with ivermectin is not recommended because of its linkage to acute toxicity and death in chelonian species (Teare and Bush, 1983).

Bacterial Diseases

Overview The presence of bacteria is a normal component of the marine turtle microbiome. Most marine turtle bacterial infections are associated with bacterial species comprising normal marine turtle flora. These bacteria can act as opportunistic pathogens in turtles that are already compromised, particularly as a result of external environmental stressors, such as cold-stunned turtles. This includes both Gram-negative and Gram-positive bacteria, although Gram-negative bacteria are isolated more frequently (Innis and Frasca Jr., 2017). Establishing links between bacterial species and marine turtle disease is challenging, as many marine bacteria will not grow in marine culture settings (Ahasan et al., 2018; Ahasan et al., 2017; Ahasan et al., 2020). However, those considered the most hazardous species associated with diseases are discussed here.

Etiology Consistent with the distribution of normal marine turtle flora, the majority of bacterial disease is also linked to Gram-negative bacteria (Innis and Frasca Jr., 2017). Several species have been linked to marine turtle diseases but experts rank the most hazardous to marine turtle health to be *Vibrio* spp., *Pseudomonas* spp., *Escherichia coli*, methicillin-resistant *Staphylococcus aureus* and *Klebsiella* spp. (Mashkour et al., 2020). *Mycobacterium* spp. have also been commonly associated with disease but are not currently considered part of the normal flora.

Host Range and Transmission All species of marine turtle can experience bacterial infections which may be a secondary, but serious, condition.

Gross and Clinical Signs A substantial range of body systems can be affected by bacterial infection. Common clinical signs associated with Gram-negative bacteria include ulcerative dermatitis, pneumonia, tracheitis, rhinitis, and stomatitis. Gram-positive infections, while less common, have been associated with pneumonia, osteomyelitis, sepsis, granulomatous dermatitis, hepatic necrosis, cholecystitis, steatitis, ulcerative dermatitis, ulcerative stomatitis, oral and skin lesions. Granulomatous lesions in the lung, liver, spleen, kidney, heart, stomach, and small intestine have been reported in marine turtles experiencing mycobacterial infection. Systemic infections, osteomyelitis and synovitis have also been associated with *Mycobacterium* spp. (Innis and Frasca Jr., 2017).

Diagnosis and Differential Diagnosis Accurate diagnosis is contingent on careful isolation of pathogenic bacteria from samples to ensure that they can be clearly separated from the normal marine turtle flora. Traditional methods of diagnosis rely on culture-based methods to identify species. However, molecular diagnostics (largely PCR) are becoming more common in the diagnosis of bacterial infections.

Treatment According to Innis and Frasca Jr. (2017), established and widespread mycobacterial infections are difficult to treat. However, marine turtles with a reduced infection, or those treated presumptively early, have improved chances of responding to treatment. It is important to notice that broad-spectrum antibiotic treatment may release a treatment cascade, as some species are dependent on gut microbes for digestion. Green turtles are hindgut fermenters, and oral antibiotics will destabilize the microbial communities needed for digestion, so will generate another problem. A future treatment method may be phage therapy, which is more targeted to the pathogenic bacteria, but not readily available (Ahasan et al., 2019).

Fungal Diseases

Overview

While fungal infections are relatively common in marine turtles, they are not thought to act as primary pathogens. Instead, these common environmental flora act as opportunistic pathogens on turtles that are already experiencing morbidity and/or when external conditions are favorable (e.g. overcrowding).

Etiology A range of fungal genera have been isolated from debilitated turtles. Experts rank *Fusarium* spp. (particularly *Fusarium solani*), *Aspergillus* spp., *Cladosporium* spp., and *Penicillium* spp. as the most hazardous to marine turtle health (Mashkour et al., 2020). Of these, *Fusarium* spp. are considered the most commonly encountered and well-studied fungal pathogen of marine turtles (Mashkour et al., 2020; Innis and Frasca Jr., 2017). However, additional species to consider include *Paecilomyces, Purpureocillium, Beauveria, Sporotrichum, Scolecobasidium, Geotrichum, Drechslera, Rhodotorula, Colletotrichum, Candida, Enterococcus, Veronaea, Ochroconis* and *Cochliobolus*.

Host Range and Transmission All species of marine turtle can host fungal infections.

Gross and Clinical Signs Fungal species considered most hazardous to marine turtles are linked to hatchling failure and challenges to captive rearing (Mashkour et al., 2020). Beyond the impact to hatchling development, there is significant variation in fungal infections manifestation. Fungal infections appear to be most commonly isolated from turtles with respiratory symptoms (e.g. pneumonia, pleuritis, respiratory tract lesions). However, fungal species have been isolated from skin lesions, intestinal lesions, bone infections, and systemic infections (see summary in Innis and Frasca Jr., 2017).

Diagnosis and Differential Diagnosis Accurate diagnosis relies on careful and appropriate sampling and culture technique, in addition to informative selection of diagnostic tests. The site of sample collection also needs to be considered in the interpretation of results; external body surfaces and/or non-sterile sites such as cloacal mucosa possess natural flora which need to be separated from pathogenic fungi through diagnostic investigations. Innis and Frasca Jr. (2017) emphasize that the cultured fungus and the fungus in the sampled lesion should correlate morphologically and/or molecularly to have pathologic relevance.

Treatment Antifungal therapy is commonly employed to treat diagnosed fungal infections. Given the opportunistic nature of most fungal infections, antifungal therapy can also be useful as a preventive in immunocompromised turtles during care. Topical treatments are effective at treating external fungal infections such as those on the skin. Localized and/or systemic treatment is typically required for internal infections. Accurate identification of the pathogenic fungus is critical to inform therapy selection. Antifungal susceptibility can also be identified through minimum inhibitory concentration (MIC) testing. While both tools can be expensive and there are available data limitations to both methods, their use is encouraged to inform antifungal therapy selection (Innis and Frasca Jr., 2017). Pharmacokinetic studies have been conducted for both itraconazole in Kemp's ridley turtles (Manire et al., 2003), and fluconazole in loggerhead (Mallo et al., 2002) and Kemp's ridley turtles (Innis et al., 2012). Some fungal infections can be effectively treated with these antifungals. However, while safe, fluconazole may not be effective in treating serious fungal infections (Innis. C et al., 2012; Innis et al., 2012; Williams et al., 2012). MIC testing can be employed to assess whether this antifungal is effective (Innis et al., 2017).

Non-Infectious Disease

Buoyancy Disorder/Floater's Syndrome

Overview Most commonly characterized by an inability to dive below the surface of the water (positive buoyancy disorder), turtles experiencing buoyancy disorder may also have difficulty ascending to the surface (negative buoyancy disorder). Afflicted turtles expend considerable energy either staying on the ocean floor to feed or reaching the surface to breathe. This condition is indicative of potential underlying pathologies and increases affected turtles' vulnerability to predation and boat strike.

Etiology Buoyancy disorder can result from a variety of causes that most commonly include gastrointestinal, coelomic, or pulmonary complications. Gastrointestinal floaters are characterized by the presence of distention due to excess gas in the gastrointestinal tract. Ileus (caused by dehydration, foreign bodies, trauma, malnutrition, disease, gastroenterocolitis) and gastrointestinal obstructions (due to ingestion of foreign bodies or other indigestible materials such as rocks) can also lead to buoyancy disorders. Pulmonary disease (most commonly pneumonia or pulmonary bullae) may elicit this disorder. In addition, gas in the coelomic cavity as a result of pulmonary tears or ruptures is characteristic of pneumocoelomic floaters. Although less common, gastrointestinal perforations can also result in pneumocoelom. Neurological disease, trauma, and decompression sickness have also been linked to this disorder (Manire et al., 2017; García–Párraga et al., 2014). It should be noted that basking on the surface of the water is a normal turtle behavior, thought to assist in rest, digestion, and thermoregulation (Manire et al., 2017; Lutcavage and Lutz, 1996). It is therefore not unusual for turtles demonstrating this behavior to be brought into care only to appear normally buoyant in captivity and to yield negative results in all diagnostic tests.

Host Range and Transmission This common, noninfectious disorder can be observed in all marine turtle species of all age classes. It is possible for floating to occur en masse (e.g. during cold–stunning events) and these events typically affect small turtles first.

Gross and Clinical Signs The inability of a turtle to ascend or descend in the water column is a clear sign of buoyancy disorder. Chronic dorsoflexion (hyperextension) of the neck in floating turtles pinches the skin between the caudal skull and cranial carapace, which often results in a cervical callus, also termed a cervical carbuncle (Mettee and Norton, 2017), (Figure 4.4). A "water line" is often visible on the carapace of chronically positively buoyant turtles (and occasionally acutely affected turtles), resulting from extended exposure of the carapace to air due to floating, thereby

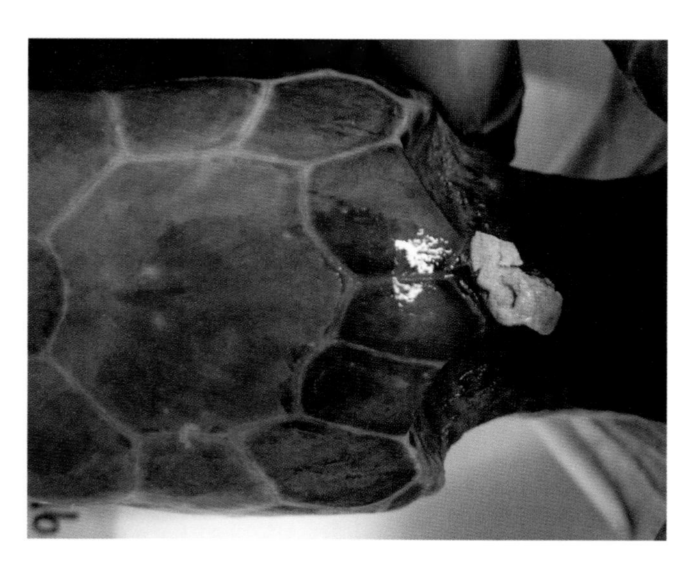

Figure 4.4 Dorsal view of a cervical callus/carbuncle resulting from an extended period of floating in a green turtle (*Chelonia mydas*). *Source:* courtesy of Erina Young, Murdoch University, Australia.

killing off epibionts in that area. This line can indicate whether the turtle is a gastrointestinal or pneumocoelomic floater (low water line on carapace; floating higher in the water column) or pulmonary disease floater (high water line on the carapace; floating lower in the water column). In some etiologies, flotation may manifest asymmetrically.

Diagnosis and Differential Diagnosis Confirmatory diagnosis of the specific etiology in each presenting turtle is essential and can be achieved through an extensive range of imaging techniques (radiography, ultrasound, endoscopy, computed tomography, magnetic resonance imaging). Gas distension in the gastrointestinal tract or gas in the coelomic cavity are indicative of this disorder. Some presentations of buoyancy disorder can be diagnosed by reduced expansion of the lungs during inspiration or compensatory increase in the size of one lung, often seen radiographically extending over the midline (Manire et al., 2017).

Treatment Treatment options vary based on the etiology of each case. Administration of intestinal motility stimulants, fluid therapy, and antibiotics for up to two weeks can resolve cases of gas distention in the gastrointestinal tract. Ileus can also be treated with intestinal motility stimulants and fluid therapy; saline enemas can be useful in nonobstructive ileus cases. Gastrointestinal floating due to foreign body ingestion may require medical management (e.g. psyllium fiber, Metamucil®, Procter & Gamble) to pass the object) or surgical intervention (removal of object). Pneumocoelomic flotation is most commonly treated by coelomocentesis, but surgical intervention may be required if a turtle does not respond to this treatment after several attempts. Lung tears and gastrointestinal perforations also require surgical intervention. The carapace water line can be monitored during care and treatment to monitor progress (Manire et al., 2017).

Trauma

Overview One of the most common reasons a turtle will be brought into a clinic for veterinary attention is traumatic injury. This includes sharp trauma, blunt trauma, constriction, and/or avulsion (Mettee and Norton, 2017), which renders the turtle unable to function and therefore obvious to fishermen and people on or near the water.

Etiology Traumatic injuries in marine turtles can be induced by a myriad of events. The most common causes of trauma include boat strike (lacerations caused by the propeller of a boat), predator encounter (Figure 4.5), entanglement in marine debris (commonly fishing line, but other types of litter can also be problematic), traditional take injuries, and entrapment in trawling/dredging equipment.

Gross and Clinical Signs Boat strike is often characterized by lacerations to the carapace but lacerations to the soft tissue, skull, and plastron can also occur (Figure 4.6). Signs of a predator encounter include bite marks, and the wound may include signs of both sharp trauma (from the predator's teeth) and blunt trauma (from the predator's jaws) (Mettee and Norton, 2017) (Figure 4.7). If the boat's propeller or predator's bite has penetrated the carapace, organs in the coelomic cavity may be exposed. Constriction from entanglement in marine debris is easily recognized. Turtles with buoyancy disorder typically develop dorsocervical carbuncles due to chronic dorsoflexion (hyperextension), which causes the skin between the skull and carapace to be chronically compressed (Mettee and Norton, 2017).

Diagnosis and Differential Diagnosis Diagnosis is readily achieved through observation of a traumatic injury. If a dorsocervical carbuncle is observed, buoyancy disorder should also be

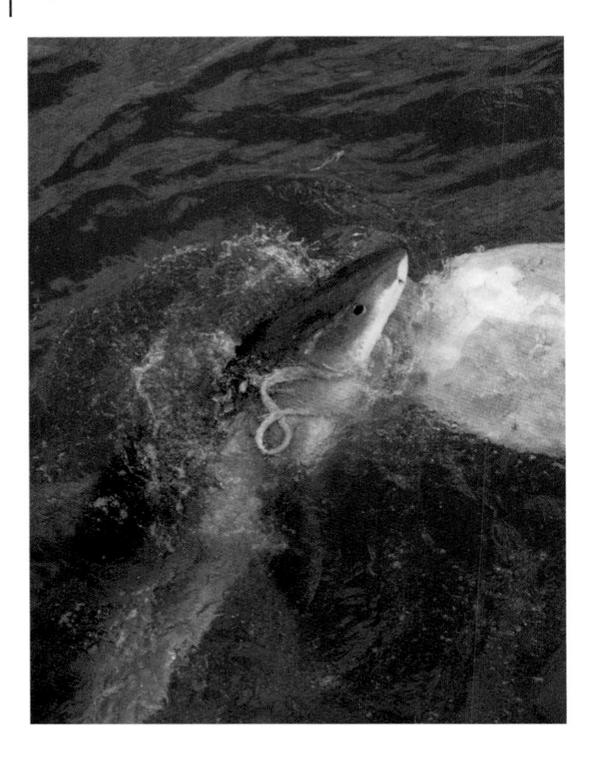

Figure 4.5 A green turtle (*Chelonia mydas*) experiencing the depredation of tiger shark (*Galeocerdo cuvier*). *Source:* Courtesy of Tristan Simpson.

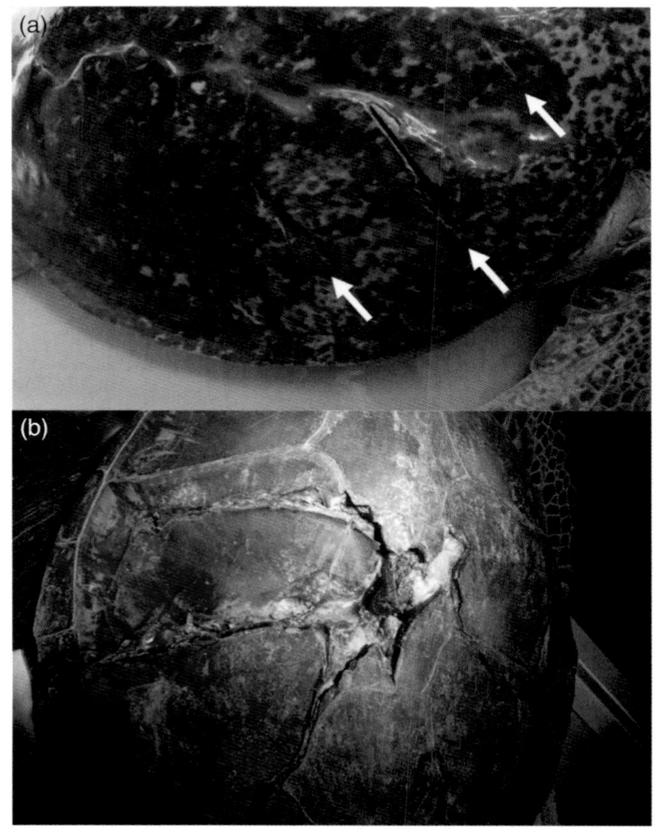

Figure 4.6 The carapace of two green turtles (*Chelonia mydas*) each with a boat-strike injury penetrating into the coelomic cavity. Common presentation is three sharp lacerations, denoted with white arrows (a), but other presentations, such as that shown in (b) can also occur. *Source:* Courtesy of Stephen Menzies, Reef HQ Aquarium, Great Barrier Reef Marine Park Authority, Australia. Annotations by K. Jones.

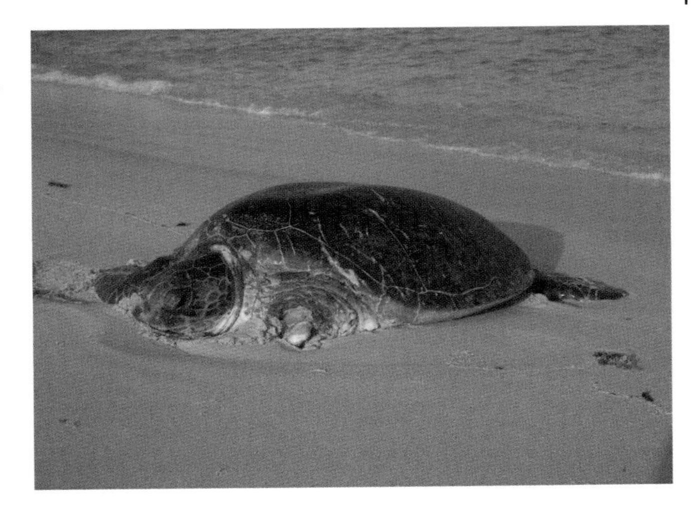

Figure 4.7 An adult green turtle (*Chelonia mydas*) with a shark bite injury to the left pectoral limb. *Source:* Courtesy of Tristan Simpson.

investigated. In some cases of entrapment in trawling/dredging equipment, turtles can develop decompression sickness (García-Párraga et al., 2014; Parga et al., 2020).

Prevention, Treatment, and Control Depending on the severity of the injury, consideration should be given to whether to treat at all. If the injury is too severe and treatment will have substantial negative impacts on welfare or long-term quality of life then euthanasia should be considered. However, if the patient is deemed a suitable candidate for treatment, the course will vary greatly depending on injury location and severity. Readers should refer to Mettee and Norton (2017) for a more comprehensive summary of treatment options for common trauma cases.

While predator encounters and natural causes are impossible to completely prevent or control, many anthropogenic causes of trauma can be minimized through public awareness and legislative action. Community engagement to increase awareness of marine turtles in the local area is highly effective. This includes education, signage, and campaigning for: i) vessel operators to keep an eye out for turtles and go slow in critical turtle habitats (e.g Go Slow – Look Out Below campaign by GBRMPA); ii) informed advice on fishing equipment selection and disposal. Mandatory use of turtle excluder devices on fishery vessels has demonstrated effectiveness in significantly reducing turtle bycatch and likely reduce associated morbidities such as decompression sickness; and iii) litter disposal.

Cold Stunning

Overview The ectothermic nature of marine turtles leads them to be heavily affected by their external environment. To facilitate optimal biological function, most marine turtle species inhabit tropical and subtropical habitats. Dramatic shifts in temperature can make them vulnerable to conditions such as cold stunning. It should be noted that rapid warming of cold-stunned turtles is more likely to lead to mortality; gradual warming, ideally through the use of more diffuse heat sources such as incubators, is recommended (Innis and Staggs, 2017; Sadove et al., 1998). To facilitate this, examination of turtles suspected of being cold stunned should be conducted in a cool room (Innis and Staggs, 2017).

Etiology Cold stunning is precipitated by decreases in water temperature beyond the natural range of turtles. Chronic cold-stunning events are typically observed in regions further from the equator and occurrence is often seasonal; rapid temperature decreases in late autumn impact turtles that failed to migrate from these foraging grounds prior to this change in season. Abnormal decreases in temperature, particularly in regions closer to the equator, is linked to acute cases of cold stunning.

Host Range and Transmission This non-infectious condition typically affects wild hard-shelled marine turtles. Reports range from singular cases to mass cold-stunning events affecting thousands of turtles (Innis and Staggs, 2017). Although it is possible for leatherback turtles to be affected by cold stunning, it is considered to be less likely, given their natural propensity to inhabit colder waters and their enhanced ability to regulate their body temperature (in comparison with hard-shelled marine turtles) (Frair et al., 1972).

Gross and Clinical Signs Lethargy is a key feature of cold-stunned turtles but other signs include inappetence, stranding, floating and/or a cessation of swimming. Bradypnea and apnea are commonly observed. Lividity and/or bruising of the plastron may also be noted in chronically cold-stunned turtles (Innis and Staggs, 2017).

Diagnosis and Differential Diagnosis The combination of gross/clinical signs with meteorological and oceanographic conditions that would facilitate cold stunning is a sound indicator of cold stunning. However, further diagnostic tools such as hematology and diagnostic imaging can be useful in identifying underlying abnormalities, guiding treatment and monitoring recovery (Innis and Staggs, 2017).

The moribund presentation of cold-stunned turtles and the clinical signs associated with the disease overlap greatly with many of the other conditions outlined in this chapter. Moreover, although thought to be incidental, turtles afflicted with this condition are often suffering from fungal, bacterial, and/or parasitic infections (Innis and Staggs, 2017). This can pose challenges in diagnosing cold stunning. To overcome this, a high emphasis must be placed on water temperature at the location of capture; oceanographic conditions such as current and wind direction should also be considered as cold-stunned turtles that are floating or have ceased swimming may be transported great distances to the site of capture.

Treatment The high dependence of this condition on the broader environment makes its prevention and control impossible. Cold-stunned turtles should be warmed slowly, with the rate of warming dependent on whether the turtle is acutely or chronically cold stunned. Where possible, initial examinations should be performed in a cool room followed by a swim test. Diffuse heat sources such as air-conditioned rooms or incubators can then be used to increase the core temperature of chronically cold-stunned turtles to 25°C by increments of 3°C/day. Treatment is also highly nuanced due to the varying clinical signs and strong associations to additional conditions and infections. Fluid therapy is administered in many cases, but the efficacy of this therapy varies greatly by case. Early administration of antifungals and antibiotics in chronically cold-stunned turtles is recommended (Innis and Staggs, 2017). Acutely cold-stunned turtles can be rehabilitated and typically released within 10 days. Chronically cold-stunned turtles often require longer time in care, with the duration of stay varying greatly by case. The turtles were free ranging and smeared in petroleum jelly to prevent flaking of shell.

Freshwater Turtles

The two main lineages of turtles living in freshwater habitats belong to the suborder Cryptodira (hidden-neck turtles) and Pleurodira (side-neck turtles). Like marine turtles, the hidden-neck turtles pull the neck and head straight back under the shell, while the side-neck turtles retract their neck and head under the shell by folding it to one side (Wilson and Swan, 2003).

Mating courtship occurs in the water in early spring. When ready to nest, females leave the water to excavate a nest hole where they lay their eggs. Once the eggs are deposited, the female fills in the nest and returns to the water, leaving the eggs to incubate on their own (Spencer and Thompson, 2003). The nesting migration could be a long, arduous trek over land, and concerned citizens occasionally bring healthy females into a clinic for rescue. Shell injury from traffic is very real though, and requires careful cleaning, reconstruction of shell, and long-term rehabilitation to allow for fractures to heal (Norton, 2005). The ability of turtles to cross over land is an important feature in their life history in response to nesting, habitat loss, food shortage, dangerous crossings, and rainfall events (Graham et al., 1996); it is also a risky activity, as it exposes them to predators and traffic trauma.

Freshwater turtles are vulnerable to many human and natural factors. They are a totem animal to First Nations people in many parts of the world, and although they are collected and consumed, such traditional harvest is not of conservation concern (Fordham et al., 2008). Modern-day habits of humans are, however, of grave concern to the survival of freshwater turtles. For example, large numbers of these turtles are accidentally caught and drowned in drum nets and crab pots and they are quite vulnerable to changes in water levels brought on by drought and human water use (Cann, 1998). Many populations of freshwater turtles are in decline as urban development causes loss of habitat and fragmentation of populations and especially nesting females are at risk of road mortality (Spinks et al., 2003; Aresco, 2005; Beaudry et al., 2008; Crawford et al., 2014). Predators are also a threat to freshwater turtles, in particular to nests and hatchlings (Thompson, 1983; Spencer and Thompson, 2005; Fordham et al., 2008).

Diseases of Freshwater Turtles: Transmission, Prevention, Treatment, and Control

Freshwater turtles, like any other animal, are susceptible to infections and transmission should be assumed to be via the water. The entry point may have been initiated by trauma, but poor environmental or captive conditions such as malnutrition or insufficient sanitation can predispose turtles to infections including abscesses, stomatitis, shell and skin disease, middle ear, and respiratory tract infection (Norton, 2005). In addition to antimicrobial treatment, it is therefore also of importance to address the living condition and diet of any captive animals and reduce spread to other individuals and wild animals by quarantine and biosecurity measures.

Bacterial Disease

Several of the bacterial species causing disease in freshwater turtles are naturally occurring environmental microorganisms that can opportunistically turn pathogenic (McKnight et al., 2020). Isolation of agents during a survey or disease investigation must therefore be assessed in context.

Several bacterial species of zoonotic potential have been reported in freshwater turtles without associated clinical signs (Hossain, 2021). The two bacterial species of common concern to pet owners are *Salmonella* spp. and *Aeromonas hydrophila*. Several studies have shown that *Salmonella* is extremely rare in free-ranging turtles (Mitchell et al., 1990; Saelinger et al., 2006), while captive populations tend to have a higher prevalence, presumably because of inappropriate husbandry conditions and stress (Mitchell et al., 1990; Stam et al., 2003).

A. hydrophila is ubiquitous in the freshwater environment and when present at low levels, it is considered a commensal. However, in weakened hosts or when environmental conditions are conducive to bacterial replication it can become an opportunistic pathogen with multiorgan involvement and high mortality rates (Pasquale et al, 1994; Ariel et al., 2017).

The softshell turtle intensive culture industry in China has revealed several cases of infections in turtles that could be of interest to other species and regions, such as Hsieh et al. (2006), who describe multiorgan infection of pond-cultured Chinese softshell turtles with *Mycobacterium marinum* as a common disease in China.

Viral Disease

There is not a vast amount of different viral diseases of freshwater turtles reported in the literature and this field will undoubtedly expand in the future. Some appear to have had sporadic significance in captive collections, including papillomavirus, and adenovirus (Doszpoly, 2013), while others have great economic impact on farmed turtles (Liu et al., 2017) or have brought an already threatened species to its knees (Chessmann et al., 2020). The arboviruses, have been investigated due to reptiles providing a reservoir for zoonotic arboviruses, but these do not cause any detectable pathology in the turtles themselves (Ariel, 2011). There are, however, viral representatives of the two major families of viruses that are repeatedly reported in turtles: the Iridoviridae and the Herpesviridae.

Ranavirus

Etiology *Ranavirus* is a genus in the Iridoviridae family represented by the type species frog virus 3 (FV3). Earlier accounts of iridovirus causing systemic infections were later classified as ranavirus in many cases. *Ranavirus* has received increasing attention due to its involvement in serious diseases of fish and amphibians, to the extent that epizootic hematopoietic necrosis virus in fish and ranavirus in general for amphibians meet the criteria for listing by the World Organisation for Animal Health (WOAH; 2016). Ranaviruses have been implicated in the worldwide decline of amphibians and mass mortalities in both aquaculture and wild fish stock.

Host Several instances of severe mortality events in turtles associated with ranavirus infections have been described in both zoological collections – mostly terrestrial tortoises (Benetka et al., 2007), free-ranging (McKenzie et al., 2019), and farmed turtles (Chen, 1999). Retrospective studies of archival material may bring even more cases to light and due to the extremely broad host range it is likely that many more species are susceptible and will be diagnosed and reported in the fullness of time.

Gross and Clinical Signs Infection targets multiple organs including the liver (Figure 4.8) stomach, esophagus, muscle, lung, spleen, and kidney, although some isolates may have a propensity for infecting the respiratory tract (Johnson et al., 2008; Allender et al., 2013).

Diagnosis Intracytoplasmic inclusion bodies can be identified in some cases and in addition to viral isolation in established cell lines (Ariel et al., 2009), diagnosis is made on the basis of immune assays and PCR targeting the major capsid protein or the polymerase gene (Holopainen et al., 2009). Immunohistochemistry techniques have been developed to demonstrate the presence of ranavirus antigens in the necrotic lesions and in individual cells (Ariel et al., 2015).

Treatment, Prevention, and Control Ranaviral infection and pathogenesis appears to be highly affected by environmental temperatures. (La Fauce et al., 2012; Allender et al., 2013) and this characteristic could be beneficially employed in a treatment situation by raising or lowering the ambient temperature of the enclosure. There are efforts under way to develop treatments against

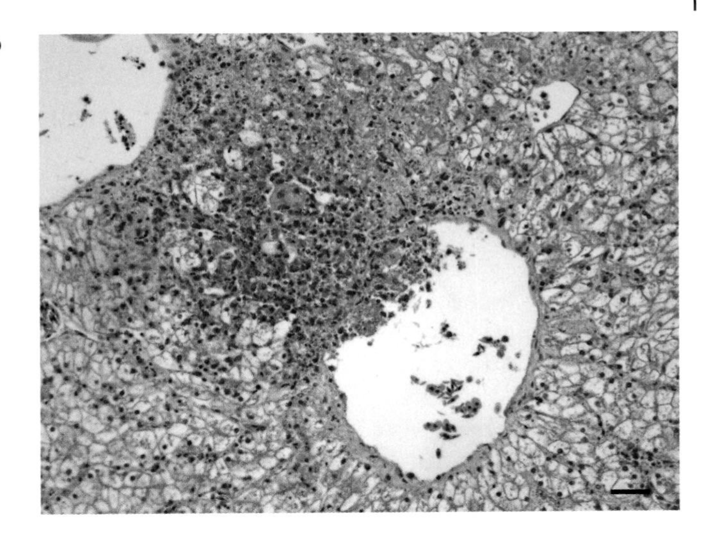

Figure 4.8 Necrotic area adjacent to a blood vessel in the liver of a freshwater turtle hatchling (*Emydura macquarii krefftii*) following intramuscular inoculation with frog virus 3 (Scale bar 40μm). *Source:* Courtesy of Wytamma Wirth.

infection, but currently general supportive care (hydration and treatment of other complications) is the mainstream approach.

The ranaviral isolates are very similar on a serological and molecular level (Pallister et al. 2007; Ariel et al., 2010) and have been reported to be able to infect hosts across classes (Moody and Owens, 1994; Mao et al., 1997; Ariel and Owens, 1997; Brenes et al., 2014). This ability of the virus has the potential to compromise prevention and control measures, since amphibians, reptiles, and fish may act as reservoir species for each other. Quarantine measures in collections and wildlife transfer should therefore consider a very large reservoir of potential carriers and multiple susceptible species.

Herpesvirus

Etiology Herpesvirus infections appear to manifest as acute signs, which may turn latent and be quiescent for the rest of the animal's life, or until the host becomes sufficiently stressed for the virus to reappear as a disease (Hoff and Hoff, 1984; Okoh et al., 2021). Chelonian herpesviruses fall into the family Herpesviridae, subfamily Alphaherpesvirinae, genus *Scutavirus* (Jungwirth, 2014; Sim, 2015).

Host Herpesvirus infection is well described in pet land tortoises as upper respiratory tract disease and necrotizing stomatitis, often associated with high mortality (Johnson et al., 2005). It is much less reported in freshwater turtles, however a herpesvirus was identified in an Australian captive freshwater turtle (*Emydura krefftii*) associated with skin lesions, but without apparent respiratory or intestinal involvement (Cowan et al., 2015).

Gross and Clinical Signs Clinical signs include nasal discharge, depression, and foaming at the mouth; pathological changes include hepatitis, stomatitis, respiratory tract infection, conjunctivitis, and central nervous system involvement (Cox, 1980; Marschang et al., 1997; Muro et al., 1998; Origgi et al., 2004; Hunt el al., 2006). A free-ranging Blandings turtle (*Emydoidea blandingii*) was recaptured with an intraoral squamous cell carcinoma (Anderson et al., 2021).

Diagnosis Eosinophilic, intranuclear inclusion bodies in cells of affected tissues are an indication that herpesvirus is involved in causing the pathology, which can also readily be confirmed with molecular diagnostics. Ossiboff et al. (2015) surveyed free-ranging populations of critically endangered bog turtles (*Glyptemys muhlenbergii*) in the United States and found that in excess of 50% were positive for herpesvirus PCR in cloacal swabs, although none of them showed clinical signs of ill health. These findings emphasize the latent lifestyle of herpesviruses and their ability to coexist with hosts without causing disease. Identification of herpesvirus in sick animals should therefore be considered with a grain of salt and careful reflection on an alternative etiology should be part of the final diagnosis.

Treatment, Prevention, and Control Optimal husbandry, supportive treatment, and potentially antiviral drugs for herpes and isolation of sick animals can reduce impact on a collection. In wild and captive animals, the disease may only be expressed under immunosuppressive conditions. The latent and subclinical nature of herpesviral infection makes prevention and control challenging.

Trionyx Sinensis Hemorrhagic Syndrome Virus

Trionyx sinensis hemorrhagic syndrome virus is a relatively recent arrival on the scene of the soft-shell turtle industry in China, with fatal outcome (Liu et al., 2017). The turtles initially show signs of hypoxia and inability to hold their neck. In experimental infection trials, this stage appeared four days post-infection. Gross symptoms included hyperemic laryngeal mucosa, an enlarged liver, and severe congestion in liver, kidney, and intestines. Histopathological changes consisted of necrosis of hepatocytes and mucosal epithelial cells, with changes to cellular architecture, nuclear dissolution, and severe congestion of capillaries in all organs (Liu et al., 2017). It appears that there could be several viruses at play in the softshell turtle industry, hampering its success, and the coming years may cast more light on this field.

Nidoviruses

Overview The most infamous nidovirus these days is the severe acute respiratory syndrome coronavirus 2 (SARS CoV-2) that is responsible for the COVID-19 pandemic. Nidoviruses are capable of infecting a wide range of both vertebrate and invertebrate hosts, often with severe and fatal outcome, and since the first discovery of nidovirus infection in snakes in 2014, the number of reported infections in reptiles is on the rise (Parrish et al., 2021).

Etiology The nidoviruses discovered in reptiles are pleomorphic, positive-strand RNA viruses in the subfamily Serpentovirineae, family Tobaviridae, suborder Tornidovirineae, order Nidovirales. Reptile nidoviruses are newly discovered and emerging as significant pathogens globally, often inflicting severe respiratory disease in captive pythons. This apparent increase may be due to a heightened awareness and better diagnostic tools, combined with close-quarter housing of collections (Marschang and Kolesnik, 2016).

Host Range and Transmission Nidoviruses have been detected in snakes and lizards with respiratory disease and without clinical signs, but the only freshwater turtle isolate was associated with high mortality in a wild population of Bellinger river snapping turtle (*Myuchelys georgesi*). This turtle is restricted to just one catchment in Australia and the disease outbreak brought this species to the brink of extinction. In captive collections of snakes, nidovirus infection can spread rapidly with great detriment, but the factors influencing the transmission and disease risk in free-living reptiles is largely unexplored (Zhang et al., 2018).

Gross and Clinical Signs Whereas nidovirus infection in snakes and lizards is reported to be associated with infection of the respiratory tract, the kidneys appeared to be the target organ of the

Bellinger river virus in freshwater turtles. Histological examination and in–situ hybridization have identified a broader cell and tissue tropism. In snakes, the early symptoms of increased mucus secretion from nostrils and mouth are followed by oral inflammation, coughing and wheezing, open–mouth breathing, and increased respiratory rate. This is accompanied by lethargy, in appetence, dehydration, and difficulty perching (Zhang et al., 2018).

Diagnosis Although the virus can grow in cell culture, the direct detection of the virus is generally via molecular detection such as real time and conventional reverse transcription PCR or in situ–hybridization (Parrish et al., 2021).

Treatment, Prevention, and Control There are no current antiviral treatments tested in reptiles, so supportive care and suitable husbandry conditions to encourage a good immune response is the best option. Good biosecurity practices in captive collections such as quarantine and screening procedures will go a long way in preventing introduction of this and other pathogens into a collection. Quarantine of sick animals, high level of hygiene, separation of equipment, and a daily husbandry procedure flowing from healthy to sick animals will reduce the spread within the collection (Parrish et al., 2021).

Fungal Disease

Fungal infections in freshwater turtles seem to mainly target the soft skin (mycotic dermatitis) or the lungs (pulmonary mycosis) associated with anorexia and mortality. Most reports are from captive animals kept in suboptimal conditions (Table 4.1). The infections are often fatal without intervention, and great emphasis should be placed on accurate diagnosis via morphological characteristics and sequence analysis, followed by suitable treatment to save remaining animals in a collection. Recently, a new onygenalean fungus, *Emydomyces testavorans*, has been described associated with slow progressing shell lesions in freshwater turtles although causality is yet to be determined (Woodburn et al., 2019 and 2021).

Parasites

Most accounts of parasites in freshwater turtles are concerned with discoveries of new parasites and prevalence studies and on no occasion do they refer to any clinical effect on wild living host animals (Goes et al., 2018). Hemogregarines, in particular, may occur in up to 100% of wild populations studied and several species of parasites are regularly reported to infect individual turtles (El Hili et al., 2021). It is therefore assumed that in most wild populations examined, a balanced relationship exists between the blood parasite, if present, and the host (Pineda-Catalan et al., 2013). External leeches are also regularly reported on freshwater turtles from the wild, with no apparent ill effect (Fediras, 2017). There is evidence that some of these may just be detritus feeders on the biome associated with the turtle (Marrone, 2016).

The prevalence of parasites in captive collections, especially captive–reared turtles, appears to be much lower, where good husbandry practice undoubtedly contributes to breaking the infection cycle (Nordmeyer et al., 2020). Parasitic infection can have a lethal outcome in captive freshwater turtles, though, as evidenced in a research collection, where over a period of several years, 16 animals died. Postmortem investigations revealed trematodiasis in all animals. Presence of spirorchiid eggs and associated granulomas in multiple organs were causing blockage of capillaries, necrosis, and bacteremia, while no adult parasites were found (Johnson et al., 1998).

Table 4.1 Fungal species recorded in freshwater turtles with reference to species of turtle and type of lesion.

Fungal species	Turtle species	Lesion	References
Emydomyces testavorans	*Actinemys marmorata*	Shell lesions	Woodburn et al. 2019; Woodburn et al. 2021; Lambert et al. 2021
Paeciliomyces lilacinus	*Trionyx sinens, Carettochelys insculpta*	Mycotic dermatitis	Li et al. 2008; Lafortune et al. 2005
Aphanomyces sinensis	*Pelodiscus sinensis*	Mycotic dermatitis	Takuma et al. 2010; Sinmuk et al. 1996
Chrysosporium sp.	*Carettochelys insculpta*	Mycotic dermatitis	Ward et al. 2012
Mucor sp.	*Trionyx ferox*	Mycotic dermatitis	Jacobson et al. 1980
Beauveria bassiniana	*Trachemys scripta*	Pulmonary mycosis	Cabo et al. 1995
Candida albicans	*Emys orbicularis*	Pulmonary candidiasis, stomatitis	Köbölkuti et al. 2016

Quarantine of new animals added to a collection until treated with antihelminthic drugs may kill adult parasites, but the damage done by eggs can still cause lethal pathology.

Crocodilians

Crocodiles, alligators, gharials, and caimans comprise the order Crocodilia. Animals within this order are typically large and semiaquatic with a tropical to subtropical distribution. Unlike many other species discussed in this chapter, crocodilians are also used by many regions in animal production systems. The need to minimize stock losses and ensure the quality of both meat and/or skin is driving the research into diseases of captive or farmed crocodilians.

Prevention and Control of Crocodilian Diseases

Disease in wild crocodilians is difficult to prevent and control but the regulated environment in captive settings lends itself to more effectively managing their health and disease. Like most production settings, high-quality feed provision, suitable stocking densities, favorable temperature gradients, and a general low-stress environment lends itself to optimal health of captive crocodilians. However, disease outbreaks are still possible and facility protocols should aim to reduce this risk where possible.

Decontamination of equipment before use in each enclosure, the use of barriers to restrict interaction between captive and wild crocodilians, and obtaining water from a clean source are recommended prevention measures (Gieger and Furmaga, 2021). Maintaining separate facilities for breeding and rearing and quarantining new animals before introducing them to a facility will likely aid in prevention. Suspected outbreaks should be controlled through disinfecting the contaminated enclosure. This includes disinfecting and draining the water in this pen. Gieger and Furmaga (2021) recommend that all pens be disinfected and have their water changed daily during this period. Outbreaks can be minimized by quarantining and treating of animals showing clinical signs of disease. Prophylactic treatment, including some antibiotics and antifungals, can further reduce the risk of outbreak.

Viral Disease

Poxviral Infections

Overview First described by Jacobson et al. (1979) in captive caimans, poxviral infection has now been reported in several genera of crocodilians. Characterized by external lesions, this infection can result in high morbidity, while mortality is typically low (Afonso et al., 2006). This disease is most significant in farmed crocodilians. Although not formally listed by the WOAH, poxviral infection is presently the only crocodilian disease for which the WOAH provides a technical disease card (Gieger and Furmaga, 2021).

Etiology This disease is caused by an infection with a poxvirus. To date, two viral strains have been genomically characterized, with one largely infecting the Nile crocodile (*Crocodylus niloticus*) and another primarily infecting the saltwater crocodile (*Crocodylus porosus*).

Host Range and Transmission Poxviral infection has been reported in captive *Caiman* spp., Nile crocodile, saltwater crocodile, and freshwater crocodile (*Crocodylus johnstoni*). Often reported in juvenile hatchling and juvenile animals less than two years of age (Gieger and Furmaga, 2021). Transmission is suspected to be facilitated by contact with skin lesions, contaminated fomites and/or water, and ingestion of contaminated feed and/or water (Gieger and Furmaga, 2021). Sarker et al. (2019) investigated infection dynamics through evolutionary genomics but noted that further research was needed.

Gross and Clinical Signs Presentation varies between hosts, with gray–white lesions that are flat to slightly depressed observed in caimans, saltwater crocodiles, and freshwater crocodiles (Ramos et al., 2002; Buenviaje et al., 2000). In Nile crocodiles, this infection manifests as raised, brown, circular, ulcerated lesions (Foggin, 1987; Huchzermeyer and Putterill, 1991; Horner, 1988). Typical lesion locations are the head, eyes, and oral mucosa, but it is possible to observe them in any location on the body. Small penetrations in the ventral coelomic scales of Nile crocodiles are characteristic of a secondary presentation of poxviral infection (Huchzermeyer et al., 2009).

Diagnosis and Differential Diagnosis Diagnosis can be confirmed through amplification of poxviral DNA using molecular biology techniques or observation of ballooning of epidermal cells, eosinophilic intracytoplasmic inclusions, and Bollinger and/or Borrel bodies in skin lesion samples (Gieger and Furmaga, 2021). Other conditions to consider as differential diagnosis include nutritional disease, conjunctivitis, mycobacteriosis, West Nile virus, dermatophilosis (brown spot disease), chlamydiosis (blindness) and respiratory infection (Gieger and Furmaga, 2021).

Treatment No specific treatment has been proposed, but the damaged tissue can be removed and/or disinfected and prophylactic treatment for secondary infections may be helpful (Gieger and Furmaga, 2021).

Systemic Lymphoproliferative Syndrome With Encephalitis

Overview Systemic lymphoproliferative syndrome with encephalitis (SLPE) is an emerging disease of captive saltwater crocodiles (Shilton et al., 2016) linked to increased mortalities in pens (Conley and Shilton, 2018).

Etiology The etiological agent of SLPE has not been confirmed. This disease has been associated with herpesviral infection, most likely crocodyline herpesvirus 2 (Hyndman et al., 2015; Shilton et al., 2016). However, this relationship needs further investigation (Conley and Shilton, 2018).

Host Range and Transmission SLPE is typically reported in juvenile saltwater crocodiles (Conley and Shilton, 2018). As an etiological link has not yet been firmly established, the mode of transmission is not yet understood.

Gross and Clinical Signs The disease is characterized by ill thrift and poor growth. Other gross clinical signs are less common, but can present as pulmonary edema, conjunctival hyperemia and/or splenomegaly (Conley and Shilton, 2018). Histological signs include lymphohistiocytic infiltrates in the brain, eye, cardiovascular system, portal tracts in the liver, pulmonary and pancreatic interstitium, and submucosa throughout the gastrointestinal tract (Conley and Shilton, 2018; Shilton et al., 2016).

Diagnosis and Differential Diagnosis Observation of these histopathological signs would support a diagnosis of SLPE. Amplification of herpesviral DNA from such cases is indicative of SLPE, but not considered a confirmatory diagnosis at present. Two other crocodilian diseases, conjunctivitis/pharyngitis and lymphonodular skin lesions, have been linked to herpesviral infection (Conley and Shilton, 2018; Hyndman et al., 2015; Shilton et al., 2016) and these should also be considered when investigating potential cases of SLPE.

Treatment No current treatment regimen has been proposed.

Adenoviral infection

Overview Adenoviral infection has been linked to mortality in farmed Nile crocodiles.

Etiology Though ultrastructural findings are indicative of adenoviral infection, the exact etiological agent has not been formally characterized.

Host Range and Transmission Captive juvenile Nile crocodiles (Pfitzer et al., 2019; Jacobson et al., 1984; Foggin, 1992; Foggin, 1987). The transmission pathway of this disease is presently data deficient.

Gross and Clinical Signs Signs of general ill health, including lethargy and emaciation have been linked to this disease (Huchzermeyer, 2002). Adenoviral infection in crocodilians is associated with hepatitis and/or enteritis (Conley and Shilton, 2018; Jacobson et al., 1984; Foggin, 1992; Foggin, 1987). Hepatic disease caused by adenoviral infection can present as liver enlargement and mottling, while thickening of the intestinal wall is characteristic of intestinal disease.

Diagnosis and Differential Diagnosis Diagnosis is presently achieved through histopathology (Conley and Shilton, 2018; Pfitzer et al., 2019). Hepatitis in Nile crocodiles has also been linked to chlamydial infection (Huchzermeyer and Limper, 1994) and the two pathogens are often found together (Huchzermeyer, 2002).

Treatment No current treatment regimen has been proposed.

West Nile Viral Disease

Overview Disease caused by West Nile virus has the potential to cause relatively high mortality in farmed crocodilians. West Nile Virus is an arbovirus spread by mosquitos (vectors) and therefore it can be spread by a range of species. This virus does not always elicit disease in infected animals but because it is a zoonotic disease that can be very serious in humans, it is a virus of concern to the WOAH.

Etiology Disease induced by infection with the West Nile virus.

Host Range and Transmission Hatchling and juvenile American alligators (*Alligator mississippiensis*) in captive settings are most severely affected by West Nile virus (Conley and Shilton, 2018; Jacobson et al., 2005; Miller et al., 2003; Nevarez et al., 2005). However, this virus also infects the Nile crocodile (Steinman et al., 2003; Simulundu et al., 2020) and saltwater crocodiles (Isberg et al., 2019). Although transmission is thought to be mosquito-borne, Habarugira et al. (2020) report on mosquito-independent transmission of this virus in saltwater crocodiles, highlighting the possibility of both mosquito- and waterborne viral transmission, in addition to vaccination strategies (Habarugira et al., 2020).

Gross and Clinical Signs Clinical signs of West Nile virus infection in crocodilians vary greatly. Weakness, lethargy, emaciation, swimming in circles, head tilt, and muscle tremors are all indicative of this disease (Nevarez, 2006). However, Conley and Shilton (2018) also note gross pathologic signs to be coelomic effusion, fibrinonecrotic colitis, oropharyngeal fibrinonecrotic inflammation, intestinal hemorrhage, and tan foci or mottling of the liver, spleen, kidneys, and/or heart. Histologic signs include heterophilic to lymphoplasmacytic meningoencephalitis with variable spinal cord involvement.

Diagnosis and Differential Diagnosis Amplification of the West Nile virus genome (or a fragment of) through reverse transcriptase PCR and isolation of the virus from the brain and spinal cord through culture-based methods is recommended for a definitive diagnosis (Nevarez, 2006). Lymphohistiocytic proliferative syndrome of alligators has been associated with West Nile virus infection (Nevarez et al., 2008).

Treatment No current treatment regimen has been proposed. However, animals that survive the course of infection will continue to thrive (Nevarez, 2006).

Parasitic Disease

Cutaneous Paratrichosomiasis

Overview Reported in both wild and captive crocodilian populations, cutaneous paratrichosomiasis is not thought to cause clinically significant disease, but lesions associated with this infection can negatively impact hide appearance (Conley and Shilton, 2018). The potential impact on commercial value makes it a disease of note in farmed crocodilians (Lott et al., 2015).

Etiology Infection with nematodes belonging to the *Paratrichosoma* genus, namely *Paratrichosoma crocodylus* and *Paratrichosoma recurvum* (Charruau et al., 2017).

Host Factors and Transmission *Paratrichosoma* spp. can afflict saltwater, freshwater, American, and Morelet's crocodiles (Conley and Shilton, 2018). Several modes of infection have been proposed, but significant gaps in the lifecycle of these nematodes have so far hampered confirmation (Charruau et al., 2017).

Gross and Clinical Signs Conley and Shilton (2018) describe gross lesions associated with cutaneous paratrichosomiasis to appear as serpentine, tightly curved to hairpin, darkly colored, "zigzag trails" on the lateral or ventral skin.

Diagnosis and Differential Diagnosis Observation of the characteristic gross signs coupled with histological findings consistent with nematode infection can be considered a reliable diagnosis. These features include clear cores containing operculated and larvated eggs located within the stratum corneum and underlying epidermal layers (Conley and Shilton, 2018). Molecular methods may also be used to characterize isolated nematodes down to the species level (Lott et al., 2015).

Other helminth infections of note include astric ascaridiasis (caused by nematode infection) and pentastomiasis (linked to pentastome infection). While these infections can make affected crocodilians susceptible to secondary infections, they do not typically cause clinical or severe disease (Conley and Shilton, 2018). They should, however, be considered in differential diagnoses.

Treatment No current treatment regimen has been proposed. Lott et al. (2015) suggested that the high genetic diversity observed in *Paratrichosoma* spp. increases the likelihood of anthelmintic resistance, further hindering treatment efforts.

Coccidiosis

Overview Coccidiosis is of particular interest to captive crocodilians because of its potential to cause mortality in afflicted animals. Case reports of this disease are well summarized in Duszynski et al. (2020).

Etiology Infection with protozoans belonging to the subclass Coccidia can elicit this disease. To date, species identification of the agent has proved challenging. While yet to be confirmed, the primary agent is morphologically similar to *Goussia* spp. (Conley and Shilton, 2018).

Host Factors and Transmission Coccidiosis has been reported in saltwater, Nile, and New Guinea crocodiles. Mode of transmission is currently unknown.

Gross and Clinical Signs Lethargy and general ill thrift are characteristic of this disease. Oocysts or sporocysts can be detected during necropsy.

Diagnosis and Differential Diagnosis Histopathological examination remains the recommended means of diagnosis; diagnosis through fecal floats and intestinal smears have proved challenging due to the fragility of the oocysts (Duszynski et al., 2020, Huchzermeyer, 2002). Histological findings consistent with coccidiosis include mural fibrosis, marked lymphohistiocytic and plasmacytic enteritis, and multifocal granulomas (Conley and Shilton, 2018).

Treatment Huchzermeyer (2002) recommends mixing sulfachloropyrazine into the feed ration.

Bacterial disease

Overview

Bacterial disease in crocodilians can elicit a range of conditions, affecting a range of body systems. Such disease is of interest to commercially produced species as it has the potential to cause skin lesions and in severe cases, mortality.

Etiology

Bacteria of major consideration in diseases of crocodilians include Mycoplasma spp., *Chlamydia* spp., *Mycobacterium* spp., dermatophilus-like bacteria, *Salmonella* spp. and *Providencia rettgeri* (Conley and Shilton, 2018; Huchzermeyer, 2002; Nevarez, 2006).

Host Factors and Transmission

Considering their natural habitat in often stagnant water, crocodiles are exposed to a multitude of bacteria in their close environment at all times. It is no wonder then that reports of bacterial disease is common in all crocodilians. This close exposure to environmental and pathogenic bacteria is especially challenging in captive pens with high density of animals. High nutritional load and aggression may be potential entry points.

Gross and Clinical Signs

A range of body systems can be affected by bacterial disease in crocodilians. Morbidity and mortality vary with species and individual cases but clinical signs can include arthritis, pneumonia, pericarditis, polyserositis, conjunctivitis, hepatitis, splenic lesions, spleen, pulmonary edema, and multifocal necrosis in the coelomic fat, skin lesions, enteritis, and systemic infection (Conley and Shilton, 2018).

Diagnosis and Differential Diagnosis

It can be challenging to separate pathogenic bacteria from the natural crocodilian flora. Moreover, some species of interest (e.g.) *Mycobacterium* spp. can be difficult to isolate (Nevarez, 2006). Diagnosis can be achieved through isolation of bacterial species using culture-based methods and/or molecular methods, combined with clinical signs which correlate to the species isolated.

Treatment

While prevention through best practice in hygiene and quarantine is recommended, outbreaks of bacterial disease may be treated with antibiotics suitable for the specific strain. Some species will be more responsive to treatment than others; *Dermatophilus congolensis* does not respond well to this form of treatment (Nevarez, 2006).

Nutritional Disease

Overview

Captive crocodilians are susceptible to a range of nutritional diseases including hypovitaminosis E, pansteatitis, hypovitaminosis A and thiamine deficiency (Conley and Shilton, 2018).

Etiology

Rancid feed and/or diets comprised of fish high in polyunsaturated fatty acids have been linked to hypovitaminosis E. Meat-only diets without vitamin A supplementation can elicit hypovitaminosis A. Multiple cycles of freezing and thawing feed can degrade thiamine in the food source. Similarly, diets high in fish can contain high levels of thiaminases which cause enzymatic destruction of thiamine. Each or both of these cases can lead to thiamine deficiency in farmed crocodilians (Conley and Shilton, 2018).

Host Factors and Transmission

All captive crocodilians are susceptible to nutritional disease. Transmission is not applicable.

Gross and Clinical Signs

Firm, yellow/brown adipose that is either discrete nodular or diffuse is characteristic of hypovitaminosis E. Depending on the location of these lesions, the hardened fat can negatively impact mobility of the tail and gastrointestinal tract motility (Conley and Shilton, 2018; Jackson and

Cooper, 1981). Squamous metaplasia is associated with hypovitaminosis A. Gross clinical signs include multiple nodules on the dorsal surface of the tongue, renal and visceral gout, and secondary tubulonephritis (Ariel et al., 1997). Signs of thiamine deficiency include lethargy, buoyancy disorder, head tilt, stargazing, limb paresis, and anisocoria (Huchzermeyer, 2003; Schoeb et al., 2002).

Diagnosis and Differential Diagnosis

Inflammation, saponification, hemorrhage, necrosis, and bands of fibrous connective tissue may be observed under histologic examination of hypovitaminosis E lesions (Conley and Shilton, 2018; Jackson and Cooper, 1981). Hypovitaminosis A can be confirmed through observation of squamous metaplasia in the lingual glands and nephron (Ariel et al., 1997). Although there are no gross lesions associated with thiamine deficiency in crocodilians, gray matter necrosis has been observed under histological examination in afflicted American alligators (Conley and Shilton, 2018).

Treatment

A thorough investigation of diet and rectification with supplements or alternative feed is recommended.

Gout

Overview

Gout is characterized by excess uric acid being deposited in joints and/or other tissues as a result of uric acid levels exceeding the renal threshold for clearance. Crocodilians can be afflicted by both articular and visceral forms of gout (Conley and Shilton, 2018).

Etiology

A range of factors contribute to gout development including stress, dehydration, high protein diets and low environmental temperature (Nevarez, 2006; Huchzermeyer, 2002).

Host Factors and Transmission

All farmed crocodilians are susceptible to gout. Transmission is not applicable.

Gross and Clinical Signs

Clinical signs of gout in live animals may be nonspecific but can include limb paresis and joint enlargement (Nevarez, 2006). White deposits, typically of a chalky to gritty consistency in and around both joints and viscera are strong indications of gout.

Diagnosis and Differential Diagnosis

Cytological methods can be employed to confirm uric acid accumulation. Observation of uric acid crystal accumulation (gout tophi) under histological investigation is also indicative of gout. In most visceral locations, gout tophi can have a sporadic distribution and minimal damage to the surrounding tissue. However, in the kidney, tophi are typically located within the tubules and/or parenchymal tissues and damage to surrounding tissue is not uncommon (Conley and Shilton, 2018).

Treatment

There may be some linkage between gout and hypervitaminosis A (Ariel et al., 1997) that should be considered along with other nutritional requirements.

Marine Iguanas

The vulnerable marine iguana (*Amblyrhynchus cristates*) is endemic to the Galápagos Islands, Ecuador. The early geological separation of this archipelago from the mainland is thought to have isolated marine iguanas from a range of pathogens, and without immunity to these they are therefore highly susceptible to pathogen-induced diseases introduced to these islands (MacLeod et al., 2020). The presence of trematodes (Pronocephalidae), bacteria (*Vibrio alginolyticus*) and mosquito bites (*Aedes taeniorhynchus*) have been reported (Bataille et al., 2012; Thaller et al., 2010; Gilbert, 1938). However, in each case the presence of these pathogens did not appear to have a hugely pathologic effect on the marine iguanas studied. An unusual mortality in 2013 was linked to infection with a novel alphaherpesvirus but this was not definitively confirmed (García-Parra et al., 2014). The paucity of reports on disease in marine iguanas has precluded further discussion of this species in this chapter, however, through close monitoring of their health, more case studies are bound to be published in the future.

Sea Snakes

Comprising the Elapidae subfamily of Hydrophiinae, true sea snakes are highly adapted to aquatic life; among several differences between true sea snakes and other elapids, key adaptations to the marine environment include their viviparous reproduction and possession of a paddle-shaped tail, valve-like nostrils, and a sublingual salt gland (Gillett et al., 2017). Sea kraits, belonging to the Laticaudinae subfamily, are semiaquatic and therefore not considered to be true sea snakes. However, it is possible that diseases afflicting sea snakes may also be reported in sea kraits, so in this context the two subfamilies are considered together. Despite this diverse group comprising over 60 individual species, reports of disease in sea snakes are limited (Udyawer et al., 2018; Gillett, 2017). This may be due to the challenges associated with studying such species in the wild (access, capture, and handling) in addition to their lack of commercial value. The scarcity of well-characterized sea snake diseases prevents a more detailed discussion in this chapter. However, the role of disease in sea snake population decline has been identified by experts as a key research question for future research (Udyawer et al., 2018). The increased interest in sea snake research will likely aid in characterizing major diseases afflicting sea snakes. Readers should note they can access a summary of case reports on this topic in section 1.8 of Gillett (2017).

Bibliography

Abreu-Grobois A, Plotkin P. 2008. Olive ridley: Lepidochelys *olivacea*. The IUCN Red List of Threatened Species, version 2022-1. International Union for Conservation of Nature and Natural Resources. Available: https://dx.doi.org/10.2305/IUCN.UK.2008.RLTS.T11534A3292503.en (accessed 6 September 2022).

Afonso CL, Tulman ER, Delhon G, et al. 2006. Genome of Crocodilepox Virus. *J Virol* 80:4978–4991.

Aguirre AA, Lutz PL. 2004. Marine turtles as sentinels of ecosystem health: is fibropapillomatosis an indicator? *EcoHealth* 1:275–283.

Ahasan MS, Kinobe R, Elliott L, et al. 2019. Bacteriophage versus antibiotic therapy on gut bacterial communities of juvenile green turtle, *Chelonia mydas*. *Environ Microbiol* 21:2871–2885.

Ahasan MS, Waltzek TB, Huerlimann R, Ariel E. 2017. Fecal bacterial communities of wild-captured and stranded green turtles (*Chelonia mydas*) on the Great Barrier Reef. *FEMS Microbiol Ecol* 93(12):fix139.

Ahasan MS, Waltzek TB, Huerlimann R, Ariel E. 2018. Comparative analysis of gut bacterial communities of green turtles (*Chelonia mydas*) pre-hospitalization and post-rehabilitation by high-throughput sequencing of bacterial 16S rRNA gene. *Microbiol Res* 207:91–99.

Ahasan MS, Waltzek TB, Owens L, Ariel E. 2020. Characterisation and comparison of the mucosa-associated bacterial communities across the gastrointestinal tract of stranded green turtles, *Chelonia mydas*. *AIMS Microbiol* 6:361–378.

Allender MC, Mitchell MA, Torres T, et al. 2013. Pathogenicity of frog virus 3-like virus in red-eared slider turtles (*Trachemys scripta elegans*) at two environmental temperatures. *J Compar Pathol* 149:356–367.

Andersson KE, Adamovicz L, Mumm LE, et al. 2021. Detection of a novel herpesvirus associated with squamous cell carcinoma in a free-ranging Blanding's turtle. *J Vet Diagnost Invest* 33:348–351.

Aresco MJ. 2005. The effect of sex-specific terrestrial movements and roads on the sex ratio of freshwater turtles. *Biol Conserv* 123:37–44.

Ariel E. 2011. Viruses in reptiles. *Vet Res* 42:100–100.

Ariel E, Freeman AB, Elliott E, et al. 2017. An unusual mortality event in Johnstone River snapping turtles Elseya irwini (Johnstone) in far north Queensland, *Australia. Aust Vet J* 95(10):355–361.

Ariel E, Holopainen R, Olesen NJ, Tapiovaara H. 2010. Comparative study of ranavirus isolates from cod (Gadus morhua) and turbot (Psetta maxima) with reference to other ranaviruses. *Arch Virol* 155:1261–1271.

Ariel E, Ladds PW, Buenviaje GN. 1997. Concurrent gout and suspected hypovitaminosis A in crocodile hatchlings. *Aust Vet J* 75:247–249.

Ariel E, Nicolajsen N, Christophersen M-B, et al. 2009. Propagation and isolation of ranaviruses in cell culture. *Aquaculture* 294:159–164.

Ariel E, Owens L. 1997. Epizootic mortalities in tilapia Oreochromis mossambicus. *Dis Aquat Organ* 29(1):1–6.

Ariel E, Wirth W, Burgess G, et al. 2015. Pathogenicity in six Australian reptile species following experimental inoculation with Bohle iridovirus. *Dis Aquat Organ* 115(3):203–212.

Barten S, Simpson S. 2019. Differential diagnoses by clinical signs: Lizards. In: Divers SJ, Stahl, SJ, ed. *Mader's Reptile and Amphibian Medicine and Surgery*, 3rd ed., 1257–1265. Philadelphia, PA: Elsevier Saunders.

Bataille A, Fournié G, Cruz M, Cedeño V, et al. 2012. Host selection and parasite infection in Aedes taeniorhynchus, endemic disease vector in the Galápagos Islands. *Infect Genet Evolut* 12:1831–1841.

Beaudry F, deMaynadier PG, Hunter ML. 2008. Identifying road mortality threat at multiple spatial scales for semi-aquatic turtles. *Biol Conserv* 141:2550–2563.

Benetka V, Grabensteiner E, Gumpenberger M, et al. 2007. First report of an iridovirus (Genus *Ranavirus*) infection in a Leopard tortoise (*Geochelone pardalis pardalis*). *Wiener Tierarztl Monatsschr* 94(9/10):243.

Boyer TH. 2019. Differential diagnoses by clinical signs: Chelonians. In: Divers SJ, Stahl, SJ, ed. *Mader's Reptile and Amphibian Medicine and Surgery*, 3rd ed., 126–1275. Philadelphia, PA: Elsevier Saunders.

Brenes R, Miller DL, Waltzek TB, et al. 2014. Susceptibility of fish and turtles to three ranaviruses isolated from different ectothermic vertebrate classes. *J Aqua Anim Health* 26:118–126.

Buenviaje G, Hirst RG, Summers PM. 2000. *Skin Diseases of Farmed Crocodiles: A Report for the Rural Industries Research and Development Corporation*. Canberra, Australia: Rural Industries Research and Development Corporation.

Cabo JFG, Serrano JE, Asensio MCB. 1995. Mycotic pulmonary disease by Beauveria bassiana in a captive tortoise. *Mycoses*, 38:167–169.

Cann J. 1998. *Australian freshwater turtles*. Singapore: Beaumont Publishing.

Casale P, Tucker AD. 2017. *The IUCN Red List of Threatened Species: Caretta caretta (amended version of 2015 assessment)* [Online]. Available: https://dx.doi.org/10.2305/IUCN.UK.2017-2.RLTS.T3897A119333622.en (accessed 6 September 2022).

Chapman PA, Cribb TH, Flint M, et al. 2019. Spirorchiidiasis in marine turtles: the current state of knowledge. *Dis Aquat Organ* 133:217–245.

Chapman PA, Owen H, Flint M, et al. 2016. Molecular characterization of coccidia associated with an epizootic in green sea turtles (*Chelonia mydas*) in south east Queensland, Australia. *PloS ONE*, 11:e0149962–e0149962.

Charruau P, Pérez-Flores JS, Labarre D. 2017. Skin parasitism by Paratrichosoma recurvum in wild American crocodiles and its relation to environmental and biological factors. *Dis Aquat Organ* 122:205–211.

Chen Z-X, Zheng JC, Jiang Y-L. 1999. A new iridovirus isolated from soft-shelled turtle. *Virus Res*, 63:147–151.

Chessman BC, McGilvray G, Ruming S, Jones HA, et al. 2020. On a razor's edge: Status and prospects of the critically endangered Bellinger River snapping turtle, *Myuchelys georgesi. Aquat Conserv* 30(3):586–600.

Coberley SS, Herbst LH, Brown DR, Ehrhart LM, et al. 2001. Detection of antibodies to a disease-associated herpesvirus of the green turtle, *Chelonia mydas. J Clin Microbiol* 39:3572–3577.

Coberley SS, Condit RC, Herbst LH, Klein PA. 2002. Identification and expression of immunogenic proteins of a disease-associated marine turtle herpesvirus. *J Virol*, 76:10553–10558.

Conley KJ, Shilton CM. 2018. Crocodilia. In: Terio KA, McAloose D, St Leger J, eds. *Pathology of Wildlife and Zoo Animals*, 855–870. Cambridge, MA: Academic Press.

Cowan ML, Raidal SR, Peters A. 2015. Herpesvirus in a captive Australian Krefft's river turtle (*Emydura macquarii krefftii*). *Aust Vet J* 93:46–49.

Cox WR, Rapley WA, Barker IK. 1980. Herpesvirus-like infection in a painted turtle (*Chrysemys picta*). *J Wildl Dis* 16:445–449.

Crawford BA, Maerz JC, Nibbelink NP, et al. 2014. Estimating the consequences of multiple threats and management strategies for semi-aquatic turtles. *J Appl Ecol* 51:359–366.

Cribb TH, Crespo–Picazo JL, Cutmore SC, et al. 2017. Elucidation of the first definitively identified life cycle for a marine turtle blood fluke (Trematoda: Spirorchiidae) enables informed control. *Int J Parasitol* 47:61–67.

Doneley B. 2018. Taxonomy and introduction to common species. In: Doneley B, Monks D, Johnson R, Carmel B, eds. *Reptile Medicine and Surgery in Clinical Practice*, 1–14. Oxford, UK: Wiley Blackwell.

Doszpoly A, Wellehan JFX, Childress AL, et al. 2013. Partial characterization of a new adenovirus lineage discovered in testudinoid turtles. *Infect Genet Evol* 17:106–112.

Doupe RG, Schaffer J, Knott MJ, Dicky PW. 2009. A description of freshwater turtle habitat destruction by feral pigs in tropical north eastern Australia. *Herpetol Conserv Biol* 4(3):331–339.

Duszynski DW, Mcallister CT, Tellez M. 2020. The Coccidia (Apicomplexa) of the Archosauria (Crocodylia: Eusuchia) of the World. *J Parasitol* 106:90–122.

El Hili RA, Achouri MS, Verneau O. 2021. Cytochrome c oxydase I phylogenetic analysis of Haemogregarina parasites (Apicomplexa, Coccidia, Eucoccidiorida, Haemogregarinidae) confirms the presence of three distinct species within the freshwater turtles of Tunisia. *Parasitol Int* 82:102306–102306.

Fediras S, Rouag R, Ziane N, et al. 2017. Prevalence of Placobdella costata (Fr. Mûller, 1846) (Hirudinida: Glossiphoniidae) on the European pond turtle (*Emys orbicularis*) in the North–East of Algeria. *Herpetol Notes* 10:3–8.

Flint M, Limpus DJ, Limpus CJ, et al. 2011. Biochemical and hematological reference intervals for Krefft's turtles Emydura macquarii krefftii from the Burnett River Catchment, Australia. *Dis Aquat Organ* 95:43–48.

Foggin CM. 1992. Disease trends on crocodile farms in Zimbabwe. *Proceedings of the 11th Working Meeting of the Crocodile Specialist Group of the Species Survival Commission*, 107–110. Gland, Switzerland: IUCN.

Foggin CM. 1987. Diseases and disease control on crocodile farms in Zimbabwe. In: Webb GJW, Manolis SC, Whitehead PJ, eds. *Wildlife management: crocodiles and alligators*, 351-–362. New South Wales, Australia: Surrey Beatty.

Fordham DA, Georges A, Brook BW. 2008. Indigenous harvest, exotic pig predation and local persistence of a long–lived vertebrate: managing a tropical freshwater turtle for sustainability and conservation. *J Appl Ecol* 45:52–62.

Frair W, Ackman RG, Mrosovsky N. 1972. Body temperature of Dermochelys coriacea: warm turtle from cold water. *Science*, 177:791–793.

Funk RS, Schnellbacher RW. 2019. Differential diagnoses by clinical signs: Snakes. In: Divers SJ, Stahl, SJ, ed. *Mader's Reptile and Amphibian Medicine and Surgery*, 3rd ed., 1249–1256. Philadelphia, PA: Elsevier Saunders.

García-Parra C, Garner MM, Wellehan Jr JFX, et al. 2014. Unusual mortality event among marine Iguanas *(Amblyrhynchus cristatus)* in the Galápagos Islands: clinical presentation and histopathologic results. Presented at the 45th Annual International Association for Aquatic Animal Medicine Conference. Gold Coast, Australia.

García-Párraga D, Crespo-Picazo JL, De Quirós YB, et al. 2014. Decompression sickness ('the bends') in sea turtles. *Dis Aqua Organ* 111:191–205.

Gibbons JW, Scott DE, Ryan TJ, et al. 2000. The Global decline of reptiles, déjà vu amphibians. *BioScience* 50:653–666.

Gieger S, Furmaga E. 2021. *The World Organisation for Animal Health (OIE) Technical Disease Card: Crocodile Poxvirus*. Available: https://www.woah.org/en/document/crocodilepox-virus-papillomatosis-in-crocodiles-infection-with (accessed 6 September 2022).

Gilbert PT. 1938. Three new trematodes from the Galapagos marine iguana *Ambly-rhynchus cristatus*. *Rep Hancock Pacific Exped* 2:91–106.

Gillett AK. 2017. *An Investigation into the Stranding of Australian Sea Snakes*. Thesis, Doctor of Philosophy, University of Queensland.

Gillett AK, Ploeg R, Flint M, Mills PC. 2017. Postmortem examination of Australian sea snakes (Hydrophiinae): anatomy and common pathologic conditions. *J Vet Diagn Invest* 29(5):593–611.

Goes VC, Brito ES, Valadão RM, et al. 2018. Haemogregarine (Apicomplexa: Adeleorina) infection in Vanderhaege's toad-headed turtle, *Mesoclemmys vanderhaegei* (Chelidae), from a Brazilian Neotropical savanna region. *Folia Parasitol* 65:1–6.

Gorbalenya AE, Enjuanes L, Ziebuhr J, Snijder EJ. 2006. Nidovirales: Evolving the largest RNA virus genome. *Virus Res* 117:17–37.

Gordon AN, Kelly WR, Lester RJ. 1993. Epizootic mortality of free-living green turtles, Chelonia mydas, due to coccidiosis. *J Wildl Dis* 29:490–494.

Graham T, Georges A, McElhinney N. 1996. Terrestrial Orientation by the Eastern Long-Necked Turtle, Chelodina longicollis, from Australia. *J Herpetol* 30:467–477.

Greenblatt RJ, Work TM, Balazs GH, et al. 2004. The Ozobranchus leech is a candidate mechanical vector for the fibropapilloma–associated turtle herpesvirus found latently infecting skin tumors on Hawaiian green turtles (*Chelonia mydas*). *Virology* 321:101–110.

Habarugira G, Moran J, Colmant AMG, et al. 2020. Mosquito-independent transmission of West Nile virus in farmed saltwater crocodiles (*Crocodylus porosus*). *Viruses* 12:198.

Haines H. 1978. A herpesvirus disease of green sea turtles in aquaculture. *Mar Fish Rev* 1:33–7.

Hargrove S, Work T, Brunson S, et al. 2016. Proceedings of the 2015 international summit on fibropapillomatosis: global status, trends, and population impacts. NOAA Technical Memorandum NMFS-PIFSC:54. Honolulu, HI: National Oceanic and Atmospheric Administration.

Hoff GL, Hoff DM. 1984. Herpesviruses of reptiles. In: Hoff GL, Frye FL, Jacobson ER, eds. *Diseases of Amphibians and Reptiles*, 159–167. Boston, MA: Springer.

Holopainen R, Ohlemeyer S, Schütze H, et al. 2009. Ranavirus phylogeny and differentiation based on major capsid protein, DNA polymerase and neurofilament triplet H1-like protein genes. *Dis of Aquat Organ*, 85:81–91.

Horner R. 1988. Poxvirus in farmed Nile crocodiles. *Vet Record* 122:459–462.

Hossain S, Heo G-J. 2021. Pet-turtles: a potential source of human pathogenic bacteria. *Arch Microbiol* 203(7):3785–3792.

Hsieh CY, Chang TC, Shen YL, et al. 2006. Pathological and PCR detection of mycobacteriosis in pond–cultured Chinese soft shell turtles, *Trionyx sinensis*. *Aquaculture* 261(1):10–16.

Huchzermeyer FW. 2002. Diseases of farmed crocodiles and ostriches. *Rev Sci Tech* 21:265–276.

Huchzermeyer FW. 2003. *Crocodiles: Biology, Husbandry and Diseases*. Oxon, UK: CABI Publishing.

Huchzermeyer FW, Gerdes GH, Foggin CM, et al. 1994. Hepatitis in farmed hatchling Nile crocodiles (Crocodylus niloticus) due to chlamydial infection. *J S Afr Vet Assoc* 65(1):20–22.

Huchzermeyer FW, Huchzermeyer KDA, Putterill JF. 1991. Observations on a field outbreak of pox virus infection in young Nile crocodiles (*Crocodylus niloticus*). *J S Afr Vet Assoc* 62(1):27–29.

Huchzermeyer FW, Wallace DB, Gerdes GH, Putterill JF. 2009. Identification and partial sequencing of a crocodile poxvirus associated with deeply penetrating skin lesions in farmed Nile crocodiles, Crocodylus niloticus. *Onderstepoort J Vet Res* 76:311–316.

Hunt CJG. 2006. Herpesvirus outbreak in a group of Mediterranean tortoises (*Testudo* spp). *Vet Clin N Am* 9:569–574.

Hyndman TH, Shilton CM, Wellehan JFX, et al. 2015. Molecular identification of three novel herpesviruses found in Australian farmed saltwater crocodiles (*Crocodylus porosus*) and Australian captive freshwater crocodiles (*Crocodylus johnstoni*). *Vet Microbiol* 181(3–4):183–189.

Innis CJ, Ceresia ML, Merigo C, et al. 2012. Single-dose pharmacokinetics of ceftazidime and fluconazole during concurrent clinical use in cold-stunned Kemp's ridley turtles (*Lepidochelys kempii*). *J Vet Pharmacol Ther* 35:82–89.

Innis CJ, Frasca Jr S. 2017. Bacterial and fungal diseases. In: Manire CA, Norton TM, Stacy BA, et al., eds. *Sea Turtle Health and Rehabilitation*, 779–790. Fort Lauderdale, FL: Ross Publishing.

Innis CJ, Frasca Jr S, Stacy B, et al. 2012. Identification and antimicrobial susceptibility of fungi isolated from marine turtles with histologically confirmed mycotic infections: 16 cases, 2005–2012. Presented at the 19th Annual Conference of the American Association of Zoo Veterinarians and Association of Reptilian and Amphibian Veterinarians. Oakland, California.

Innis CJ, Harms CA, Manire CA. 2017. Therapeutics. In: Manire CA, Norton TM, Stacy BA, et al, eds. *Sea Turtle Health and Rehabilitation*, 497–526. Fort Lauderdale, FL: Ross Publishing.

Innis CJ, Staggs LA. 2017. Cold–stunning. In: Manire CA, Norton TM, Stacy BA, Innis CJ, et al, eds. *Sea Turtle Health and Rehabilitation*, 675–687. Fort Lauderdale, FL: Ross Publishing.

Isberg SR, Moran JL, De Araujo R, et al. 2019. First evidence of Kunjin strain of West Nile virus associated with saltwater crocodile (*Crocodylus porosus*) skin lesions. *Aust Vet J* 97(10):390–393.

Jackson OF, Cooper JE. 1981. Nutritional diseases. In: Cooper JE, Jackson OF, eds. *Diseases of the Reptilia*, 2ned ed., 409–428. London, UK: Academic Press.

Jacobson ER, Calderwood MB, Clubb SL. 1980. Mucormycosis in hatchling Florida softshell turtles. *J Am Vet Med Assoc* 177(9):835–837.

Jacobson ER, Gardiner CH, Foggin CM. 1984. Adenovirus-like infection in two Nile crocodiles. *J Am Vet Med Assoc* 185(11):1421–1422.

Jacobson ER, Gaskin JM, Roelke M, Greiner EC, et al. 1986. Conjunctivitis, tracheitis, and pneumonia associated with herpesvirus infection in green sea turtles. *J Am Vet Med Assoc* 189(9):1020–1023.

Jacobson ER, Ginn PE, Troutman JM, et al. 2005. West Nile virus infection in farmed American alligators (*Alligator Mississippiensis*) in Florida. *J Wildl Dis* 41:96–106.

Jacobson ER, Harman GR, Maxwell LK, Laille EJ. 2003. Plasma concentrations of praziquantel after oral administration of single and multiple doses in loggerhead sea turtles (*Caretta caretta*). *Am J Vet Res* 64:304–309.

Jacobson ER, Popp JA, Shields RP, Gaskin JM. 1979. Poxlike skin lesions in captive caimans. *J Am Vet Med Assoc* 175(9):937–940.

Johnson CA, Griffith JW, Tenorio P, Hytrek S, et al. 1998. Fatal trematodiasis in research turtles. *Comp Med* 48:340–343.

Johnson AJ, Pessier AP, Wellehan JFX, Brown R, et al. 2005. Identification of a novel herpesvirus from a California desert tortoise (*Gopherus agassizii*). *Vet Microbiol* 111:107–116.

Johnson AJ, Pessier AP, Wellehan JFX, Childress A, et al. 2008. Ranavirus infection of free–ranging and captive box turtles and tortoises in the United States. *J Wildl Dis* 44:851–863.

Jones K, Ariel E, Burgess G, Read M. 2016. A review of fibropapillomatosis in Green turtles (*Chelonia mydas*). *Vet J* 212:48–57.

Jungwirth N, Bodewes R, Osterhaus ADME, et al. 2014. First report of a new alphaherpesvirus in a freshwater turtle (*Pseudemys concinna concinna*) kept in Germany. *Vety Microbiol* 170(3–4):403–407.

Kobolkuti LB, Czirjak GA, Spinu M. 2016. Effects of malnutrition and improper captive maintenance on European pond turtle (*Emys orbicularis*): a case report. *J Anim Plant Sci* 26:874–879.

La Fauce K, Ariel E, Munns S, et al. 2012. Influence of temperature and exposure time on the infectivity of Bohle iridovirus, a ranavirus. *Aquaculture* 354:64–67.

Lafortune M, Wellehan JFX, Terrell SP, et al. 2005. Shell and systemic hyalohyphomycosis in Fly River turtles, Carettochelys insculpta, caused by Paecilomyces lilacinus. *J Herpeto Med Surg* 15(2):15–19.

Lambert MR, Hernández–Gómez O, Krohn AR, et al. 2021. Turtle shell disease fungus (*Emydomyces testavorans*): first documented occurrence in California and prevalence in free-living turtles. *Icthyol Herpetol* 109(4):958–962.

Li X-L., Zhang C-L, Fang W-H, Lin F-C. 2008. White-spot disease of Chinese soft-shelled turtles (Trionyx sinens) caused by *Paecilomyces lilacinus*. *J Zhejiang Univ Sci B* 9:578–581.

Liu L, Cao Z, Lin F, et al. 2017. The histopathological characteristics caused by *Trionyx sinensis* hemorrhagic syndrome virus (TSHSV) and comparative proteomic analysis of liver tissue in TSHSV-infected Chinese soft-shelled turtles (*Pelodiscus sinensis*). *Intervirology* 60:19–27.

Lott MJ, Hose GC, Isberg SR, et al. 2015. Genetics and infection dynamics of *Paratrichosoma sp.* in farmed saltwater crocodiles (*Crocodylus porosus*). *Parasitol Res* 114:727–35.

Lutcavage ME, Lutz PL. 1996. Diving physiology. In: Lutz PL, Musick JA, Wyneken J, eds. *The Biology of Sea Turtles*, 277–296. Boca Raton, Fla: CRC Press.

MacLeod A, Nelson KN, Grant TD. 2020. *Amblyrhynchus cristatus (errata version published in 2020). The IUCN Red List of Threatened Species 2020 e.T1086A177552193*. https://dx.doi.org/10.2305/IUCN.UK.2020-2.RLTS.T1086A177552193.en (accessed 6 September 2022).

Mallo KM, Harms CA, Lewbart GA, Papich MG. 2002. Pharmacokinetics of fluconazole in loggerhead sea turtles (*Caretta caretta*) after single intravenous and subcutaneous injections, and multiple subcutaneous injections. *J Zoo Wildl Med* 33:29–35.

Manire C, Montgomery N. 2014. Intestinal Coccidia resembling Caryospora spp. in green and loggerhead sea turtles: Occurrence and effective treatment. Presented at the International Association of Aquatic Animal Veterinarians 45th Annual Conference, Gold Coast, QLD, Australia.

Manire CA, Norton TM, Walsh MT, Campbell LA. 2017. Buoyancy Disorders. In: Manire CA, Norton TM, Stacy BA, Innis CJ, et al, eds. *Sea Turtle Health and Rehabilitation*, 689–705. Fort Lauderdale, FL: Ross Publishing.

Manire CA, Rhinehart HL, Pennick GJ, et al. 2003. Steady-state plasma concentrations of itraconazole after oral administration in Kemp's ridley sea turtles, *Lepidochelys kempi*. *J Zoo Wildl Med* 34(2):171–8.

Manire CA, Stacy BA, Kinsel MJ, et al. 2008. Proliferative dermatitis in a loggerhead turtle, *Caretta caretta*, and a green turtle, *Chelonia mydas*, associated with novel papillomaviruses. *Vet Microbiol* 130:227–237.

Mao J, Hedrick RP, Chinchar VG. 1997. Molecular characterization, sequence analysis, and taxonomic position of newly isolated fish iridoviruses. *Virology* 229(1):212–220.

Marrone F, Sacco F, Kehlmaier C, et al. 2016. Some like it cold: the glossiphoniid parasites of the Sicilian endemic pond turtle *Emys trinacris* (Testudines, Emydidae), an example of 'parasite inertia'? *J Zoo Syst Evol Res* 54:60–66.

Marschang RE, Gravendyck M, Kaleta EF. 1997. Herpesviruses in tortoises: investigations into virus isolation and the treatment of viral stomatitis in *Testudo hermanni* and *T. graeca*. *J Vet Med B* 44:385–394.

Marschang RE, Kolesnik E. 2016. Detection of nidoviruses in live pythons and boas. *Tierarztl Prax Ausg K Kleintiere Heimtiere* 45:22–26.

Mashkour N, Jones K, Kophamel S, et al. 2020. Disease risk analysis in sea turtles: a baseline study to inform conservation efforts. *PloS One* 15:e0230760.

Mashkour N, Jones K, Wirth W, Burgess G, et al. 2021. The Concurrent Detection of Chelonid Alphaherpesvirus 5 and Chelonia mydas Papillomavirus 1 in Tumored and Non-Tumored Green Turtles. *Animals* 11(3):697.

Mashkour N, Maclaine A, Burgess GW, Ariel E. 2018. Discovery of an Australian Chelonia mydas papillomavirus via green turtle primary cell culture and qPCR. *J Virol Methods* 258:13–23.

McKenzie CM, Piczak ML, Snyman HN, et al. 2019. First report of ranavirus mortality in a common snapping turtle *Chelydra serpentina*. *Dis Aquat Organ* 132(3):221–227.

McKnight DT, Zenger KR, Alford RA, Huerlimann R. 2020. Microbiome diversity and composition varies across body areas in a freshwater turtle. *Microbiology* 166:440–452.

Mettee SM, Norton TM. 2017. Trauma and Wound Care. In: Manire CA, Norton TM, Stacy BA, et al, eds. *Sea Turtle Health and Rehabilitation*, 657–674. Fort Lauderdale, FL: Ross Publishing.

Miller DL, Mauel MJ, Baldwin C, et al. 2003. West Nile virus in farmed alligators. *Emerg Infect Dis* 9:794–799.

Mitchell JC, McAvoy B. 1990. Enteric bacteria in natural populations of freshwater turtles in Virginia. *Virginia J Sci* 41:233–242.

Mitchell JC, Pague CA, Gibbons JW. 1990. Body size, reproductive variation, and growth in the slider turtle, at the northeastern edge of its range. In: Avery HW ed. *Life History and Ecology of the Slider Turtle*, 146–151. Washington, DC: Smithsonian Institution Press.

Moody NJG, Owens L. 1994. Experimental demonstration of the pathogenicity of a frog virus, Bohle iridovirus, for a fish species, barramundi Lates calcarifer. *Dis Aquat Organ* 18:95–102.

Mortimer JA, Donnelly M. 2008. *The IUCN Red List of Threatened Species: Eretmochelys imbricata*. https://dx.doi.org/10.2305/IUCN.UK.2008.RLTS.T8005A12881238.en (accessed 6 September 2022).

Muro J, Ramis A, Pastor J, Velarde R, et al. 1998. Chronic rhinitis associated with herpesviral infection in captive spur-thighed tortoises from Spain. *J Wildl Dis* 34:487–495.

Nevarez J. 2006. Crocodilian Differential Diagnosis. *Reptile Med Surg* 705–714.

Nevarez JG. 2019. Differential diagnoses by clinical crocodilians. In: Divers SJ, Stahl, SJ, ed. *Mader's Reptile and Amphibian Medicine and Surgery*, 3rd ed., 1276–1282. Philadelphia, PA: Elsevier Saunders.

Nevarez JG, Mitchell MA, Kim DY, et al. 2005. West Nile virus in alligator, *Alligator mississippiensis*, ranches from Louisiana. *J Herpetol Med Surg* 15:4–9.

Nevarez JG, Mitchell MA, Morgan T, et al. 2008. Association of West Nile virus with lymphohistiocytic proliferative cutaneous lesions in American alligators (*Alligator mississippiensis*) detected by RT-PCR. *J Zoo Wildl Med* 39:562–566.

Nordmeyer SC, Henry G, Guerra T, et al. 2020. Identification of blood parasites in individuals from six families of freshwater turtles. *Chelonian Conserv Biol* 19:85–94.

Norton TM. 2005. Chelonian emergency and critical care. *Semin Avian Exotic Pet Med* 14(2):106–130.

Okoh GSR, Horwood PF, Whitmore D, Ariel E. 2021. *Herpesviruses in reptiles. Front Vet Sci* 8:642894–642894.

Origgi FC. 2012. Testudinid Herpesviruses: a review. *J Herpetol Med Surg* 22:42–54.

Origgi FC, Romero CH, Bloom DC, et al. 2004. Experimental transmission of a herpesvirus in Greek tortoises (*Testudo graeca*). *Vet Pathol* 41(1):50–61.

Ossiboff RJ. 2018. Serpentes. In: Terio KA, McAloose D, St. Leger J, eds. *Pathology of Wildlife and Zoo Animals*, 897–919. Philadelphia, PA: Elsevier Saunders.

Ossiboff RJ, Raphael BL, Ammazzalorso AD, et al. 2015. Three novel herpesviruses of endangered Clemmys and Glyptemys turtles. *PloS One* 10:e0122901.

Pallister J, Gould A, Harrison D, Hyatt Aet al. 2007. Development of real-time PCR assays for the detection and differentiation of Australian and European ranaviruses. *J Fish Dis* 30:427–438.

Parga ML, Crespo-Picazo JL, Monteiro D, et al. 2020. On-board study of gas embolism in marine turtles caught in bottom trawl fisheries in the Atlantic Ocean. *Sci Rep* 10:5561–5561.

Parrish K, Kirkland PD, Skerratt LF, Ariel E. 2021. Nidoviruses in reptiles: a review. *Front Vet Sci* 8:733404–733404.

Pasquale V, Baloda SB, Dumontet S, Krovacek K. 1994. An Outbreak of *Aeromonas hydrophila* Infection in Turtles (*Pseudemis scripta*). *Appl Environ Microbiol* 60:1678–1680.

Pfitzer S, Boustead KJ, Vorster JH, et al. 2019. Adenoviral hepatitis in two Nile crocodile (*Crocodylus niloticus*) hatchlings from South Africa. *J S Afr Vet Assoc* 90:e1–e4.

Pineda-Catalan O, Perkins SL, Peirce MA, et al. 2013. Revision of Hemoproteid genera and description and redescription of two species of chelonian Hemoproteid parasites. *J Parasitol* 99:1089–1098.

Ramos M, Coutinho S, Matushima E, Sinhorini I. 2002. Poxvirus dermatitis outbreak in farmed Brazilian caimans (Caiman crocodilus yacare). *Aust Vet J* 80:371–372.

Rebell G, Rywlin A, Haines H. 1975. A herpesvirus-type agent associated with skin lesions of green sea turtles in aquaculture. *Am J Vet Res* 36:1221–4.

Red List Standards and Petitions Subcommittee. 1996. *The IUCN Red List of Threatened Species: Natator depressus*. https://dx.doi.org/10.2305/IUCN.UK.1996.RLTS.T14363A4435952.en (accessed 6 September 2022).

Rowe CL. 2008. "The calamity of so long life": life histories, contaminants, and potential emerging threats to long-lived vertebrates. *Bioscience* 58:623–631.

Sadove S, Pisciotta R, Digiovanni R. 1998. Assessment and initial treatment of cold-stunned sea turtles. *Chelonian Conserv Biol* 3:84–86.

Saelinger CA, Lewbart GA, Christian LS, Lemons CL. 2006. Prevalence of Salmonella spp in cloacal, fecal, and gastrointestinal mucosal samples from wild North American turtles. *J Am Vet Med Assoc* 229:266–268.

Sarker S, Isberg SR, Moran JL, et al. 2019. Crocodilepox virus evolutionary genomics supports observed poxvirus infection dynamics on saltwater crocodile (*Crocodylus porosus*). *Viruses* 11:1116.

Schoeb TR, Heaton-Jones TG, Clemmons RM, et al. 2002. Clinical and necropsy findings associated with increased mortality among American alligators of Lake Griffin, Florida. *J Wildl Dis* 38:320–37.

Seminoff JA. 2004. *The IUCN Red List of Threatened Species: Chelonia mydas*. https://dx.doi.org/10.2305/IUCN.UK.2004.RLTS.T4615A11037468.en (accessed 6 September 2022).

Shilton CM, Jerrett IV, Davis S, et al. 2016. Diagnostic investigation of new disease syndromes in farmed Australian saltwater crocodiles (*Crocodylus porosus*) reveals associations with herpesviral infection. *J Vet Diagn Invest* 28:279–290.

Sim RR, Norton TM, Bronson E, et al. 2015. Identification of a novel herpesvirus in captive Eastern box turtles (Terrapene carolina carolina). *Vet Microbiol* 175:218–223.

Simulundu E, Ndashe K, Chambaro HM, et al. 2020. West Nile virus in farmed crocodiles, Zambia, 2019. *Emerg Infec Dis* 26:811–814.

Sinmuk S, Suda H, Hatai K. 1996. Aphanomyces infection in juvenile soft-shelled turtle, Pelodiscus sinensis, imported from Singapore. *Mycoscience* 37:249–254.

Spencer R-J, Thompson MB. 2003. The significance of predation in nest site selection of turtles: an experimental consideration of macro- and microhabitat preferences. *Oikos* 102:592–600.

Spencer R-J, Thompson MB. 2005. Experimental analysis of the impact of foxes on freshwater turtle populations. *Conserv Biol* 19:845–854.

Spinks PQ, Pauly GB, Crayon JJ, Bradley Shaffer H. 2003. Survival of the western pond turtle (*Emys marmorata*) in an urban California environment. *Biol Conserv* 113:257–267.

Stacy BA, Chapman PA, Stockdale-Walden H, et al. 2019. Caryospora-Like coccidia infecting green turtles (*Chelonia mydas*): an emerging disease with evidence of interoceanic dissemination. *Front Vet Sci* 6:372.

Stacy BA, Foley AM, Greiner E, et al. 2010. Spirorchiidiasis in stranded loggerhead *Caretta caretta* and green turtles Chelonia mydas in Florida (USA): host pathology and significance. *Dis Aquat Organ* 89:237–259.

Stacy BA, Werneck MR, Walden HDS, Harms CA. 2017. Parasitology. In: Manire CA, Norton TM, Stacy BA, et al., eds. *Sea Turtle Health and Rehabilitation*, 727–747. Fort Lauderdale, FL: Ross Publishing.

Stam F, Römkens TEH, Hekker TAM, Smulders YM. 2003. Turtle-associated human salmonellosis. *Clin Infect Dis* 37:e167–e169.

Steinman A, Banet-Noach C, Tal S, et al. 2003. West Nile virus infection in crocodiles. *Emerg Infect Dis* 9:887–889.

Takuma D, Sano A, Wada S, et al. 2010. *Aphanomyces sinensis* sp. nov., isolated from juvenile soft–shelled turtle, *Pelodiscus sinensis*, in Japan. *Mycoscience* 52:119–131.

Teare JA, Bush M. 1983. Toxicity and efficacy of ivermectin in chelonians. *J Am Vet Med Assoc* 183:1195–7.

Thaller MC, Ciambotta M, Sapochetti M, et al. 2010. Uneven frequency *of Vibrio alginolyticus* group isolates among different populations of Galápagos marine iguana (*Amblyrhynchus cristatus*). *Environ Microbiol Rep* 2:179–184.

Thompson MB. 1983. Populations of the Murray river tortoise, Emydura (Chelodina): the effect of egg predation by the red fox, *Vulpes vulpes. Aust Wildl Res* 10(2):363–371.

Udyawer V, Barnes P, Bonnet X, et al. 2018. Future directions in the research and management of marine snakes. *Front Mar Sci* 5:399.

Uetz P, Freed P, Aguilar R, Hošek J, eds. 2021. *The Reptile Database*. http://www.reptile-database.org (accessed 6 September 2022).

Upton SJ, Odell DK, Walsh MT. 1990. *Eimeria caretta* sp.nov. (Apicomplexa: Eimeriidae) from the loggerhead sea turtle, *Caretta caretta* (Testudines). *Can J Zool* 68:1268–1269.

Zhang J, Finlaison DS, Frost MJ, et al. 2018. Identification of a novel nidovirus as a potential cause of large scale mortalities in the endangered Bellinger River snapping turtle (*Myuchelys georgesi*). *PloS One*, 13:e0205209.

Walden HDS, Greiner EC, Jacobson ER. 2020. Parasites and parasitic diseases of reptiles. In: Jacobson ER, Garner MM, eds. *Infectious Diseases and Pathology of Reptiles: Color Atlas and Text, Diseases and Pathology of Reptiles Volume 1*, 859–968. Boca Raton, FL: CRC Press.

Wallace BP, Tiwari M, Girondot M. 2013. *The IUCN Red List of Threatened Species: Dermochelys coriacea*. https://dx.doi.org/10.2305/IUCN.UK.2013-2.RLTS.T6494A43526147.en (accessed 6 September 2022).

Ward JL, Hall K, Christian LS, Lewbart GA. 2012. Plasma biochemistry and condition of confiscated hatchling pig-nosed turtles (Carettochelys insculpta). *Herpetol Conserv Biol* 7(1):38–45.

Wibbels T, Bevan E. 2019. *The IUCN Red List of Threatened Species: Lepidochelys kempii*. https://dx.doi.org/10.2305/IUCN.UK.2019-2.RLTS.T11533A155057916.en (accessed 6 September 2022).

Williams SR, Sims MA, Roth-Johnson L, Wickes B. 2012. Surgical removal of an abscess associated with Fusarium solani from a Kemp's ridley sea turtle (Lepidochelys kempii). *J Zoo Wildl Med* 43:402–406.

Wilson SK, Swan G. 2003. *A Complete Guide to Reptiles of Australia*. Sydney, Australia: New Holland.

Woodburn DB, Kinsel MJ, Poll CP, et al. 2021. Shell lesions associated with *Emydomyces testavorans* infection in freshwater aquatic turtles. *Vet Pathol* 58:578–586.

Woodburn DB, Miller AN, Allender MC, et al. 2019. *Emydomyces testavorans*, a New Genus and Species of Onygenalean Fungus Isolated from Shell Lesions of Freshwater Aquatic Turtles. *J Clin Microbiol* 57(2): e00628–18.

Appendix 4.1

Etiology of amphibian diseases

Reptiles	Etiology (most likely)
Sudden death	Bacterial septicemia, water quality issues (hydrogen sulfide), toxicosis (heavy metal, copper, herbicide, pesticide), parasites, trauma, electrocution, handling stress, malnutrition, viral infection, aneurysms
Poor growth	Nutritional deficiency, stress/water quality issues, insufficient caloric intake, heavy parasitism, underfeeding, high temperature, heart disease, chronic inflammation, neoplasia, renal disease, maladaptation to captivity, postpartum female
Anorexia	Sepsis, improper temperature/environment, dystocia, neoplasia, CNS disease, respiratory disease, GI disease, renal disease, tongue damage/oral disease, normal in gravid females of some species, normal in males of some species during breeding season, brumation
Icterus/green discoloration, generalized	Prehepatic, hepatic, post–hepatic causes as per mammals
Uncoordinated swimming or gait/ nervousness/ buoyancy issues	Generalized infectious disease, pneumonia, fungal infection (Ophidiomyces–S), electrocution, spinal trauma, toxicosis (medications, chemicals, heavy metals, environment), osteomyelitis, CNS disease, water quality issues, thiamine deficiency (S), parasitism, otitis/endolymphatic duct inflammation, nutritional deficiency (hypocalcemia, vitamin B deficiency, biotin deficiency, vitamin E/ selenium deficiency), renal disease, neoplasia, joint luxation, hyperthermia, freezing, hypoglycemia (C), West Nile Virus (C)
Inability to submerge	Pneumonia, emaciation, neoplasia, gas accumulation in GI tract or coelom
Gasping/dyspnea:	
Lung disease	Pneumonia (bacterial, viral, parasitic – nematodes, pentastomes, aspiration/ drowning), neoplasia, edema
Anemia[a]	Blood loss, hemoparasites, chronic disease, poor nutrition
Tracheitis/nasal blockage	Mucus, foreign body
Oral disease	Stomatitis, neoplasia, foreign body
Pleuroperitoneal expansion	Ascites, neoplasia, peritonitis
Skin:	
Petechiae	Sepsis
Hemorrhage, necrosis, ulcers	Trauma, parasite migration, virus infection – herpesvirus (T, C), ranavirus (T), poxvirus (C), West Nile virus (C)], thermal burn, poor water quality, sepsis, parasitic (Spirorchiid blood flukes (T), shell osteomyelitis (T), *Dermatophilus* (C), sloughing due to iatrogenic hypervitaminosis A, bacterial infection (aerobic/anaerobic), emaciation
Parasites	Ectoparasites, encysted parasites, blood flukes (T), marine leeches (T)
Crusts	Bacterial, fungal, parasitic disease, burns, dysecdysis, dermatophilosis (C)
Wrinkling	Dehydration, dysecdysis (S), emaciation, acariasis, hypovitaminosis C (S)

(*Continued*)

Reptiles	Etiology (most likely)
Nodules/lumps	Granulomas – bacterial, fungal (*Ophidiomyces*, S), parasitic (Spirorchiid blood flukes (T), encysted parasites, virus – Poxvirus (C), neoplasia, rib fractures, unresorbed fetal yolk (S), gut impactions/feces (S), gravid female (S), endolymphatic calcium accumulation, keratin cysts, aneurysms, fibropapillomatosis tumors (sea turtle), gas supersaturation, piecemeal skin shedding (T), skin tags, aural abscess
Serpigenous/ zigzag lesion	Paratrichosoma parasitism (C)
Sloughed scutes (T)	Bacteria/fungal infection, renal failure, nutritional deficiency, can also be normal
Macules	Poxvirus (C)
Respiratory:	
Nasal discharge	Pneumonia, gastritis (source of discharge), *Mycoplasma* (T), virus (T) (herpesvirus, ranavirus, adenovirus, reovirus, paramyxovirus), coccidians (T), chlamydiosis (T), foreign bodies, oronasal fistula
Pneumonia	Bacteria – *Mycoplasma* (C), virus, parasite, fungal
Nasal erosion/ swelling	Upper respiratory disease, mycobacteriosis
Mouth:	
Hemorrhage/ ulcers/necrosis	Bacterial septicemia, trauma, stomatitis, coagulopathy, toxins, anemia, virus infection
Increased mucus/exudate	Bacterial infection, sepsis, parasitism, esophagitis, gastritis, tracheitis, pneumonia, virus (herpes)
Gas bubbles	Gas supersaturation
Nodules	Granulomas, gingival hyperplasia, dental neoplasia, parasitic cyst
Overgrowth of the beak (T)	Nutritional disease, protein deficiency/excess
Edema	Bacterial infection, uremia from renal disease
Eye:	
Exophthalmia/ swelling	Bacterial septicemia, gas bubble disease/supersaturation, neoplasia, granulomas, blocked lacrimal duct (S), periorbital swelling – venous congestion (heart disease, renal disease, aneurysms, infection), hypovitaminosis A (T), foreign bodies, chlamydiosis (C), herpesvirus (CT)
Ulcers/ hemorrhage	Fungus, bacterial septicemia, viral infection, trauma, blindness
Corneal edema/ cloudiness	Poor water quality, conspecific aggression, bacterial, viral, fungal, or parasitic disease, retained spectacles (S, L), subspectacular fluid accumulation (S, L), impending shed (S), recent brumation (S), hypovitaminosis A, lipid infiltration (arcus lipoides corneae – aging change), freezing
Ophthalmitis	Trauma, hematogenous spread of pathogens
Cataract	Age-related change, low brumation temperature (S, L)
Microphthalmia/ enophthalmia	Chronic ophthalmitis, congenital, narrow palpebral fissure, thiamine deficiency (T), emaciation, dehydration, hypotension (sepsis)
Lens luxation	Trauma
Enucleation	Trauma (predator, stocking density too high), severe ophthalmitis
Nodules	Granulomas (bacteria, fungi, parasite)

Reptiles	Etiology (most likely)
Muscle:	
Atrophy	Emaciation, denervation
Liquefaction/ necrosis	Bacterial infection
Nodules/ swelling	Granulomas, neoplasia, encysted parasites
White foci	Necrosis
Skeleton:	
Deformity	Fracture, osteomyelitis, congenital, metabolic bone disease, tail loss (defensive autotomy, L)
Lameness	Osteomyelitis, arthritis (*Mycoplasma*), muscle disease, fractures, metabolic bone disease, gout, pseudogout, trauma, neoplasia, spondylosis, fibrous osteodystrophy/metabolic bone disease (rare in T)
Shell Disease (T)	Trauma, bites, calcinosis circumscripta, improper temperatures, bacteria (*Beneckea chitonovora*), fungi
Soft/abnormal shell (T)	Hyperparathyroidism (nutritional), bacteria, fungi, congenital
Abdomen/coelom:	
Enlarged (general)	Neoplasia, overweight, egg binding/dystocia/mucometra, GI impaction/disease, peritonitis, cardiovascular/hepatic disease leading to ascites, renal disease, other causes of hypoproteinemia, parasites, gastritis (S), gas distention from putrefied ingesta, fecal impaction, organomegaly, granulomas, uroliths
Ascites	Bacterial septicemia, liver failure, renal failure, heart disease, neoplasia, hypoproteinemia
Peritonitis, nodular/ granulomatous	Bacteria, parasites, fungus, neoplasia
Petechiae	Bacterial septicemia
Gas	Gut rupture, body wall perforation, inflammation with gas-producing microbes or fungi
Liver:	
Nodules	Bacteria, myxozoan infection (biliary), encysted parasites, fungi, neoplasia
Stomach:	
Nodules	Granulomas (fungi, bacteria, parasites), neoplasia
Mucosal thickening	Protozoans (cryptosporidians, S)
Intestine:	
Hyperemia/ hemorrhage	Bacterial septicemia (*Salmonella*)
Necrosis	Bacteria, parasites (coccidians)
Prolapse (colon, cloaca, oviduct, phallus, bladder)	Spinal disease, poor muscle tone, gastroenteritis, impactions, intussusception, constipation
Nodules	Granulomas (fungi, bacteria, parasites), neoplasia

(*Continued*)

Reptiles	Etiology (most likely)
Reproductive:	
Dystocia	Obesity, nutrition, dehydration, primipara, abnormal eggs, improper temperatures, improper cage/environment, oviduct infection/torsion/compression, ectopic egg, oviduct prolapse, nutritional hyperparathyroidism (T), hypovitaminosis A (T), hypocalcemia

[a] Reptile membranes are typically more pale than those of mammals.
(C), Crocodilians; CNS, central nervous system; GI, gastrointestinal; (L), Lacertilia/lizards; (S), Serpentes; (T), Testudines/turtles. *Sources:* Barten and Simpson (2019); Boyer (2019); Funk et aql. (2019); Nevarez (2019); Ossiboff (2018).

5

Aquatic Birds

Nicole M. Nemeth

Parasitic Diseases of Major Taxa

Macroparasite infections in aquatic birds are common and most often incidental; substantial parasite burdens may contribute to morbidity and mortality. Mites, lice, cestodes, trematodes, and nematodes are most often detected in some species (Buckles, 2018; Stidworthy and Denk, 2018; Forrester and Spaulding, 2003).

Ectoparasites

Ectoparasites include nasal leeches (*Theromyzon* spp.) in the nares, nasal sinuses, or tracheal lumen of some duck species. Affected individuals may have discharge from nares, cloudy corneas, and/or globe collapse (Davies et al., 2008; Fenton et al., 2018). Chewing lice, *Mallophaga* spp., and mites may be evident on feathers; the latter may also infest the subcutis and nasal cavity. Chiggers can cause dermatitis. Myiasis may occur in nestlings and adults of some species (Fenton et al., 2018).

Metazoan Parasites

Eustrongylides and numerous ascarids can be in segments of the alimentary tract, especially in piscivorous aquatic bird species (e.g. *Eustrongylides ignotus* in the ventriculus of Ciconiiformes; *Eustrongylides tubifex* in esophagus and proventriculus of mergansers; Figure 5.1). Abnormally high nematode load or aberrant parasite migration are rare, but may cause morbidity and mortality due to gastrointestinal perforation or rupture, which can lead to coelomitis and sepsis (e.g., *Anisakis* spp., *Contracaecum* spp., *Baylisascaris* spp.; Figure 5.2). Differentials include penetrating foreign bodies.

In waterfowl, *Amidostomum* and *Epomidiostomum* spp. reside between the ventricular koilin and mucosa, whereas the spirurids *Streptocara* and *Echinuria* spp. parasitize the proventricular lumen; these nematodes may cause damage to the gastrointestinal lining and/or impair gastrointestinal motility. Aquatic birds are definitive hosts of acanthocephalans (thorny-headed worms) in the small intestine (Figure 5.3); large burdens can lead to emaciation, gastrointestinal nodules,

Pathology and Epidemiology of Aquatic Animal Diseases for Practitioners, First Edition.
Edited by Laura Urdes, Chris Walster, and Julius Tepper.

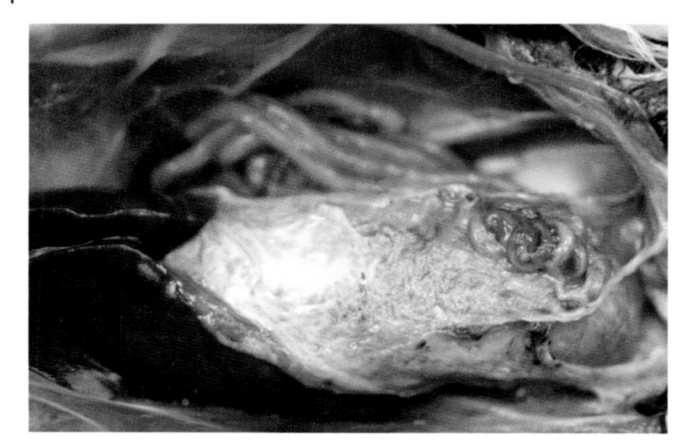

Figure 5.1 Great blue heron. Caudal coelomic cavity with *Eustrongylides* sp. embedded in fibrinous adhesions over the gastrointestinal serosa. *Source:* Courtesy of the Southeastern Cooperative Wildlife Disease Study.

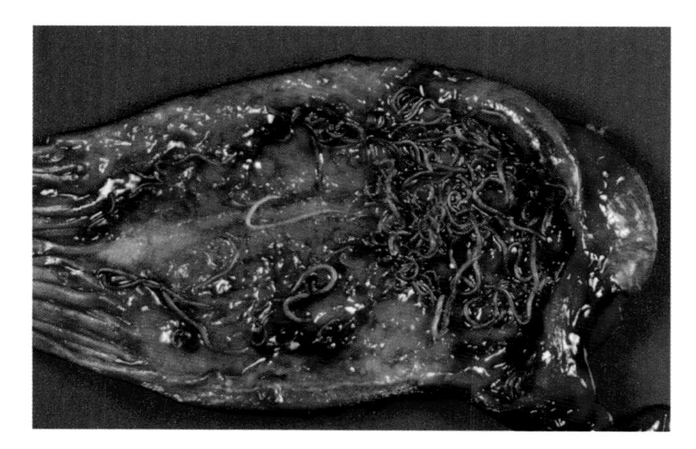

Figure 5.2 Double crested cormorant. Proventriculus with moderate load of *Contracecum* species parasites. *Source:* Courtesy of the Southeastern Cooperative Wildlife Disease Study.

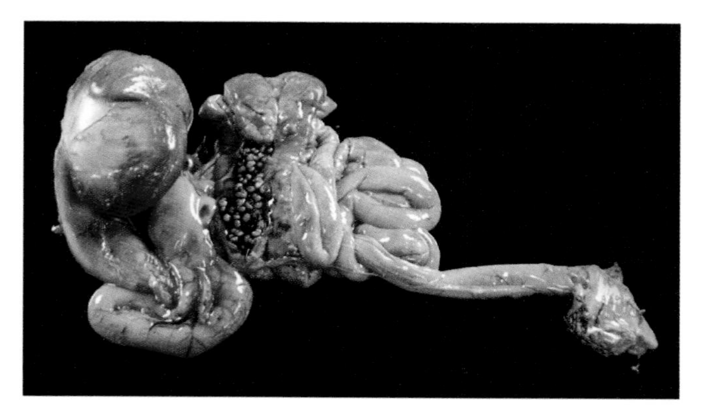

Figure 5.3 Common eider with a heavy load of acanthocephalans (thorny-headed worms) in the small intestine. *Source:* Courtesy of the Southeastern Cooperative Wildlife Disease Study.

serositis, and death (Fenton et al., 2018). Parasite identification can be confirmed by morphologic assessment by light microscope. Differentials include gastrointestinal foreign body, bacterial enteritis and coccidial enteritis; however, visualization of high loads of alimentary tract nematodes helps to differentiate them.

Hemoprotozoans and Intracellular Protozoans

Penguins are highly susceptible to fatal malaria (50–80% mortality) caused by *Plasmodium* spp. (most commonly, *Plasmodium relictum*); young and immunosuppressed birds are most susceptible. Transmission, and thus disease detection, is seasonal, as these protozoans are transmitted by mosquitoes. Clinically, there may be sudden death, anemia (e.g. pale mucous membranes), vomiting, anorexia, depression, and isolation. More severe disease manifestations may include ataxia, seizures, and paralysis.

Diagnosis is by light microscopy of blood smears or impression smears of spleen or liver, revealing parasitemia (intraerythrocytic parasites), although death may preclude parasitemia in some cases. Serology and polymerase chain reaction (PCR) of blood have been used with some success. Gross findings may include pulmonary edema and hydropericardium, as well as splenomegaly and hepatomegaly; spleen, liver, and heart exhibit mononuclear cell inflammation. Meronts in endothelial cells may lead to occlusion and rupture of blood vessels and focal necrosis. These organisms may be evident in macrophages and endothelial cells of multiple organs (lungs, heart, liver, and spleen) by histopathology. Respiratory and circulatory complications are often the ultimate cause of death (Buckles, 2018).

A variety of aquatic taxa are susceptible to renal or intestinal coccidiosis (primarily, *Eimeria*, but also *Isospora*, *Wenyonella* and *Tyzzeria* spp.), which is often incidental (e.g. in loons, shags, gannets, double-crested cormorants, geese, and other waterfowl). However, fatal disease may occur, especially in young birds, and has been documented in a variety of species (e.g. shearwaters, cranes, and lesser scaup). Clinically, disease may include lethargy, diarrhea, bloodstained vent, emaciation, and sudden death. Gross examination may reveal poor nutritional condition, yellow-tinged fat and muscle, distended, and possibly hemorrhagic and/or thickened intestines, with pale nodules and impacted cloaca and pericloacal fecal/urate accumulation. Kidneys may be enlarged and chalky (urate deposition). Microscopically, kidneys have mononuclear cell inflammation with gametocytes and oocysts in collecting ducts and renal epithelia (Fenton et al., 2018; Stidworthy and Denk, 2018).

Infections with *Sarcocystis* spp. (e.g., *Sarcocystis rileyi*) are generally subclinical in waterfowl and grossly resemble rice-like grains within the skeletal muscle (Figure 5.4). Microscopically, these are bradyzoite-filled protozoal cysts within myocytes. Usually, there is no associated inflammatory cell response, unless the protozoal cysts degenerate and rupture (Fenton et al., 2018). Rarely, *Sarcocystis*

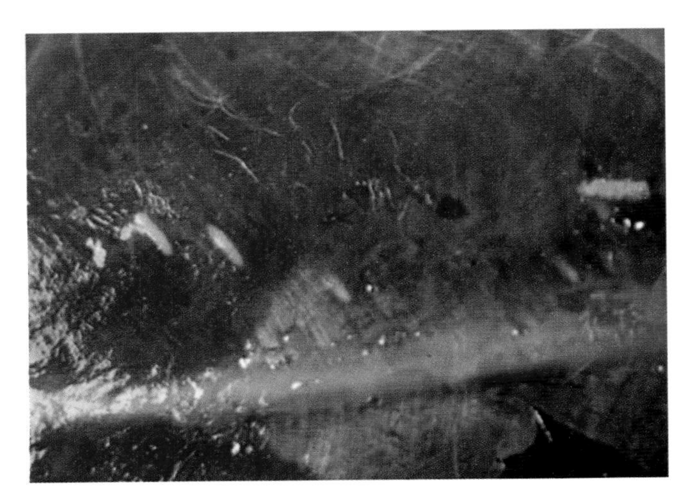

Figure 5.4 Duck (species unspecified). *Sarcocystis* species protozoan cysts in the pectoral muscle. *Source:* Courtesy of the Southeastern Cooperative Wildlife Disease Study.

spp. access the brain, causing neurologic disease and corresponding inflammation. The schizonts are evident by histopathology; immunohistochemistry and PCR can confirm the diagnosis (Spalding et al., 2002).

Viral Diseases

The information below provides some of the most common viruses to cause disease among aquatic birds and it is not meant to provide an exhaustive list. For example, circoviruses can cause morbidity and mortality in gulls and several herpesvirus or herpesvirus-like infections have been reported in African penguins, loons and flamingos (Buckles, 2018; Stidworthy and Denk, 2018).

Avian Poxvirus Disease

Overview and Etiology

Virus from the family Poxviridae, genus Avipoxvirus which infects most avian species (e.g., penguins, tropicbirds, pelicans, petrels, shearwaters, albatross, flamingos) and can manifest as dry (cutaneous) and wet (diphtheric) forms. Young birds may be more susceptible to severe disease.

Signs and Diagnosis

Severe disease can lead to emaciation, lethargy, secondary bacterial infections, and disorientation. Impaired vision and dysphagia may occur, depending on anatomic location of the lesions (Figure 5.5). Rarely, lesions may also be in lungs, leading to dyspnea. Gross lesions include proliferative, crusty, tan-yellow, irregular, sometimes, ulcerated nodules on nonfeathered or paucifeathered skin (e.g. around beak, eyelids, facial mucocutaneous junctions, legs, pericloacal) or between feather tracts in other areas (e.g. wings, neck) or in the oral and upper alimentary tract mucosa (Buckles, 2018; Fenton et al., 2018; Stidworthy and Denk, 2018). Diagnosis is confirmed with histopathology (characteristic intracytoplasmic, eosinophilic inclusion bodies, known as Bollinger bodies, epithelial hyperplasia, and ballooning degeneration) or by PCR testing of affected skin or mucosa (Buckles, 2018; Stidworthy and Denk, 2018).

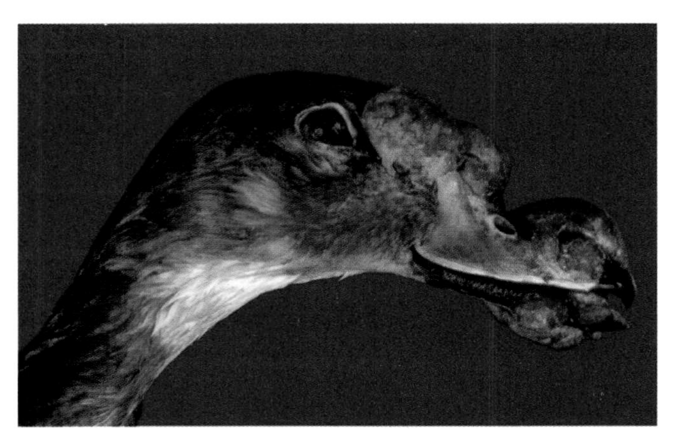

Figure 5.5 Wood duck. Avian poxvirus infection in the skin over the face and beak and oral mucosa. *Source:* Courtesy of the Southeastern Cooperative Wildlife Disease Study.

Differential Diagnoses

Differentials include chronic bacterial infections of the skin, for which the etiology is often difficult to determine due to chronicity. Oral poxviral lesions can resemble those of candidiasis. Some poxviral infections self-resolve but severe infections are less likely to do so and prognosis should be weighed against the stress of long-term treatment, which consists of supportive care.

Treatment/Management

No treatment is available.

Duck Virus Enteritis ("Duck Plague")

Overview and Etiology

Virus from the family Herpesviridae, genus Anatid alphaherpesvirus 1. The infection can lead to acute disease with high mortality rates in ducks (especially in Muscovy ducks), geese, and swans. While disease can occur any time of year, it is most often diagnosed in spring and early summer (US Geological Survey, 1999a).

Signs and Diagnosis

The disease may manifest as sudden death. Grossly, hemorrhage may be present in the heart (Figure 5.6) and mesentery; the full-length of the alimentary tract, the gut-associated lymphoid tissue (GALT), the liver and pancreas may undergo necrosis. Button-like lesions in the gut (consisting of segmental GALT hemorrhage and necrosis) and hepatomegaly with necrosis are characteristic (Hansen and Gough, 2007; Fenton et al., 2018). Hemorrhage in the gut may progress to plaques and ulcerations overlain with diphtheritic membranes (Figure 5.7; Wobeser, 1997a; Fenton et al. 2018). Microscopically, together with hemorrhage and necrosis, there may be intraepithelial, intranuclear, and sometimes intracytoplasmic, eosinophilic inclusion bodies in cells of multiple

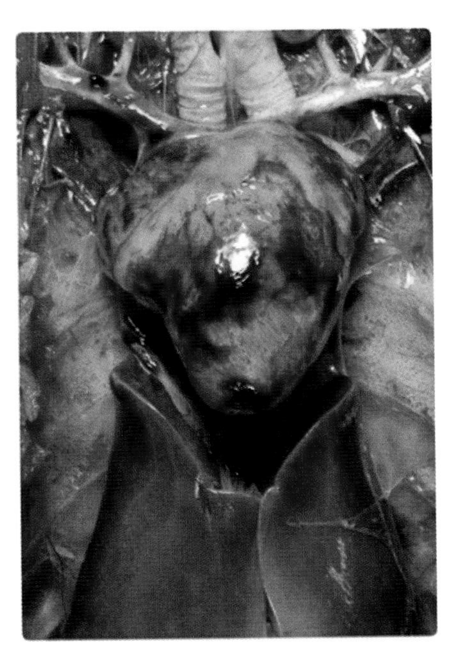

Figure 5.6 Muscovy duck with cardiac hemorrhages due to duck virus enteritis. *Source:* Courtesy of the Southeastern Cooperative Wildlife Disease Study.

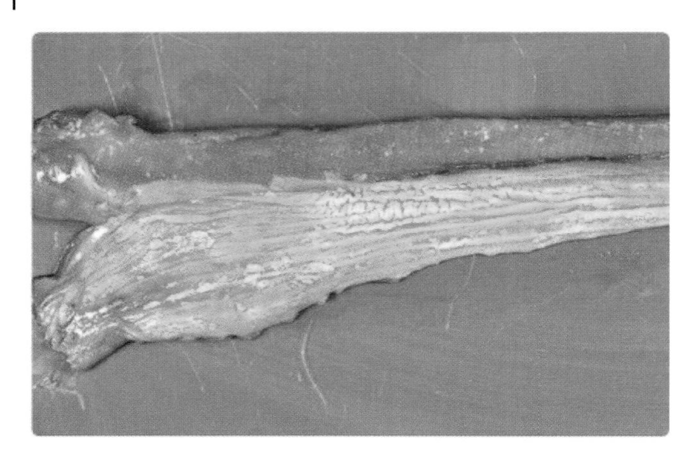

Figure 5.7 Muscovy duck with ulcerations covered in fibrin and diphtheritic membranes in the crop and esophagus due to duck virus enteritis. *Source:* Courtesy of the Southeastern Cooperative Wildlife Disease Study.

tissues, most notably, of the gastrointestinal epithelium and hepatocytes (Hansen and Gough, 2007). Diagnosis is by virus isolation or PCR of liver or other affected tissues (Fenton et al., 2018).

Differential Diagnoses

Differential diagnoses may include severe coccidian infections, *Pasteurella multocida* infection and clostridial enterotoxemia. Treatment consists of supportive care. The virus is highly contagious, so suspect infected individuals should be isolated from other birds.

Treatment/Management

No treatment is available.

Avian Influenza

Overview and Etiology

Avian influenza viruses (genus *Alphainfluenzavirus*, family Orthomyxoviridae) are most commonly reported to infect waterfowl and shorebirds, which are natural reservoirs of low pathogenicity avian influenza viruses (AIV) type A (AIAV). However, these viruses also can infect other aquatic birds (e.g. egrets, herons, pelicans, and flamingos).

Signs and Diagnosis

Low pathogenic AIV infections are subclinical and often involve oral and/or cloacal viral shedding. However, highly pathogenic AIV can cause systemic infections that may lead to acute death, neurologic disease (e.g. tremors, torticollis, opisthotonos, lethargy, swimming in circles, seizures), as well as non-specific signs such as fluffed feathers, diarrhea, and nasal discharge. The course of disease often is rapid and fatal, and thus otherwise healthy birds often are in good nutritional condition. Gross lesions may be absent or may include hepatosplenomegaly, multiorgan, multifocal (pinpoint to larger, irregular foci) necrosis in liver, pancreas (Figure 5.8), spleen, and less commonly in adrenal gland and heart, sometimes with hemorrhage, pulmonary congestion and edema, and cerebral and cerebellar hyperemia, congestion, edema, and/or malacia (Figure 5.9; Ellis et al., 2004; Stallknecht et al., 2007). Histopathology may include nonsuppurative inflammation and necrosis, which are most severe in brain, pancreas, and liver, but can also be in adrenal gland and lymphoid tissue in spleen and disseminated (e.g. gastrointestinal). Diagnosis is by virus isolation or immunohistochemistry of affected tissues (Fenton et al., 2018).

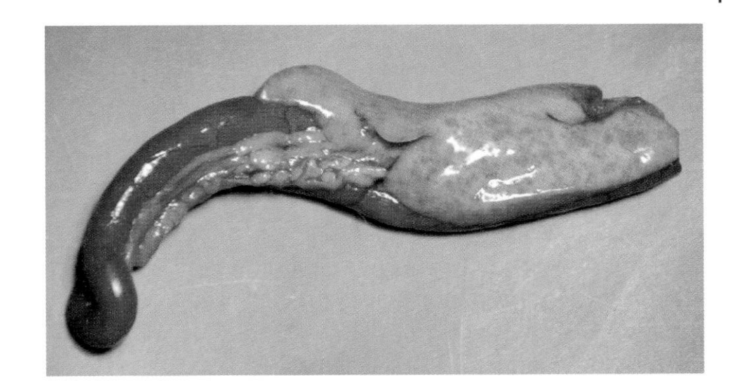

Figure 5.8 Hooded merganser. Multiple, pinpoint, discolored (necrotic) foci in the pancreas due to highly pathogenic influenza A virus infection. *Source:* Courtesy of the Southeastern Cooperative Wildlife Disease Study.

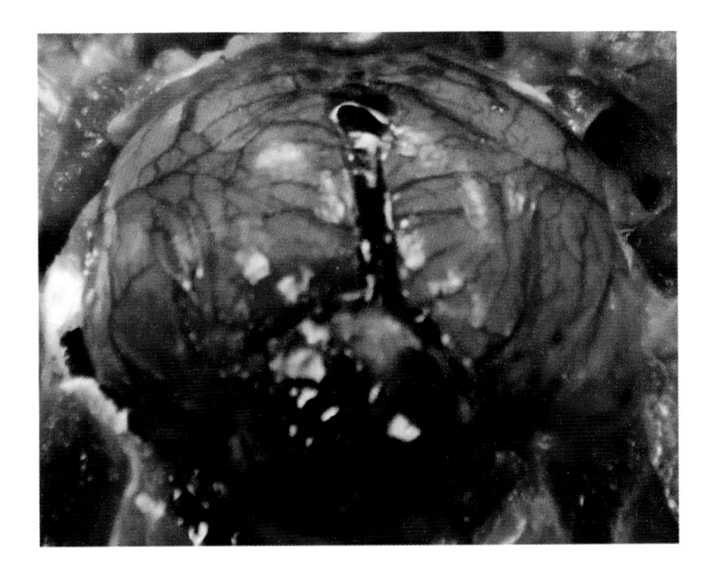

Figure 5.9 Lesser scaup. Marked vascular congestion in the meninges overlying the cerebrum and marked hyperemia (reddening) of the cerebellum due to highly pathogenic influenza A virus infection. *Source:* Courtesy of the Southeastern Cooperative Wildlife Disease Study.

Differential Diagnoses

Differentials include paramyxoviral infections, but host species range for these viruses is more limited compared with highly pathogenic AIV.

Treatment/Management

Treatment consists of supportive care. As AIVs are highly contagious, suspected infected individuals should be isolated from other birds. Highly pathogenic IAVs can be zoonotic. The disease is reportable to the World Organisation for Animal Health (WOAH) and other federal and regional authorities, depending on location of detection.

West Nile Disease

Overview and Etiology

Viruses from the family Flaviviridae, genus *Flavivirus* are able to cause fatal infections in numerous aquatic bird species, including scaup, mallards, and other ducks, geese, penguins, loons, pelicans, herons, grebes, cormorants, flamingos, and gulls (Steele et al. 2000). Because the virus is transmitted by mosquitoes, disease detection generally is seasonal.

Signs and Diagnosis

Most infections are subclinical; however, when evident, signs are often nonspecific to neurological disease, consisting of lethargy, dyspnea, vomiting, and diarrhea. When present, neurological signs may include ataxia, head tilt, head tremors, seizures, and hind limb paresis or paralysis. Gross lesions are often absent or they may include pale streaks or foci in the myocardium and splenomegaly. Histopathology varies based on the disease progression, but in fatal infections there may be myocardial necrosis (acute cases) or nonsuppurative myocarditis and meningoencephalitis (in subacute to chronic cases). Diagnosis is by microscopic lesions concurrent with immunohistochemistry, virus isolation, or reverse transcriptase PCR (rtPCR) of affected tissues (for virus isolation or PCR, pooled brain, heart, and kidney samples are recommended; Cox et al., 2015; Buckles, 2018; Stidworthy and Denk, 2018).

Differential Diagnoses

For neurologic disease, include eastern equine encephalitis virus and aquatic bird *Bornavirus* (host species range for aquatic bird *Bornavirus* is more limited than West Nile virus), paramyxoviruses and highly pathogenic AIV infections may have similar clinical presentations and histopathology. Numerous other paramyxoviruses infect avian aquatic species subclinically; their clinical and pathologic effects remain poorly understood.

Treatment/Management

No treatment is available.

Eastern Equine Encephalitis

Overview and Etiology

Virus from the family Togaviridae, genus *Togavirus* is similar to West Nile virus in that transmission is maintained in bird–mosquito sylvatic cycles; thus, disease detection is generally seasonal. Fatal infections have been reported in great egret, whooping crane, and penguins (Dein et al., 1986; Fenton et al., 2018; Stidworthy and Denk, 2018).

Signs and Diagnosis

Clinical disease may include anorexia, lethargy, vomiting, recumbency, hind-limb paresis, and paralysis (Wobeser, 1997a; Fenton et al., 2018). Gross lesions are often absent but may include myocardial pallor, pericardial fluid, hepatomegaly, splenomegaly, and ascites (Stidworthy and Denk, 2018). Microscopically, liver, spleen, lung, and meninges may have nonsuppurative inflammation and necrosis, with possible spinal cord edema (Wobeser, 1997a; Fenton et al., 2018). Diagnosis is by histopathology concurrent with immunohistochemistry, virus isolation or rtPCR of affected tissues (e.g. brain, heart, spleen; Fenton et al., 2018).

Treatment/Management

No treatment is available.

Newcastle Disease

Overview and Etiology

Avian paramyxovirus-1 from the family Paramyxoviridae, genus *Avulavirus* is infective for many aquatic avian species (e.g., ducks, geese); Infection is usually subclinical.

Signs and Diagnosis

The infection may cause neurologic disease, diarrhea, and death in domestic geese, Muscovy ducks, and gulls. Affected birds may also be weak, be unable to fly, and have unilateral wing or leg paralysis. Several species (e.g. double-crested cormorant and American white pelican) are susceptible to substantial disease outbreaks. There are no specific gross lesions but histopathology may include nonsuppurative encephalitis and myelitis, with neuronal degeneration, as well as hemorrhage and necrosis in the gastrointestinal tract, pancreas, and the lymphoid tissue. Diagnosis is by histopathology concurrent with immunohistochemistry of the affected tissue(s), virus isolation or PCR of cloacal swabs (Buckles, 2018; Fenton et al., 2018).

Differential Diagnoses

Differentials include highly pathogenic AIVs, eastern equine encephalitis virus and West Nile virus.

Treatment/Management

No treatment is available.

Wellfleet Bay Virus Disease

Overview and Etiology

Virus from the family Orthomyxoviridae, genus *Quaranjavirus* can cause disease and death in common eiders (Allison et al., 2015).

Signs and Diagnosis

Grossly, affected birds may have pale foci in the liver (Figure 5.10) and pancreas, and hepatomegaly and splenomegaly corresponding microscopically with necrosis. Diagnosis is by histopathology combined with immunohistochemistry, virus isolation or rtPCR of affected tissues. Serology may also be helpful (Fenton et al., 2018).

Treatment/Management

Not available.

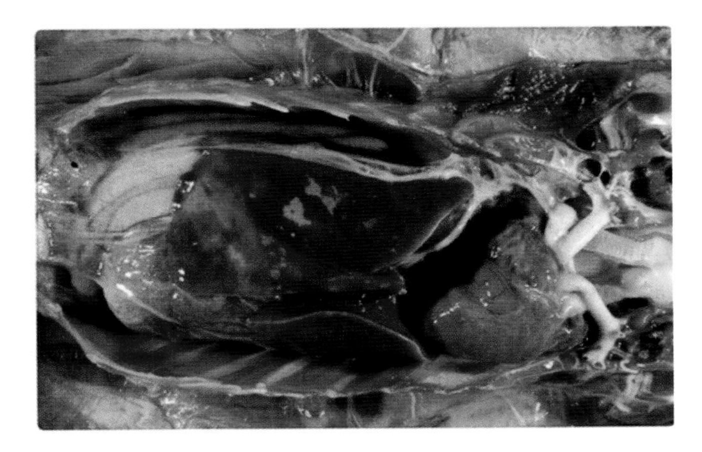

Figure 5.10 Common eider. Necrotizing hepatitis due to Wellfleet Bay virus infection. *Source:* Courtesy of the Southeastern Cooperative Wildlife Disease Study.

Aquatic Bird Bornavirus 1 Disease

Overview/Etiology

Viruses from the family Bornaviridae, genus *Orthobornavirus* are infective for various waterfowl species (e.g. Canada geese and trumpeter swans).

Signs and Diagnosis

Clinical disease may include weakness, lethargy, lameness, and neurologic signs (e.g., ataxia, hypermetria, torticollis, head tremors, stargazing, opisthotonos, impaired vision). Grossly, affected birds may have esophageal or crop impaction. Microscopically, there is nonsuppurative inflammation in the spinal cord, peripheral nerves, and myenteric ganglia/nerves, and less commonly in adrenal gland and the surrounding blood vessels, or nerve ganglia in the gastrointestinal tract serosa or muscularis (Delnatte et al., 2013). Diagnosis is by histopathology combined with immunohistochemistry or rtPCR of the brain (Fenton et al., 2018).

Treatment/Management

As for the above viral diseases, treatment consists of supportive care. Specific treatment is not available.

Bacterial Diseases of Major Taxa

The information below provides some of the most common bacteria to cause disease among aquatic birds and it is not meant to provide an exhaustive list. For example, enteric bacterial pathogens of aquatic birds include *Escherichia coli*, *Klebsiella* spp., *Salmonella* spp. and *Clostridium* spp. Clostridial enterotoxemia can lead to odorous diarrhea and peracute to acute death in penguins, which are usually found dead in good nutritional condition.

Salmonellosis

Overview and Etiology

Caused by either *Salmonella typhimurium*, or *Salmonella anatis* in penguins, salmonellosis ranges from subclinical to clinical disease (e.g. diarrhea, pasty vent, lethargy, drooped wings) and can cause die-off in mute swans, ducks, American coots, gulls, cattle egrets, and others (Daoust and Prescott, 2007; Fenton et al., 2018).

Signs and Diagnosis

Gross lesions in acute disease may include hepatomegaly and splenomegaly, with pale (necrotic) foci that can progress to inflammatory nodules ("paratyphoid nodules") in liver, spleen, skeletal muscles, subcutis, and brain. Affected birds may also have caecal plugs, fibrinous pericarditis, peritonitis, air sacculitis, and ulcerative enteritis (Wobeser, 1997b; Fenton et al., 2018). Histopathology includes myriad Gram-negative bacilli associated with inflammation and necrosis. Diagnosis is by history, gross pathology, and histopathology, combined with bacterial culture and/or PCR testing of the affected organs, most commonly, the liver (Fenton et al., 2018).

Differential Diagnoses

Differential diagnoses include coccidial enteritis, other bacteria (including clostridial disease).

Treatment/Management
Treatment is with antimicrobials and supportive care. Zoonotic precautions should be taken.

Mycobacteriosis (Tuberculosis)

Overview/Etiology
Mycobacteriosis (tuberculosis) is caused by *Mycobactyerium* spp., most commonly *Mycobactyerium avium* complex species such as *M. avium* sub. *avium* and *M. avium* sub. *intracellulare* and *Mycobactyerium genavense*. Commonly, infections are diagnosed in zoo or captive collections, but they have been documented in free-ranging penguins, pelicans, flamingos, and other wild aquatic birds.

Signs and Diagnosis
Disease is often chronic. Grossly, affected birds may be emaciated with pale nodules in the liver (Figure 5.11) and less commonly in spleen, intestine, and/or lungs, and hepatomegaly or splenomegaly (Wobser, 1997b; Buckles, 2018; Fenton et al., 2018). Birds may have pericarditis, air sacculitis, and less frequently, bone involvement (Wobeser, 1997b). Microscopically, these correspond to yellow-gray, nodular foci (granulomas) that may contain intracellular and extracellular, acid-fast bacilli. Secondary amyloidosis can occur. Diagnosis by impression smears and staining for cytology, histopathology, and mycobacterial culture, with confirmation by PCR (Buckles, 2018; Stidworthy and Denk, 2018).

Differential Diagnoses
Differential diagnoses include aspergillosis, nocardiosis, and salmonellosis (Fenton et al., 2018).

Treatment/Management
Management is via antimicrobials and supportive care. Zoonotic precautions should be taken.

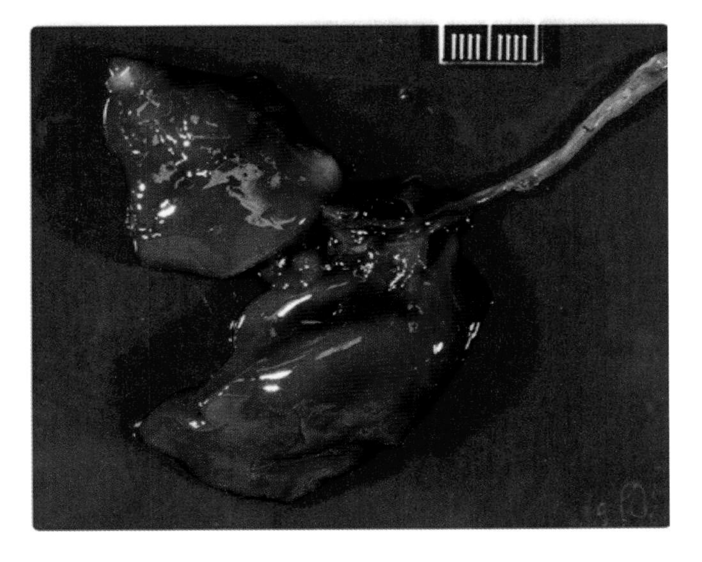

Figure 5.11 Blue-winged teal. Granulomatous hepatitis associated with *Mycobacterium avium* infection. *Source:* Courtesy of the Southeastern Cooperative Wildlife Disease Study.

Pasteurellosis

Overview and Etiology

Infection by *Pasteurella multocida* is the cause of avian cholera, which affects many aquatic species (e.g., penguins, pelicans, cormorants, loons, grebes, petrels, and others) and can potentially cause substantial disease outbreaks. In wild waterfowl, peracute mortality due to septicemia is most common; birds are generally found dead in good nutritional condition.

Signs and Diagnosis

When found alive, signs may appear neurologic (e.g., ataxia, disorientation, head tilt). Grossly, there are petechial hemorrhages evident on the surfaces of heart, liver and spleen, and hyperemic intestines. Histopathology reveals necrosis and inflammation in the spleen and liver, with Gram-negative coccobacilli. Diagnosis is by history and histopathology, concurrent with immunohistochemistry or bacterial culture; confirmation is by PCR; choice samples include heart blood, liver, bone marrow, or other affected tissues (Fenton et al., 2018). Several other bacteria within the same family (Pasteurellaceae) can cause similar presentation, including peracute death; these include Bisgaard taxon 40 strains, which have caused fatal, disseminated bacterial infections in common (*Sterna hirundo*) and sandwich terns (*Thalasseus sandvicensis*), as well as rhinoceros auklets (*Cerorhinca monocerata*) (Knowles et al., 2019; Niedringhaus et al., 2021). These infections may be predisposed by stressful events, such as migration or severe weather.

Differential Diagnoses

Differentials include viral and bacterial infections (e.g. duck virus enteritis, clostridial enterotoxemia) and pathogens causing sudden death (e.g. highly pathogenic avian influenza virus, *Erysipelothrix rhusiopathiae*, *Streptococcus zooepidemicus*).

Treatment/Management

Treatment is via antimicrobials and supportive care. Zoonotic precautions should be taken.

Chlamydiosis

Overview and Etiology

Chlamydia spp. (e.g. *Chlamydia psittaci*) infection can cause disease in penguins, fulmars, shearwaters, pelicans, and others.

Signs and Diagnosis

Affected birds have anorexia, lethargy, and pale, green droppings. Grossly, there is hepatomegaly and splenomegaly, with inflammation and necrosis associated with intracellular organisms, which are highlighted via histochemical stains (e.g., Giemsa, Gimenez, modified Gimenez PVK stain, and Macchiovello). Diagnosis is by histopathology paired with immunohistochemistry or bacterial culture/isolation from the affected tissue, feces or swabs, confirmed by PCR (Stidworthy and Denk, 2018).

Treatment/Management

Treatment is via antimicrobials and supportive care. Zoonotic precautions should be taken.

Infection with *Reimerella anatipestifer*

Overview/Etiology

Infection with *Reimerella anatipestifer* can cause die-off due to septicemia in various species of free-ranging ducks, geese and swans.

Signs and Diagnosis

The infection may be subclinical or it may lead to green diarrhea, ocular discharge, neurologic signs (e.g. weakness, lethargy, ataxia, swimming in circles; Wobeser, 1997b). Grossly, affected birds may have splenomegaly, exudative and fibrinous inflammation, with deposition on multiple serosal surfaces, including tracheal mucosa, ovary, lung, sinusal mucosa, heart, liver, kidney, brain, meninges, and joints. Histopathology reveals fibrinous exudate on serosal surfaces with intracellular and extracellular Gram-negative bacilli, and possibly thrombosis. Diagnosis is by gross and microscopic findings paired with bacterial culture/isolation from heart blood, brain, liver, spleen, kidney, lung, and air sacs; multiple tissues should be submitted for the diagnosis to be established (heart blood and brain are preferred; Fenton et al., 2018).

Differential Diagnoses

Differential dagnoses vary by host species and include duck virus enteritis and salmonellosis.

Treatment/Management

No treatment is available.

Fungal Diseases of Major Taxa

Aspergillosis

Overview and Etiology

Aspergillus spp. (e.g., *Aspergillus fumigatus*, *Aspergillus flavus*) can infect most, if not all, avian species. Among aquatic birds, aspergillosis, which is sometimes fatal, has been reported in loons, pelicans, gannets, albatross, sea ducks, eiders, and swans. The disease is often associated with immunosuppression, malnutrition, young age, coinfections, and physiologic stressors.

Signs and Diagnosis

The disease can manifest acutely, but more often it is chronic. Clinically, diseased birds may present with weakness, inability to fly, open mouth breathing/dyspnea, tachypnea, and cyanosis. Gross lesions of acute disease may include dark red, edematous lungs (i.e., congestion, hemorrhage) and small, pale, nodular foci (granulomas) in the lungs (Figure 5.12). Chronic disease may correspond to thickened and cloudy air sacs, with fungal plaques (blue, olive-green, brown, or black, velvety if conidia) and hepatomegaly and/or splenomegaly. Fungi invade blood vessels and can disseminate to the liver, kidney, adrenal glands, and other tissues and organs. Microscopically, affected tissues have heterophilic and granulomatous inflammation, with characteristic fungal hyphae (basophilic to transparent, 3–6 μm in diameter, septate, thin, and parallel-walled with dichotomous acute angled branching; Buckles, 2018; Fenton et al., 2018; Stidworthy and Denk, 2018). Diagnosis is by characteristic gross and histopathology; Grocott–Gomori's methenamine silver stain and periodic acid Schiff reaction highlight the fungus microscopically. The fungal species can be identified through fungal culture and molecular testing (Fenton et al., 2018).

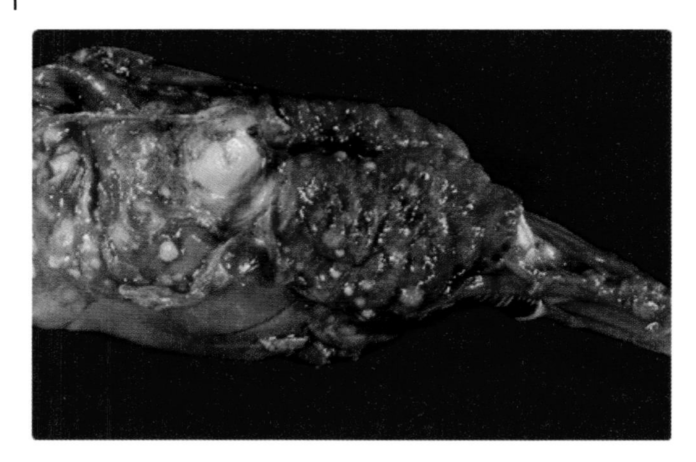

Figure 5.12 Laughing gull. Lungs, air sacs, and gastrointestinal serosa are obscured by multifocal fungal granulomas (*Aspergillus* sp.). *Source:* Courtesy of the Southeastern Cooperative Wildlife Disease Study.

Differential Diagnoses

Differential diagnoses include mycobacteriosis, nocardiosis, other fungal infections (e.g. *Mucor* spp.; many of these differ morphologically) and chronic reaction to inhaled foreign material.

Treatment/Management

Treatment includes antifungals and supportive care; however, late in the disease process, prognosis is poor. The low rate of recovery should be considered with the treatment associated stress in this case.

Candidiasis

Overview and Etiology

Candida albicans, a yeast-like fungi, although rarely reported in aquatic birds, can infect and cause disease (candidiasis) in many (if not all) taxa of aquatic birds, which broadly have included gulls, terns, ducks, geese, and shorebirds. This disease is more often seen in captive-reared or housed birds. The source of infection is likely contaminated environments, followed by ingestion of the yeast.

Signs and Diagnosis

Clinically, birds may appear in general poor condition, poor nutritional condition, with lethargy. Grossly, the oral cavity, crop, and esophagus may have white to pale tan or gray, rough and/or thickened plaques or nodules along the mucosal surface, sometimes with associated ulceration (US Geological Survey, 1999f). Diagnosis can be made by scraping the surface of mucosal lesions with identification of the thin-walled, ovoid budding yeasts, for which pseudohyphae or filamentous hyphae may be evident; organisms also may be evident by histopathology and highlighted by periodic acid Schiff and methenamine silver stains, with confirmation via PCR or culture.

Non-Infectious Diseases of Major Taxa

Trauma

Overview and Etiology

Trauma is a common cause of death among birds and other wildlife, especially those that live in close proximity to humans. Entanglement in, or ingestion of debris, waste/trash, fishing gear

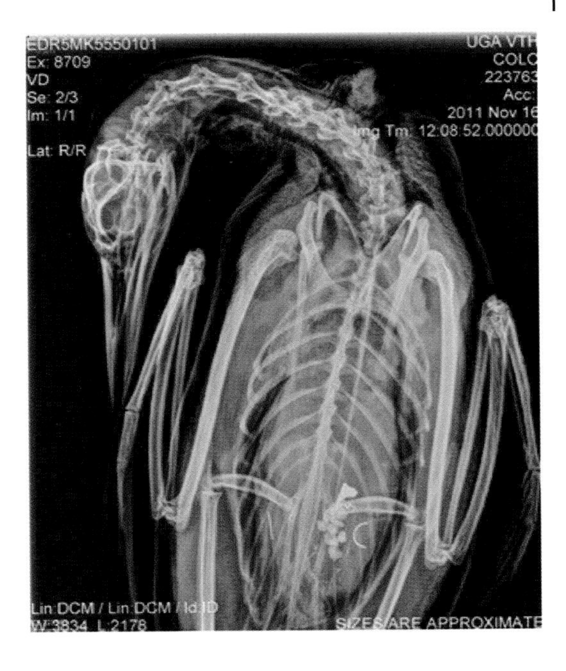

Figure 5.13 Common loon. Radiograph revealing ingested fishing tackle within the gastrointestinal tract, visible in the caudal coelomic cavity. *Source:* Courtesy of the Southeastern Cooperative Wildlife Disease Study.

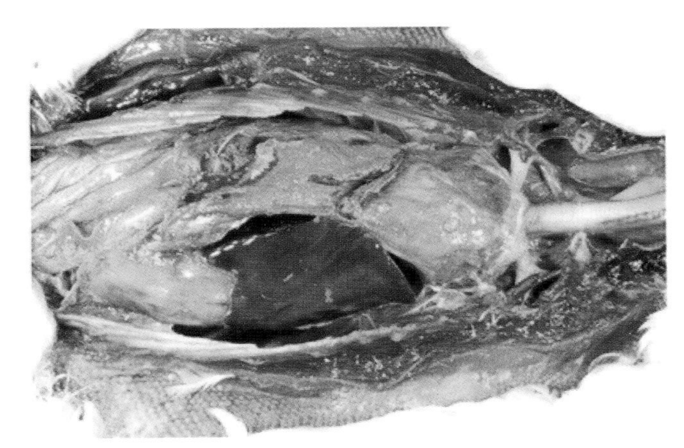

Figure 5.14 Common loon. Necrotizing coelomitis with fibrin overlying a liver lobe, associated with ingestion of wire. *Source:* Courtesy of the Southeastern Cooperative Wildlife Disease Study.

(Figure 5.13), and other objects can cause injuries and associated morbidity and mortality (Figure 5.14). In some cases, entanglements can lead to drowning, especially in marine species (e.g. albatross, petrel, boobies, frigate birds).

Signs and Diagnosis

Birds that undergo acute trauma or trauma-associated drowning are often found in good nutritional condition, with food in the alimentary tract; they may have clear watery fluid in air sacs or distal trachea, fluid or debris in pulmonary airways, oozing of white, frothy fluid from cut surfaces and congested vasculature. Predation is another cause of trauma in aquatic birds (Figure 5.15), including from invasive or feral species, such as mongoose, rats, and cats (Stilworthy and Denk, 2018). Gunshot (Figure 5.16) and collisions with stationary or moving objects are additional sources of trauma that can lead to debilitation and death. Radiographs can assist in confirming the diagnosis.

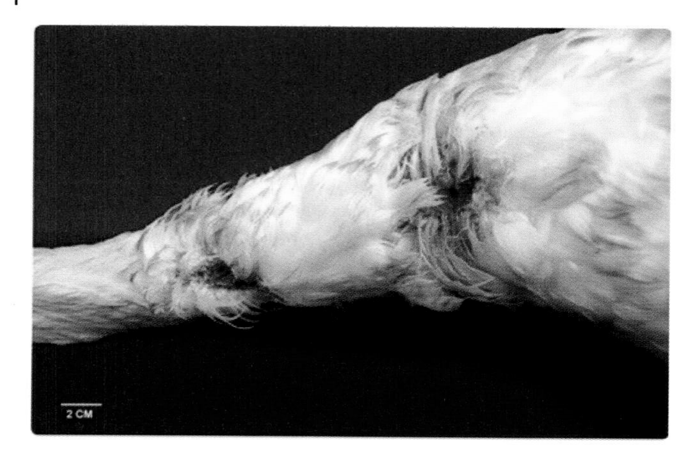

Figure 5.15 Trumpeter swan with trauma along the neck from predator-induced bite (puncture) wounds. *Source:* Courtesy of the Southeastern Cooperative Wildlife Disease Study.

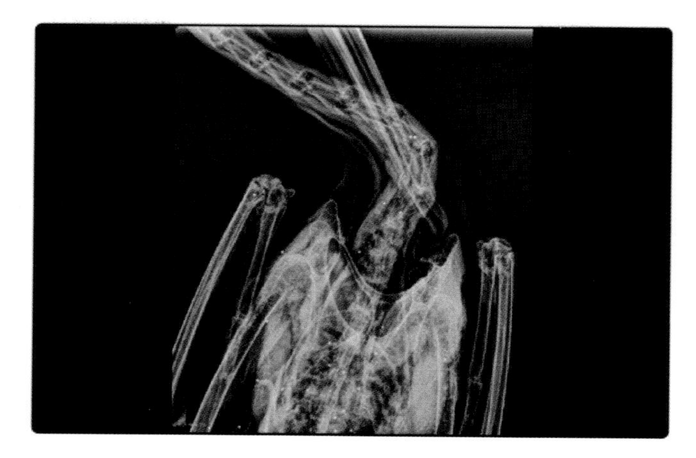

Figure 5.16 American white pelican. Radiograph revealing multiple pellets leading to gunshot trauma. *Source:* Courtesy of the Southeastern Cooperative Wildlife Disease Study.

Starvation

Overview and Etiology

Starvation is commonly observed among aquatic birds, and most often, it is attributed to malnutrition or starvation due to depleted or poor access to food resources (e.g., aquatic invertebrates, vertebrates, and vegetation). Many wild aquatic bird species are susceptible, especially those that depend on marine ecosystems (e.g., penguins, puffins), migratory species that depend on resources across broad geographic regions and immature birds (Stidworthy and Denk, 2018). Starvation and malnutrition can lead to mass mortality events that are exacerbated by adverse weather events, altered environmental and climatic conditions (e.g. oceanic currents or temperatures affecting distribution and quantity of food resources), overharvesting of aquatic resources by humans (leading to nutrient poor resources) and other factors.

Signs and Diagnosis

Starving birds lack subcutaneous and visceral adipose reserves and have skeletal muscle atrophy, prominent or sharp keel bone (Figure 5.17), shrunken liver, empty alimentary tract, and are often concurrently dehydrated. Microscopically, serous atrophy of fat may be evident around the heart and in the bone marrow, whereas the liver presents with hepatocellular atrophy

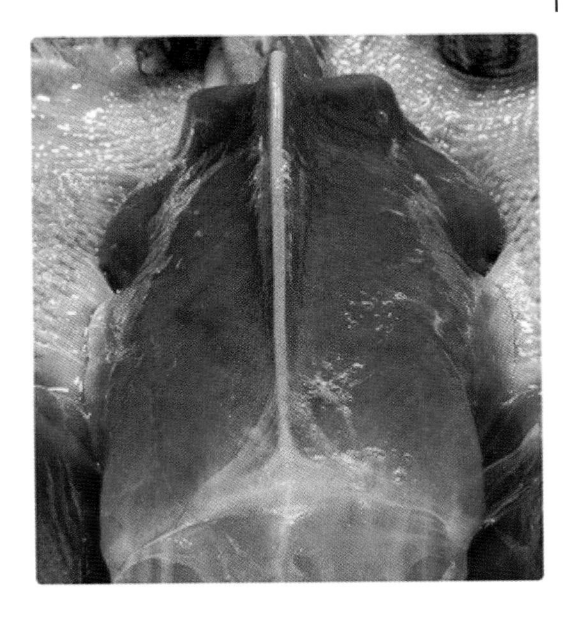

Figure 5.17 Emaciation in a common eider, showing prominent keel bone and atrophied pectoral muscles. *Source:* Courtesy of the Southeastern Cooperative Wildlife Disease Study.

(Fenton et al., 2018). Gross evaluation of fat content in the bone marrow (in nonpneumatic long bones) can support the diagnosis. Emaciated animals are more susceptible to infections, toxicosis, and hypothermia owing to the lack of energy reserves to find cover, and especially in conjunction with physiologically stressful events, such as migration and adverse weather events (Stidworthy and Denk, 2018).

Starvation also may be associated with ingestion of plastics, which can block or otherwise impede digestion; alternately, starvation may predispose to ingestion of less appropriate food items, such as plastics. The presence of plastics in marine environments is an emerging and urgent problem that affects a large proportion of many species of aquatic wildlife. A comprehensive review of microplastics in marine vertebrates revealed that 50.4% of seabirds studied were affected by microplastics (Ugwu et al., 2021). Another study evaluated ingestion of marine debris (mostly plastic) in the gastrointestinal tracts of numerous coastal and pelagic avian species in the southwest Atlantic ocean and observed 30% of examined individuals of 11 species had debris; the species with greatest quantities of ingested debris included Atlantic yellow-nosed albatross (*Thalassarche chlororhynchos*), Cory's shearwater (*Calonectris borealis*), Manx shearwater (*Puffinus puffinus*), brown booby (*Sula leucogaster*), and Magellanic penguin (*Spheniscus magellanicus*) (Vanstreels et al. 2021). Plastics cause harm in a variety of ways, including entanglements, as well as via direct ingestion of plastic debris (e.g. bottles, containers, nets, fishing line) or via ingestion of animals at lower trophic levels. In addition, encounters by wildlife with plastic and other waste can lead to entanglement, drowning, suffocation, and lacerations and other wounds (Figure 5.18). Plastic waste management, including prevention of plastics reaching marine environments, is imperative to prevent the worsening of the vast quantities of plastics continually entering oceans globally (Alzugaray et al., 2020).

Careful evaluation of the entire gastrointestinal tract during necropsy is necessary and it is important to document the presence of plastics; however, some microplastics are not grossly or microscopically visible and thus require more advanced techniques for detection (e.g. density separation, pyrolysis, gas chromatography/mass spectrometry, Raman spectroscopy, and Fourier transform infrared spectrometry; Ugwu et al., 2021).

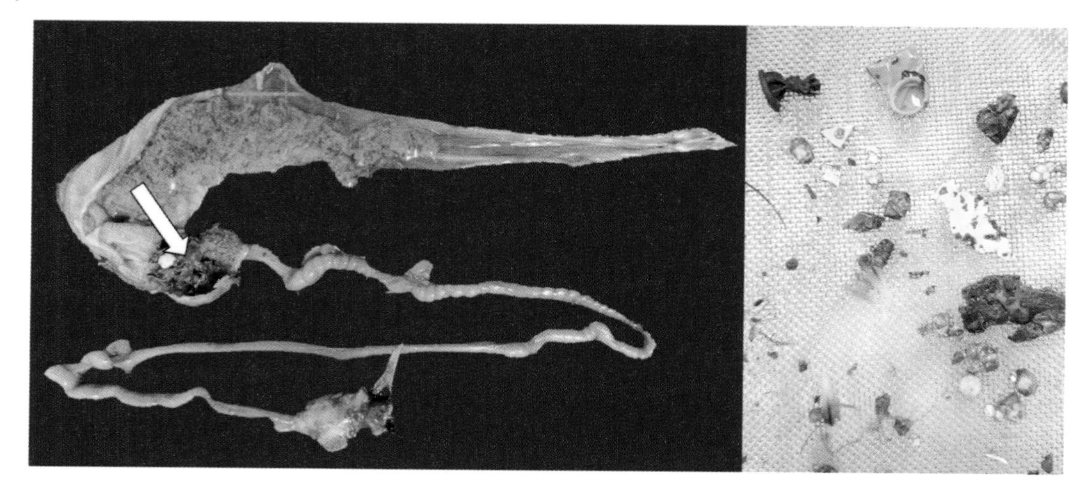

Figure 5.18 Left: Plastic debris within the ventriculus (arrow) of an adult male soft-plumaged petrel (*Pterodroma mollis*) that died of starvation. *Source:* Courtesy of Allan Poltronieri Santos, IPRAM. Right: Plastic and other anthropogenic debris removed from the gastrointestinal tract of a southern giant petrel (*Macronectes giganteus*). *Source:* Courtesy of Luciana Gallo, IBIOMAR, CONICET.

Aside from emaciation, nutritional imbalances are rarely diagnosed and reported in wild birds. Hypovitaminosis A has been documented in waterfowl that primarily ingest grains with lack of green vegetation. This condition can also second starvation. Clinically affected birds, especially young birds, may have stunted growth, ataxia, and paresis/paralysis. Gross lesions may entail thickened oral mucosa and excessive keratin in the skin. These lesions correspond microscopically to epidermal hyperkeratosis and epithelial squamous metaplasia. Differentials for oral lesions include candidiasis and avian pox (Fenton et al., 2018). Vitamin E deficiency is most commonly diagnosed in piscivorean birds (e.g., herons, egrets, storks) due to poor diet, which may include rancid fish (i.e., oxidized fatty acids). Grossly and histologically, fat is variably expanded by inflammation (steatitis; Figure 5.19). Necrotic and mineralized muscle tissue grossly may exhibit pale streaks (Fenton et al., 2018).

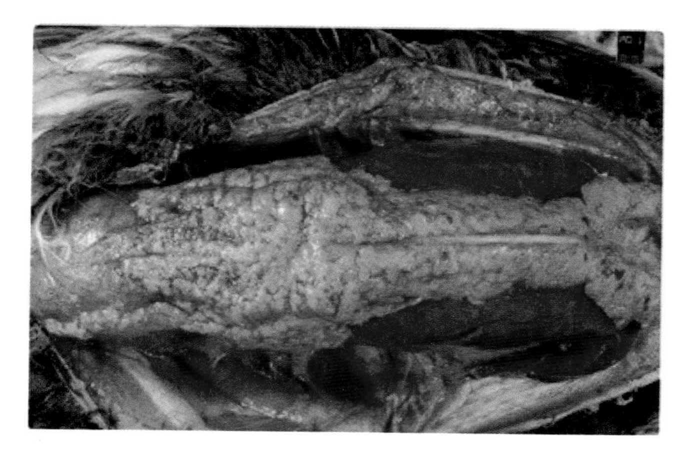

Figure 5.19 Great blue heron. The pectoral muscles and abdominal viscera are covered in a thick band of inflamed adipose tissue (steatitis, potentially associated with vitamin E deficiency). *Source:* Courtesy of the Southeastern Cooperative Wildlife Disease Study.

Gout or Hyperuricemia

Overview and Etiology

Gout is more commonly diagnosed in captive birds, but it can affect wild aquatic birds and is usually associated with, and considered secondary to, impaired renal function. Dietary factors (e.g. high protein or hypovitaminosis A) may be contributing factors of the disease. Uric acid accumulation in kidneys can also occur with severe dehydration.

Signs and Diagnosis

Grossly, there are white gritty or chalky deposits (urates) on the surface of organs (e.g. kidneys, heart) and/or in the joints. The kidneys may be bilaterally enlarged and pale. Histopathology reveals urate crystals in the affected tissues, together with inflammation and necrosis, and with fibrosis in chronic cases (Wobeser, 1997e).

Ingestion of Foreign Bodies

Overview and Etiology

Plastics, metals, sharp food items, such as fish bones or exoskeleton (Figure 5.20) can obstruct or cause damage to the lining of the gastrointestinal tract, leading to disease and starvation.

Signs and Diagnosis

Clinical signs may include dehydration, anorexia, weight loss, lethargy, weakness, extended molt, coelomic distention, regurgitation, vomiting, and diarrhea to scant feces. Necropsy may

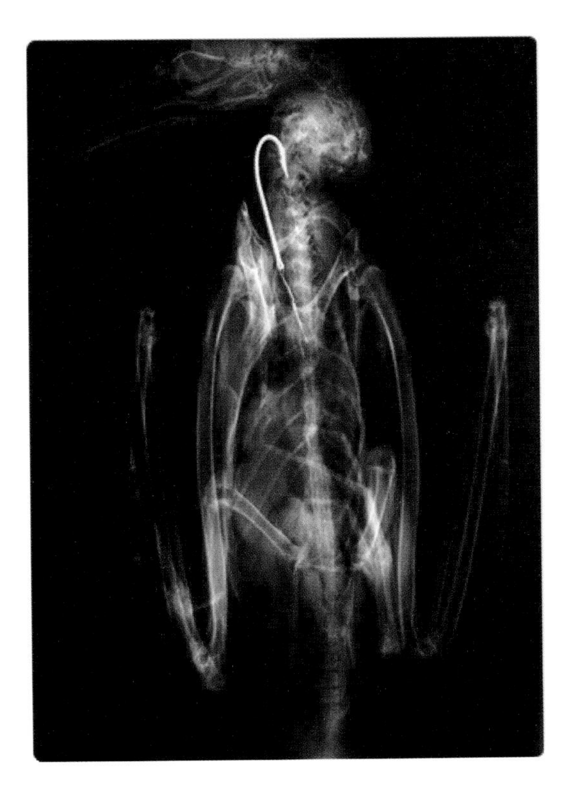

Figure 5.20 Gannet. Radiograph revealing ingested fishhook in the esophagus.
Source: Courtesy of the Southeastern Cooperative Wildlife Disease Study.

reveal mild inflammation, erosion, and ulceration in affected areas of the digestive tract walls. With severe damage, the wall may perforate and lead to coelomitis and sepsis. Ingestion of plastics (macro and microplastics) has become more commonly detected among pelagic species (e.g. albatrosses, petrels, shearwaters) (Stidworthy and Denk, 2018). Aside from overt damage to the gastrointestinal tract described above, the long-term health effects of plastic ingestion in aquatic birds are poorly understood. Esophageal impaction is frequently reported in Canada geese and can be associated with lead toxicosis, excess or dry plant-based feed (soybeans, cowpeas, green plants), discarded fishing line, nematode infection (Amidostomum spp.), aquatic bird *Bornavirus* infection, and mycotoxicosis. Grossly, the mid-cervical esophagus is markedly distended by a dense bolus of food (Fenton et al., 2018). Radiographs can assist in confirming the presence and location of some materials, which are often lodged in the proventriculus.

Amyloidosis (Protein Misfolding Disease)

Overview and Etiology

Amyloidosis is most commonly reported in waterfowl. It occurs spontaneously or concurrently with other chronic diseases, such as infections and neoplasia.

Signs and Diagnosis

Grossly, the liver is enlarged, tan to orange and friable; the spleen may also be enlarged. As a result, both organs are susceptible to fracture and hemorrhage. Diagnosis generally is made by the characteristic microscopic appearance, as smooth, pale pink material that disrupts and replaces normal cellular architecture in the liver, spleen, kidney, and less commonly, in the intestine or other organs. In light microscopy, the material is pink to orange, and it may exhibit apple-green birefringence under polarized light. Congo red stain is less useful to highlight the material in birds compared with mammals; thioflavin T stain may highlight amyloid via fluorescent microscopy. The gold standard diagnostic modality for confirmation is electron microscopy (Fenton et al., 2018).

Exertional Myopathy

Overview and Etiology

Exertional myopathy can occur in birds with a history of high-stress pursuit and/or capture. Grossly, large muscle groups may exhibit pale streaks that microscopically correspond to myocyte degeneration and necrosis, sometimes, with mild inflammation. This condition may lead to acute or delayed death (Fenton et al., 2018).

Pododermatitis ("Bumblefoot")

Overview and Etiology

Pododermatitis can occur in many aquatic bird species, and it is more commonly diagnosed in captive compared with free-ranging birds. Bacterial infection can occur following pressure sores (e.g. inflammation, necrosis, and fibrosis) on the plantar surface of the feet, and is facilitated by small breaches in the skin. Inciting causes can include bacteria, such as *Staphylococcus aureus*, *Escherichia coli*, *Proteus mirabilis*, *Enterococcus* spp., *Pseudomonas* spp., *Clostridium* spp., or fungi.

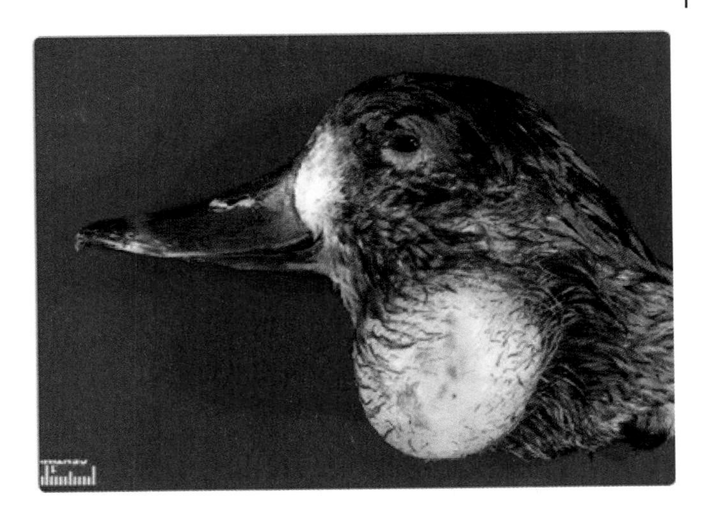

Figure 5.21 Ring-necked duck. Fibroma along the cranial neck of a hunter-harvested duck.
Source: Courtesy of the Southeastern Cooperative Wildlife Disease Study.

Signs and Diagnosis

The infection can progress to osteomyelitis, tenosynovitis, and systemic amyloidosis (Wobeser, 1997b; Stidworthy and Denk, 2018; Fenton et al., 2018). Grossly, skin on the plantar surfaces of the feet (often bilateral) may have cracks or fissures, epidermal erosions, or ulcers, with underlying diffuse to nodular thickening. Microscopically, subacute lesions may include hyperplasia and dysplasia of the epidermis, to more chronic lesions of keratinocytic hydropic degeneration, epidermal hyperplasia, and dyskeratosis, chronic lymphohistiocytic to granulomatous inflammation, sometimes with discrete granulomas, granulation tissue, and bacterial colonies at various levels of the affected epidermis and dermis (Wyss et al., 2015). Diagnosis is by visualization of Gram-positive cocci associated with the lesions (via Gram stain), concurrent with bacterial culture and PCR (Fenton et al., 2018).

Spontaneous Neoplasia

Overview and Etiology

Neoplasias are rarely reported in wild aquatic birds. Broadly, neoplasias include lymphomas, neuroendocrine, hepatic and ovarian tumors, melanoma (e.g. in penguins), gastrointestinal adenocarcinoma, squamous cell carcinoma, and cholangiocarcinoma (Buckles, 2018; Stidworthy and Denk, 2018). Neurofibrosarcoma, liposarcoma, spindle cell sarcoma, hepatocellular carcinoma, lymphoma, fibroma (Figure 5.21), testicular tumors (seminoma), and chondrosarcoma have been diagnosed in a variety of waterfowl (e.g. ducks, swans, geese) and gulls (Fenton et al., 2018).

Toxicoses of Major Taxa

Heavy Metal Intoxications

Lead Toxicosis

Overview and Etiology Lead toxicosis is common among many species of aquatic birds, especially those that tend to ingest shiny objects (e.g. fishing tackle and lead shot) from the floor of water

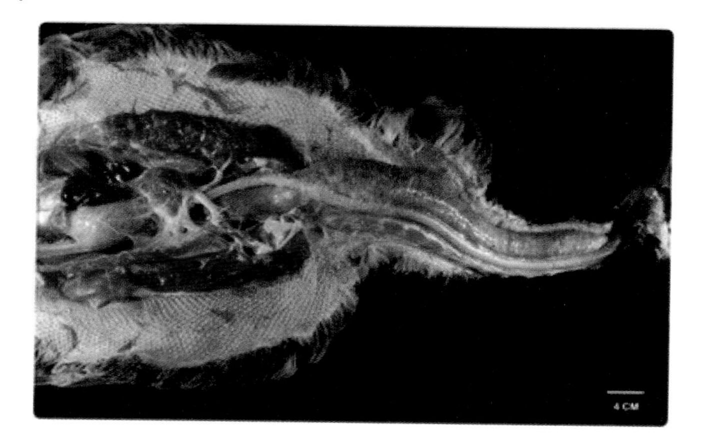

Figure 5.22 Canada goose. Esophageal–proventricular impaction resulting from lead toxicosis. *Source:* Courtesy of the Southeastern Cooperative Wildlife Disease Study.

bodies (e.g. loons, diving ducks, penguins). Lead-based objects may be evident on radiographs, and they may be recoverable from the alimentary tract. The risk lies with the toxins being able to leach out and be absorbed into the bloodstream.

Signs and Diagnosis Clinically, affected birds may exhibit abnormal posture (drooped wings), inability to fly, bright green droppings, and pasty vent. Acutely intoxicated birds are often in good nutritional condition. Bloodwork may reveal hypochromic anemia, hemolytic anemia (acute cases) and leukocytopenia (chronic cases; Fenton et al. 2018). Often, there are no gross lesions, but chronically affected birds may have muscle atrophy, lack of adipose reserves, subcutaneous edema of the head and mandible (e.g. geese and swans), food impaction (stasis) in the esophagus and proventriculus (Figure 5.22), distended gall bladder, erosions in ventricular lining, myocardial pallor, hydropericardium, and nephromegaly. Microscopically, there may be myocardial and hepatocellular degeneration, hepatic cord atrophy, prominent intracellular hemosiderin, renal tubular degeneration and necrosis, muscle degeneration, necrosis and atrophy, lymphoid atrophy, and demyelination in the central and peripheral nervous systems. Rarely, characteristic acid-fast, intranuclear "lead inclusions" may be evident in the renal tubular epithelium (Buckles, 2018; Fenton et al., 2018; Stidworthy and Denk, 2018). Diagnosis is by assessment of blood lead concentrations (antemortem), liver or kidney lead levels via toxicological tests (postmortem); if liver is not available, bone can be used to assess for chronic lead exposure.

Differential Diagnoses As for many of the following toxicoses, include toxicosis with other heavy metals and organophosphates and carbamates, botulism, and neurotropic viruses.

Treatment/Management Treatment includes attempts at chelation therapy and supportive care and endoscopy or surgery may be indicated to remove remaining lead sources from the alimentary tract (Huang and Mayer, 2019).

Zinc Toxicosis

Overview and Etiology Zinc toxicosis is rarely diagnosed. It can occur with ingestion of zinc-containing materials (e.g. pennies/coins, galvanized metal, fertilizer, paint); thus, diving ducks are prone (Fenton et al., 2018).

Signs and Diagnosis Clinically, birds may exhibit lethargy, weakness, anorexia and weight loss, anemia, polyuria/polydipsia, hemoglobinuria, regurgitation, diarrhea, and neurologic signs. Clinical pathology findings may include leukocytosis and hypochromic regenerative anemia, as well as biochemistry abnormalities (e.g. elevated levels of lactate dehydrogenase, aspartate aminotransferase, bile acids, and creatine phosphokinase; Huang and Mayer, 2019). Gross findings may be minimal. Microscopic changes primarily involve ventriculus and pancreas. Acute cases may have pancreatic zymogen depletion, acinar cell atrophy and necrosis, while chronic cases present with pancreatic fibrosis, exocrine regeneration, ductular hyperplasia, ventricular degeneration and necrosis, which can be transmural. Diagnosis is by histopathology, location of the zinc-containing products (via radiographs or necropsy), and toxicological testing of liver or kidney to assess the zinc levels in these organs (Fenton et al., 2018).

Treatment/Management Treatment includes supportive therapy, anticonvulsants, chelation therapy and antibiotics/antifungals. Endoscopy or surgery may be indicated to remove the zinc source from the alimentary tract (Huang and Mayer, 2019).

Mercury Toxicosis

Overview and Etiology Mercury toxicosis has been documented in aquatic species that feed on fish and shellfish. It can be associated with some industrial-related land use. Methylmercury can cross the blood–brain barrier, leading to central nervous system and reproductive disorders and disease, manifested by infertility and embryonic death.

Signs and Diagnosis Clinical signs may include weakness, impaired mobility, anorexia, and altered vocalization. Gross lesions are often absent; histopathology may include spinal cord demyelination, possibly, liver and kidney degeneration, and necrosis in some species (Fenton et al., 2018; Stidworthy and Denk, 2018). Diagnosis is by toxicologic testing of kidney or liver (Fenton et al., 2018).

Organophosphates and Carbamates

Overview and Etiology

Organophosphates and carbamates are used in insecticides and pesticides. They inhibit release of acetylcholinesterase at the neuromuscular junction. Acetylcholinesterase breaks down some neurotransmitters; thus, its inhibition leads to perpetual excitation. Toxicosis can lead to acute die-off in numerous species of birds.

Signs and Diagnosis

Clinically, birds experience hyperexcitability (acute) to eventual depression and weakness (within three days), muscle tremors, excessive lacrimation and salivation, epistaxis, bronchospasm, dyspnea, bradycardia, miosis, paralysis, opisthotonos, and gastrointestinal signs (e.g. diarrhea, emesis); respiratory paralysis may lead to death (US Geological Survey, 1999b; Fenton et al., 2018). Gross lesions are non-specific (e.g multiorgan hyperemia and petechiae); affected birds are often in good nutritional condition with abundant food in the proximal alimentary tract. Microscopically, there may be vascular congestion and mild hemorrhage in the brain (Wobeser, 1997c; Fenton et al., 2018). Diagnosis is by history of recent pesticide use in the region, clinical signs, and toxicological tests (e.g. cholinesterase screening of whole blood or cerebrum sample). Decreased brain cholinesterase activity indicates exposure. The chemical compounds can be identified in feed, gastrointestinal contents or liver metabolites via gas chromatography/mass spectrometry (Fenton et al., 2018).

Treatment/Management

With carbamate toxicosis, neurochemical changes are reversible, but this is not the case with organophosphate toxicosis. Treatment of respiratory signs is with atropine and neuromuscular toxicosis with intravenous pralidoxime (O'Malley and O'Malley, 2018).

Per/Polyfluoroalkyl Substances

Per/polyfluoroalkyl substances (PFAS) are fluorinated compounds found in many human-made materials (e.g. clothes, food containers, firefighting foam, paper, anti-stick coating on appliances and carpets) that bioaccumulate in the environment and often end up in water bodies. PFAS are becoming increasingly detected in aquatic (especially marine) birds and other wildlife, in which they pose a health threat. PFAS may be ingested via water (especially for species that feed close to the surface or topwater) or prey (especially species at higher trophic levels due to toxin bioaccumulation). Although overt health effects that cause gross and microscopic lesions are poorly documented, some PFAS are known carcinogens and can cause oxidative damage that affects physiological processes including reproduction, as well as impair development of the central nervous and immune systems (van der Schyff et al., 2020).

Biotoxins from Harmful Algal Blooms

Overview and Etiology

Biotoxins from harmful algal blooms often cause disease in aquatic birds in summer, when waters are warm; species that eat fish and invertebrates are most susceptible (Landsberg et al., 2007; Stidworthy and Denk, 2018; Gibble et al., 2021). Some of these organisms (e.g. *Karenia brevis*) produce neurotoxins (brevetoxins) that may be ingested or inhaled and manifest as subclinical to fatal neurologic disease, which may predispose to the development of other diseases such as bacterial infection (Niedringhaus et al., 2021). Species that frequent coastal areas and feed on pelagic prey (e.g. cormorants, shags) and filter feeders (e.g. flamingos) are especially susceptible. Large die-off events involving multiple species may result. Marine dinoflagellates, diatoms, and freshwater cyanobacteria can produce a variety of toxins (e.g. domoic acid, saxitoxins, brevetoxins, anatoxins, microcystins, lyngbyatoxins) under certain environmental conditions. Toxins are ingested after bioaccumulation in water or prey (Buckles, 2018; Stidworthy and Denk, 2018). Herons and egrets are susceptible to toxicosis due to a toxin-producing cyanobacteria that may include microcystin, with a potential dietary role (i.e. low vitamin E).

Signs and Diagnosis

Clinical signs are often neurological and include disorientation, ataxia, paresis, paralysis, constricted pupils, torticollis, tremors, and seizures, but may also include tachycardia, dyspnea, vomiting, diarrhea, ocular and nasal discharge, and weakness; death may occur due to drowning or respiratory complications. There are no characteristic gross or microscopic lesions, but there may be edema, hyperemia and hemorrhage in the trachea and lungs, hemorrhage or mucus in the intestine, and skeletal muscle necrosis and hemorrhage. Grossly, affected birds may have abundant, firm, subcutaneous and intracoelomic adipose which, microscopically, indicates necrosis, and heterophilic and histiocytic inflammation type (Figure 5.19; Neagari et al., 2011). Microcystin toxicosis may include jaundice with liver necrosis and hemorrhage (Wobeser, 1997d; Fenton et al., 2018; Stidworthy and Denk, 2018). Diagnosis requires detection of toxins in environmental samples (e.g. water) and/or gastrointestinal contents or liver of affected birds by toxicologic tests (high-performance liquid chromatography, enzyme-linked immunosorbent assay, LISA; Fenton et al., 2018). Diagnosis of many of the above toxicoses is complicated by the fact that quantified toxic thresholds to determine exposure compared with toxicosis, as well as the spectrum of disease manifestations from acute to chronic (which may be subtle yet important), are not yet well characterized.

Treatment/Management

No treatment is available.

Avian Vacuolar Myelinopathy

Overview and Etiology

Avian vacuolar myelinopathy has been diagnosed in numerous waterfowl species (e.g. coots, ducks, geese) and it is believed to result from exposure to a toxin produced by an epiphytic cyanobacterium (*Aetokthonos hydrillicola*), associated with aquatic vegetation (Bidigare et al., 2009).

Signs and Diagnosis

There are no characteristic gross lesions; affected birds may be in good nutritional condition. Diagnosis is by history of being found in or around lakes that contain this plant, seasonality (late fall to winter), rapid onset of neurologic signs (e.g. ataxia, difficulty flying and swimming, head sway, and ascending paralysis), and characteristic histopathology. The latter includes bilaterally symmetric vacuolation (intramyelinic edema) in white matter of the brain and spinal cord (Rocke et al., 2002).

Differential Diagnoses

Differential diagnoses includes neurotropic viruses, bacterial sepsis, and neurotoxins.

Treatment/Management

Currently, there is no treatment aside from supportive care. An avian bioassay has been developed for detection of the toxin and confirms presence of the toxin in tissues (e.g. brain, skeletal muscle) of affected animals; however, this testing is not yet commercially available (Breinlinger et al., 2021).

Botulism

Overview and Etiology

Botulism is caused by neurotoxins (types A–G) produced by the bacterium *Clostridium botulinum*. It is typically seasonal (approximately July to September in many areas of the United States and Canada). Type C botulism can lead to die-off in American white pelicans, and it has been reported in loons, cormorants, grebes, fulmars, and albatross. Type E botulism affects more commonly piscivorous birds, such as loons and grebes. Similar to algal blooms, botulism occurs seasonally (late summer to early fall), based on environmental conditions, such as warm water temperature and presence of decaying organic matter (Fenton et al., 2018; Stidworthy and Denk, 2018).

Signs and Diagnosis

Botulinum toxin inhibits neurotransmission by blocking acetylcholine release, leading to neurologic signs (such as weakness, paresis, and flaccid paralysis, "limber neck," paralysis of nictitating membranes, inability to fly or swim, and possible drowning (Fenton et al., 2018; Stidworthy and Denk, 2018). There are no characteristic gross or microscopic findings (Fenton et al., 2018). Diagnosis is by history, clinical signs, ruling out other potential etiologies (e.g. trauma, infections), and toxicologic testing to confirm toxin in feed, blood (serum), liver, or gastrointestinal contents. The mouse bioassay is the gold standard test. Alternatives, where available, are antigen capture ELISA for type C toxin in serum and PCR for toxin genes (Fenton et al., 2018; Stidworthy and Denk, 2018).

Differential Diagnoses

Differentials include other toxins, such as heavy metals (e.g. lead) and mycotoxins. Careful examination of locational and environmental aspects is crucial to pinpointing the diagnosis.

Treatment/Management

Some species have a better prognosis for recovery from botulism (e.g. waterfowl species) when provided supportive care, including shade and abundant, clean, fresh water in a low-stress environment. Botulinum antitoxin is available. Coots, shorebirds, gulls, and grebes appear to have a reduced chance of recovery from botulism (US Geological Survey, 1999c).

Mycotoxicosis

Overview and Etiology

Micotoxins are produced by fungi (e.g. aflatoxins, trichothecenes) and toxicosis results from ingestion of fungal toxins in moldy feed (e.g., corn). Outbreaks have been described in geese and ducks.

Signs and Diagnosis

Clinically, there may be impaired growth, poor reproductive output, and/or sudden death (Wobeser, 1997d; Fenton et al., 2018). Gross lesions are variable; acute aflatoxicosis may lead to enlarged, pale liver, renal and pancreatic hemorrhage, hydropericardium, and ascites. More chronic manifestations include firm, shrunken liver, with reticular pattern of fibrosis (Wobeser, 1997d). Diagnosis is by toxicological testing of feed, including apparently normal and moldy feed if possible, and chemical analysis of gastrointestinal contents, if feed is not available (Fenton et al., 2018).

Treatment/Management

Treatment is by removal of the toxic feed; supplemental vitamins, minerals, protein, and lipids, as well as activated charcoal, may help alleviate the effects of mycotoxin (Hoerr, 2020).

Oiling of Aquatic Birds

Overview and Etiology

Oiling occurs from accumulation on feathers and skin and, sometimes ingestion, of petroleum (hydrocarbon-containing) products. It can be fatal if thermoregulation and buoyancy are affected (i.e. risk of drowning), leading to intoxication from ingestion or inhalation (Fenton et al., 2018).

Signs and Diagnosis

Clinically, oiling can manifest as neurologic disease (from hyperexcitation to depression, tremors, ataxia) and respiratory disease (e.g. tachypnea, shallow respiration, dyspnea), as well as weakness, nasal discharge, and dehydration (Osweiler, 2020). It may also lead to anemia, immunosuppression, and reproductive problems, including embryonic mortality (Wobeser, 1997d; Fenton et al., 2018). Grossly, birds may be emaciated with evidence of oil products on feathers and skin; they may have pulmonary congestion and hemorrhage, gastrointestinal hemorrhage, lymphoid depletion, and enlarged, pale liver. Histopathology is non-specific and may include pulmonary fluid or debris in airways, ventricular ulceration, hemosiderosis, hepatic lipidosis, adrenal necrosis and urate deposits in the kidney. Diagnosis is by collective observations of environmental data, physical presence or odor of oil on birds, and evidence of concurrent emaciation, weakness, and pulmonary or gastrointestinal damage. Chemical analysis may help identify hydrocarbons in tissues (lung, liver, and kidney) oil products in the gastrointestinal contents on external or internal tissues (Fenton et al., 2018; Osweiler, 2020).

Treatment/Management

If oil has been ingested, activated charcoal may assist in removing contaminants and additives to the petroleum products (albeit not the petroleum itself); supplemental oxygen may aid in respiration (with purging of ventilators to rid them of accumulated volatile compounds). Animals with petroleum-induced damage of pulmonary tissues are highly susceptible to bacterial pneumonia that necessitates broad-spectrum antibiotics. Mild soap/detergents with frequent rinsing should be used to remove oil from skin and feathers (Osweiler, 2020).

Salt Toxicosis

Salt toxicosis is rarely reported in birds, but may occur when birds have limited access to fresh water and/or are subjected to high saline environments to which they are not accustomed. Ingested salt (sodium chloride) can lead to hypernatremia and associated neuronal changes in the brain that may include cell shrinkage, and cerebral hemorrhage and edema. Other lesions also are non-specific and may include hyperemia of the brain surface, visceral hemorrhages, gout (mineralization) on viscera, corneal erosions, and pulmonary edema. Salt can also encrust on feathers and affect mobility, leading to overexertion (e.g. extertional myopathy) and even drowning (US Geological Survey, 1999e). Diagnosis is made through history, clinical signs, assessment for sodium chloride antemortem (serum, cerebrospinal fluid), or in brain tissue or suspect food/water/ingested material. Supportive care includes gradually restoring hydration and electrolyte balance over several days, with continuous assessment of serum sodium concentration as a guide (Thompson, 2018).

Disease Epidemiology in Aquatic birds

Based on the diverse taxonomy (Longshaw et al., 2021) widespread distribution of aquatic birds, as well as high degree of mobility (i.e., flight), disease control and prevention including of large or widespread disease outbreaks often are challenging. In some cases, collection and removal of infected carcasses is practiced and may reduce environmental contamination. Remining healthy birds may be dispersed or relocated to non-outbreak areas and if species are of conservation concern, rehabilitation may be attempted. If these methods are employed, timely response is critical

(United States Geological Survey, 1999d). Land management practices, such as reducing output of potentially toxic chemicals as well as organic compounds, especially into water sources or into run-off, may help manage some of the above diseases (e.g., botulism, numerous toxicoses; United States Geological Survey, 1999c). Although vaccines for some of the above pathogens have been established for use in poultry and may be used in valued zoo collections and other captive settings (e.g., West Nile virus), their use generally is not logistically feasible in free-ranging birds. Among the diseases discussed above, West Nile fever and eastern equine encephalitis are WOAH listed notifiable diseases under the "Multiple species diseases, infections and infestations" category. Under the "Avian diseases and infections" listed diseases that may be encountered in the category of aquatic birds include, avian chlamydiosis, avian mycoplasmosis (Mycoplasma gallisepticum and M. synoviae), duck virus hepatitis, Newcastle disease (avian paramyxovirus-1), fowl typhoid (*Salmonella gallinarum and S. pullorum*; although these Salmonella spp. are not the expected species from aquatic wild birds, they are listed here for completeness), avian influenza viruses, and influenza A viruses of high pathogenicity (WOAH, 20220).

Migratory aquatic birds provide unique epidemiological challenges in tracking disease maintenance and spread as well as potential management, because some species (e.g., waterfowl) travel long distances and congregate at high densities on water bodies at stopover, breeding, or overwintering sites. Such a scenario provides abundant opportunities for sharing of infectious agents and toxins, especially because birds are often immunosuppressed and energetically challenged (e.g., avian influenza viruses, avian paramyxoviruses, *P. multocida*, *Clostridium botulinum* toxin; Stallknecht et al., 2007).

A summary of major clinical–pathologic presentation and system-specific differential diagnoses of aquatic birds is presented in Appendix 5.1.

References

Allison AB, Ballard JR, Tesh RB, et al. 2015. Cyclic avian mass mortality in the northeastern United States is associated with a novel orthomyxovirus. *J Virol* 89:1389–1403.

Alzugaray L, Di Martino M, Beltramino L, et al. 2020. Anthropogenic debris in the digestive tract of a southern right whale (*Eubalaena australis*) stranded in Golfo Nuevo, *Argentina. Mar Pollut Bull* 161(Pt A):111738.

Bidigare RR, Christensen SJ, Wilde SB, Banack SA. 2009. Cyanobacteria and BMAA: Possible linkage with avian vacuolar myelinopathy (AVM) in the south-eastern United States. *Amyotroph Lateral Scler* 10(Suppl 2):71–73.

Breinlinger S, Phillips TJ, Haram BN, et al. 2021. Hunting the eagle killer: a cyanobacterial neurotoxin causes vacuolar myelinopathy. *Science* 371(6536):eaax9050.

Buckles EL. 2018. Phoenicopteriformes. In: Terio KA, McAloose D, St. Leger J, eds. *Pathology of Wildlife and Zoo Animals*. San Diego, CA: Academic Press, pp. 683–692.

Cox SL, Campbell GD, Nemeth NM. 2015. Outbreaks of West Nile virus in captive waterfowl in Ontario, Canada. *Avian Pathol* 44(2):135–141.

Daoust P-Y, Prescott JF. 2007. Salmonellosis. In: Thomas NJ, Hunter DB, Atkinson CT, eds. *Infectious Disease of Wild Birds*. Ames, IA: Blackwell, pp. 270–288.

Davies RW, Govedich FR, Moser WE. 2008. Leech parasites of birds. In: Atkinson CT, Thomas NJ, Hunter DB, eds. *Parasitic Diseases of Wild Birds*. Ames, IA: Wiley-Blackwell, pp. 501–511.

Dein JF, Carpenter, JW, Clark GG, et al. 1986. Mortality of captive whooping cranes caused by eastern equine encephalitis virus. *J Am Vet Med Assoc* 189:1006–1010.

Delnatte P, Ojkic D, DeLay J, et al. 2013. Pathology and diagnosis of avian bornavirus infection in wild Canada geese (*Branta canadensis*), trumpeter swans (*Cygnus buccinators*) and mute swans (*Cygnus olor*) in Canada: a retrospective study. *Avian Pathol* 42:114–128.

Ellis TM, Bousfield RB, Bissett LA, et al. 2004. Investigation of outbreaks of highly pathogenic H5N1 avian influenza in waterfowl and wild birds in Hong Kong in late 2002. *Avian Pathol* 33(5):492–505.

Fenton H, McManamon R, Howerth EW. 2018. Anseriformes, Ciconiiformes, Charadriiformes, and Gruiformes. In: Terio KA, McAloose D, St. Leger J, eds. *Pathology of Wildlife and Zoo Animals*. San Diego, CA: Academic Press, pp. 693–716.

Forrester DJ, Spalding MG. 2003. *Parasites and Diseases of Wild Birds in Florida*. Gainesville, FL: University Press of Florida.

Friend M, Franson JC, eds. *Field Manual of Wildlife Diseases*. Biological Resources Division Information and Technology Report 1999-001. Washington, *DC: Printing Office*.

Gibble CM, Kudela RM, Knowles S, et al. 2021. Domoic acid and saxitoxin in seabirds in the United States between 2007 and 2018. *Harmful Algae* 103:101981.

Hansen WR, Gough RE. 2007. Duck plague (duck virus enteritis). In: Atkinson CT, Thomas NJ, Hunter DB, eds. *Infectious Disease of Wild Birds*. Ames, IA: Wiley-Blackwell, pp. 87–107.

Hoerr FJ. 2020. Mycotoxicoses in poultry. In: *Merck Veterinary Manual*. Rahway, NJ: Merck & Co. https://www.merckvetmanual.com/poultry/mycotoxicoses/mycotoxicoses-in-poultry?query=mycotoxins#v44844471 (accessed September 2022).

Huang J, Mayer J. 2019. Lead and zinc toxicity in birds. *Today's Vet Pract* 9(1):72–76.

Knowles S, Bodenstein BL, Berlowski-Zier BM, et al. 2019. Detection of Bisgaard taxon 40 in rhinoceros auklets (*Cerorhinca monocerata*) with pneumonia and septicemia from a mortality event in Washington, USA. *J Wildl Dis* 55(1):246–249.

Landsberg JH, Vargo GA, Flewelling LJ, Wiley FE. 2007. Algal biotoxins. In: Thomas NJ, Hunter DB, Atkinson CT, eds. *Infectious Disease of Wild Birds*. Ames, IA: Blackwell, pp. 431–455.

Longshaw M, Baumgartner W, Becker Welsh T, et al. 2021. Taxonomy, anatomy and physiology. In: Urdeș L, Walster C, Tepper J, eds. *Fundamentals of Aquatic Veterinary Medicine*. Ames, IA: Wiley Blackwell, pp. 30–49.

Neagari Y, Arii S, Udagawa M, et al. 2011. Steatitis in egrets and herons from Japan. *J Wildl Dis* 47(1):49–55.

Niedringhaus KD, Shender LA, DiNuovo A, et al. 2021. Mortality in common (*Sterna hirundo*) and sandwich (*Thalasseus sandvicensis*) terns associated with bisgaard taxon 40 infection on Marco Island, Florida, USA. *J Comp Pathol.* 184:12–18.

O'Malley GF, O'Malley R. 2018. Organophosphate poisoning and carbamate poisoning. In: *Merck Veterinary Manual*. Rahway, NJ: Merck & Co. https://www.merckmanuals.com/professional/injuries-poisoning/poisoning/organophosphate-poisoning-and-carbamate-poisoning (accessed 4 September 2022).

Osweiler GD. 2020. Overview of petroleum product poisoning. In: *Merck Veterinary Manual*. Rahway, NJ: Merck & Co. https://www.merckvetmanual.com/toxicology/petroleum-product-poisoning/overview-of-petroleum-product-poisoning?query=oiling (accessed 4 September 2022).

Rocke TE, Thomas NJ, Augspurger T, Miller K. 2002. Epizootiologic studies of avian vacuolar myelinopathy in waterbirds. *J Wildl Dis* 38(4):678–684.

Spalding MG, Yowell CA, Lindsay DS, et al. 2002. Sarcocystis meningoencephalitis in a northern gannet (Morus bassanus). *J Wildl Dis* 38(2):432–437.

Stallknecht DE, Nagy E, Hunter DB, et al. 2007. Avian Influenza. In: Thomas NJ, Hunter DB, Atkinson CT, eds. *Infectious Disease of Wild Birds*. Ames, IA: Blackwell, pp. 108–130.

Steele KE, Linn MJ, Schoepp RJ, et al. 2000. Pathology of fatal West Nile virus infections in native and exotic birds during the 1999 outbreak in New York City, New York. *Vet Pathol* 37:208–224.

Stidworthy MF, Denk D. 2018. Sphenisciformes, Gaviiformes, Podicipediformes, Procellariiformes, and Pelecaniformes. In: Terio KA, McAloose D, St. Leger J, eds. *Pathology of Wildlife and Zoo Animals*. San Diego, CA: Academic Press, pp. 649–682.

Thompson LJ. 2018. Sodium chloride (salt). In: Gupta RC, ed. *Veterinary Toxicology*, 3rd ed. San Diego, CA: Academic Press, pp. 461–464.

Ugwu K, Herrera A, Gómez M. 2021. Microplastics in marine biota: a review. *Mar Pollut Bull* 169:112540.

US Geological Survey. 1999a. Duck plague. In: Friend M, Franson JC, eds. *Field Manual of Wildlife Diseases*. Biological Resources Division Information and Technology Report 1999-001. Washington, DC: Printing Office, pp. 141–152.

US Geological Survey. 1999b. Organophosphorous and carbamate pesticides. In: Friend M, Franson JC, eds. *Field Manual of Wildlife Diseases*. Biological Resources Division Information and Technology Report 1999-001. Washington, DC: Printing Office, pp. 287–294.

US Geological Survey. 1999c. Avian botulism. In: Friend M, Franson JC, eds. *Field Manual of Wildlife Diseases*. Biological Resources Division Information and Technology Report 1999-001. Washington, DC: Printing Office, pp. 271–282.

US Geological Survey. 1999d. Disease Control Operations In: Friend M, Franson JC, eds. *Field Manual of Wildlife Diseases*. Biological Resources Division Information and Technology Report 1999-001. Washington, DC: Printing Office, pp. 19–48.

US Geological Survey. 1999e. Salt In: Friend M, Franson JC, eds. *Field Manual of Wildlife Diseases*. Biological Resources Division Information and Technology Report 1999-001. Washington, DC: Printing Office, pp. 347–348.

US Geological Survey. 1999f. Candidiasis In: Friend M, Franson JC, eds. *Field Manual of Wildlife Diseases*. Biological Resources Division Information and Technology Report 1999-001. Washington, DC: Printing Office, pp. 135–136.

van der Schyff V, Kwet Yive NSC, Polder A, et al. 2020. Perfluoroalkyl substances (PFAS) in tern eggs from St. Brandon's Atoll, Indian Ocean. *Mar Pollut Bull* 154:111061.

Vanstreels RET, Gallo L, Serafini PP, et al. 2021. Ingestion of plastics and other debris by coastal and pelagic birds along the coast of Espírito Santo, Eastern Brazil. *Mar Pollut Bull* 173(Pt B):113046.

Wyss F, Schumacher V, Wenker C, et al. 2015. Pododermatitis in captive and free-ranging greater flamingos (Phoenicopterus roseus). *Vet Pathol* 52:1235–1242.

Wobeser GA. 1997a. Other viruses. In: *Diseases of Wild Waterfowl*, 2nd ed. New York, NY: Plenum Press, pp. 43–54.

Wobeser GA. 1997b. Other bacteria, mycoplasmas, and *Chlamydiae*. In: *Diseases of Wild Waterfowl*, 2nd ed. New York, NY: Plenum Press, pp. 71–91.

Wobeser GA. 1997c. Pesticides, PCBs, and related chemicals. In: *Diseases of Wild Waterfowl*, 2nd ed. New York, NY: Plenum Press, pp. 179–188.

Wobeser GA. 1997d. Other toxic substances. In: *Diseases of Wild Waterfowl*, 2nd ed. New York, NY: Plenum Press, pp. 189–208.

Wobeser GA. 1997e. Miscellaneous diseases. In: *Diseases of Wild Waterfowl*, 2nd ed. New York, NY: Plenum Press, pp. 211–224.

World Organisation for Animal Health. 2022. *Animal Diseases*. Paris, France: WOAH. https://www.woah.org/en/what-we-do/animal-health-and-welfare/animal-diseases (accessed 4 September 2022).

Appendix 5.1

Avian clinicopathologic presentations with differential diagnoses

It should be noted that in many avian cases, illness is advanced before the appearance of clinical signs, and that these signs are often non-specific (e.g. emaciation, lethargy, anorexia, fluffed feathers, diarrhea). This may give the appearance of sudden death when the disease (including infections) may have initiated days to weeks earlier.

Clinicopathologic presentations	Differential etiologic diagnoses
Sudden death	Infection: bacterial – *Pasteurella multocida*, *Streptococcus* spp., *Salmonella* spp., *Erysipelas rhusiopathiae* septicemia; clostridial enterotoxemia, and others; protozoal: *Plasmodium* spp. (malaria), *Eimeria*/*Isospora* spp., *Sarcocystis* spp., *Toxoplasma* spp. and others; viral – highly pathogenic influenza A viruses, paramyxoviruses (virulent Newcastle disease virus, duck viral enteritis virus, eastern equine encephalitis virus, Wellfleet Bay virus, and others); toxicosis – e.g. mycotoxins, harmful algal biotoxins, *Clostridium botulinum* toxins, cyanide, pesticides e.g. organophosphates/carbamates; traumatic injury (acute or chronic); stress/exertional myopathy
Emaciation (e.g. decreased adipose reserves; muscle atrophy)	Starvation (inadequate resource availability or ability to forage for a variety of causes), heavy gastrointestinal parasite load, chronic infections (viral: West Nile virus, herpesvirus, eastern equine encephalitis, paramyxoviruses, Wellfleet Bay virus, aquatic bird *Bornavirus*, adenovirus, and others; bacterial: *Mycobacterium* spp., *Chlamydia* spp., *Salmonella* spp. and others; protozoal: *Sarcocystis* spp., *Toxoplasma gondii*; *Hemoprotozoa* and others), chronic toxin exposure (lead, zinc, algal biotoxins/harmful algal bloom e.g., domoic acid, saxitoxins, and others); denervation due to traumatic injury; nutritional deficiency; decreased vision/foraging due to poxviral or other proliferative, facial, skin or oral/upper alimentary tract lesions (*Capillaria* spp., *Trichomonas* spp.), amyloidosis (affected organs diffusely, tan-orange; often secondary to other disease)
Poor growth in nestlings/immature birds	Stress, malnutrition/starvation, vitamin deficiency (hypovitaminosis A), heavy parasitism, alimentary tract foreign body, chronic toxins (mycotoxins, lead and other heavy metals, and other environmental contaminants)
Anemia (e.g., weakness, thinned blood, tissue pallor)	Hemoprotozoa (*Plasmodium* spp., *Atoxoplasma* spp., and others), hemorrhage from traumatic injury, heavy metal (lead/zinc) toxicosis, anticoagulant (rodenticide) toxicosis

(*Continued*)

Clinicopathologic presentations	Differential etiologic diagnoses
Central nervous system disease variably involving brain, meninges, spinal cord (neurologic signs - e.g., ataxia, disorientation, torticollis, seizures, depression, partial or complete paralysis, paresis)	Traumatic injury, infections (viral: highly pathogenic influenza A viruses, West Nile virus, eastern equine encephalitis virus, aquatic bird *Bornavirus*, paramyxoviruses and others, hemorrhage; bacteria: *Pasteurella multocida*, Bisgaard taxon 40, *Riemerella anatipestifer*, *Salmonella* spp., inflammatory or malacic foci; protozoa: *Toxoplasma gondii*, *Sarcocystis* spp., hemoprotozoa; other parasites: *Baylisascaris* spp.; disseminated fungal: *Aspergillus* spp.), toxicosis (many cause nonspecific lesions such as cerebral and cerebellar congestion; e.g. organophosphate/carbamate pesticides, chlorinated hydrocarbons, lead, zinc, mercury, salt, harmful algal biotoxins e.g. brevetoxins, domoic acid, botulism toxin, saxitoxin, aetokthonotoxin – causative toxin of avian vacuolar myelinopathy, white matter vacuolation of cerebrum and cerebellum evident histologically). Gross lesions in the brain often are uncommon aside from hemorrhage/congestion; many of the above etiologies may only be visualized histologically. It should be recognized that generalized/systemic infectious disease, nutritional deficiency, starvation, stress, exhaustion, and other factors may appear clinically similar to neurologic signs
Integumentary disease (hyperemia, crusting, proliferative)	Ectoparasite infestation (leeches, mites, chiggers, louse, fly larvae, ticks), infections (viral: poxvirus, nodular hyperplasia; bacterial: staphylococcal pododermatitis and others; fungal: *Trichophyton* sp. and others), traumatic injury, neoplasia (squamous cell carcinoma, lipoma, lymphoma, melanoma, and others), xanthoma, chronic response to traumatic injury (scabbing and scarring), soiling of feathers with environmental debris (salt encrustation, oil, soap)
Intracoelomic lesions	Ascites due to cardiomyopathy, hepatopathy, neoplasia-associated lymphatic obstruction, malnutrition/hypoproteinemia; inflammatory effusion from infection/inflammation (*Salmonella* spp., *Mycobacterium* spp. and others), or ascending urogenital infections including nephritis, hepatitis, pancreatitis, and reproductive tract inflammation or abnormal egg laying/breakage, septicemia, carcinomatosis (very rare), systemic mycosis (*Aspergillus* spp.); mycotoxicosis; hemocoelom (from trauma, body wall trauma/perforation, gastric or duodenal perforation, neoplasia); parasitic granulomas or cysts, neoplasia (carcinomas, leiomyoma, mesothelioma and others); intracoelomic steatitis (microcystins/low vitamin E)
Joint disease and skeletomuscular injury/inflammation/pallor:	
Arthritis	Infection (bacterial: *Mycoplasma* spp., *Staphylococcus aureus*, and others; fungal), advanced age (chronic use arthritis), traumatic injury, skeletal malformations (congenital, response to injury, healed infections (osteomyelitis)
Skeletal muscle pallor (necrosis or fibrosis)	Vitamin deficiency (vitamin E – pale streaks), exertional myopathy (pale streaks), harmful algal biotoxins (necrosis, hemorrhage); traumatic injury (acute – hemorrhage; subacute to chronic – inflammation; chronic – fibrosis/scarring), parasites (multifocal firmness, pallor e.g. *Sarcocystis* spp. aka "rice breast")

Clinicopathologic presentations	Differential etiologic diagnoses
Upper respiratory tract (infraorbital sinus, choana, larynx, trachea, syrinx):	
Crusting/discharge around nares	Serous, mucoid, mucopurulent – nasal, sinus, or tracheal parasites (respiratory mites, chiggers, trematodes, nematodes, leeches, fly larvae), infection (bacterial: *Streptococcus* spp., *Mycoplasma* spp.; viral: poxvirus – rare in this anatomic region, herpesviruses and others; fungi: (e.g. *Aspergillus* spp.), nutritional defect (e.g., hypovitaminosis A), choanal atresia or other congenital/ anatomic deformities (rare)
Hemorrhage (from nares or around choana)	Traumatic injury, ulceration from proliferative skin disease (mites or other parasites, poxviral infection, or neoplasia – rare), parasites (respiratory mites, nematodes or other metazoan parasites, mycoses: e.g. aspergillosis), pulmonary or gastric hemorrhage (from ulcers or other injury ulcers)
Inflammation	Response to traumatic injury, infection (bacterial: *Mycoplasma* spp., *Avibacterium* spp., secondary bacterial infection to poxviral infection, and Herpes-like or herpesviruses causing tracheitis)
Dyspnea/stridor/rales	Foreign body obstruction/inhalation (fishing gear, fish bones or other prey related parts, oil from oiling incidents), parasitic granuloma/ parasites or other infections (viral: poxvirus – rare in respiratory tract; bacterial: *Riemerella anatipestifer*, and others; fungi: *Aspergillus* spp.), neoplasia (chondrosarcoma, squamous cell carcinoma, and others), algal biotoxins (excessive oronasal secretions, traumatic injury), nutritional defect (hypovitaminosis A)
Lower respiratory tract (lung and air sacs):	
Pneumonia	Infection (bacterial: *Salmonella*, *Mycobacterium* spp. – airsacculitis, *Riemerella anatipestifer* – pneumonia, and others; viral: highly pathogenic influenza A viruses, avian paramyxoviruses, adenoviruses, and others; parasites: hemoprotozoa, *Toxoplasma gondii*, respiratory mites, and others; fungal: *Aspergillus* spp. – may include hemorrhage if acute), aspiration of foreign material (e.g. water, ectoparasites)
Hemorrhage and edema	Traumatic injury, infection (bacterial septicemia, viral: highly pathogenic influenza A viruses, avian paramyxoviruses and others; protozoal: hemoprotozoans and others), toxicosis (harmful algal biotoxins, oil and gas hydrocarbons, salt, and others); aspiration, drowning, asphyxiation, congestive heart failure – rare, euthanasia artifact – pentobarbital euthanasia
Nodules	Granulomas due to infections (parasites, bacterial: *Mycobacterium* spp. and others; fungal: *Aspergillus* spp., poxvirus – rare in respiratory tract), neoplasia (primary or metastatic, including carcinoma, adenocarcinoma, lymphoma)
Respiratory paralysis	Toxins such as organophosphates and carbamates, *Clostridium botulinum* – flaccid neck paralysis, can lead to drowning

(*Continued*)

Clinicopathologic presentations	Differential etiologic diagnoses
Upper alimentary tract (oral cavity, beak, pharynx, crop, esophagus, proventriculus, ventriculus):	
Hemorrhage, ulceration, and/or necrosis	Infections including septicemia (bacterial: *Salmonella* spp. – crop/esophagus inflammation; *Riemerella anatipestifer* – fibrinous serositis; viral: poxvirus, duck virus enteritis virus or other herpesviruses; protozoal: *Trichomonas* spp.; nematodes: *Capillaria* spp., *Amidostomum* sp., and others; trematodes and others), traumatic injury (foreign bodies, e.g. fishing gear, fish bones or other prey parts, plastics/trash), toxicosis (lead, zinc-ventricular erosions; organophosphates and carbamates – excessive salivation), oiling (gastrointestinal hemorrhage), algal biotoxins (excessive oronasal secretions, hemorrhage); uremia (from gout); stress; neoplasia-associated (squamous cell carcinoma, adenocarcinoma and others)
Nodules or thickened mucosa	Infections (bacterial: *Salmonella* spp., *Mycobacterium* spp., and others; viral: poxvirus; parasitic: see above; fungi/yeast: *Candida albicans* plaque-like foci) or chronic/healed traumatic injury (from sharp objects, see above); neoplasia (squamous cell carcinoma, leiomyoma, lymphoma); vitamin deficiency (hypovitaminosis A, thickened mucosa)
Crop/esophageal impaction and food stasis	Viral infection (aquatic bird *Bornavirus*, poxvirus, and others); lead toxicosis; severe parasite infection (*Trichomonas*, *Capillaria* spp., or others), mycotoxins, obstruction (foreign body), congenital defects (pyloric stenosis), dietary (high proportion of dry, vegetative material)
Beak abrasion, tissue defects (missing tissue) or excessive growth	Traumatic injury; nutritional deficiency; viral: induced beak overgrowth (picornavirus – documented in some birds e.g. passerines, but not yet aquatic species)
Lower alimentary tract: small and large intestine, ceca(e):	
Impaction (with or without wall rupture)	Heavy parasite load (nematodes, trematodes, cestodes, acanthocephalans), foreign bodies (see above), mycotoxins, abundant dry feed or other cause of dehydration (e.g. lack of water access or generalized illness leading to decreased mobility), lead toxicosis, neoplasia (see above)
Abnormal droppings (e.g. discolored, dry or watery)	Dark feces: melena from hemorrhage due to intestinal infection (adenovirus, *Salmonella* spp., coccidians, and others), trauma, gastrointestinal ulceration or perforation (from stress, parasite-induced damage, or other foreign body-induced trauma), neoplasia (adenocarcinoma, lymphoma, and others); bright green urates: anorexia, debilitation (from many causes), toxicosis (lead or zinc), viral or bacterial infection (highly pathogenic influenza A viruses, *Chlamydia* spp. – rare, *Riemerella anatipestifer*, and others); watery/loose feces: excessive drinking/swallowing (behavioral, during drowning), protein-losing enteropathy from a variety of causes (infection, inflammation – *Salmonella* spp., adenovirus, heavy gastrointestinal parasite burden and others), stress, neoplasia; dry feces: dehydration from infections, toxicosis, lack of food/water (from immobility due to traumatic injury or other), neoplasia

Clinicopathologic presentations	Differential etiologic diagnoses
Vomiting/regurgitation	Infection (hemoprotozoa, protozoa, coccidians, hemorrhagic, bacteria – *Salmonella* spp. – enteritis, cecal plugs; clostridial enterotoxemia; viruses-duck virus enteritis, West Nile virus, eastern equine encephalitis virus, highly pathogenic influenza A viruses; fungi/yeast – *Candida albicans*, *Aspergillus* spp. – very rare in distal tract, and others), toxicosis (lead, zinc, organophosphates and carbamates, harmful algal biotoxins, and others), foreign bodies (see above), heavy parasite load (nematodes)
Impaction (with or without wall rupture)	Heavy parasite load (nematodes, trematodes, cestodes, acanthocephalans), foreign bodies (see above), mycotoxins, abundant dry feed, or other cause of dehydration (lack of water access or generalized illness leading to decreased mobility), lead toxicosis, neoplasia (see above)
Eye:	
Corneal ulcers	Infection (fungal: *Aspergillus* spp.; bacterial, viral –rare), traumatic injury, hyposalinity, salt toxicity, ultraviolet light-induced damage, chemical or smoke exposure; common gross artifact if carcass has been frozen
Conjunctivitis	Infection (bacterial: *Mycoplasma* spp., viral – poxvirus and others); traumatic injury, secondary swelling (fluid retention), nutritional defect (hypovitaminosis A)
Skeletal muscle:	
Atrophy	Emaciation, lack of use due to generalized illness, denervation/traumatic injury, chronic myositis, myopathy (chronic exertional myopathy), congenital deformity/malnutrition (immature birds)
Necrosis and/or hemorrhage	Traumatic injury, septicemia, exertional myopathy (pallor), septicemia, vitamin deficiency (vitamin E, pale streaks), harmful algal biotoxins – necrosis, hemorrhage
Nodules/inflammation	Parasitic granulomas (protozoa: *Sarcocystis* spp.; cestodes, nematodes), heterophilic granulomas (from bacterial infection), healing/fibrosis following traumatic injury, neoplasia
Cardiovascular:	
Hemorrhage, necrosis, inflammation (e.g. pale foci or streaking)	Infection (protozoal: *Sarcocystis* spp., *Toxoplasma gondii* inflammation; bacterial: *Streptococcus* spp., *Staphylococcus* spp., *Listeria monocytogenes* – rare, myocarditis; *Pasteurella multocida* hemorrhage, *Salmonella* spp., fibrinoheterophilic pericarditis; *Mycobacterium* spp., pericarditis; *Riemerella anatipestifer*, myocarditis; viral: West Nile virus, highly pathogenic influenza A viruses, duck virus enteritis – hemorrhage, equine encephalitis virus – less common; hemoprotozoal), nutritional myopathy, toxicosis (lead, myocardial pallor – necrosis or fibrosis, hydropericardium), neoplasia (lymphoma)
Nodules	Granulomas (from bacterial, fungal or parasitic infection), neoplasia (carcinoma metastases)
Hydropericardium	Lead toxicosis, mycotoxins, viral infection (highly pathogenic influenza A viruses), bacterial infection (septicemia, see above)

(*Continued*)

Clinicopathologic presentations	Differential etiologic diagnoses
Mineralization (surface)	Gout (chalky material on pericardium); atherosclerosis (thickening and plaques, sometimes with mineralization, in large artery walls), secondary to inflammation from infection(see above)
Kidney:	
Renomegaly	Infection (bacterial: *Leptospira* spp., *Escherichia coli*/coligranulomas, *Salmonella* spp.; protozoal: coccidians, *Eimeria* spp.; viral and others), neoplasia (lymphoma), uremia/gout (chalky material –mineral on visceral surfaces, including kidney), amyloidosis, toxicosis (zinc), congenital defect, urinary tract blockage
Cystic change	Congenital defects (may also include hypoplasia, dysplasia, aplasia), hydronephrosis, parasitic and other infections, neoplasia
Necrosis, pallor and/or hemorrhage	Infection (bacterial, viral, parasitic including coccidiosis, *Eimeria* spp., see above), acute infarct (from infection or traumatic injury; chronic infarcts will appear as sunken areas), neoplasia-associated (see above), amyloidosis, mycotoxins (petechiae)
Granulomas/nodules	Infection (bacterial, fungal, parasites-cestodes, trematodes, nematodes), neoplasia (urogenital carcinoma-uncommon), hypoplasia, dysplasia
Spleen and disseminated lymphoid tissue:	
Splenomegaly-common nonspecific/reactive finding; and/or pallor (necrosis), hemorrhage	bacterial: *Salmonella* spp., *Mycobacterium* spp., *Listeria monocytogenes* – rare, *Escherichia coli*, *Staphylococcus* spp., *Chlamydia* spp. – rare, *Riemerella anatipestifer*, *Pasteurella multocida*, coligranuloma and others; fungal: *Aspergillus* spp.; parasitic: *Tri/Tetratrichomonas* spp., hemoprotozoa, trematodes, schistosomes – *Heterobilharzia* spp.; amyloidosis; oiling (hepatomegaly), neoplasia – lymphoma; toxicosis (zinc), marked vascular congestion (barbiturate euthanasia artifact); lymphoid hyperplasia (reactive, neoplastic)
Splenic nodules	Granulomas (bacterial, fungal, parasitic), hematoma, hyperplasia, neoplasia (lymphoma, disseminated carcinoma/adenocarcinoma and others)
Liver and pancreas:	
Hepatomegaly (common non-specific/reactive finding in birds, pallor – necrosis, hemorrhage)	Infection (see causes above for splenomegaly), toxicosis (microcystin, mycotoxins – petechial hemorrhage, zinc – pancreas), amyloidosis, lipidosis (pale orange-yellow, enlarged, greasy liver due to excessive nutrition or starvation/cachexia), glycogenosis (exogenous or endogenous corticosteroids), neoplasia (lymphoma, carcinoma; metastases), toxicosis (microcystins – jaundice, hepatic necrosis and hemorrhage, acute mycotoxicosis – hemorrhage), infarct/hemorrhage from traumatic injury or bacterial emboli, nutmeg liver pattern from hypoxia (congestive heart failure, severe pneumonia); oiling (hepatomegaly); hemosiderosis (starvation, nutritional, hemorrhage, iron storage defect), fibrosis (from parasite damage, chronic mycotoxicosis), neonatal status (normal, from yolk ingestion)

Clinicopathologic presentations	Differential etiologic diagnoses
Nodules	Granulomas (parasitic, bacterial: *Mycobacterium* spp. and others, mycotic), encysted parasites, post-necrotic scarring (from past injury), biliary ectasia (trematodes and others), hyperplasia, fibrosis or biliary hyperplasia (repair following inflammation or necrosis from past injury), neoplasia – rare (hepatocellular carcinoma, cholangioma/cholangiocarcinoma, pancreatic carcinoma/adenocarcinoma, disseminated tumors e.g. lymphoma)
Shrunken, firm, dark	Atrophy (cachexia), hemosiderosis (iron accumulation), fibrosis, mycotoxins (acute – pale, enlarged liver; chronic – firm, shrunken liver)
Reproductive tract:	
Nodules or focal/multifocal areas of pallor	Parasitic granulomas or cysts, inflammatory response due to egg rupture, or ascending infection, or disseminated infection affecting reproductive tract, neoplasia (leiomyomas, adenocarcinoma, lymphoma and others)
Dystocia, fetal (in ovo) demise or eggshell thinning	Obesity, malnutrition, dehydration, malpositioning in egg (difficult hatch), suboptimal temperature or other environmental factors, oviduct or intracoelomic infection (bacterial), torsion, compression, ruptured egg(s), oviduct prolapse, toxicosis (chlorinated hydrocarbon insecticides – eggshell thinning/failure to hatch), hypovitaminosis A, hypocalcemia

6

Aquatic Mammals

Pádraig Duignan

The etiology and clinical signs for diseases of mammals are listed in Appendix 6.1.

Parasitic Diseases of Major Taxa

Protista (Ciliates, Flagellates, Amoebae and Apicomplexa)

Etiology, Host Range and Transmission

Hematophagus megapterae is a common ciliate identified from the baleen plates of humpback (*Megaptera novaengliae*), fin (*Balaenoptera borealis*), and blue (*Balaenoptera musculus*) whales. Ciliates are also common in the upper respiratory tract of several odontocete cetaceans (dolphins) and are sometimes identified in feces, including *Kyaroikeus cetarius, Planilamina ovata, Planilamina magna, Balantidium* and other uncharacterized species. Ciliates may also be epiphytic on cyamids (Crustacea, Amphipoda) attached to the skin of baleen whales. Flagellates are taxonomically diverse and the genera identified from aquatic mammals include *Giardia, Trypanosoma, Leishmania, Trichomonas, Cryptobia, and Jarrelia. Giardia* spp. are found in the gastrointestinal tract of a wide variety of hosts worldwide.

Many different species and subspecies are recognized and they have a direct life cycle with resistant infective stages ingested from the environment. Asexual reproduction occurs in the host but sexual reproduction has not been described. Trypanosomes (*Trypanosoma* and *Leishmania* spp.) have an indirect life cycle involving an arthropod and a mammal. *Jarellia atramenti* or a related flagellate and *Cryptobia* spp. have been isolated from blowhole secretions of odontocetes in care (Poynton et al. 2001; Sweeney et al. 1999). A novel genus, *Planilamina* n. gen., with two species, was described from the blowholes of captive bottlenose dolphins and false killer whales, *Pseudorca crassidens* (Ma et al., 2006). *Chilomastix* or *Hexamita*-like flagellates have been found in the feces of a bowhead whale (*Balaena mysticetus*) harvested in Alaska and Indo-Pacific bottlenose dolphins (*Tursiops aduncus*) from the Red sea. Uncharacterized trichomonads have been identified on the mucosal epithelium and in crypts in the stomach and duodenum of California sea lions (*Zalophus californianus*) in rehabilitation. Amoebae are pathogens of global importance and include *Entamoeba histolytica* and *Dientamoeba fragilis*. Free-living amoebae, such as *Naegleria fowleri,*

Pathology and Epidemiology of Aquatic Animal Diseases for Practitioners, First Edition.
Edited by Laura Urdes, Chris Walster, and Julius Tepper.

Acanthamoeba spp., and *Balmuthia mandrillaris,* may cause significant disease as opportunistic pathogens. Most amoebae are commensal and part of the gastrointestinal tract biome (Heckmann et al., 1987; Hermosilla et al., 2016).

The Apicomplexa associated with systemic infection include *Toxoplasma gondii, Sarcocystis neurona, Neospora caninum,* related uncharacterized parasites, and the hemosporidia (e.g. *Babesia* and *Plasmodium* spp.). Apicomplexa that are only associated with enteric infection include the genera *Cystoisospora* (*Isospora*), *Eimeria*, and *Cryptosporidium*. *T. gondii* is a single species with many genotypes, for which felids (domestic and wild cats) are the asymptomatic definitive host. Any homeothermic vertebrate can act as an intermediate host of *T. gondii* by ingesting sporulated oocysts shed in cat feces that contaminate the environment or that are ingested by a paratenic host, such as filter-feeding (clams, mussels) or grazing (snails, limpets) mollusks. The infection has been recorded in many marine mammal species worldwide from the poles to the tropics, with higher rates of infection in the tropics, where felid populations are higher. Sea otters (*Enhydra lutris*) are a good example of how infection in a marine species is linked to contamination of the environment from terrestrial runoff (land to sea transmission). In California, exposure rates for *T. gondii* and/or *S. neurona* in necropsied southern sea otters ($\geq$ 78%) and seropositivity (> 71%) are much higher than in northern sea otters from Alaska, where there are fewer cats (Miller et al., 2020). Toxoplasmosis has also been documented in phocids, otariids, odontocetes, sirenians, and freshwater mustelids like river otters and mink. While seropositivity has been documented in free-ranging polar bears from Alaska, Greenland, and Norway, clinical disease has not yet been detected (Dubey et al., 2021). However, congenital infection was diagnosed by histopathology in a neonatal polar bear in a German zoo (cited by Dubery et al., 2021). Toxoplasmosis has not been described in mysticete whales.

The genus *Sarcocystis* has several species, identified from aquatic mammals, including *S. neurona, Sarcocystis canis, Sarcocystis pinnipedi* and *Sarcocystis arctosi*. There are also uncharacterized *Sarcocystis* spp. An *S. neurona*-like pathogen is the most commonly described for marine mammals. It was first documented as a cause of placentitis and abortion in Pacific harbor seals, *Phoca vitulina richardsii* (Lapointe et al., 1998). The life cycle is similar to that of *T. gondii* with New World opossums (*Didelphis virginianus* and *Didelphis albiventris*) as the definitive hosts. *Neospora caninum* and other uncharacterized *Neospora* spp. are also closely related to *T. gondii* and there is potential for serologic cross-reactivity. In contrast to *T. gondii*, the definitive hosts are canids. Otherwise, the life cycle is similar to that of *Toxoplasma* and *Sarcocystis* spp., as is the breadth of potential intermediate hosts and the potential for vertical transmission causing reproductive failure. While infection is widespread in wildlife, documentation of clinical neosporosis is rare. Incidental infection, as detected by molecular diagnostics (polymerase chain reaction, PCR), have been reported from phocids, otariids, and odontocetes but not in mysticetes, sea otters, or polar bears (Huggins et al., 2015).

Haemosporidia are apicomplexans that include the pathogenic genera *Babesia* and *Plasmodium*. They have a life cycle that includes a hematophagus arthropod such as a mosquito or tick. Evidence for infection of marine mammals is lacking but a survey of wild asymptomatic American river otters (*Lontra canadensis*) in North Carolina found a high prevalence of a unique Piroplasma in erythrocytes (Birkenheuer et al., 2006). Enteric apicomplexans that infect aquatic mammals include the genera *Eimeria, Cystoisospora* and *Cryptosporidium* and most species are host specific. All have a simple direct life cycle with infection resulting from ingestion of oocysts that are shed in feces. At least five species of *Eimeria* have been described, including *Eimeria phocae* in North Atlantic harbor seals (*Phoca vitulina vitulina*; Hsu et al., 1974; McClelland, 1993; van Bolhuis et al., 2007), *Eimeria weddelli* and *Eimeria arctowskii* in Antarctic crabeater

(*Lobodon carcinophagus*) and leopard seals (*Hydrurga leptonyx*; Drozdz, 1987). *Eimeria trichechi* is found in Amazonian manatees (*Trichechus inunguis*; Lainson et al., 1983), while Florida manatees (*Trichechus manatus latirostris*) have *Eimeria manatus* (Upton et al., 1989).

Clinical and Gross Signs

The clinical significance for most protists is unknown. Infection of the upper respiratory tract of cetaceans by ciliates is common, and although they feed on erythrocytes their pathogenicity is unknown. They are often found in association with bacteria or helminth parasites, such as the trematode *Nasitrema* spp. In immunocompromised hosts, ciliates may act as opportunistic pathogens causing dermatitis, cellulitis, pneumonia, and lymphadenitis, as described for Atlantic bottlenose dolphins (*Tursiops truncatus*) infected with the cetacean morbillivirus (Schulman and Lipscomb, 1999). Unidentified ciliates are also associated with dermatitis and pneumonia in stranded and debilitated cetaceans, but their role as primary pathogens is unknown (Woodward et al., 1969; Peterson and Hoggard, 1996; Choi et al., 2003; Van Bressem et al., 2008; Lair et al., 2016). Flagellates have been identified in phocids, otariids, odontocetes, mysticetes, and sirenians from a range of contaminated and pristine environments, but their role in clinical disease is unknown. Trypanosomes may be medically important in humans as a cause of sleeping sickness and Chagas disease, but their role in marine mammal health is less clear. There is one report of Chagas-like myocarditis in a captive polar bear (*Ursus maritimus*) in Mexico (Jaime-Andrade et al., 1997). *Leishmania* spp. cause cutaneous or systemic pathology in humans and terrestrial animals bitten by sand flies, the intermediate hosts. Systemic infection was reported for a stranded Mediterranean monk seal (*Monachus monachus*) with concurrent parapox infection (Toplu et al., 2007). The flagellates identified in California sea lion intestines were associated with crypt abscesses and mixed bacterial populations suggestive of a dysbiosis. Fecal screening has identified *Entamoeba* spp. in whales but the clinical significance is not known (Heckmann et al., 1987; Hermosilla et al., 2016).

The Apicomplexa are the most pathogenic protozoa for aquatic mammals. Once ingested, *T. gondii* traverses the gastrointestinal tract and disseminates widely in the body as rapidly dividing tachyzoites. This can be acutely fatal for fetuses or immunocompromised individuals. Once an immune response is initiated, the tachyzoites transform to bradyzoites and form tissue cysts in the brain, myocardium, or skeletal muscle, where they may persist without causing substantial inflammation for months to years. Clinical toxoplasmosis may recrudesce later in response to decreased immune competence, as seen with certain systemic infections (morbillivirus infection or bacterial septicemia), physiological state (pregnancy, lactation), malnutrition or old age. Toxoplasmosis results in nonsuppurative meningomyeloencephalitis with perivascular lymphocytic cuffing and meningitis, multifocal gliosis throughout the brain and spinal cord (Figure 6.1a,b) associated with large thin-walled cysts that are packed with thousands of elongate spindaloid curved bradyzoites (Figure 6.1c). The tissue cysts are clearly visible on histology using hemoxylin and eosin (H&E) stain, but tachyzoites are not easily identified without immunohistochemistry using *T. gondii* antiserum (Figure 6.1d).

Intermediate hosts for *Sarcocystis* spp. are infected by ingesting sporocysts shed by asymptomatic definitive hosts, or through consuming infected meat. Following ingestion, asexually produced merozoites spread systemically, enter host cells, and proliferate to form schizonts and, finally, tissue cysts. As with *T. gondii*, fatal disseminated infection including meningoencephalitis is a cause of death. Among aquatic mammals, river and sea otters, phocids, otariids, odontocetes of the eastern North Pacific have been identified as intermediate hosts, with tissue cysts detected in the central nervous system, heart, and skeletal myocytes of fatally and incidentally infected

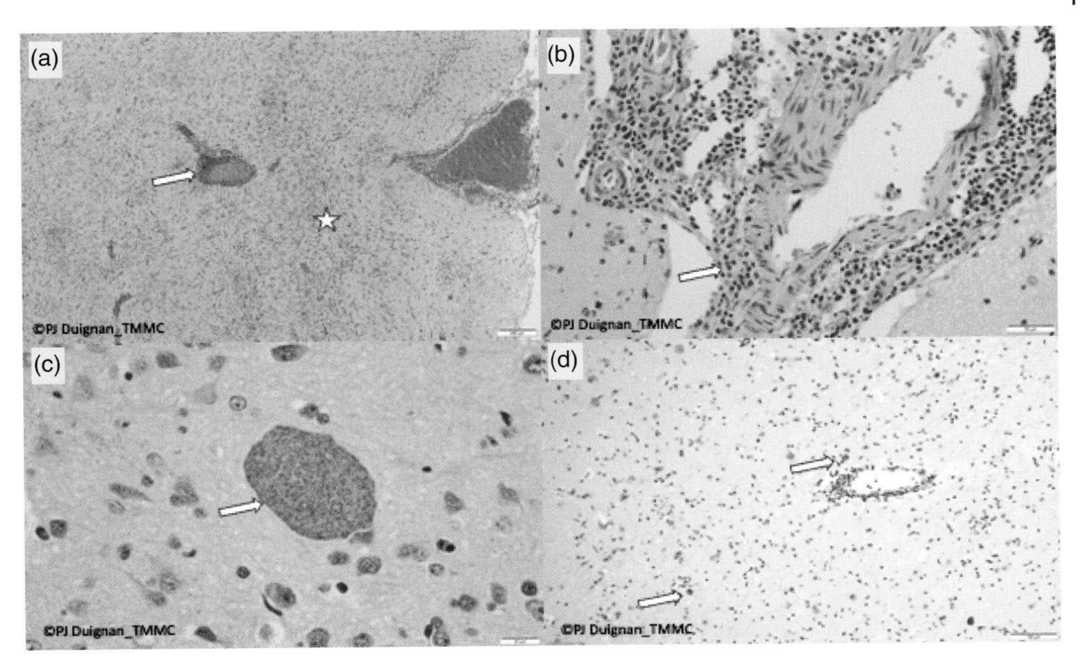

Figure 6.1 Southern sea otter (*Enhydra lutris nereis*). (a) Cerebrum, nonsuppurative meningoencephalitis, lymphocytic perivascular cuffing (white arrow) and diffuse gliosis (star). *Toxoplasma gondii* infection. H&E stain. (b) Cerebrum and meninges, lymphoplasmacytic infiltration (arrow), *T. gondii* infection, H&E stain. (c) Brain, thin-walled protozoal tissue cyst (arrow), *T. gondii*, H&E stain. (d) Hippocampus, multifocal immunolabelling (arrows) of *T. gondii* parasites throughout tissues, immunohistochemical staining, and hematoxylin counterstain.

animals. An unusual polyphasic rhabdomyositis that has similarities to immune-mediated myositis in dogs and humans has been described for California sea lions with systemic apicomplexan infection (Carlson-Bremer et al., 2012; Seguel et al., 2019). Clinically affected animals present with a suite of signs that vary depending on the muscle groups most affected (Figure 6.2a,b). Some animals appear lethargic and emaciated, as is seen with malnutrition. Others exhibit severe involvement of the muscles of mastication and striated muscle of the esophagus; these animals present with megaesophagus and emaciation, often with a slack mandible and angular appearance of the dorsal head due to muscle atrophy. Other animals present with dyspnea and respiratory stridor (Whoriskey et al., 2021). At necropsy, they usually have severely atrophied laryngeal, intercostal, diaphragmatic, and pectoral muscles (Figure 6.2c,d,e,f,g). The myositis is lymphohistiocytic with myonecrosis and continuing regeneration (Figure 6.2). At the periphery of lesions, T lymphocytes may be observed invading the sarcolemma of myocytes and major histocompatibility complex II antigen can be detected in myocytes, suggesting an immune-mediated pathogenesis (Seguel et al., 2019). Higher burdens of tissue cysts, and higher *S. neurona* antibody titers are observed in sea lions with rhabdomyositis than in those with other causes of mortality (Figure 6.2h,i).

S. pinnipedi is an endemic and largely asymptomatic parasite of Arctic ringed (*Phoca hispida*) and bearded (*Erignathus barbatus*) seals. However, it was associated with an epidemic of fatal hepatitis in gray seals (*Halichoerus grypus*) in Maritime Canada (Haman et al., 2015 cited in Miller et al., 2018). *S. arctosi* and uncharacterized *S. canis*-like protozoa have been implicated in hepatitis in polar bears (Gardner et al., 1997). Fatal hepatitis caused by *S. canis* was diagnosed in a Steller's

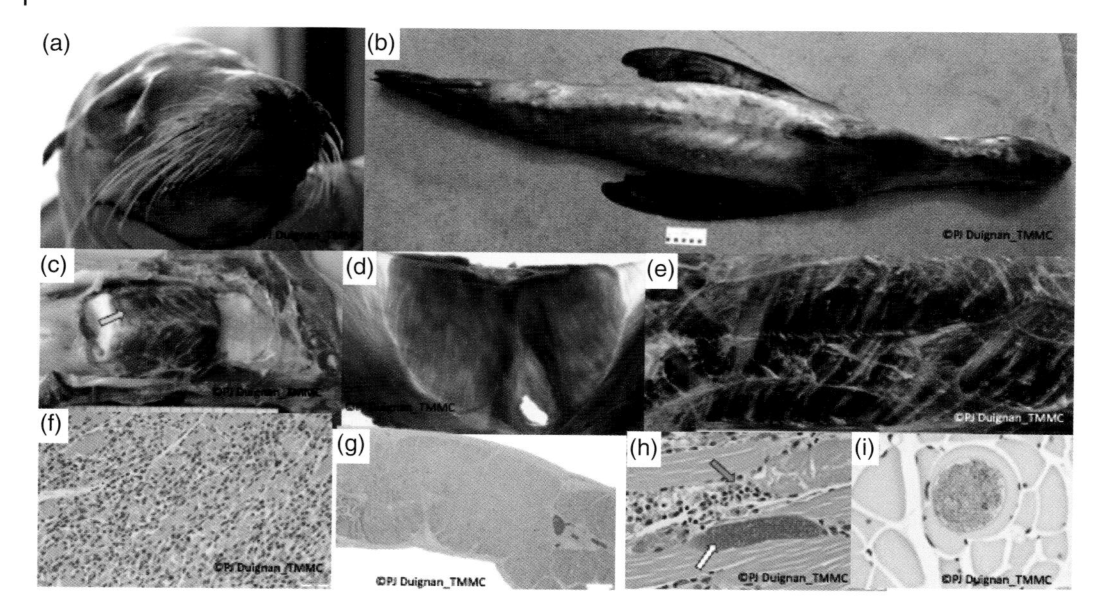

Figure 6.2 California sea lion (*Zalophus californianus*). (a) Marked atrophy of the cranial and facial muscles, polyphasic rhabdomyositis. (b) Same animal as (a), showing severe diffuse skeletal muscle atrophy. (c) Polyphasic rhabdomyositis, larynx showing atrophy and streaking of the dorsal cricoarytenoideus muscles. (d) Polyphasic rhabdomyositis, diaphragm showing atrophy (translucency) and streaking. (e) Polyphasic rhabdomyositis, superficial pectoral muscle showing multifocal streaking and generalized atrophy. (f) Polyphasic rhabdomyositis, histopathology of skeletal muscle showing marked lymphocytic and histiocytic infiltration with acute myonecrosis (hypereosinophilic fibers) and continuing regeneration (more basophilic myofibers with large centralized nuclei), H&E stain. (g) Diaphragm, showing full thickness myositis (pale blue staining), H&E stain. (h) Polyphasic rhabdomyositis, skeletal muscle showing a mature *Sarcocystis neurona* tissue cyst (white arrow) and interstitial infiltration of lymphocytes and histiocytes (blue arrow). H&E stain. (i) Skeletal muscle with *S. neurona* tissue cyst. Immunohistochemical staining showing positive reaction (brown stain) with *S. neurona* antibody.

sea lion (*Eumetopias jubatus*) found dead in Glacier Bay, Alaska (Welsh et al., 2014). A wide range of marine mammal species from phocids to Mysticetes, but excluding sirenians, commonly have uncharacterized *Sarcocystis* spp. tissue cysts in skeletal muscle and myocardium without pathology (Miller et al., 2018).

Enteric apicomplexan infections, such as *Eimeria phocae*, are usually incidental. However, in a rehabilitation setting with crowding of young animals and poor hygiene, outbreaks of enterocolitis can occur with acute death due to dysentry and dehydration, or more chronically, from anorexia and emaciation.

Diagnosis

Ciliates, flagellates and amoebae can be diagnosed from wet mounts or cytology preparations of respiratory tract swabs or sputum from live patients with signs of respiratory disease. Special stains, such as Wright–Giemsa and silver stains, can be used to aid detection or organisms. Fecal flotation with microscopic examination can be used for oocysts of enteric protozoa or flagellates, such as *Girardia*. Fluoroscopy can be used to distinguish between species and to rule out nonpathogenic organisms via species-specific antisera. However, similar organisms are frequently identified in animals without clinical illness. Protozoa are often observed in histological preparations of skin or respiratory tract lesions, but the association between the organism and lesion is usually unknown.

Toxoplasmosis and sarcocystosis are diagnosed in live patients via serology (agglutination, enzyme-linked immunoassay, and Western blots), available through commercial laboratories in endemic areas. At postmortem examination, histopathology, immunohistochemistry, PCR, and sequencing are used to identify species and genotype (Zhang et al., 2019). PCR is regarded as the gold standard for definitive confirmation of infection and species identification, but diagnosis of protozoal disease and confirmation of protozoal-associated mortality requires histopathology, often supported by immunohistochemistry. Transmission electron microscopy (TEM) is useful for identification of life stages in tissues and for characterization of novel species (Miller et al., 2018).

Differential Diagnoses

For respiratory tract and gastrointestinal tract infections, the differential list includes bacteria, viruses, mollicutes, fungi, and metazoan parasites. *T. gondii* and *Sarcocystis* spp. infections often result in acutely fatal systemic disease with neurological signs, such as seizures, central blindness and ataxia, for which viral infections or neurotoxins should be considered.

Treatment/Management

For animals in managed care, the first consideration for enteric and respiratory protozoa is to limit transmission. For enteric pathogens the goal should be to reduce fecal contamination of the environment. Protozoal oocysts are often highly resistant to commercial disinfectants. The infective dose is usually low, the life cycle is direct, fecal–oral, and animals in rehabilitation facilities are frequently immunocompromised, malnourished and have comorbidities, making them even more susceptible to opportunistic infections and disease. Oral sulfonamides (sulfaquinoxaline, sulfamethoxazole) and amprolium have been used to treat enteric infections (Miller et al., 2018).

For systemic apicomplexans (*T. gondii, S. neurona* and *N. caninum*), treatment options depend on whether the host is a stranded marine mammal in a rehabilitation hospital or a long-term display animal in a managed care setting. For the former, the severity of brain, spinal cord, or skeletal muscle lesions is generally so severe at the time of stranding that euthanasia may be the most humane option once the diagnosis is confirmed. Attempts at treatment with medications (such as ponazuril) and supportive care are costly, prolonged (months) and often end in failure (Whoriskey et al., 2021). For animals in managed care, diagnosis may occur at an earlier stage of infection if clinical signs of disease are noted early, and prompt treatment can result in clinical resolution. Oral medications licensed for treatment of equine protozoal myelitis have been used off-label for marine mammals. Ponazuril has been used to treat sarcocystosis in sea otters (5 mg/kg PO once daily), harbor seals and sea lions (10 mg/kg PO every 24 hours for at least 28 days) with variable success (Miller et al., 2018; Whoriskey et al., 2021).

Prevention of systemic protozoal disease of animals in managed care requires exclusion of potential definitive and intermediate hosts (cats, opossums, birds, rodents, and arthropods) from animal enclosures and food preparation or storage areas. Feeding live prey should be discouraged and, while freezing (−20°C) does not kill all oocysts or sporocysts, it can greatly reduce the tissue burden. For free-ranging coastal marine mammals, reducing the contamination of their habitat by land-based pathogens is key, but it requires significant effort to restore estuarine habitat, reduce contamination of waterways by feces from definitive hosts (e.g. cats and opossums), and/or eliminate introduced feral definitive hosts from key habitat areas for endangered and rare species like southern sea otters and Hawaiian monk seals (*Monachus schauinslandi*).

Trematoda: Digenia

Etiology, Host Range, and Transmission

At least 14 families of digenians (flukes) are found in all taxa of aquatic mammals except polar bears. They typically have a heteroxenous life cycle involving one or more intermediate hosts such as mollusks or fish, and sometimes a paratenic host. Sites of infection in the definitive host for the adult digenian varies by species. The digestive tract, including the bile ducts, gall bladder, pancreatic ducts, stomach, intestine, cecum, and buccal cavity are most commonly infected. The respiratory tract is favored by other species, including the cranial sinuses, nasal cavities, eustachian tubes, middle ear, lower airways, and lungs.

Clinical and Gross Signs

Infection may be inconsequential or cause significant pathology and death. Aberrant parasite migration can result in invasion of the cerebrum with fatal consequences in odontocetes and otariids (Geraci and St. Aubin, 1987; Degollada et al., 2002; Fauquier et al., 2004). Some species, such as *Ascotyle longa* and *Pseudamphistomum truncatum,* have zoonotic potential (Periera et al., 2013; Niemanis et al., 2016). Only digenians of clinical significance are described here.

Sea otters are often infected by the digenian *Microphallus pirum*, which normally infects seabirds and has crustaceans as an intermediate host (Figure 6.3). Otters living in suboptimal habitats may consume the same crustaceans in large numbers, resulting in heavy parasite burdens that can be associated with fatal enteritis (Mayer et al., 2003). *Microphallus pirum* and *Profilicollis* spp. acanthocephalan parasites of sea otters share the same intermediate crustacean hosts (e.g. sand crabs; *Emerita analoga*), so high enteric loads of both parasites often co-occur (Mayer et al., 2003). The digenian of pinnipeds (*Orthosplanchnus fraterculus*) can cause chronic fibrosing cholecystitis in northern sea otters.

Digenians in pinnipeds are generally found in the gastrointestinal tract and associated tissues such as the biliary system and pancreatic ducts. As with sea otters, avian-associated species, such as *Microphallus* spp. and *Apophallus* (*Pricetrema*), rarely cause pathology except in extremely high burdens, when enteritis may ensue. In South American sea lions (*Otaria flavescens*), very high burdens of potentially zoonotic *Ascotyle longa* have been reported without clinical consequences (Periera et al., 2013). California sea lions are commonly infected by *Zalophotrema* spp. that can

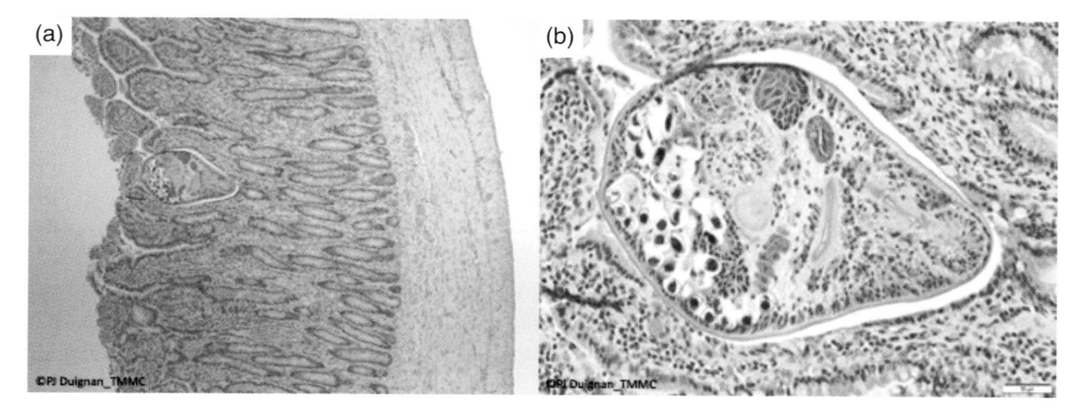

Figure 6.3 Southern sea otter, jejunum with section through a fluke, *Microphallus* sp. or *Plenosoma* spp. (Digenea, Trematoda), embedded in the mucosa, with minimal tissue reaction, H&E stain. (a) Low power view. (b) High power view, showing mature trematode.

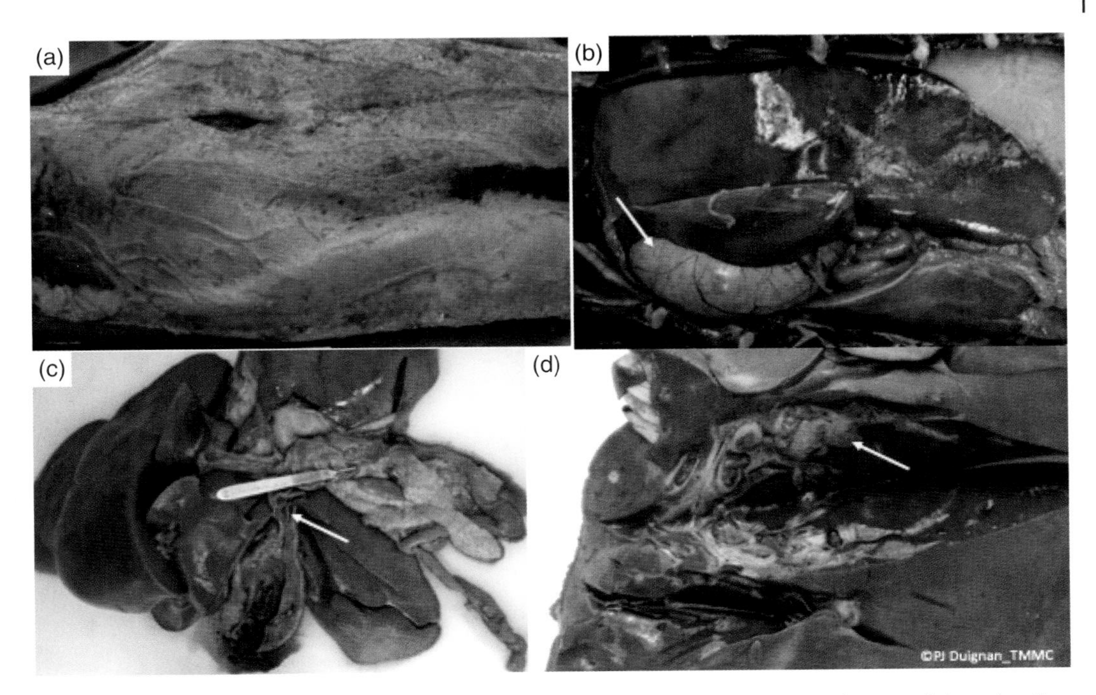

Figure 6.4 California sea lion, (a) ventral abdominal skin reflected to show diffuse icterus of the subcutis and blubber. (b) Markedly distended gall bladder (arrow). (c) Liver and gall bladder opened to show a thickened convoluted bile duct (arrow) that is partially occluded at the duodenal papilla (point of scalpel handle). (d) Incised liver showing marked thickening (fibrosis) and ectasia of bile ducts containing large numbers of liver flukes (*Zalophotrema hepaticum*, Trematoda) and viscous bile.

cause cholangiocystitis with marked biliary hyperplasia, fibrosis and lymphoplasmacytic inflammation in older animals (Figure 6.4). Secondary bacterial infection can result in hepatitis, pancreatitis, or abscessation. Galapagos sea lions (*Zalophotrema wollebaeki*) may be infected by an avian digenian (*Philophthalmus zalophi*), which is found in the orbit and causes conjunctivitis (Dailey et al., 2005). Occasionally, fatal cholangiohepatitis has been reported for various aquatic or amphibious mammals in Europe and Asia, including gray seals in the Baltic Sea, river otters (*Lutra lutra*) and introduced North American mink, *Mustela vision* (Neimanis et al., 2016). A common denominator for these hosts is the ingestion of freshwater cyprinid fish, the intermediate host for the trematode *Pseudamphistomum truncatum*. Clinical indications of severe cholangiohepatitis include evidence of hepatic failure on clinical chemistry, abdominal pain, anorexia, diarrhea, posterior paresis, polydipsia, photophobia and, in advanced cases, icterus, and neurologic signs (e.g. head weaving) attributable to hepatic encephalopathy.

Cetaceans may also have digenian parasites in their gastrointestinal tract, bile and pancreatic ducts, and respiratory tract. As with pinnipeds, most infections are subclinical. *Braunina*, *Pholeter*, and *Synthesium* spp. induce incidental fibrotic nodules in the gastrointestinal mucosae of odontocetes. Of greater significance is infection of the bile ducts and pancreatic ducts by *Campanula* spp., which can result in debilitating or fatal hepatic and pancreatic cirrhosis (Migaki et al., 1971; Dailey and Stroud, 1978; Geraci and St. Aubin, 1987; Siebert et al., 2001; Jauniaux et al., 2002). Odontocetes are also host to *Nasitrema* spp., which inhabits the cranial sinuses, where it may cause mild sinusitis. However, on occasion, parasites can migrate along the auditory nerve and into the brain, where they cause VIIIth cranial neuritis and extensive cerebral hemorrhage and malacia, which can result in stranding or death (Dailey and Walker, 1978; O'Shea et al., 1991; Morimitsu et al., 1987, 1992; Degollada et al., 2002). *Hunterotrema* spp. are found in the lungs of odontocetes, where they may cause pneumonia and sometimes fatal aberrant migration to the brain.

Sirenians harbor a wide diversity of digenians, but few are pathogenic. *Pulmonicola* spp. inhabit the nasal cavities and lungs of Florida manatees, where they may cause pneumonia (Buergelt et al., 1984). *Nudacotyle* spp. infection can cause hemorrhagic enteritis (Beck and Forrester, 1988). Other species (*Faredifex* spp., *Lankatrema* spp., *Labicola* spp. and *Moniligerum* spp.) have been associated with gastrointestinal abscesses or nodules (Dailey et al., 1988). In dugongs (*Dugong dugon*), the digenian *Opistotrema* spp. causes fibrinopurulent rhinitis with secondary bacterial infection (Blair, 1981).

Diagnosis

Detection of characteristic thick-walled (variably gold or brown-pigmented and operculated) trematode eggs in feces, nasal or pulmonary secretions or exudate can facilitate confirmation of patent, subclinical infections. Associated abnormalities on clinical chemistry include marked elevation of liver enzymes (aspartate aminotransferase and alanine transaminase) and inflammatory indicators, such as elevated leukocyte counts (leukocytosis or leukopenia) and decreased maturity of circulating granulocytes (left shift).

Differential Diagnoses

For hepatobiliary trematodes, other causes of hepatopathy should be ruled out, such as bacterial infection, viruses (adenoviruses), congenital defects (vascular shunts), other parasites (e.g. *Sarcocystis* spp.), or toxins (e.g. microcystins). Neurological signs that may result from cerebral migration, hemorrhage and malacia, include seizures and obtundation. Other conditions that can cause similar signs include meningoencephalitis (e.g. morbilliviruses, toxoplasmosis, sarcocystosis, brucellosis, and other bacterial infections), toxins (e.g. domoic acid, saxitoxin), or cranial trauma.

Treatment and Management

Most respiratory and gastrointestinal trematodes are part of the normal biome of free-ranging aquatic mammals and do not require treatment. Captive marine mammals are usually fed prefrozen food that is assumed to be free of viable parasites. If fresh or live prey are fed, periodic prophylaxis may be instituted. Similarly, should treatment be necessary based on clinical signs and a confirmed diagnosis, digenian trematodes are susceptible to praziquantel, which has been used to treat dolphins for *Nasitrema* infection (10 mg/kg PO once). Praziquantel is also used in pinnipeds to treat trematodiasis and cestodiasis (5 mg/kg intramuscularly, IM, or PO twice, or 10 mg/kg IM or PO once; Gulland et al., 2018).

Cestoda

Etiology, Host Range, and Transmission

Cestodes (tapeworms) have a heteroxenous life cycle. Aquatic mammals can serve as definitive hosts for genera within the Tetrabothriidae and Diphyllobothriidae, with the parasite residing usually in the intestine. Aquatic mammals can also be the intermediate host for several genera of the families Phyllobothriidae (*Phyllobothrium* and *Monorygma* spp.) and Lecanicephalidae (*Polypocephalus* spp.), of which encysted larvae are found in blubber, on serosal surfaces in the abdominal cavity, the parietal and visceral peritoneum, on membranes such as the mesentery and mesometrium. Sharks are thought to be the definitive host for these cestodes (Aznar et al., 2007).

Several species of *Diphyllobothrium* and *Diplogonoporous* are zoonotic (Scholtz and Kuchta, 2016). Anthroponotic disease has been described in Mediterranean monk seals and Cape fur seals (*Arctocepohalus pusillus pusillus*) by the human tapeworm (*Taenia solium*) probably contracted through exposure to sewage.

Clinical and Gross Signs

Intestinal cestodes are rarely associated with clinical signs or significant pathology (Figure 6.5a). Dailey and Stroud (1978) described nodular granulomas on the intestinal mucosa of cetaceans associated with the attachment sites of *Strobicephalus triangularis*, possibly causing obstruction (Figure 6.5b). Large boluses of *Diphylloborthrium* spp. obstructed the intestines of a young, emaciated beluga whale (*Delphinapterus leucas*) stranded in the St. Lawrence estuary (Measures et al., 1995). A similar association between poor body condition and growth rate with heavy *Diphyllobothrium* burdens was suggested for Hawaiian monk seals, (Reif et al., 2006).

Small *Phyllobothrium* cysts (up to 1 cm diameter) are common in the ventral and perineal blubber of pinnipeds and odontocetes. When these cysts occur in high densities (Figure 6.6a), they could negatively impact thermoregulation. Degenerate cysts can also result in pyogranulomatous inflammation and abscessation (Figure 6.6b). *Monorygma* are typically large cysts (2–3 cm diameter), and in high numbers they may act as space-occupying lesions in the pelvic cavity (Figure 6.6c,d). As with *Phylloborthrium*, degenerate cysts may incite a local inflammation. Sea otters, particularly the more piscivorous northern subspecies, are definitive hosts for *Diphyllobothrium* and *Diplogonoporus* spp., but usually without clinical consequences. Cestodes have not been reported for free-living polar bears or sirenians. In a study on cape fur seals, cysts were found in various organs, including the brain, and death followed seizures (De Graaf et al., 1980).

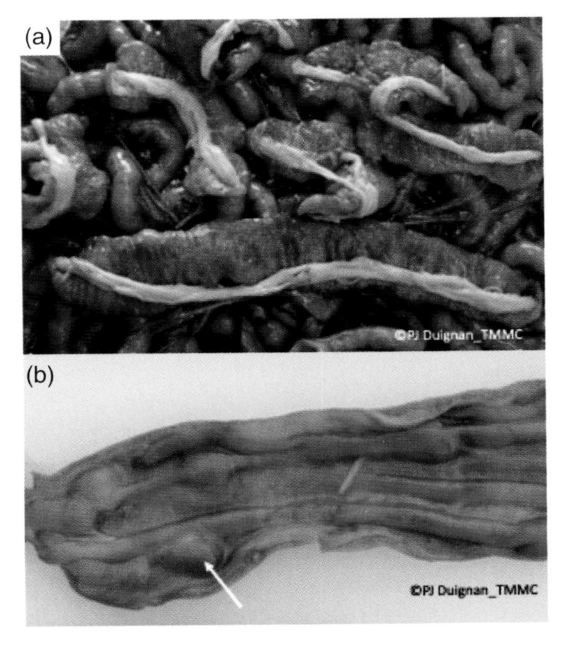

Figure 6.5 Striped dolphin, *Stenella coeruleoalba*. (a) Jejunum with heavy burden of tapeworms (*Tetrabothrius* spp. Cestoda). (b) Colon with mucosal nodules (arrow) associated with the cestode *Strobicephalus triangularis*.

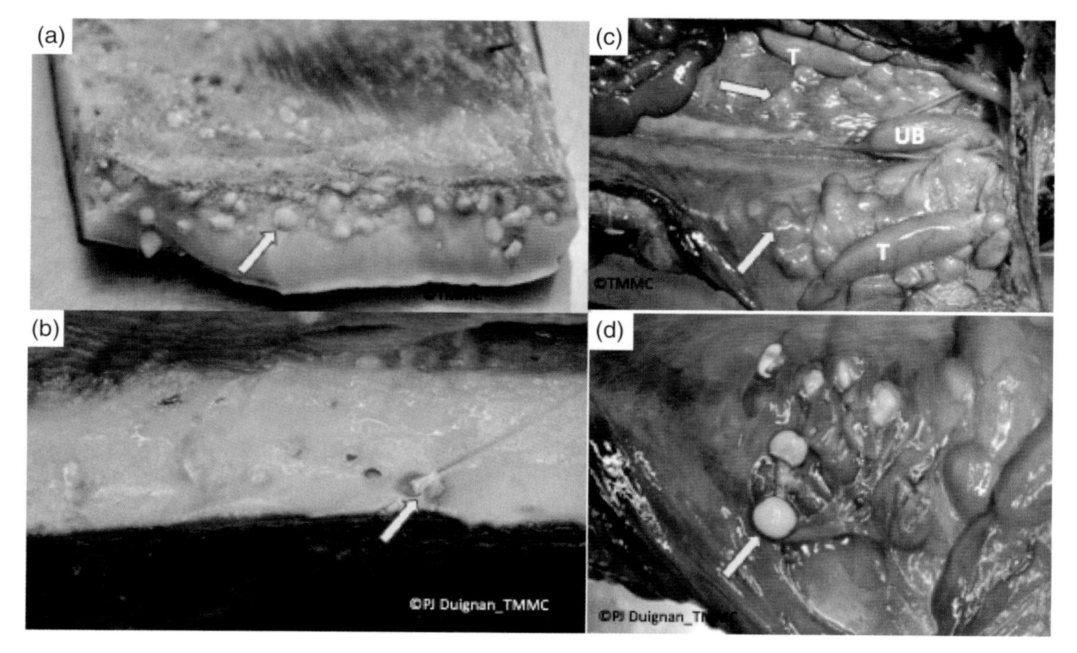

Figure 6.6 (a) Striped dolphin, skin and hypodermis (blubber), multifocal yellow-white cysts (arrow), plerocercoids (larval stage) of a cestode (*Phyllobothrium* spp.). (b) Pygmy sperm whale (*Kogia breviceps*), skin and blubber with multifocal gritty white nodules (granulomas) associated with degenerate cestode plerocercoids (arrow). (c) Striped dolphin, peritoneum with multifocal fluid-filled nodules (arrows), plerocercoids of a cestode *Monorygma* spp. adjacent to the testes (T) and urinary bladder (UB). (d) Striped dolphin as in (c), showing the larval cestodes from opened cysts (arrow).

Diagnosis

Intestinal cestodiasis is diagnosed via direct fecal examination, fecal flotation, or observation of cestode strobila on the pelage, substrate or in a pool.

Differential Diagnoses

Rarely, intestinal cestodes cause intestinal impaction or obstruction. Other potential causes include foreign body ingestion (e.g. rocks, large fish bones, fishing gear, or other foreign bodies), intestinal accidents (volvulus, intussusception), ileus, or gastrointestinal neoplasia.

Treatment and Management

As for digenian trematodes, intestinal tapeworms are normal biota in free-ranging aquatic mammals and rarely cause significant clinical disease. Animals maintained in captivity and fed prefrozen prey are generally not exposed to viable parasite life stages. Where treatment is required, praziquantel may be used (Odontoctes: 2 mg/kg PO once; pinnipeds: 5 mg/kg IM or PO twice daily, or 10 mg/kg IM or PO once; sea otters: 5 – 25 mg/kg PO or subcutaneously, SC, repeat in 2 weeks, 6 mg/kg IM once; sirenians: 10–20 mg/kg PO once).

Acanthocephala

Etiology, Host Range, and Transmission

Thorny-headed worms of aquatic mammals belong to the family Polymorphidae and are usually found in the intestine. *Bolbosoma* spp. are the predominant parasites of cetaceans, while

Corynosoma spp. and *Profillicollis* spp. are the predominant species found in pinnipeds and sea otters. No acanthocephalans have been described for sirenians or polar bears. Their life cycle requires a crustacean intermediate host and some species may use fish as paratenic hosts.

Clinical and Gross Signs

The multihooked proboscis of acanthocephalans allows them to anchor to the intestinal mucosa, causing focal hemorrhage, inflammation, and fibrosis. *Bolbosoma balanae* was associated with transmural intestinal abscesses in a stranded emaciated juvenile gray whale (*Eschrichtius robustus*) in California (Dailey et al., 2000), while *Bolbosoma capitatum* was associated with ulcerative enteritis in false killer whales (*Pseudorca crassidens*) in Japan (Kikuchi, 1993). However, unless infection is extremely heavy, acanthocephalans are usually tolerated by the host with minimal clinical consequences. In young or immune-compromised animals, heavy infestations can be associated with emaciation, malnutrition, enteritis and anemia, or intestinal perforation and peritonitis (Mayer et al., 2003). Southern sea otters are an exception to the rule in that they are highly susceptible to developing verminous peritonitis due to *Profillicollis* spp. infection (Figure 6.7). These are endemic parasites of marine birds that have sand crabs or spiny mole crabs (*Emerita analoga* and *Blepharipoda occidentalis*, respectively) as intermediate hosts. Acanthocephalan peritonitis was found to be a significant primary cause of death or comorbidity in stranded southern sea otters in California (Kreuder et al., 2003; Miller et al., 2020), and it is a major cause of nutritional stress for the species (Estes et al., 2003). For juvenile and subadult animals, *Profillicollis* peritonitis accounted

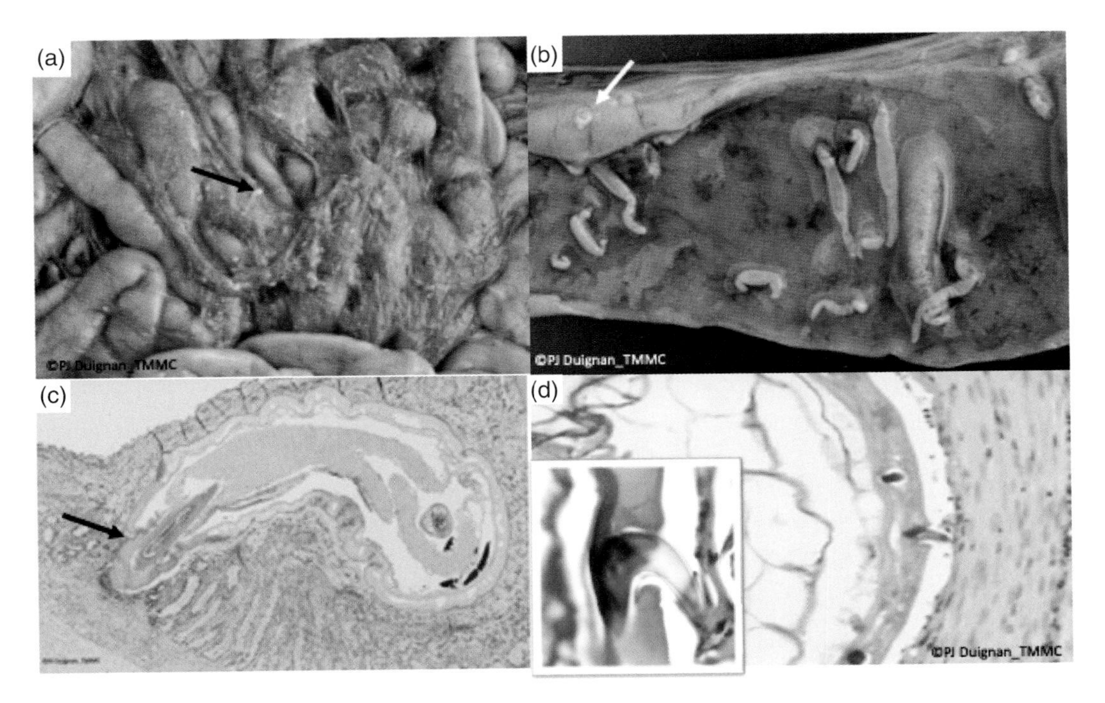

Figure 6.7 Southern sea otter. (a) small intestine, omentum and mesentery, fibrinous inflammation with numerous degenerating parasites (*Profillicollis* spp., Acanthocephala, arrow). (b) Jejunum with acanthocephalans attached to the mucosa and traversing the intestinal wall (arrow). Note the focal hemorrhage at attachment sites. (c) Jejunum with acanthocephalan (*Profillicollis* spp.) embedded in the mucosa (arrow), H&E stain. (d) Jejunum with acanthocephalan beneath the tunica muscularis. Note the hook on the proboscis and magnified in the inset image, H&E stain.

for up to 40% of deaths. Most otters with fatal acanthocephalan peritonitis (61%) also have bacterial peritonitis as a concurrent cause of death or sequela (Miller et al., 2020). Fatal acanthocephalan peritonitis also co-occurred with enteritis, enterocolitis or proctitis. Concurrent intestinal disease (possibly of bacterial and/or viral origin), was observed in 20% of acanthocephalan peritonitis cases, compared with 7% of otters without this condition (Miller et al., 2020). Seasonally, acanthocephalan peritonitis mortality is most prevalent in late spring and early summer (Miller et al., 2020). By contrast, sea otters are the definitive host for *Corynosoma enhydri* acanthocephalans; these parasites do not perforate through the intestines, and the infection rarely causes clinical signs or pathology.

Diagnosis

Eggs with thick multilayered walls encasing an acanthor can be identified by fecal flotation or sedimentation techniques in some, but not all, hosts; for example, *Profilicollis* spp. infections are usually nonpatent in sea otters, while *Corynosoma enhydri* infections produce copious eggs that can be detected on fecal flotation. Adult acanthocephlans are sometimes shed in feces of live animals or can be collected at necropsy; species are distinguished based on morphological characteristics (Mayer et al., 2003; Kuzmina et al., 2018).

Differentials

For intestinal nodules, other helminth parasites such as digenian trematodes should be considered. Fibrinous peritonitis can also be caused by bacterial infection or gastrointestinal tract perforation by a foreign body.

Treatment and Management

For captive animals, the simplest way to prevent infection is by avoiding feeding high risk prey items such as sand crabs to sea otters. Ensuring that all food is frozen and thawed prior to feeding is an excellent method of preventing infection by both helminth and protozoan parasites. For treatment, albendazole can be used, at 100 mg/kg PO twice a day for 3 days, repeated every 2 weeks for four to six rounds of treatment.

Nematoda

Etiology, Host Range, and Transmission

Nematodes are the largest and most diverse group of helminths in aquatic mammals and the group with the greatest potential to cause morbidity and mortality. Some are host specific and can infect any host that consumes potential intermediate hosts. Many nematode parasites also have zoonotic potential secondary to consumption of intermediate hosts carrying infective larval stages (McClelland, 2002; Lehnert et al., 2010). Some nematodes, such as *Anisakis* spp., use paratenic hosts (fish) to bridge the gap between krill (which serves as hosts for infective third stage larvae) and krill-eating fish that are consumed by cetaceans (Hays et al., 1998). Vertical transmission is an alternative transmission strategy used by some nematodes, such as lungworms and hookworms. Marine mammals may also become accidental hosts, sometimes with fatal consequences, for nematodes of terrestrial mammals. As an example, *Capillaria hepatica*, a nematode of rats that can also be zoonotic, can cause severe, fatal necrotizing hepatitis and fibrinous peritonitis in sea otters (Miller et al., 2020a).

Another land-based nematode that has been reported as an opportunistic pathogen for pinnipeds in California is *Pelodera strongyloides*; hair follicle infection in harbor seals was associated with mild dermatitis and alopecia (McHuron et al., 2013A), while incidental follicular infection has been observed in California sea lions (Duignan, unpublished). *Pelodera strongyloides* is a facultatively parasitic free-living soil nematode that invades the hair follicles of mammals through direct contact of skin with contaminated material. The infection is most commonly described in livestock and dogs, but it has also been reported in rodents, a black bear, and humans. The infection may be associated with intense pruritus, erythema, alopecia, and folliculitis. Of interest, two researchers involved in capture and sampling of harbor seals developed dermatitis after three days of fieldwork at the same location where all four *P. strongyloides*-infected harbor seals were captured. Dermatitis in affected humans was characterized by an intensely pruritic papillary rash on the arms, shoulders, abdomen, and legs. The rash developed by the third day following the capture and resolved one week later without medical intervention (McHuron et al., 2013). Because histological diagnosis of *P. strongyloides* infection in the harbor seals was made months after the capture, confirmation of *P. strongyloides*-associated dermatitis in capture personnel was not possible. However, this ubiquitous facultative parasite should be considered as a differential for pruritic skin rashes that develop in humans following marine mammal capture and handling activities in the future. Although these parasites can be zoonotic, the most likely source of infection was extended through contact with contaminated soil during the seal capture activities.

Clinical and Gross Signs

Genera of the Anisakidae family (*Anisakis, Pseudoterranova, Contracaecum, Phocascaris, Heterocheilus, Paradujardinia*) are common in the stomach or proximal small intestine of cetaceans, pinnipeds, and sirenians. In stranded California sea lions, *Pseudoterranova* and *Contracaecum* spp. are commonly associated with gastric or proximal intestinal ulcers (Migaki et al., 1971). The nematodes are usually attached in large numbers to the exposed submucosa and are surrounded by a raised rim of granulation tissue; owing to the gross appearance of these lesions, they are often described as "volcano ulcers" (Figure 6.8). Occasionally, there is secondary bacterial infiltration and abscessation in the gastric wall. Rarely, the ulcers perforate the *tunica muscularis* and serosa. Such perforations are usually sealed by the omentum, but they may occasionally lead to peritonitis and death. Why infection has a fatal outcome in some animals is unknown, but it may be related to aberrant migration, higher parasite loads, or maladapted, malnourished, or immune-compromised hosts (Greig et al., 2005).

Metastrongylus spp. or lungworms are a diverse group that can be highly pathogenic in pinnipeds and odontocetes, but less so in *Mysticetes*, sirenians, and polar bears (Greig et al., 2005; Fauquier et al., 2009; Lehnert et al., 2014; Lair et al., 2016). They are absent from sea otters, probably as a consequence of their diet. The adult parasites may be found in the cranial sinuses, major airways, or alveolar parenchyma, while larval migration may also involve the circulatory system and lymphatics. One of the most pathogenic is *Otostrongylus circumlitus*, a large lungworm of northern phocids. This parasite has an indirect life cycle involving development of infective third-stage larvae in the intestinal wall of finfish (Bergeron et al., 1997). Larval migration from the gastrointestinal tract to the lung involves the portal circulation to the liver, then the caudal vena cava, the right atrium and ventricle, and finally, passing via the pulmonary arteries to the lung (Figure 6.9). Hepatic migration can be associated with necrosis and granulomatous inflammation. Intravascular migration may cause arteritis, thrombosis, and thromboembolism, resulting in fatal pulmonary infarction or disseminated intravascular coagulation (DIC; Yang et al., 2018; Wessels et al., 2019). Even in well-adapted hosts such as harbor or ringed seals (*Pusa hispida*), heavy *O. circumlitus* burdens in the bronchi and bronchioles can cause significant obstruction, negatively affecting overall fitness, diving ability, foraging, growth, survival, and recruitment (Onderka, 1989;

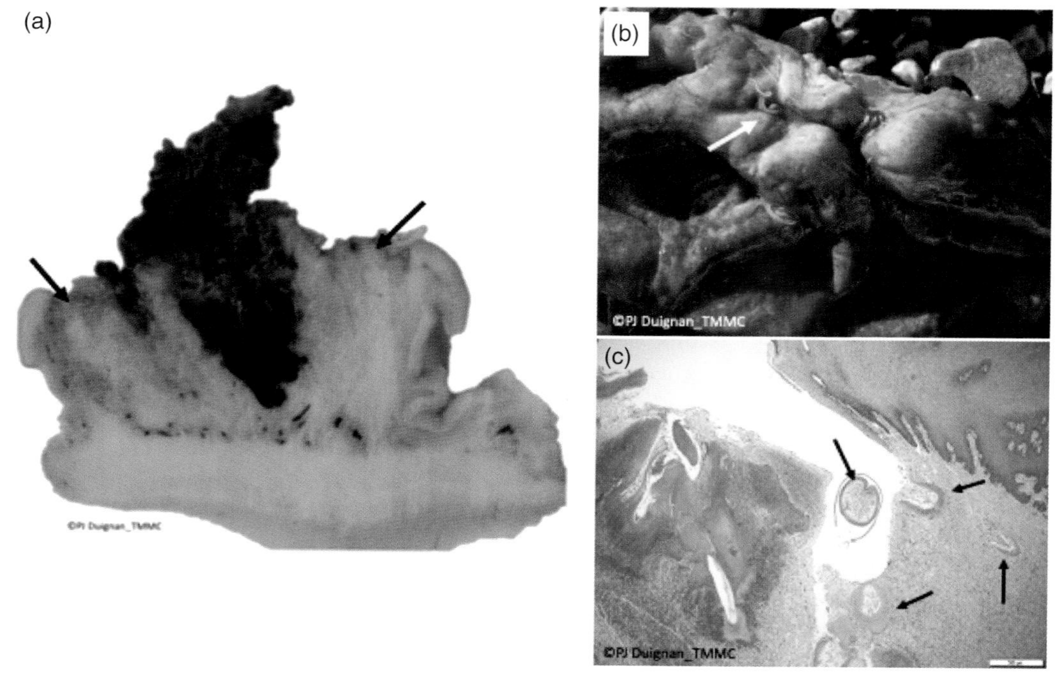

Figure 6.8 (a) California sea lion, stomach wall sectioned through a "volcano ulcer" showing the thick ring of granulation tissue (arrows) and the erupting center composed of numerous nematodes (Ascaroidea), necrosis and hemorrhage (black tissue). Formalin-fixed tissue. (b) Narwhal, *Monodon monoceros*, second gastric compartment mucosa with numerous "volcano" ulcers and nematodes (arrow). (c) Narwhal, first gastric chamber with "volcano" ulcer and multiple sections through nematodes extending into the granulation tissue below the ulcer (arrows), H&E stain.

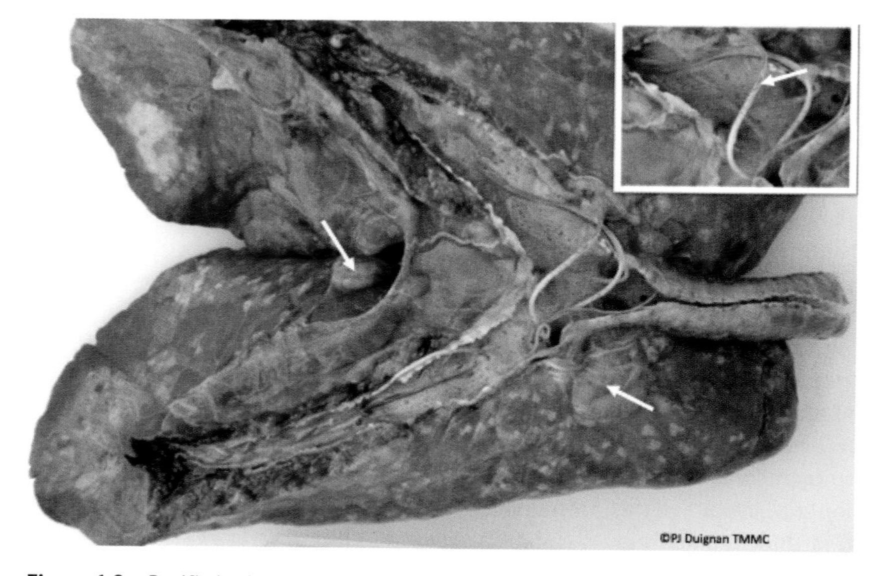

Figure 6.9 Pacific harbor seal (*Phoca vitulina*) lungs with bronchi opened to show numerous mature metastrongylid nematodes (*Otostrongylus circumlitus*) and excess frothy catarrhal exudate. The lungs are over inflated, diffusely congested, with focal consolidation (note the tan mass in the caudal–medial aspect of the left lung), and lymphadenopathy (tracheal and mediastinal lymph nodes, arrows). Inset shows that the nematodes have a reproductive tract (arrow).

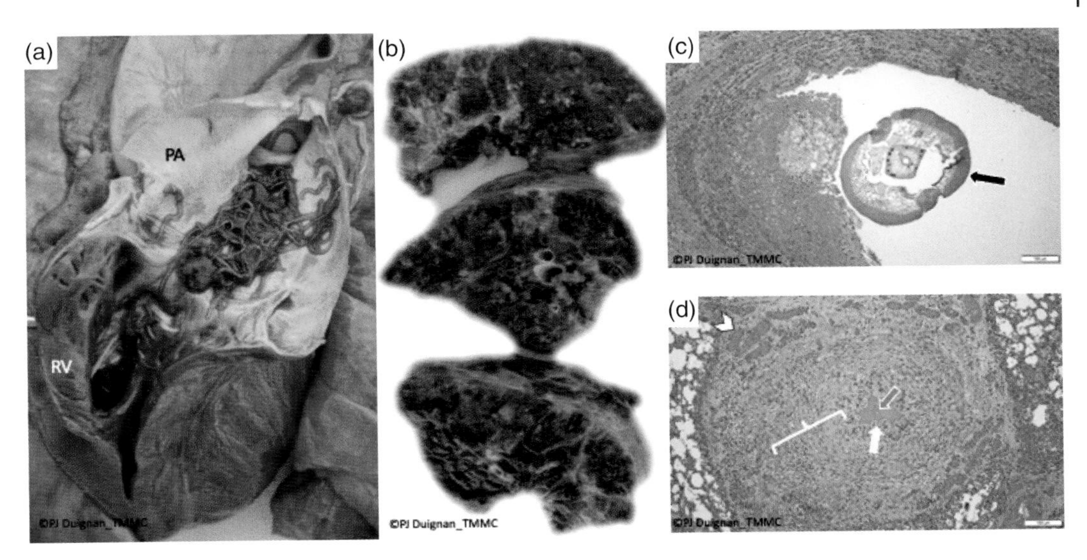

Figure 6.10 Northern elephant seal (*Mirounga angustirostris*). (a) Right ventricle (RV) and pulmonary artery (PA) opened to show a heavy burden of nematodes (*Otostrongylus circumlitus*). (b) Serial section of one lung lobe showing extensive hemorrhage indicative of diffuse pulmonary infarction. (c) Histological section of lung showing immature *O.circumlitus* (arrow) in the lumen of a pulmonary arteriole, H&E stain. (d) Pulmonary arteriole with concentric laminar medial hypertrophy (delimited by bracket) and vacuolation, endothelial cell hypertrophy (white arrow), luminal stenosis (blue arrow) and post-stenotic capillary dilatation (arrowhead). Neutrophils are transmigrating through the arteriolar tunica media and adventitia.

Gosselin et al., 1998). The northern elephant seal (*Mirounga angustirostris*) appears to be less adapted to *O. circumlitus* infection; DIC, pulmonary infarction, and hemorrhage are common causes of death for stranded weanlings in California (Gulland et al., 1997; Kaye et al., 2017; Yang et al., 2018).

At necropsy, *O. circumlitus* is most common in the right ventricle and pulmonary arterial tree, where the nematodes are often associated with areas of pulmonary infarction (Figure 6.10a,b). However, adult nematodes are rarely found in the bronchi and bronchioles. On histology, there is pulmonary arterial medial hypertrophy, luminal stenosis, intravascular thrombi that sometimes contain intra-arterial nematodes, and occasional endarteritis or periarteritis (Figure 6.10c,d; Yang et al., 2018). In contrast, the pulmonary arterial lesions observed in northeastern Atlantic gray seals (*Halichoerus grypus*) include circumferential intimal proliferation, subintimal granulomatous inflammation and deposition of Splendore–Höeppli-like material associated with intravascular nematodes (Wessels et al., 2019). Pulmonary infarction, hemorrhage, and death can be the end result in both species.

Parafilaroides spp. are lungworms commonly found in otariids and phocids worldwide. Although these parasites are much smaller than *O. circumlitus*, their life cycle is similar (Dailey, 1970). Adults and larvae reside in alveoli and smaller bronchioles; infection is associated with variable granulomatous inflammation. Larval migration through the liver may cause focal necrosis and inflammation, while arterial migration by *Piranthus decorus* can cause pulmonary arteritis and thrombosis in Guadalupe fur seals (*Arctocephalus townsendi*; Seguel et al., 2018). In California sea lions, infection is observed in stranded animals of all age classes, and the intensity of infection varies from mild to severe. In severe infections, verminous bronchopneumonia is characterized by goblet-cell hyperplasia in bronchioles, leading to airway obstruction by mucopurulent exudate admixed with

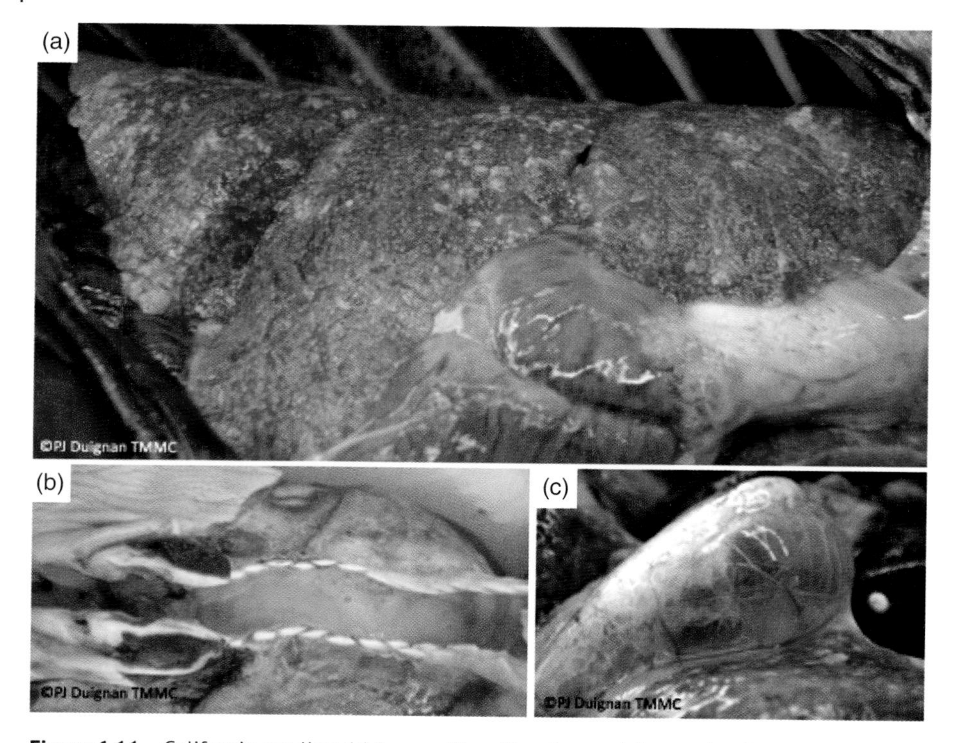

Figure 6.11 California sea lion. (a) Lung with miliary tan nodules randomly scattered throughout. Granulomatous bronchopneumonia caused by the metastrongylid lungworm *Parafilaroides decorus*. (b) Bronchus opened to show viscous mucopurulent exudate filling the lumen. (c) Thoracic cavity showing severe mediastinal emphysema (distended air-filled bullae).

P. decorus larvae and adults. The parenchyma often has a miliary pattern of consolidation with pyogranulomatous inflammation, atelectasis, and alveolar emphysema (Figure 6.11a). The airway exudate can vary from frothy, to catarrhal, to mucopurulent (Figure 6.11b); in severe cases, airway obstruction results in mediastinal and pleural emphysema (Figure 6.11c).

On histology, adult nematodes within the alveolar parenchyma rarely incite a marked inflammatory response, but areas of larval infection are associated with granuloma formation. Verminous bronchopneumonia is often complicated by opportunistic bacterial infection and other parasites, such as respiratory mites, *Orthohalarachne diminuata* (Figure 6.12).

The respiratory nematodes of odontocetes are members of the Pseudaliidae family (*Stenurus* spp., *Halocercus* spp., *Pseudalius* spp., *Torynurus* spp., *Pharurus* spp., *Skrjabinalius* spp.). They are commonly found in the cranial sinuses and surrounding the tympanoperiotic (ear) bones (Figure 6.13a,b), but they are not known to cause significant inner ear pathology (Lehnert et al., 2014; Morell et al., 2017). They are also found in nasal passages, major airways, and alveolar parenchyma. As with pinnipeds, the host response to infection varies from incidental to severe; heavy burdens can cause verminous bronchopneumonia (Figure 6.13,c,d) and can be a primary or contributory cause of death, often in association with opportunistic bacteria, fungi, or protozoa. The life cycles are less well understood, but experimental infection confirmed that *Pharurus pallasii* of the cranial sinuses of belugas use fish as intermediate or paratenic hosts (Houde et al., 2003). In the North Sea, larvae of three species of Pseudaliidae that infect harbor porpoises (*Phocoena phocoena*) were found in wild fish (Lehnert et al., 2010). Transplacental or

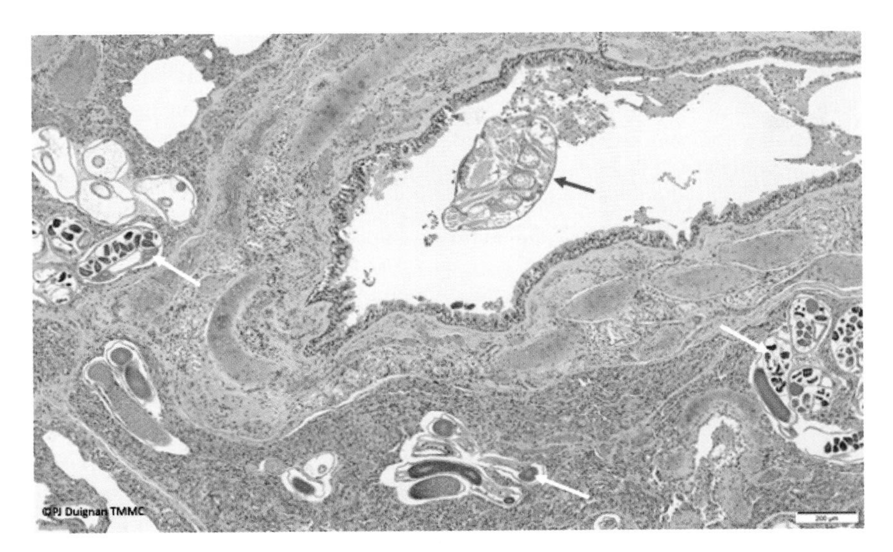

Figure 6.12 California sea lion, lung, bronchiole containing a mite, *Orthohalarachne diminuta*, (blue arrow) and the surrounding parenchyma has several mature nematodes (*P. decorus*) surrounded by granulomatous inflammation (white arrow).

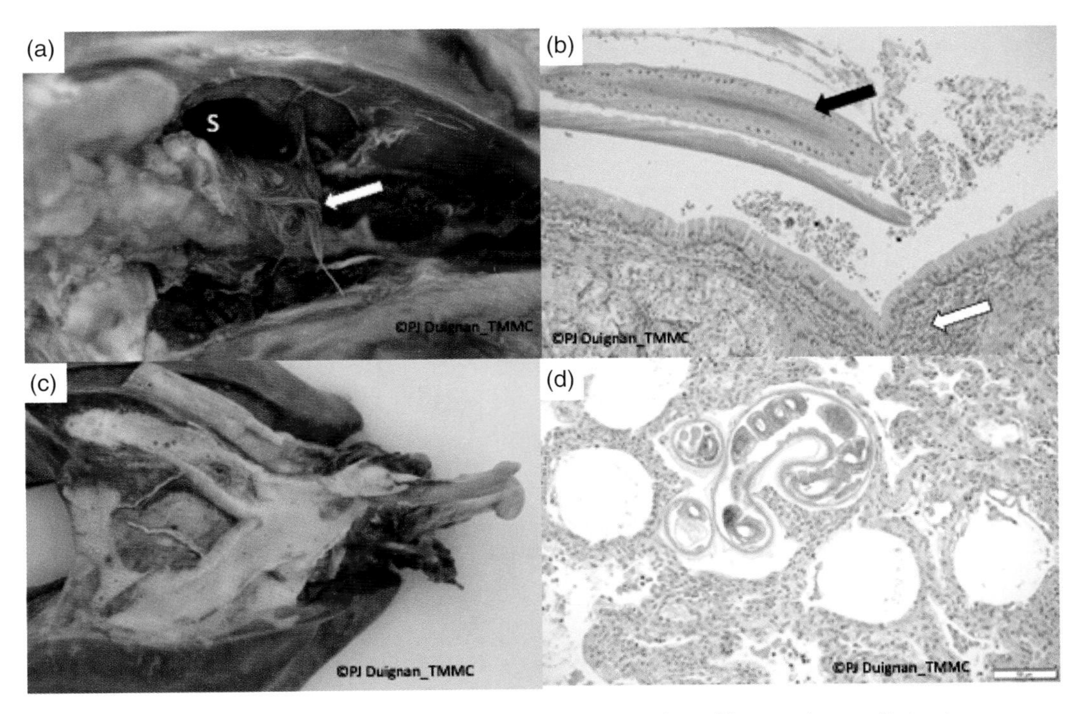

Figure 6.13 (a) Harbor porpoise (*Phocoena phocoena*), pterygoid sinus (S) opened ventrally to show numerous nematodes (*Stenurus* spp., arrow). (b) Narwhal, pterygoid sinus with luminal nematode (black arrow) and minimal submucosal lymphoplasmacytic inflammation (white arrow). (c) Harbor porpoise, lungs with bronchi opened to show a large number of mature nematodes (*Stenurus* spp.) and frothy mucoid exudate. (d) Narwhal, lung with mature nematode (*Holocercus monoceris*) in the parenchyma and minimal inflammatory response.

transmammary transmission was demonstrated for *Halocercus lagenorynchi* in bottlenose dolphins (*Tursiops truncatus*; Dailey et al., 1991), and neonatal infection consistent with vertical transmission has been recorded for many odontocete species, worldwide (Measures, 2018). Infection of the cranial sinuses and middle ear result in mild to moderate chronic mixed leukocytic submucosal inflammation, epithelial hyperplasia, or squamous metaplasia, and rarely, purulent inflammation or hemorrhage (Faulkner et al., 1998; Siebert et al., 2001; Houde at al., 2003; Lehnert et al., 2005; Measures, 2018). There is no empirical evidence that pseudaliids of the cranial sinuses cause auditory neuritis or invade the brain (Morell et al., 2017; Measures, 2018). In contrast, verminous pneumonia is a significant cause of death in stranded odontocetes (Jepson et al., 2000; Siebert et al., 2001; Jauniaux et al., 2002; Fauquier et al., 2009; Lair et al., 2016). The bronchointerstitial verminous pneumonia observed in odontocetes is histologically similar to that in pinnipeds, and it can include catarrhal bronchitis, bronchiolitis, granulomatous alveolitis, occasional edema, and hemorrhage in more acute cases, alveolar, interstitial and bullous emphysema, and chronic fibrotic granulomas. Pulmonary arteritis, endocarditis, and thrombosis was described in harbor porpoises infected with *Pseudalius infexus* (Jepson et al., 2000; Jaunaiux et al., 2002).

Hookworms (*Uncinaria* spp.) are found in many otariids and some phocids, with distinct clades present in the northern and southern hemispheres and at least seven distinct species identified via phylogenetic characterization (Nadler et al., 2013). These nematodes are not host specific and *Uncinaria leucasi*, the first species described, parasitizes both northern fur seals (*Callorhinus ursinus*) and Steller sea lions in the North Pacific. Studies of northern fur seals and New Zealand sea lions (*Phocarctos hookeri*), Australian sea lions (*Neophoca cinerea*), and South American fur seals (*Arctocephalus australis*) revealed that hookworms have a direct life cycle, with both horizontal and vertical transmission (Olsen and Lyons, 1962: Castinel et al., 2007a, Marcus et al., 2014; Seguel et al., 2017a), but the lactogenic route appears to be the most significant route of transmission. Pups are hosts to adult nematodes, which are hematophagous in the small intestine (Figure 6.14a). Eggs are passed in feces and third-stage larvae are released into the substrate, where they penetrate the skin of new hosts of both sexes and all ages. The larvae encyst

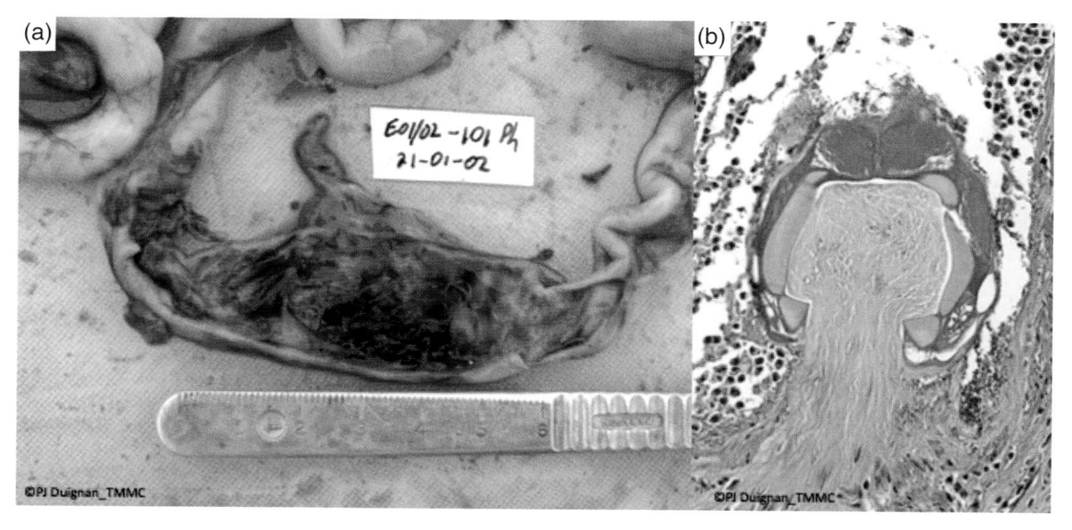

Figure 6.14 New Zealand sea lion (*Phocarctos hookeri*). (a) Jejunum with numerous nematodes (hookworm, *Uncinaria* spp.) and mucosal hemorrhage (black content). (b) Histological section of the jejunum showing the pharynx of *Uncinaria* spp. attached to the mucosa. H&E stain.

indefinitely in host tissue, particularly in the ventral blubber, and only complete the cycle if they have encysted in tissues of a breeding female. When an infected, pregnant fur seal or sea lion returns to the rookery the following season, the larvae are hormonally reactivated via parturition, migrate to the mammary gland, and enter the milk. Nursing pups are infected as soon as they suckle, thus completing the life cycle. Patent infections in infected pups last up to three months, when these hosts generally develop immunity to the parasites. For pups, the outcome of infection depends on the infective dose, individual host genetics, population size and density, the substrate of the rookery, and the local microclimate (Lyons et al., 2005; Castinel et al., 2007a; Acevedo-Whitehouse et al., 2009). Mortality can be as high as 70% in some California sea lion rookeries while, for New Zealand sea lions, northern fur seals, Australian sea lions, and South American fur seals, rates may vary between 15% and 50% of total pup mortality (Castinel et al., 2007b; Lyons et al., 2011; Seguel et al., 2013; Marcus et al., 2014). Observed pathology in pups reflects the hematophagous feeding strategy of adult nematodes, facilitated by secretion of anticoagulant proteins that induces chronic iron deficiency anemia. In California and New Zealand sea lions, variations in a single nuclear polymorphism are directly associated with the severity of hookworm-induced anemia (Acevedo-Whitehouse et al., 2006, 2009). Parasitic feeding sites in the intestinal mucosa (Figure 6.14b) also provide a portal for opportunistic bacterial infection, and the combination of mechanical trauma and host inflammatory response can result in villous blunting, malabsorption, and reduced pup growth (Chilvers et al., 2009; Seguel et al., 2017a). Pups that die from hemorrhagic enteritis are often in excellent body condition; the intestines are usually distended with blood and there is a high hookworm burden. In some cases, hookworms can penetrate into the peritoneal cavity, resulting in fibrinosuppurative peritonitis (Castinel et al., 2007b; Spraker et al., 2007; Seguel et al., 2017a). While *Uncinaria* spp. hookworm infections have been identified in several phocids such as ringed, northern and southern elephant seals, and Mediterranean monk seals no significant pathology has been observed.

Crassicauda spp. and *Placentonema* spp. are fascinating spirurid nematodes that infect cetaceans and likely have crustacean intermediate hosts. Fourteen species of *Crassicauda* have been described including *C. crassicauda, C. giliakiana, C. anthonyi, C. bennetti, C. grampicola, C. boopis, C. magna, C. tortilis, C. delamureana, C. fuelleborni, C. costata* and *C. carbonelli*. Key infection sites may include the kidneys (*C. giliakiana, C. anthonyi, C. bennetti, C. boopis, C. tortilis, C. delamureana, C. costata*), reproductive system (*C. crassicauda, C. carbonelli, C. fuelleborni*), pterygoid sinuses (*C. grampicola*) or subcutaneous tissues and "gillslit" glands of pygmy sperm whales, *Kogia breviceps* (*C. magna*), (Jabbar et al., 2015; Keenan-Bateman et al., 2016, 2018; Marcer et al., 2019). Adult nematodes vary from 1 to 7 m in length; the cephalic end of the worm is usually anchored within a tissue or organ, causing local inflammation, while the caudal end is free in a duct where eggs can be released to the exterior, as demonstrated for *C. magna* infection in pygmy sperm whales (Figure 6.15).

C. grampicola is found in the mammary glands and lactiferous ducts of mature female odontocetes (Figure 6.16). It is likely to have a direct life cycle, by passing their eggs to the calf via milk consumption. The infection may cause mastitis and it compromises neonatal survivorship by reducing milk quantity or quality (Geraci et al., 1978).

C. grampicola is also found in the cranial sinuses, where it may induce mucosal ulceration, inflammation, hemorrhage, cranial neuritis, and osteolysis (Figure 6.17a,b) (Dailey and Stroud, 1978; Pascual et al., 2000, van Bressem et al., 2006, 2020). The lesions are more prevalent and extensive in younger hosts, and heavy infestation may be a significant cause of mortality (Balbuena and Simpkin, 2014; van Bressem et al., 2020). Males of the Mediterranean pilot whales (*Globicephala melas*) are susceptible to *C. carbonelli*, residing in the penile urethra (Raga and

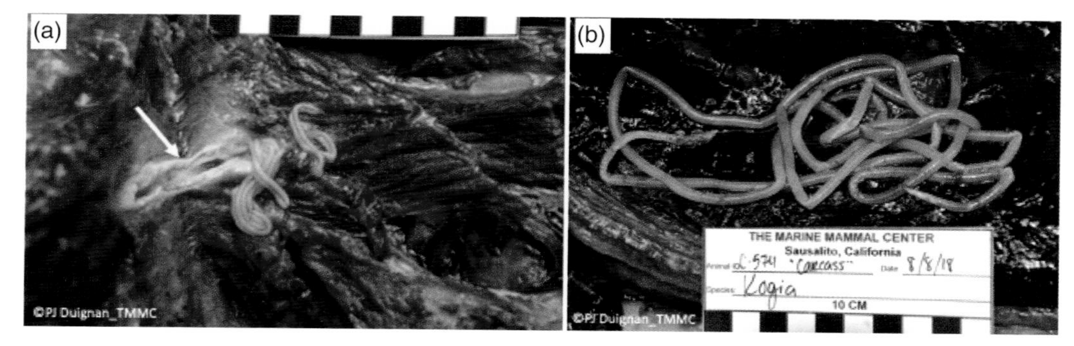

Figure 6.15 Pygmy sperm whale. (a) Skin and blubber removed to expose the duct of the exocrine gill gland on the side of the head (arrow). The large nematode within the gland duct is likely *Crassicauda magna*. (b) Lateral thoracic fascia containing an embedded adult *Crassicauda* spp. (Nematoda).

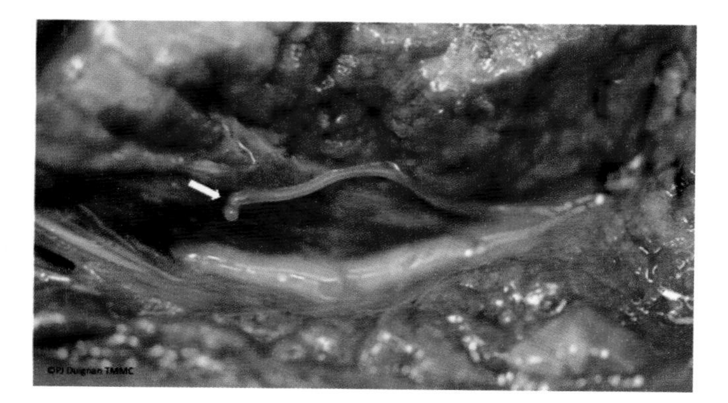

Figure 6.16 Harbor porpoise, adult female mammary gland; a mature female *Crassicauda* spp. (Nematoda) is visible in the main lactiferous duct. Note the subterminal constriction at the caudal end (arrow), around which the caudal end of the male is usually coiled.

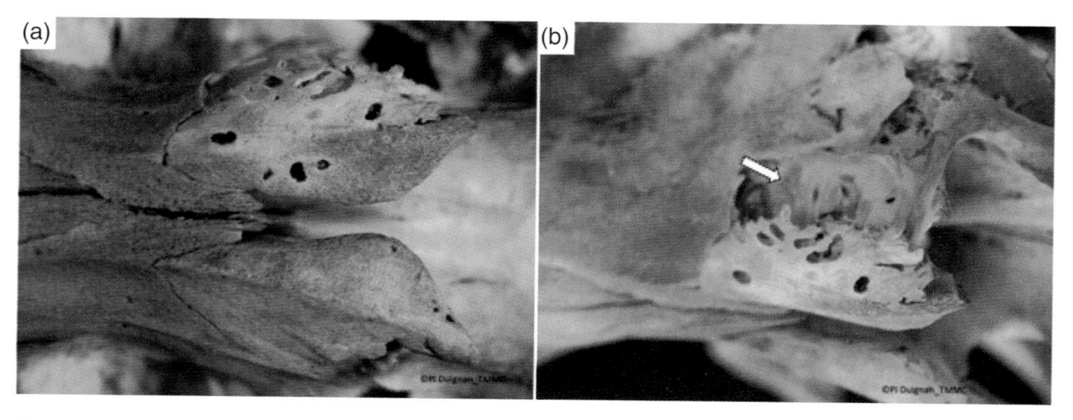

Figure 6.17 Indo-Pacific humpback dolphin, *Sousa chinensis*. (a) Cranium, ventral view of the pterygoid bones (rostral to left and caudal to right). The left bone (top) has numerous irregularly shaped fenestrations, with smooth rounded edges penetrating the bone into the space that would have enclosed the pterygoid sinus in life. (b) Lateral view of the same cranium with the pterygoid sinus space indicated by the arrow. This is an example of *Crassicauda* spp. (Nematoda)-induced cranial osteolysis. *Source:* Specimen PEM N487 courtesy of Dr. G. Hofmeyr, Port Elizabeth Museum, South Africa.

Balbuena, 1990). The cephalic end of the parasite is deeply embedded in the *corpus cavernosum* of the penis, where it causes focal granulomatous inflammation and hemorrhage; the caudal end of *C. carbonelli* is free within a duct that communicates with the urethra. *C. boopis* infects the kidneys of baleen whales and some beaked whales, where it can cause thrombophlebitis, renal infarction and systemic thromboembolism. The cephalic end of this nematode is embedded in a reniculus, where it causes focal necrosis and inflammation, while the caudal end is free to shed eggs into the ureter. While *C. boopis* is common in fin whales (*Balaenoptera physalus*) of the North Atlantic, pathogenicity is equivocal (Lambertsen, 1986; Lempereur et al., 2017). In the North Pacific ocean, *C. boopis* infects the kidneys of humpback whales (*Megaptera novaengliae*; Duignan, unpublished observation). However, in Cuvier's beaked whales (*Ziphius cavirostris*) in New Zealand (Duignan et al., 1999) and the eastern North Atlantic (Diaz-Delgado et al., 2016), this parasite causes extensive renal necrosis and arteriosclerosis, which likely causes stranding in severely affected individuals. In Stejneger's beaked whales (*Mesoplodon stejnegeri*) crassicaudiasis was associated with systemic amyloidosis in two adults that were part of a mass stranding in the Sea of Japan (Tajima et al., 2007, 2015). The largest spirurid, *Placentonema gigantisima* (up to 9 m in length), inhabits the uterus and placenta of sperm whales (*Physeter macrocephalus*), with no apparent pathologic consequences (Lambertsen, 1997).

Acanthocheilonema spirocauda (seal heartworm) is a filaroid nematode found in the right ventricle and pulmonary artery of northern hemisphere phocids (Figure 6.18a). The life cycle is indirect; circulating microfilariae are likely ingested by hematophagous seal lice (*Echinophtherius horridus*), mosquitoes or simuliids and transferred mechanically to a new host following development into third-stage larvae (Geraci et al., 1981; Leidenberger et al., 2007; Lehnert et al., 2016).

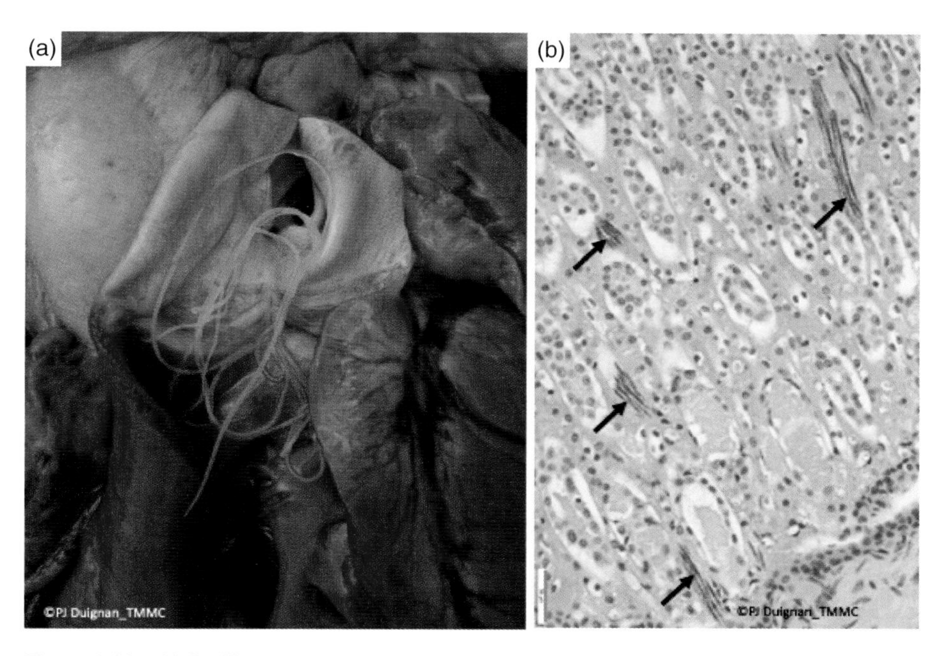

Figure 6.18 (a) Pacific harbor seal, heart, right ventricle and pulmonary trunk opened to show long slender nematodes, seal heartworm *Acanthocheilonema spirocauda* (Nematoda), in the lumen. (b) California sea lion, renal papilla, showing numerous nematode larvae (arrows) in capillaries. *Acanthocheilonema odenhali* (Nematoda).

Adults may be present in low numbers without pathologic consequences, but high burdens can be associated with arteritis and pulmonary embolism (Lehnert et al., 2007a). In otariids, *Acanthocheilonema odenhali* is frequently found in the perimuscular fascia of California sea lions and in the subcutis of northern fur seals, without inciting an inflammatory response (Kuzmina et al., 2018). Larvae (microfilariae) are common in blood smears and histological sections with no apparent inflammation (Figure 6.18b).

Trichinella nativa is an Arctic-adapted nematode that is of greatest significance as a zoonotic infection in humans who consume undercooked skeletal muscle from polar bears, walrus, belugas, or some phocids (Forbes, 2000). Affected people can develop severe myositis, but infection rarely causes clinical signs in aquatic mammals. Rarely, polar bears can exhibit myositis, eosinophilia, and occasional central nervous system involvement (Dailey, 2001).

Diagnosis

The clinical signs observed in animals with clinically significant infections such as verminous pneumonia or hemorrhagic enteritis, in combination with relevant epidemiologic data (age class, season, habitat etc.) and ancillary clinical examination (auscultation, radiography, hematology, serum chemistry), aid diagnosis. Patent nematode infections of the gastrointestinal system or respiratory tract can be confirmed based by the presence of characteristic eggs or larvae in the feces or sputum. Prepatent infections can be more challenging but for some, such as *Parafilaroides decorus* lungworm in otariids, novel molecular tests can facilitate diagnosis (Williams et al., 2020).

Differential Diagnoses

For the animals exhibiting dyspnea, differentials for verminous pneumonia include bacterial or viral (e.g. morbilliviruses, influenza viruses) infections and systemic mycoses (e.g. aspergillosis, blastomycosis, cryptococcoses, coccidioidomycosis). Differentials for gastrointestinal nematode parasitism include other parasites (e.g. cestodes, protozoa, trematodes), various bacterial enteritides, viral infection, and dysbiosis. Hookworm enteritis usually manifests as either sudden death (severe acute infections) or anemia in more chronic cases. For pups that die unexpectedly in rookeries, crush trauma caused by conspecific adults would be the first differential, but septicemia secondary to bite wounds should also be considered. For cases with anemia, consider malnutrition, gastric ulceration, bone marrow or other hematopoietic pathology, protozoal parasites, or specific nutritional deficiencies (e.g. minerals or trace elements).

Treatment and Management

For animals in managed care, the same principles apply as for other helminth parasites. Avoid infection by feeding only high-grade, prefrozen food, to kill intermediate stages of the parasites. For pinnipeds, odontocetes, and manatees, ivermectin (0.2 mg/kg or 200 µg/kg IM, SQ, once, repeat in two weeks if needed) is commonly used to treat nematode infections, and it is also efficacious against arthropods (lice and mites) in pinnipeds, sea otters, and polar bears. Fenbendazole (10 mg/kg PO once or repeated up to five days) has also been used for nematode infections of pinnipeds and small odontocetes. Anthelminthic treatment for nematodes that reside in the lungs or blood vessels carries the risk of inducing an overwhelming inflammatory response or tissue infarction caused by large numbers of dying nematodes. Anti-inflammatory medication and supportive therapy should be included in addition to anthelminthic therapy, or as an alternative.

Arthropods

Etiology, Host Range, and Transmission

Respiratory mites (family Halarachnidae) of the genus *Orthohalarachne* are common in otariids and walruses, while mites of the genus *Halarachne* are found in phocids and northern and southern sea otters. These parasites appear to spread directly between hosts, likely through nursing or contact between sympatric species at haul-out sites. For example, southern sea otters in California are infected by *Halarachne halichoeri*, a classical nasal mite of harbor seals, and infection rates are highest in areas where both species are in close contact (Pesapane et al., 2018). A history of prior captive care is also a significant risk factor for sea otter nasopulmonary mite infestation, suggesting that these parasites can spread between animals in rehabilitation and zoological settings (Shockling Dent et al., 2019).

Crustacean ectoparasites or epibionts are most common on cetaceans and sirenians. They include barnacles (Cirripedia), amphipods (Cyamidae or whale lice), parasitic copepods (*Penella* spp.), and commensal copepods (*Balaenophilus* spp.) (Figure 6.19). Barnacles such as *Xenobalanus globicipitis* are common obligate commensals on mysticete cetaceans, less so on odontocetes and sirenians, and least common on pinnipeds. However, increased burdens can occur on debilitated animals of multiple species (Kane et al., 2008). Cyamids (at least 26 species) are common on cetaceans and are frequently located in anatomic areas with the greatest protection from being dislodged by surface contact or water movement, such as the axilla, blowhole, genital and mammary slits, and around cranial callosities; they are often associated with skin defects or wounds, where they feed on dead or sloughed skin (Schell et al., 2000).

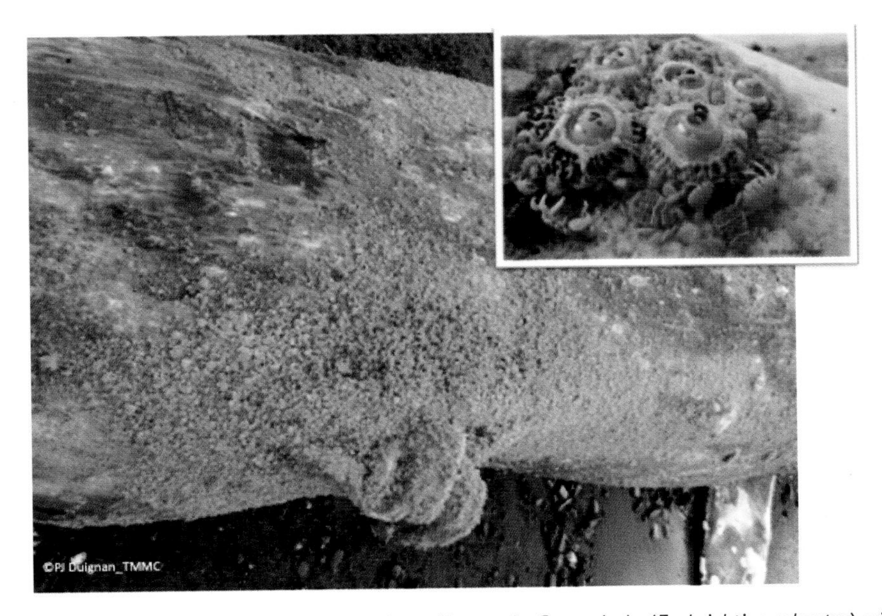

Figure 6.19 Malnourished, stranded yearling male Gray whale (*Eschrichtius robustus*) with a heavy burden of ectoparasites including barnacles and whale lice (Cyamidae) around the genital region and extending dorsally. The inset shows a higher magnification view of a cluster of barnacles on the skin, surrounded by numerous cyamids.

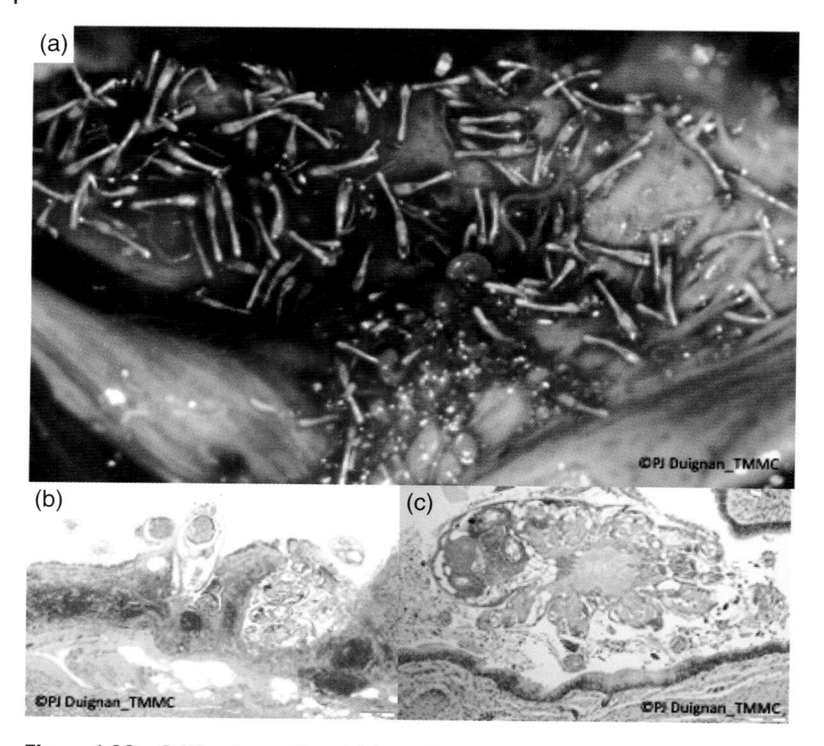

Figure 6.20 California sea lion. (a) Juvenile male with generalized crusting dermatitis and numerous sucking lice, *Echinophthirius horridus*, in the hair coat. (b) *Echinophthirius horridus* from the same case. (c) Skin section, sebaceous ducts in the dermis are dilated and filled with mites, *Demodex zalophi*. H&E stain.

Clinical and Gross Signs

Clinical signs range from sneezing and mucus discharge to dyspnea. Light infestations result in minor irritation, goblet cell hyperplasia, and excess mucus production, but heavy infestation can be associated with erosion, ulceration, and squamous metaplasia of the nasal mucosa (Figure 6.20a,b). Eroded respiratory epithelium can compromise the normal mucociliary escalator of the respiratory tract, facilitating secondary bacterial infection. Mites are detectable deep in the bronchiolar tree via bronchoscopy and histopathology (Figures 6.12 and 6.20c) and can be associated with pathology. Concurrent *Orthohalarachne diminuata* and β-hemolytic streptococcal infection was implicated in an epidemic of bronchopneumonia in South American fur seals, possibly exacerbated by stress caused by increased temperatures over the 2016 breeding season in Chile (Sequel et al., 2018). In California sea lions, *O. diminuata* is frequently observed in the bronchioles, and it likely contributes to the bronchointerstitial pneumonia caused by *Parafilaroides decorus* nematodes and bacteria, such as *Streptococcus phocae* (Figure 6.12). In a case–control study, infected otters were 14 time more likely to have respiratory disease if they had nasal mites (Pesapane et al., 2018; Shockling Dent et al., 2019).

Sucking lice (Anoplura, Echinophthiriidae) are ectoparasites of pinnipeds and river otters that can cause anemia in heavily infested pups (Dailey, 2001; Leonardi and Palma, 2013; Marcus et al., 2015). Transmission is both vertical between mothers and pups and horizontally between pups. Three nymphal life stages occur on the host and all are hematophagous. In addition to causing anemia and dermatitis (Figure 6.21a,b), lice may act as vectors for other pathogens, such as

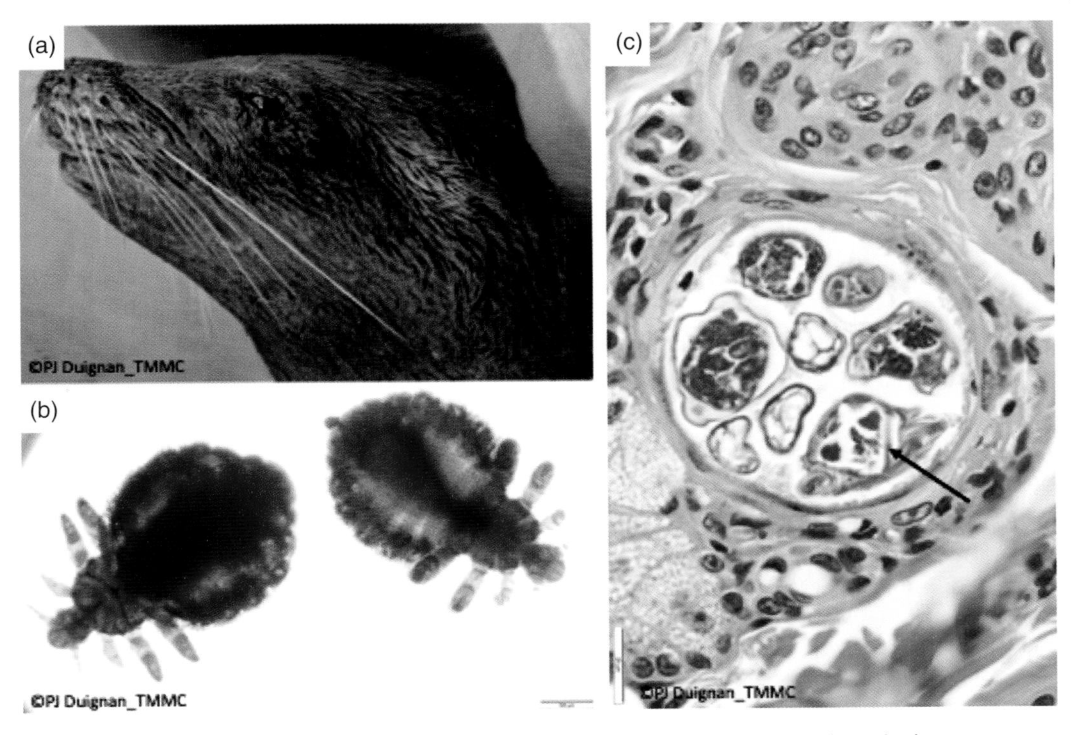

Figure 6.21 California sea lion. (a) Nasopharynx opened to show numerous cigar-shaped mites, *Orthohalarachne attenuata*, attached to the mucosa. (b) Histological section of the nasopharynx with mites embedded within the markedly ulcerated and inflamed respiratory mucosa, H&E stain. (c) Lung showing a bronchiole containing *O. diminuta mite* in the lumen. H&E stain.

nematodes or viruses. *Echinophthirius horridus* is thought to vector the heart worm (*Acanthocheilonema spirocauda*) of harbor seals. *Lepidophthirus macrorhinhi* infests southern elephant seals (*Mirounga leonina*), and it was found to contain an alphavirus against which the hosts had antibodies but no discernible pathology (Linn et al., 2001).

Demodex and *Sarcoptes* spp. mites infect the hair follicles and sebaceous gland ducts (Figure 6.21c) or the cornified layer of the skin, and have been associated with pruritis, hyperkeratosis, and alopecia in pinnipeds (Nutting and Dailey, 1980; Dailey, 2001; Kuzmina et al., 2018). Demodectic mange has also been reported in southern sea otters; in that study, intrafollicular mites were observed in the integument of 55% of examined sea otters, and 20% had clinical demodicosis (Javeed et al., 2021). The presence of multiple densely packed intrafollicular mites generally was associated with pigmentary incontinence, ectatic follicles, lymphoplasmacytic perifolliculitis, and neutrophilic and lymphoplasmacytic dermal inflammation. Other findings included epidermal hyperplasia, orthokeratotic hyperkeratosis of epidermis and follicular epithelium, concurrent pyoderma, and cell necrosis. Perioral integument, especially of the chin, had the highest prevalence of mites and the highest mite density, suggesting facial contact as a means of mite transmission.

Rather than acting as parasites, whale lice (Cyamidae) probably play a more symbiotic role by debriding exfoliated epidermis and cleaning tissue debris from wounds. As with true lice, infestation is likely transmitted vertically from mother to calf, and all life stages remain on the host. The infestation appears to be higher in moribund cetaceans and may indicate chronic debilitation (Lehnert et al., 2007b, 2021). Penellids are elongate copepods, the head of which is usually deeply embedded in the blubber of baleen whales, where they induce a minor local inflammatory response. Rarely, they can attach to pinnipeds, such as the northern elephant seals, and cause more severe dermatitis (Dailey et al., 2002).

Diagnosis

Diagnosis is based on observation of ectoparasitic lice in the pelage of pinnipeds or signs of respiratory tract discharge in these or sea otters. Under anesthesia, live mites can be observed in the external nares or on the nasal planum, and by endoscopy in the trachea or bronchi.

Differential Diagnoses

For pinnipeds with heavy lice infestations, bacterial or mycotic causes of dermatitis should be considered, but close examination of the pelage should reveal the ectoparasites. For severe respiratory tract infections by mites, other forms of respiratory infection should be considered (bacterial, viral, mycotic), and combined infections by multiple pathogen types can occur.

Treatment and Management

For pinnipeds and river otters, lice and mite transmission occurs through direct contact, so management of infection across groups of animals housed together is important. Ivermectin is efficacious to treat lice and mites in pinnipeds (0.2 mg/kg or 200 µg/kg IM, SQ once, repeat in two weeks if needed) and sea otters (0.1–0.5 mg/kg SC or PO, repeated at two weeks if necessary; 0.3 mg/kg intranasally).

Bacterial Diseases

Leptospirosis

Etiology, Host Range, and Transmission

Leptospira interrogans serovar *Pomona* was first recognized as the cause of an epidemic among California sea lions in Northern California and Oregon during the autumn of 1970 (McIlhattan et al., 1971); this same serovar has since been implicated in seasonal outbreaks and periodic epidemics that occur at three to five year intervals. Since the 1980s, leptospirosis has been the most significant cause of stranding among California sea lions admitted to the Marine Mammal Center in Sausalito, California (Gerber et al., 1993; Greig et al., 2005). During an epidemic in Northern California, in 2017–2018, the mortality rate for sea lions admitted to the center approached 60%. Genetic typing has shown that over a 30-year period, all the sea lion isolates belong to a clade that is distinct from those infecting terrestrial animals (Zuerner and Alt, 2009) and isolates from sympatric northern elephant seals belong to yet another distinct clade (Delaney et al., 2014). However, disease is less frequent in elephant seals and no leptospirosis epidemics have been recorded. Pathogenic *Leptospira* spp. colonize the kidneys and are shed in the urine. They can proliferate in aquatic environments, infect new hosts via contact with skin or mucous membranes, and then disseminate hematogenously. Once immunity develops, leptospires disappear from the bloodstream, but they may remain in the kidneys for years. Chronic asymptomatic shedders are believed to maintain endemic infection in the population (Prager et al., 2013).

The ecology of leptospirosis in Northern California is likely influenced by climate and oceanographic variables. From 2013 to 2017, an unprecedented absence of cases was noted, suggesting that *Leptospira* ceased circulating. During the same period, antibody titers and prevalence declined to low levels, and animals born between 2013 and 2016 were seronegative. This apparent decline in cases was followed by a small outbreak in 2017, and a major epidemic in 2018. The age distribution of cases in these more recent outbreaks included a much higher proportion of older animals, when compared with the previous endemic period; this pattern is consistent with pathogen reemergence and spread in a naïve population following an extended period of apparent absence. This extended period of reduced *Leptospira* exposure may have been driven by concurrent, severe oceanographic anomalies, through the combined effects of reduced fecundity and increased pup mortality, and altered age- and sex-specific habitat use, which changed population mixing and transmission dynamics. By 2017, conditions were likely ideal for reemergence: births had replenished the number of susceptible naïve animals, and oceanographic conditions normalized, likely shifting movement patterns back to those conducive to *Leptospira* transmission (Prager et al., 2019).

Clinical and Gross Signs

Clinically affected sea lions are depressed, assume a tucked fetal position (abdominal pain), are polydipsic, hyporexic to anorexic, and may present with melena. Clinical pathology includes azotemia, hyperphosphatemia, hypernatremia, and variable leukocytosis. A consistent necropsy finding is enlarged pale kidneys which, on section, have diffusely pale expanded cortices that contrast markedly with congested or hemorrhagic corticomedullary junctions (Figure 6.22a,b). On histology, the classic lesion is tubulointerstitial nephritis characterized by acute tubular necrosis with formation of luminal casts containing leptospires detectable by silver staining or immunohistochemistry. In animals that survive longer, tubular regeneration is a feature. The inflammatory response is primarily lymphocytic and plasmacytic infiltration into the interstitium of the cortex, but variable numbers of neutrophils and macrophages are also present (Figure 6.22c,d,e;

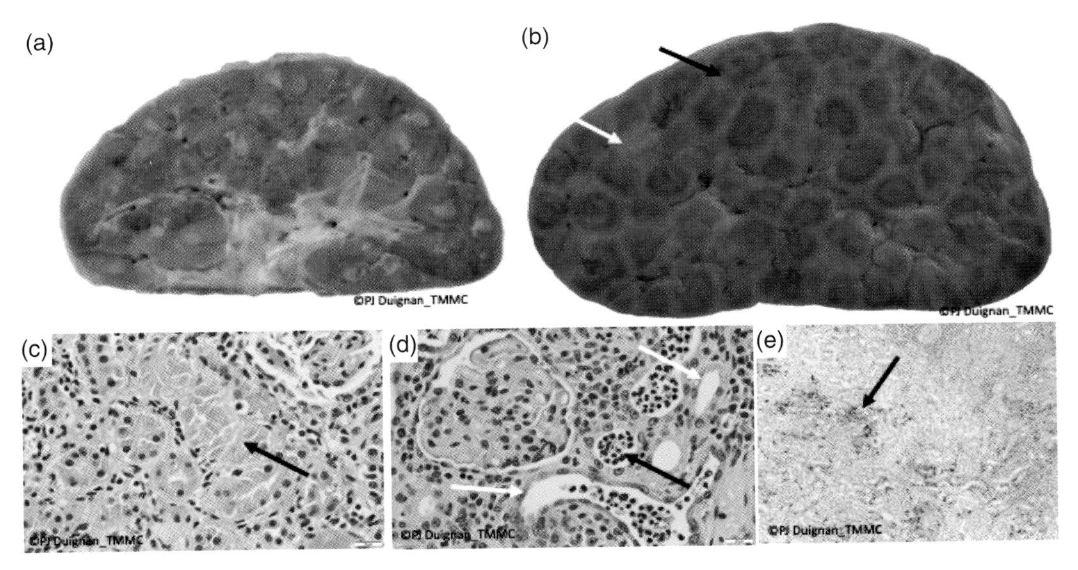

Figure 6.22 California sea lion. (a) Sagittal section of a normal kidney. Note the renicular structure. (b) Sagittal section of a swollen kidney with expanded pale tan cortices (white arrow) and congestion or hemorrhage at the corticomedullary junctions (black arrow). Leptospirosis (*Leptospira interrogans* sv. *Pomona*). (c) Kidney cortex showing acute tubular necrosis, leptospirosis (arrow). H&E stain. (d) Kidney cortex showing tubular casts (black arrow) and tubular epithelial regeneration (white arrow). Note that glomeruli are unaffected, H&E stain. (e) Kidney, immunohistochemical stain: red-stained leptospires are visible in renal tubules and interstitium (arrow).

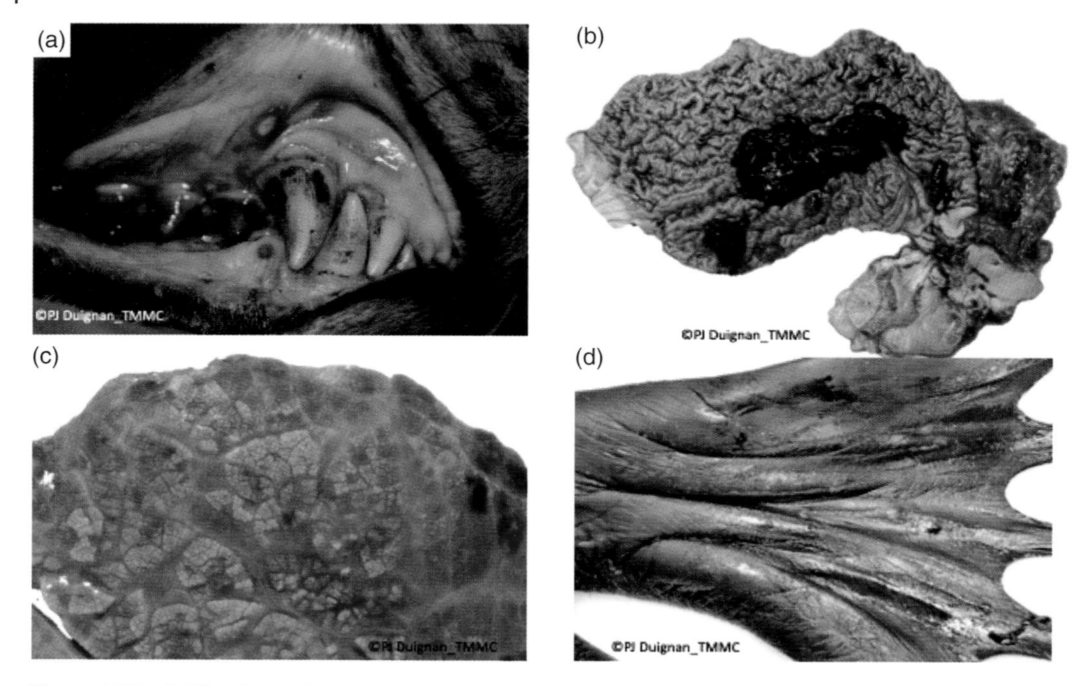

Figure 6.23 California sea lion, leptospiral uremic syndrome. (a) Oral and gingival mucosa with numerous ulcers. (b) Stomach, gastric ulcers with hemorrhage (black content). (c) Lung with marked interstitial and interlobular edema. (d) Pelvic flipper, plantar aspect, epidermal ulceration, and erosion.

Duignan et al., 2019). Pathogenesis of the renal damage is not well understood, but it is likely that it is immune mediated (Acevedo-Whitehouse et al., 2018). As a consequence of the renal pathology, many sea lions develop uremic syndrome with ulceration of the buccal, urogenital, or gastric mucosae (Figure 6.23a,b). The last often results in fatal gastric hemorrhage. Many have severe diffuse pulmonary edema (Figure 6.23c) and secondary bacterial pneumonia, while others develop a necrotizing dermatitis with degloving of the flipper integument (Figure 6.22d; Duignan et al., 2019).

Leptospirosis epidemics have not been recorded among sea otters, but fatal infection has been reported in northern sea otters, in Washington state (Knowles et al., 2020). Affected animals exhibited cyanotic oral mucous membranes, renal swelling, congestion, or pale streaks on the cut surface of renal lobules, hematuria, dehydration, lymphadenopathy, pulmonary congestion, and rarely, adrenal hemorrhage and congestion. Histopathology was similar to that reported for sea lions, with lymphoplasmacytic tubulointerstitial nephritis, intraluminal spirochetes and immunoreactivity to leptospiral antigens in the renal tubules and interstitium.

Diagnosis

Diagnosis can be based on clinical presentation, serum chemistry values (azotemia), and renal ultrasound (hyperechoic cortices). Serology (microscopic agglutination test), urine culture, and PCR are excellent confirmatory tests (Whitmer et al., 2019).

Differential Diagnoses

Sea lions presenting with apparent abdominal pain (tucked fetal position) could have other causes of acute abdominal pain, such as pyelonephritis, pyometra, neoplasia, gastric perforation, intestinal volvulus, gastric torsion, or trauma. Serum chemistry and renal ultrasound can facilitate diagnosis.

Treatment and Management

Treatment should be based on patient body size, tractability, and prognosis (Whitmer et al., 2021); it consists of parenteral fluids, antimicrobials, gastric protectants, and electrolyte supplementation with lactated Ringer's solution, 100 ml/kg/day SQ for up to 10 days. All animals receive a single dose of a third-generation cephalosporin 6.6 mg/kg IM upon admission. Oxytetracycline (20 mg/kg IM once every three days) is administered to anorexic animals. Other animals receive doxycycline (5 mg/kg PO twice daily) in herring. Histamine H2-receptor antagonists or H2-blockers are administered up to seven days, for gastric ulceration (e.g. famotidine 1 mg/kg SQ, IM, or PO once daily for three to seven days). In hypokalemic animals, potassium is supplemented in lactated Ringer's solution to a total potassium content of 24 mEq/l. Hospitalized animals receive freshwater *ad libitum* and are offered frozen-thawed herring two to three times daily, which includes a multivitamin supplement with vitamin C, daily, PO. During large epidemics involving subadult and adult sea lions with variably severe clinical presentations, hospital staff and facilities can be quickly overwhelmed. To facilitate triage, classification and regression tree analysis was conducted based on data from the Marine Mammal Center to optimize treatment success (Whitmer et al., 2021).

Infection in California sea lions is endemic in Northern California. Prevention of intraspecific transmission and zoonotic infection in captive care facilities requires isolation of suspected clinical cases, and good hygiene with regular disinfection.

Brucellosis

Etiology, Host Range, and Transmission

Two species of *Brucella* with a global distribution, *Brucella ceti* and *Brucella pinnipedialis*, have been described based on their host association with cetaceans and pinnipeds, respectively (Foster et al., 1996, 2007; Lynch et al., 2011a; Nymo et al., 2011; Guzman-Verri et al., 2012; Buckle et al., 2017). Although the mode of transmission is unknown, these bacteria are likely shed in body fluids or secretions, similar to brucellosis in terrestrial mammals, with fetal fluids at calving/pupping being a likely source of high numbers of bacteria. Vertical transmission may also occur in utero, as well as through bacterial contamination of milk. In addition to exposure to fetal fluids, another potential mode of horizontal transmission may be sexual contact. Lungworms may act as paratenic hosts in pinnipeds and cetaceans as proposed for *Parafilaroides* spp. of harbor seals (Garner et al., 1997). In Europe and New Zealand, human infections have been contracted through necropsies and from laboratory isolated marine brucellae (McDonald et al., 2006; Tryland, 2018). In Peru, two cases of potential community-acquired human neurobrucellosis were also associated with infection by marine *Brucella* spp. strains (Sohn et al., 2003).

Clinical and Gross Signs

While many cetacean species carry *Brucella ceti* without apparent disease, diverse lesions have been attributed to infection, including endometritis and placentitis leading to fetal distress and abortion (Figure 6.24a), blubber abscesses, meningoencephalitis (Figure 6.24b), hepatic necrosis, lymphoid necrosis, myocarditis, osteoarthritis (Figure 6.23c,d), orchitis, mastitis, and pneumonia (Miller et al., 1999; Ohishi et al., 2003; Tachibana et al., 2006; Daglish et al., 2008; Gonzales-Barrientos et al., 2010; Colegrove et al., 2016; Buckle et al., 2017). Fatal disseminated infections have been described in Atlantic white-sided dolphins, *Lagenorhynchus acutus* (Foster et al., 2002; Dagleish et al., 2007). In terrestrial mammals, brucellosis is a significant cause of reproductive failure; the same is likely for cetaceans. In both captive and free-ranging odontocetes, brucellosis has been identified as the etiology of necrotizing and suppurative placentitis and endometritis

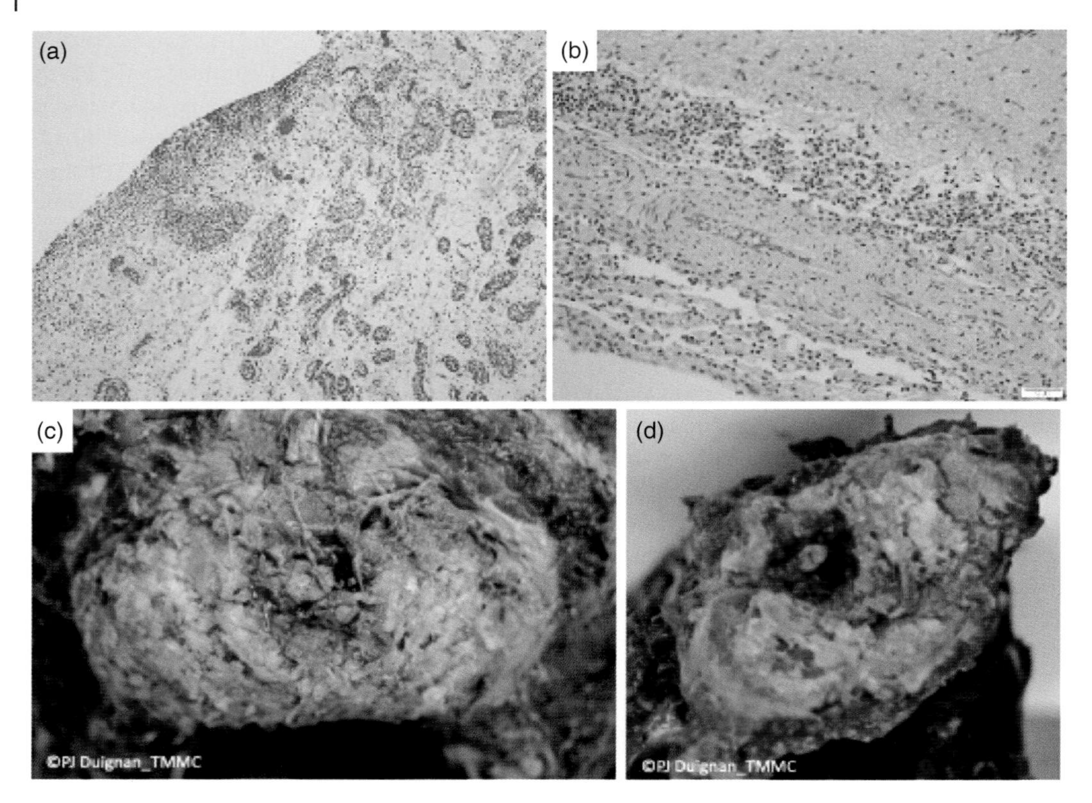

Figure 6.24 (a) Bottlenose dolphin (*Tursiops truncatus*), uterus, lymphoplasmacytic endometritis associated with *Brucella ceti* infection. Photo courtesy of Dr. Jeffrey Curtiss, formerly University of Illinois, USA. (b) Bottlenose dolphin, lymphoplasmacytic meningitis, *Brucella ceti*. *Source:* Photo courtesy of Dr. Jeffrey Curtiss, formerly University of Illinois, USA. (c, d) Striped dolphin, chronic atlanto-occipital arthritis, *B. ceti* infection.

with intralesional bacteria in placental and uterine exudate (Miller et al., 1999; Gonzales-Barrientos et al., 2010; Buckle et al., 2017). Although gross lesions are rare in aborted fetuses or stillborn calves, pulmonary lesions attributable to fetal distress can be observed on histopathology, including alveolar and interstitial pneumonia, and meconium aspiration (Colegrove et al., 2016; Buckle et al., 2017). Even in autolyzed carcasses, *B. abortus* antigen can be detected in lung tissue via immunohistochemistry (Buckle et al., 2017). *Brucella* spp. infection is also associated with granulomatous epididymitis and orchitis in adult male Bryde's whales (*Balaenoptera edeni*) and harbor porpoises.

The most common and severe lesions in odontocetes with brucellosis are often in the central nervous system, with a predilection for the brainstem, cerebellum, medulla oblongata, and spinal cord. An increased volume of cerebrospinal fluid (CSF) may contain mononuclear leukocytes and sloughed ependymal cells. Ependymitis, choroiditis, and leptomeningitis often results in reduced CSF drainage, leading to acquired hydrocephalus. On histology, the myelomeningoencephalitis is mainly lymphoplasmacytic, and is associated with neuronal loss (particularly cerebellar Purkinje cells), satellitosis, spongiosis, miliary gliosis, and perivascular edema. Other potential lesions include arteriolar fibrinoid necrosis with perivascular leukocytic infiltration, hemorrhage or edema. Along with the reproductive tract and CNS, the third most common site of infection in cetaceans is the musculoskeletal system. Discospondylitis has been described in harbor porpoises, and fibrinopurulent osteoarthritis and degenerative arthritis are reported from stranded striped dolphins (*Stenella coeruleoalba*) and short-beaked common dolphins (*Delphinus delphis*) from California, and Atlantic white-sided dolphins from the North Atlantic (Figure 6.24c,d). Guzman-Verri et al. (2012) also described *Brucella* species-associated valvular endocarditis in a striped dolphin.

The significance of *B. pinnipedialis* as a cause of pathology in aquatic mammals is unresolved (Tryland et al., 2018). Although numerous studies confirm seroreactivity against marine brucellae in phocids (Forbes et al., 2000; Nielsen et al., 2001, 2005; Tryland et al., 2005, 2012; Zarnke et al., 2006; Nymo et al., 2011, Jensen et al., 2013; Lambourn et al., 2013), otariids (Mackereth et al., 2005; Roe et al., 2010; Lynch et al., 2011a; Tryland et al., 2012; Duncan et al., 2014a), polar bears (Tryland et al., 2001; O'Hara et al., 2010), and river and sea otters (Foster et al., 1996; Hanni et al., 2003), there is little evidence of pathology associated with infection. Granulomatous osteoarthritis and myelitis associated with an uncharacterized marine *Brucella* sp. was documented in a southern sea otter that also had concurrent *Toxoplasma gondii* encephalitis (Miller et al., 2017). Three *Brucella* spp. PCR-positive northern sea otters were also detected at Bering Island, Russia, but no associated pathology was noted (Burgess et al., 2017).

Diagnosis

Diagnosis of infection in aquatic mammals ideally requires bacterial isolation or molecular identification of bacterial genome. Because of significant zoonotic potential, culture should only be carried out in a laboratory with the appropriate level of biosecurity (minimum biosafety level 2 or 2+). Farrell's medium is recommended for *Brucella* spp. isolation, using an extended incubation period of up to two weeks in a slightly CO_2-enriched environment. Serology (agglutination test) is useful for epidemiological investigations. Gross pathology and histopathology are necessary to characterize the significance of infection. Immunohistochemistry or immunofluorescence using *B. abortus* antiserum has been used to diagnose some suspected cases. PCR and sequencing are also used for confirmation of the infection and to characterize the identity of infective strains. All diagnostic modalities have benefits and challenges (Foster et al., 2002; Godfroid 2002; Poester et al., 2010; Guzman-Verri et al., 2012; Wu et al., 2014; Tryland et al., 2018).

Differential Diagnoses

For abortion or embryonic death in marine mammals, other bacteria, mollicutes, viruses and toxins should also be considered. Meningoencephalitis may also be caused by other bacteria, viruses, or protozoa. Chronic arthritic lesions in Brucella-infected odontocetes have few other differential diagnoses, but mollicutes (e.g. *Mycoplasma* spp.) should be considered. Due to the difficulty of confirming *Brucella* spp. infection, cases of arthritis caused by this bacterium are likely underdiagnosed.

Treatment and Management

Treatment has not been described for cetaceans where infection is more likely to have clinical significance. For dolphins in captive breeding programs, establishing the status of infection in the group via serologic screening is advisable. Isolation of potentially infected animals at calving could reduce the risk of horizontal transmission.

Coxiella burnetti

Etiology, Host Range, and Transmission

Coxiella burnetti, a Gram-negative bacterium, is the causative agent of Q fever, which is also an important zoonosis. Most commonly reported from terrestrial ungulates, coxiellosis was first diagnosed as a cause of placentitis and abortion in a Pacific harbor seal in California (Lapointe et al., 1999). Because this bacterium has many similarities to *Brucella* in its tropism for infecting the reproductive tract, factors that affect transmission for *Brucella* may also apply to *Coxiella*.

Clinical and Gross Signs

In addition to causing placentitis and abortion in a Pacific harbor seal, *C. burnetti* was also detected in the placenta of a Steller sea lion from Washington state with placentitis (Kersh et al., 2010). Serologic surveys in marine mammals of the north-east Pacific revealed a high prevalence of antibodies in harbor seals, Steller sea lions and northern fur seals, suggestive of endemic infection (Kersh et al., 2012; Minor et al., 2013). *C. burnetti* was also identified via PCR in the placenta of harbor porpoises, harbor seals, and Steller sea lions (Kersh et al., 2010). This bacterium was investigated as a potential cause of the declining population of northern fur seal; a high seroprevalence was observed in the population, in association with a high proportion of PCR-positive placentas, but no gross or microscopic evidence of placentitis was found (Duncan et al., 2012, 2014b). As with pinnipeds, serologic surveys of northern sea otters found high levels of seropositivity, but no evidence of pathology (Duncan et al., 2015). Current evidence suggests that *C. burnetti* infection is widespread in marine mammals of the north-east Pacific, but large-scale effect on the population dynamics through fetal death and abortion is not documented.

Diagnosis

In the affected harbor seal and Steller sea lion, placentitis was diagnosed on histopathology and confirmed via bacterial culture. Subsequent surveys employed serology (immunofluorescent antibody test), PCR, histopathology, and immunohistochemistry, using *C. burnetti* antiserum (Kersh et al., 2012; Minor et al., 2013).

Differential Diagnoses

Brucellosis and leptospirosis are other bacterial infections that could cause abortion or reproductive failure. Mollicutes (*Mycoplasma* or *Ureoplasma* spp.) are also possible causes, together with some viral infections (morbilliviruses) and toxins.

Treatment and Management

There are no documented cases where *C. burnetti* was successfully treated in an aquatic mammal. As the bacteria are likely shed in fluids or secretions from the reproductive tract, minimizing exposure to fetal fluids or placentas is advisable to prevent bacterial transmission to other captive animals or humans.

Vibriosis

Etiology, Host Range, and Transmission

Vibrio spp. are Gram-negative motile bacteria that are ubiquitous in marine and brackish environments. While some species are pathogenic, the significance of culture results should be interpreted with caution. This is particularly important where skin lesions are attributed to these organisms (Fujioka et al., 1988; Buck et al., 1991). Marine species include *Vibrio vulnificus, Vibrio parahemolyticus, Vibrio alginolyticus, Photobacterium damsalae* subsp. *damsalae* (formerly *Vibrio damsela), Vibrio anguillarum and Vibrio fluvialis*. The human pathogen *Vibrio cholerae* has been isolated from Indo-Pacific humpback dolphins (*Sousa chinensis*) exposed to sewage-contaminated waters

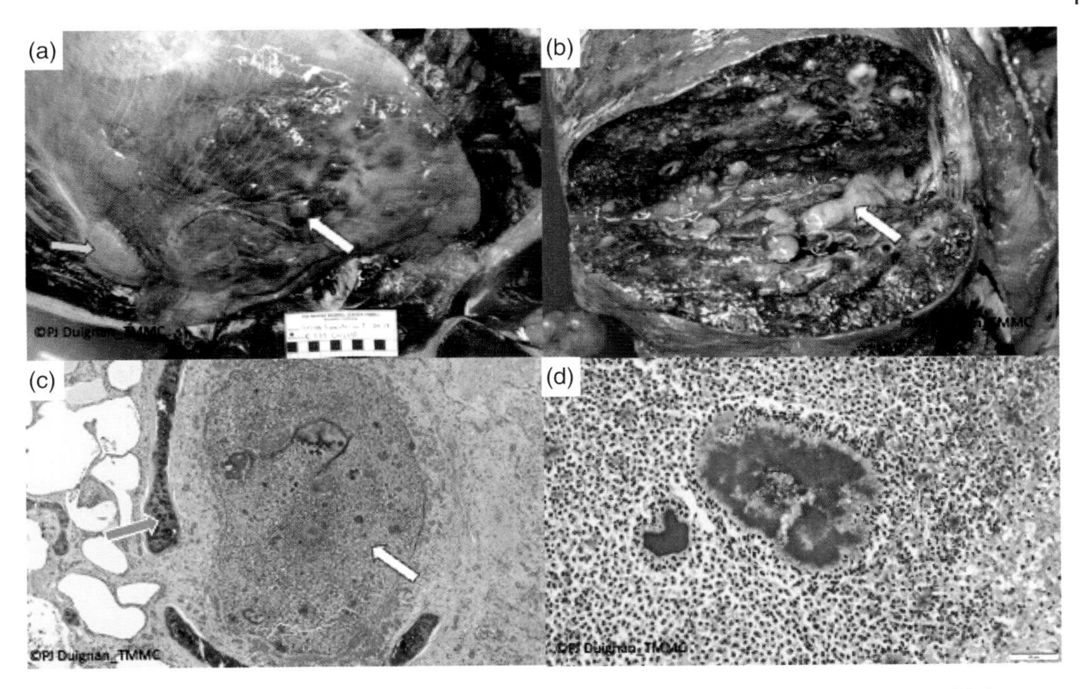

Figure 6.25 Bottlenose dolphin, adult male. (a) Lung with cranial ventral consolidation and multiple nodules (white arrow) due to vibriosis. The yellow arrow indicates the pleural lymph node. (b) Lung incised to show viscous purulent exudate (arrow) from abscesses and bronchioles. (c) Lung histology showing bronchiectasis with the lumen occluded by dense pyogranulomatous exudate containing numerous basophilic granules (white arrow). Bronchiolar cartilage is indicated (blue arrow). (d) Higher power view of the bronchiolar exudate showing that the granules are dense colonies of bacteria (*Vibrio alginolyticus* was isolated in pure culture) surrounded by palisading leukocytes. The exudate is composed of neutrophils and some macrophages.

(Parsons and Jefferson, 2000). There is concern for an increase in fatal vibriosis in coastal marine mammals living close to centers of urbanization and in polar marine habitats as sea temperatures rise (Miller et al., 2010a; Goertz et al., 2013).

Clinical and Gross Signs

V. alginolyticus in mixed infection with other vibrios such as *V. parahemolyticus* can cause fatal suppurative bronchopneumonia, septicemia, and meningoencephalitis in captive and free-living dolphins (Di Renzo et al., 2017, Duignan unpub; Figure 6.25). *V. parahemolyticus* and *V. cholerae* were isolated from a beluga whale that died from septicemia following capture for display purposes (Buck et al., 1989). Similar *Vibrio* spp. have been isolated from stranded pinnipeds and feces of free-ranging animals in California and Hawaii without disease associations (Littnan et al., 2006; Hughes et al; 2013; Greig et al., 2014). Isolates have also been obtained from stranded California sea lions, harbor seals, and elephant seals at the Marine Mammal Center with gastritis, enteritis, septicemia, abscesses, and pneumonia (Thornton et al., 1998). Mixed bacterial infections that included *Vibrio* spp. were obtained at necropsy from dugongs that died from pneumonia (Nilesen et al., 2013). *Vibrio* spp. have also been isolated from feces and tissues of sea otters, but their pathological significance is less well characterized.

Diagnosis

Culture and identification of the organism from affected tissues or exudate is the best way to diagnose infection. Gross and histopathology in fatal cases will assist in identifying whether infection was the primary or a contributory cause of death.

Differentials

Other forms of systemic bacterial infection should be ruled out by culture and potential underlying viral disease (e.g. morbillivirus infection) by histopathology and/or immunohistochemistry or PCR.

Treatment and Management

Bacterial culture and sensitivity should be performed to help optimize antibacterial therapy for managed care animals. Cases in free-ranging marine mammals are generally fatal and are diagnosed postmortem. Given that potentially pathogenic *Vibrio* spp. are ubiquitous in the aquatic environment, prevention is best achieved via good husbandry, regular wellness checks, and hygiene in animal holding and food preparation areas.

Pasteurellosis

Etiology, Host Range, and Transmission

The Pasteurellaceae are a large family of bacteria. Although many are commensal in the respiratory tract of mammals and birds, some are important opportunistic pathogens for captive and free-ranging aquatic mammals.

Clinical and Gross Signs

Pasteurella multocida and *Mannheimia haemolytica* (formerly, *Pasteurella haemolytica*) have been isolated from captive bottlenose dolphins and belugas with septicemia (Sweeny and Ridgway, 1975; Tryland et al., 2018). Foster et al. (1998) isolated *Actinobacillus scotiae* from a harbor porpoise that stranded in Scotland with septicemia. In pinnipeds, *Pasteurella multocida* was isolated in pure culture from adult Pacific harbor seals that stranded with neurological signs and suppurative meningitis and pneumonia at necropsy (Duignan, personal communication); this bacterium is also occasionally isolated in mixed culture from abscesses in stranded California sea lions. The Pasteurellaceae *Otariodibacter oris* and *Bisgaardia* spp. are part of the normal flora of the pinniped oral cavity, but can be pathogenic in infected bite wounds. *Otariodibacter oris* was isolated in pure culture or in combination with *Arcanobacterium pyogenes* and *Streptococcus phocae* from abscesses and a case of osteomyelitis in California sea lions, while *Bisgaardia* genomospecies one was isolated in pure culture from a harbor seal abscess (Hansen et al., 2013). *Bisgaardia hudsonensis* has been isolated from clinically normal phocids, but also from a gray seal with septicemia and malnourished harbor seals with pulmonary hemorrhages (Foster et al., 2011a). Nielsen et al. (2013) isolated *P. multocida* in mixed culture from the lungs of a dugong with pneumonia.

Diagnosis

Pasteurellaceae can be isolated in culture and species confirmed via antigen testing, as well as PCR and sequencing (Hansen et al., 2013). Histopathology is important to determine the significance of bacterial isolates for necropsy cases.

Differential Diagnoses

Differential diagnoses include other bacteria with potential to cause septicemia, pneumonia, or meningoencephalitis. Differentiate with culture and standard microbial typing techniques.

Treatment and Management

In captive management, for Pasteurellaceae infection in marine mammals, culture and antimicrobial sensitivity should be used to select the most appropriate antimicrobial therapy. In stranded animals, cases are often diagnosed postmortem in animals with fatal septicemia.

Enterobacteriaceae

Enterobacteriaceae are a large family of Gram-negative bacteria that encompasses both commensal enteric flora and significant pathogens. It includes the genera *Klebsiella, Salmonella, Shigella, Escherichia, Proteus, Enterobacter, Serratia*, and *Citrobacter*. Many of these bacteria produce vasoactive endotoxins that can damage vascular endothelium and cause rapidly fatal endotoxic shock.

Klebsiellosis

Etiology and Transmission

Hypermucoviscous (HMV) *Klebsiella pneumoniae* was first recognized as a significant marine mammal pathogen when it caused two successive epidemics at the largest breeding colony of New Zealand sea lions in the Auckland Islands during 2002 and 2003 (Castinel et al., 2006, 2007b). *K. pneumoniae*, together with *Salmonella* spp. and hookworm enteritis, was implicated in a mortality spike in California sea lions in breeding colonies on San Miguel Island that began in 2001 (Spraker et al., 2007). These bacteria are environmentally resistant, making horizontal transmission the most likely method of spread in colonies or in captive care facilities (Soto et al., 2020). HMV and non-HMV *K. pneumoniae* has also recently been reported as a cause of mortality in southern sea otters in California (Chang et al., 2021).

Clinical and Gross Signs

Sea lion pups less than two months of age were affected by an acute syndrome that variously included necrotizing dermatitis of the face and head, necrosuppurative cellulitis of the flippers, disseminated abscesses, suppurative pneumonia, pleuritis, peritonitis, polyarthritis, meningitis, and encephalitis (Figure 6.26). Many of the affected pups were in excellent body condition. The HMV *K. pneumoniae* epizootics resulted in three times higher mortality of New Zealand sea lion pups than mean losses during preceding years (Castinel et al., 2007b). Retrospective studies on archival necropsy samples from seasons prior to 2002 failed to recover *K. pneumoniae*, suggesting that this bacterium was introduced to the colony from elsewhere. After the 2003 breeding season, mortality rates for pups returned to normal, but *K. pneumoniae* was cultured from additional cases in 2004 and 2005 (Castinel et al., 2007b). Pup mortality returned to baseline levels in the year 2006 and remained within normal limits for another three seasons (Roe et al., 2015). Preliminary characterization of HMV *K. pneumoniae* isolates obtained from pups in years 2002 through 2005, showed that isolates were clonal and indistinguishable from an isolate from an adult male New Zealand sea lion that died from septicemia on the Otago Peninsula of New Zealand's South Island, in 2004. All pup-origin HMV *K. pneumoniae* isolates were also negative for antimicrobial resistance factors (extended-spectrum beta-lactamases), which would have been expected if the sea lions had been recently infected from a human source, and sea lion isolates were distinct from the *K. pneumoniae* serotypes isolated from human patients in New Zealand hospitals (Castinel et al., 2007b). Further characterization of the isolates confirmed it was the HMV-K2 serotype that first appeared in humans in east Asia in the mid-1980s (Shon et al., 2013; Roe et al., 2015). At the

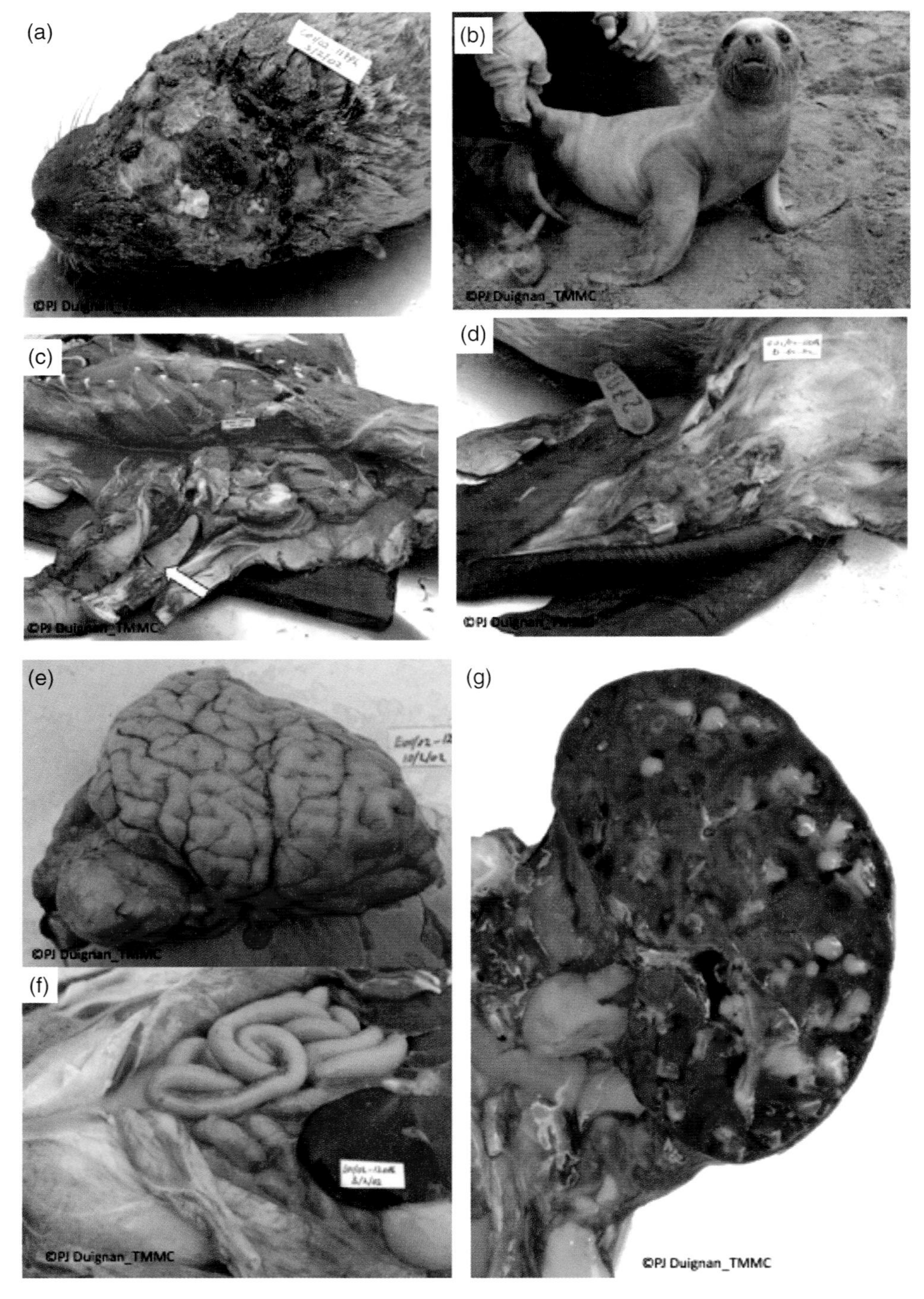

Figure 6.26 New Zealand sea lion Hypermucoviscous (HMV) *Klebsiella pneumoniae* epidemic. (a) Pup with necrotizing cranial and facial dermatitis. (b) Massively swollen and fluctuant right pectoral flipper. (c) Necrosuppurative myositis and osteomyelitis of the pectoral flipper of the pup in (b). The necrotic radial bone with separation at the distal epiphysis is indicated (arrow). (d) Suppurative carpal arthritis and cellulitis of the fore flipper (different case to the pup in (b). (e) Brain extracted to show suppurative meningitis. (f) Abdominal cavity with abundant yellow exudate, suppurative peritonitis. (g) California sea lion, juvenile, suppurative pyelonephritis, HMV *K. pneumoniae* isolated.

present time, two decades since it first appeared as a pathogen in the New Zealand sea lion population, HMV *K. pneumoniae* appears to have become endemic, causing mortalities each breeding season (Roe, personal communication).

For California sea lions breeding on San Miguel Island in Southern California, a marked increase in pup mortality was noted in the year 2001 compared with the previous 15 years of population monitoring. Investigations initiated in the year 2002 identified a hookworm enteritis/bacteremia syndrome associated with *Uncinaria* spp., *K. pneumoniae* and *Salmonella* spp. co-infections (Spraker et al., 2007). The primary lesions were suppurative peritonitis, polyarthritis, pleuritis, hepatitis, pneumonia, and meningitis. It is not known whether the serotypes of *K. pneumoniae* isolated from the San Miguel sea lion pups was the HMV K2 serotype. Later studies of California sea lions that stranded on the central California coast revealed that HMV *K. pneumoniae* was a sporadic cause of mortality in juveniles through adults. Infected animals commonly exhibit pneumonia, pleuritis, pyothorax, pyelonephritis, and liver or lung abscesses (Figure 6.26g; Jang et al., 2010; Seguel et al., 2017b). Results of these latter studies suggest that *K. pneumoniae*-associated pathology differs between New Zealand and California sea lions, affecting only pups for the former and older animals in the latter (Seguel et al., 2017b; Colegrove et al., 2018). However, lesions described for California sea lion pups on San Miguel Island were similar to the suite of lesions described in New Zealand sea lion pups over the same time period (2002–2003; Castinel et al., 2007b; Spraker et al., 2007).

In contrast, sporadic HMV *K. pneumonia* infections in California sea lions from central California typically affect older animals that strand in areas far away from the Southern California breeding colonies (Jang et al., 2010; Seguel et al., 2017b; Whitaker et al., 2018). While HMV *K. pneumoniae* is a rare cause of death for adult New Zealand sea lions, an isolate indistinguishable from the sea lion pup epizootic strain was the cause of death for an adult male New Zealand sea lion found dead on the New Zealand mainland, far away from the Auckland Islands where the epizootics occurred in pups, demonstrating that fatal HMV *K. pneumoniae* infection was not limited to pups, as is the case for California sea lions (Castinel et al., 2007b; Lenting et al., 2019).

HMV *K. pneumonia* is an emerging pathogen in human medicine. Many human strains exhibit antibiotic resistance; the bacteria can spread quickly in non-immunocompromised patients, and can cause life-threatening community-acquired infection in younger healthy hosts (Shon et al., 2013). It is concerning that HMV *K. pneumoniae* infections emerged almost simultaneously in two widely separated sea lion species in the North Pacific and Southern Ocean. While infection in California sea lions is not too surprising, given their proximity to the highly developed California coastline, it is more surprising that it has been introduced to New Zealand's relatively pristine and remote sub-Antarctic islands, where it is having a measurable impact on an endangered species (Wilkinson et al., 2006; Roe at al., 2015).

All HMV *K. pneumoniae* infections in southern sea otters were assessed as either the primary cause of death or as a direct result of the primary cause of death (Chinn et al., 2021). Affected southern sea otters exhibited bronchopneumonia, tracheobronchitis and/or pleuritis, enteritis, *Profilicollis* spp. acanthocephalan peritonitis, septic peritonitis, and septicemia. All SSO HMV *K. pneumoniae* isolates were capsular type K2, the serotype most associated with fatal infections in CSLs. Although the bacterial screening period extended from 1998 through 2007, all four HMV *K. pneumoniae*-infected southern sea otters stranded during 2005.

Diagnosis

Most HMV *K. pneumoniae* cases are diagnosed at necropsy and are often associated with fatal pulmonary abscesses and pyothorax. Although the presentation is generally characteristic, diagnosis should be confirmed by aerobic culture and typing.

Differential Diagnoses

Less common causes of pyothorax in sea lions are *Nocardia* spp., *Streptococcus phocae* and *Pasteurella multiocida* infections, which should be excluded via bacterial culture.

Treatment and Management

In humans, HMV *K. pneumoniae* is often acquired as a nosocomial infection, which can be prevented by good hospital hygiene. For marine mammals, this bacterium can be isolated from biofilms in pens and pools, but it can be controlled by commercial disinfectants (Soto et al., 2020). Marine mammal isolates also demonstrate susceptibility to all antibiotics used in veterinary medicine.

Salmonellosis

Etiology, Host Factors, and Transmission

Salmonella spp. are frequently isolated from the gastrointestinal tract or feces of free-ranging and stranded aquatic mammals (Gilmartin et al., 1979; Foster et al., 1999; Thornton et al., 1998; Fenwick et al., 2004; Davison et al., 2010). The epidemiology of infection is complex with asymptomatic carriers, persistence of the bacterium in sewage and sea water, cycling of infection between marine and terrestrial animals and humans (Polo et al., 1999; Palmgren et al., 2000; Fenwick et al., 2004). Marine mammals may acquire infection from human effluent, but zoonosis has also been documented (Duignan, 2000).

Clinical and Gross Signs

The clinical significance of *Salmonella* infection or isolates obtained from aquatic mammals is not always clear. Stoddard et al. (2005) isolated *Salmonella* spp. from liver in California sea lions, harbor seals and elephant seals suspected to have died from septicemia, but no lesions were described in these cases. *Salmonella enterica* serovar *Newport* is a frequent isolate from marine mammals worldwide, having been identified in necropsy surveys of free-ranging pinnipeds from California's Channel Islands (Gilmartin et al., 1979), South Georgia (Palmgren et al., 2000), and New Zealand's Auckland Islands (Fenwick et al., 2004). On the US Pacific coast, *S. enterica* serovar *Newport* was isolated from a harbor porpoise that died from septicemia, and from a killer whale calf that died from omphalophlebitis (Norman et al., 2005; Colegrove et al., 2010). *Salmonella enterica* serovar *typhimurium* was isolated from a wildlife carer in New Zealand who was hospitalized with enteritis. The same serovar was isolated from a fur seal pup that had died from septicemia and hepatic necrosis, while in rehabilitation under the care of the human patient (Duignan, 2000).

Diagnosis

As for other bacterial infections, isolation and identification of the organism is the most reliable means of detecting *Salmonella* spp. infection. Owing to the complex epidemiology, the significance of infection should always be verified via gross necropsy and histopathology.

Differentials

Other bacterial infections that can cause septicemia, enteritis, or hepatitis should be considered.

Treatment and Management

For captive animals, maintain good hygiene and sanitation in animal holding and food preparation facilities, as well as storage areas. Maintain biosecurity and exclude rodents and wild birds from pens and food preparation areas. Culture and sensitivity can be used to identify appropriate antimicrobials for affected animals.

Melioidosis

Etiology, Host Factors, and Transmission

Burkholderia pseudomallei causes melioidosis in captive cetaceans (mainly odontocetes) and pinnipeds in Asia, where the organism is endemic in humans and animals. It is also found in warm waters of Northern Australia, southern Europe, India, Central and South America, and the Middle East (So et al., 1984; Liong et al., 1985; Kinoshita,2008; Canales et al., 2020).

Clinical and Gross Signs

Two distinct lesion patterns are noted; acute septicemia, which occurs most commonly, and chronic diffuse granulomatous inflammation, which is seen less frequently. Acute infection is nonspecific and manifests as anorexia, lethargy, and dyspnea. Dolphins with fatal septicemia may exhibit disseminated pyogranulomas and abscesses. Histopathology reveals necrohemorrhagic bronchopneumonia, necrotizing hepatitis, splenitis, and lymphadenitis, with intralesional Gram-negative bacilli.

Diagnosis

Bacterial culture and DNA sequencing are recommended to confirm melioidosis. Enzyme-linked immunosorbent assay (ELISA) serology using a lipopolysaccharide-specific monoclonal antibody has also been validated for dolphin serum (Thepthai et al., 2005).

Differential Diagnoses

For acute septicemia, other bacterial infections should be ruled out via culture and/or molecular diagnostics (DNA sequencing).

Treatment and Management

Where melioidosis is endemic, the organism is present in soil. *Burkholderia pseudomallei* has a wide host range, making control a challenge. Death from septicemia can also occur acutely with poor response to therapy. Culture and sensitivity testing will assist with antibacterial selection.

Campylobacteriosis

Etiology, Host Factors, and Transmission

Campylobacteriosis is an important food-borne enteritis in humans. A novel *Campylobacter* spp. was isolated from New Zealand sea lion pups and adults that died in an epidemic during the 1998 breeding season (Duignan, 1999).

Clinical and Gross Signs

The New Zealand sea lion epidemic was characterized by eruption of epidermal nodules and ulcers associated with neutrophilic vasculitis on adults, while pups died from acute septicemia. Approximately 50% of pups died at the main breeding rookery during the epidemic (Duignan, 1999; Stratton et al., 2001). This mortality pattern did not recur at the rookery during the following year, and *Campylobacter* spp. infection was not detected over subsequent intensive mortality surveys (Castinel et al., 2007b).

Another novel species, *Campylobacter insulaengigrae*, was isolated in Scotland from harbor seals and harbor porpoises, but the clinical significance was not reported (Foster et al., 2004). Both *C. insulaengigrae* and *Campylobacter jejuni* were isolated from weanling northern elephant seals in California, but no associated clinical signs or pathology were reported (Stoddard et al., 2007).

Diagnosis
Culture and molecular characterization should be performed from suspect lesions.

Differentials
Other causes of septicemia should be considered.

Treatment and management
Treatment has not been described for aquatic mammals. Culture and sensitivity testing could be used to guide therapy. Good hygiene and biosecurity for captive facilities can facilitate exclusion of potential wildlife carriers and minimize risk of transmission to captive animals.

Erysipelosis

Etiology, Host Factors, and Transmission
Erysipelothrix spp., including *Erysipelothrix rhusiopathiae*, are Gram-positive to Gram-variable, non-acid-fast bacilli, ubiquitous in the marine environment worldwide. *E. rhusiopathiae* is common in fish skin mucus, posing a potential source of infection for aquatic mammals and humans (van Bressem et al., 2008; Opriessnig et al., 2013). These bacteria can be commensals or opportunistic pathogens in marine animals. They are also zoonotic pathogens. In the Arctic, erysipelosis is an emerging epidemic disease in terrestrial wildlife (Mavrot et al., 2020; Tomaselli et al., 2022).

Clinical and Gross Signs
Septicemic erysipelosis is rare in pinnipeds, with one case described during rehabilitation of a stranded juvenile hooded seal, *Cystophora cristata* (Dunn et al., 2001). Prior to the development of vaccination and antibiotic treatment protocols, the bacterium was a significant cause of septicemia and mortality in captive cetaceans, and occasionally in stranded animals (Dunn et al., 2001; Nollens et al., 2016). Two presentations are recognized: acute infection, characterized by non-specific clinical signs such as lethargy, followed by sudden death (Kinsel et al., 1997); at necropsy, there are serosanguinous cavitary effusion, serosal petechiae and ecchymoses, lymphadenomegaly and splenomegaly, and epidermal sloughing; on histology, there is necrotizing lymphadenitis and hepatitis with large numbers of Gram-positive rods and neutrophilic infiltration. The second presentation is dermatological and is mostly described in captive bottlenose dolphins and belugas, which present with gray rhomboidal skin plaques, anorexia, and an inflammatory leukogram (van Bressem et al., 2008). These epidermal lesions are associated with dermal vasculitis and resemble diamond-skin disease of pigs with erysipelosis.

Diagnosis
Acute infection can result in death with few premonitory signs. In contrast, the presence of rhomboidal skin lesions of chronic erysipelosis in dolphins are conducive to erysipelosis diagnosis. The bacterium is often easily cultured from lesions, food fish, and the environment on standard media. Species can be confirmed by PCR. It may be difficult to detect in chronic cases (Fidalgo et al., 2000).

Differentials

For sudden death in captive dolphins, rule out other causes of septicemia.

Treatment and Management

Because *E. rhusiopathiae* is present in the mucous slime on fish skin, removal of the external mucus layer of food fish helped to reduce infection in captive dolphins. The epidermal disease presentation in dolphins can be treated with antibiotics. The septicemic form can also be treated with antibiotics, but the clinical course is often short, and signs are minimal and non-specific, characterized by depression and anorexia. Acutely affected animals usually die, hence diagnosis is established postmortem. Commercial swine recombinant vaccines confer protective immunity to captive dolphins, with minimal risk of adverse reactions (Nollens et al., 2016). Effective immunization required three initial doses, followed by an annual booster (Lacave et al., 2019).

Nocardiosis

Etiology, Host Factors, and Transmission

Nocardia spp. are Gram-positive, facultative intracellular aerobic organisms, ubiquitous in soil, fresh water, and the marine environment. Several species are pathogenic in marine mammals worldwide, including *Nocardia asteroides, Nocardia farcinia, Nocardia brasiliensis, Nocardia cyriacigeorgica, Nocardia levis* and *Nocardia paucivorans* in cetaceans, and *N. asteroides, N. farcinia, N. brasiliensis* and *Nocardia otitisdiscavarium* in pinnipeds (St. Leger et al., 2009; Gehring et al., 2013). The infection has been reported for 10 different odontocete species with no apparent species predilection, and two phocid seal species, a leopard seal (*Hydrurga leptonyx*), and hooded seals (*Cystophora cristata*; St. Leger et al., 2009). Among phocids, juvenile hooded seals appear to be the most susceptible (St. Leger et al., 2009). It is a rare fatal infection in free-ranging Pacific harbor seals in Northern California. The infection is thought to occur via inhalation, inoculation, or ingestion.

Clinical and Gross Signs

Depending on the route of infection, initial lesions may be in the skin (via inoculation) or respiratory tract (via inhalation). Pyogranulomatous pneumonia is the most common presentation in odontocetes with progression to systemic lesions, such as granulomatous meningoencephalitis, osteomyelitis, splenitis, lymphadenitis, and myocarditis (Degollada et al., 1996; St. Leger et al., 2009). In pinnipeds, granulomatous inflammation occurs in the lungs, pleura, lymph nodes, liver, spleen, kidneys, brain, and skin (Figure 6.27a,b,c). Typical branching bacterial chains can be visualized by Gram stains or culture (Figure 6.27d,e).

Diagnosis

Nocardia spp. can be cultured on blood agar under aerobic or microaerophilic conditions, at 37°C, for 2–10 days, producing characteristic growth of Gram-positive chains (Figure 27e); PCR and sequencing can be used to differentiate species (St. Leger et al., 2009). Most cases are diagnosed postmortem. On histology, the organisms stain poorly with H&E and exhibit variable staining with Gram stain. These bacteria are most easily observed using modified acid-fast (e.g. Fite's) or silver stains (e.g. Grocott-Gomori's methenamine silver).

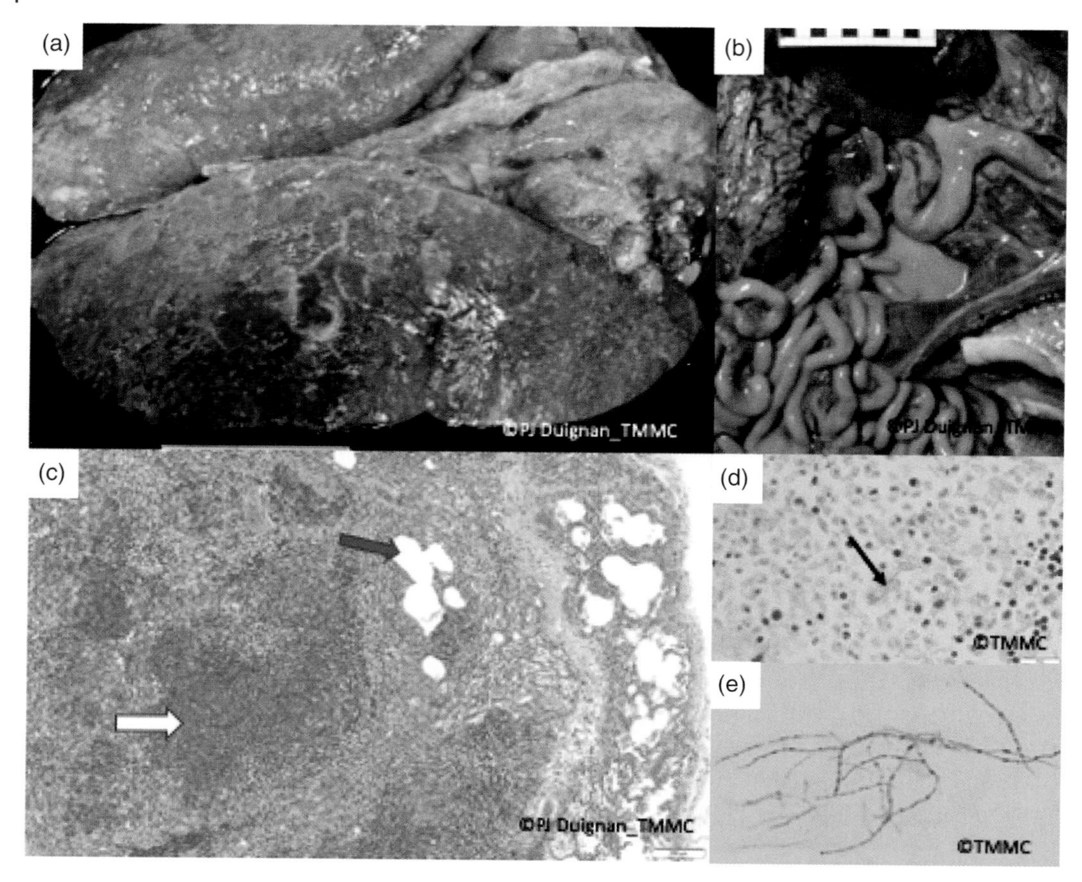

Figure 6.27 Pacific harbor seal. (a) Lungs with diffuse pulmonary consolidation, fibrinous pleuritis and marked mediastinal and interlobular emphysema, *Nocardia* spp. (b) Peritoneal cavity from (a), showing opaque yellow exudate. (c) Lung histopathology from (a), showing severe pyogranulomatous pneumonia effacing the alveolar parenchyma (white arrow) with foci of alveolar emphysema (blue arrow). H&E stain. (d) Pleural impression smear from (a), showing elongated branching bacterial chains typical of *Nocardia* spp. (arrow). Wright–Giemsa stain. (e) *Nocardia* spp. in culture on a blood agar plate under microaerophilic conditions. Source: Photo courtesy of C. Rios, Marine Mammal Center.

Differential Diagnoses

Nocardiosis should be considered a differential for respiratory or neurologic disease in cetaceans or pinnipeds. Numerous bacteria and fungi can cause disseminated pyogranulomas and abscesses. Lesions should be cultured using media selective for both bacteria and fungi for suspect cases.

Treatment and Management

Nocardiosis in humans is a chronic infection that is difficult to treat, often requiring months of antimicrobial therapy. There are few reports of therapy in aquatic mammals. A captive beluga whale calf with an axillary abscess was treated initially with broad-spectrum antibiotics. Following isolation of *N. paucivorans* and sensitivity testing, trimethoprim sulfadiazine was administered. However, the calf developed pancytopenia that persisted for five weeks (Gehring et al., 2013). Trimethoprim sulfadiazine has also been linked with bone marrow suppression and pancytopenia in bottlenose dolphins and killer whales.

Other Pyogenic Bacteria

Clinical and Gross Signs

Abscesses and suppurative inflammation are common findings at necropsy for stranded marine mammals. In terrestrial mammals, *Trueperella (Arcanobacterium) pyogenes* is a common cause of abscesses. In pinnipeds, the related *Arcanobacterium phocae* is commonly isolated from stranded pinnipeds of the North Atlantic, while *Arcanobacterium pluranimalium* has been isolated from harbor porpoises (Lawson et al., 2001). *A. phocae* is also commonly isolated from pyogenic infections and abscesses in California sea lions, northern elephant seals, harbor seals, common dolphins and sea otters, in California (Ready et al., 2021). Isolates are often mixed and may include β-hemolytic streptococci, *Staphylococcus aureus*, *Corynebacterium* spp., *Pseudomonas* spp., *Aeromonas* spp., *Edwardsiella* spp., *Klebsiella* spp., and some of the Enterobacteriaceae covered above. *Streptococcus phocae* is a β-hemolytic commensal of the upper respiratory tract in some animal species and is frequently isolated from cases with pneumonia, septicemia, endocarditis, and abscesses (Thornton et al., 1998; Ready et al., 2021). Its broad host range encompasses fish, pinnipeds, cetaceans, and mustelids, with *S. phocae* being currently recognized as an important opportunistic pathogen of marine species worldwide. In an epidemiological survey, *S. phocae* was isolated from 40.5 % of fresh dead southern sea otters examined 2004 through 2010, and skin trauma of any type was a significant risk factor for infection (Bartlett et al., 2016). Sea otters infected with *S. phocae* were more likely to present with abscesses or bacterial septicemia at necropsy. A survey of marine mammal pathology cases from the NE Pacific and Canadian Arctic concluded that *S. phocae* was an opportunistic pathogen in otherwise debilitated animals (Taurisano et al., 2018). Supporting this hypothesis, *S. phocae* was recognized as an important opportunist in the dolphins infected by immunosuppressive cetacean morbillivirus (CeMV) in the eastern Atlantic (Diaz-Degolado et al., 2017).

In dogs, *Streptococcus canis* is a common cause of pneumonia and septicemia. The pathogenesis of infection in dogs involves super-antigens produced by group A *S. canis*, which bind to major histocompatibility complex-II molecules, eliciting a cytokine storm and resulting in vascular leakage, edema, hemorrhage, hypotension, coagulopathy, shock, and multiple organ failure (Fulde and Valentin-Weigand, 2012). Similar pathophysiological mechanisms are likely for *S. Phocae*-infected aquatic mammals. *Streptococcus iniae* is a commensal of fish which can also cause vegetative endocarditis. Captive or free-living cetaceans may be exposed to this bacterium in their prey. Localized infections have been documented, including pneumonia, pleuritis, pyothorax, dermatitis ("golf ball disease"), myositis, and panniculitis (Bonar and Wagner, 2003; Bonar et al., 2007). In the NW Atlantic, *Streptococcus marimammalium* has been found incidentally in the respiratory tract of gray seals and harbor seals, but little is known of its pathogenic potential (Lawson et al., 2005).

Diagnosis

Diagnosis is by culture and identification of the bacterium from exudate, abscesses, or inflamed tissues.

Differential Diagnoses

Most pyogenic bacteria cause similar gross lesions; consideration of host factors, examination of cytology from impression smears and assessment of epidemiological factors may help to narrow the differential list while results from bacterial culture and histopathology are pending.

Treatment and Management

Broad-spectrum antibiotics are the treatment of choice until culture and sensitivity results are available. The outcome may depend on the site of infection, bacterial load, disease severity and comorbidities, such as malnutrition and trauma (Ready et al., 2021).

Mycobacteriosis

Etiology, Host Factors, and Transmission

Mycobacteria are a diverse group of Gram-positive, acid-fast organisms that can be marine saprophytes, opportunistic pathogens or true (primary) pathogens. Species that occasionally cause granulomatous inflammation in marine mammals include *Mycobacterium cheloniae, Mycobacterium fortuitium, Mycobacterium chitae, Mycobacterium marinum, Mycobacterium abscessus* and *Mycobacterium mageritense* (Tryland et al., 2018). Highly pathogenic mycobacteria are known as the *Mycobacterium tuberculosis* complex, which includes *Mycobacterium tuberculosis* of humans, *Mycobacterium bovis* of cattle and other mammals, and *Mycobacterium pinnipedii*, found mainly in otariids in the southern hemisphere (Bernardelli et al., 1996; Cousins et al., 2003). Zoonotic transmission from infected pinnipeds to animal keepers has been documented (Thompson et al., 1993; Kiers et al., 2008). In New Zealand, *M. pinnipedii* has been isolated from cattle, suggesting sea to land transmission (Cousins et al., 2003). Mycobacteria may be shed by infected animals in sputum, respiratory aerosols, feces, and urine.

Clinical and Gross Signs

Saprophytic mycobacteria can cause pneumonia, granulomatous dermatitis, panniculitis, pleuritis, and lymphadenitis sporadically in cetaceans, manatees, and pinnipeds. *M. pinnipedii* is known to cause disseminated granulomas and death in Australian sea lions, Australian fur seals (*Arctocephalus pusillus doriferus*), New Zealand sea lions and fur seals (*Arctocephalus forsteri*), South American sea lions and fur seals (*Arctocephalus australis*) and sub-Antarctic fur seals (*Arctocephalus tropicalis*; Forshaw and Phelps, 1991; Bastida et al., 1999; Bernadelli et al., 1996; Hunter et al., 1998; Boardman et al., 2014). Pinnipeds with tuberculosis may be asymptomatic or display non-specific signs, such as anorexia, weight loss, and lethargy. One New Zealand sea lion was diagnosed postmortem with severe systemic *M. pinnipedii* infection, after being observed for 30 minutes hauled out, dyspneic, and emaciated at Sandy Bay breeding colony (Duignan, personal observation). Although the lungs are often affected in pinnipeds, coughing is rarely observed. The severity of infection varies from relatively small caseous granulomas in peripheral or hilar lymph nodes to fulminant disseminated granulomatous pneumonia, pleuritis, and generalized peripheral lymphadenitis (Figure 6.28a,b,c). Granulomas are often mineralized. The respiratory tract and thorax are the most commonly affected sites, but granulomas may also be found in the liver, kidneys, spleen, reproductive tract, mammary glands, and abdominal lymph nodes (Roe et al., 2019; Lindsay and Gray, 2021). Microscopic examination reveals granulomas characteristic for *M. tuberculosis* complex, with low to moderate numbers of organisms visible on acid fast stains (Figure 6.28,d,e,f).

Tuberculosis is rarely diagnosed in cetaceans. A Hector's dolphin, (*Cephalorhynchus hectori)* found dead in New Zealand with granulomatous pneumonia, lymphadenitis and lymphangitis was confirmed to have *M. pinnipedii* infection (Roe et al., 2019).

Diagnosis

Clinical signs in pinnipeds are often mild or non-specific. A zoological park in Europe housing South American sea lions conducted an antemortem study to compare three commercial serologic

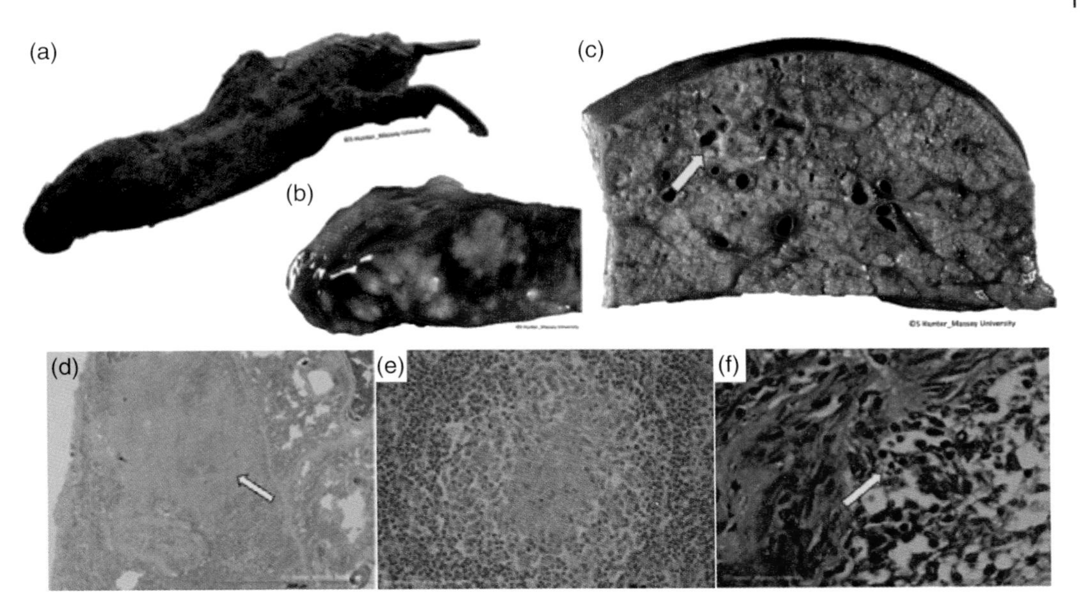

Figure 6.28 New Zealand sea lion, adult male. (a) Generalized severe emaciation, adipose and skeletal muscle atrophy. (b) Lymph node, multifocal granulomatous lymphadenitis with patchy mineralization (white foci); tuberculosis. (c) Lung, cut section shows a pale area of granulomatous inflammation adjacent to a bronchiole (arrow). Tuberculosis, *Mycobacterium pinnipedii* granulomatous pneumonia. (d) Lung, histopathology showing lobular granulomatous inflammation with mineralization (arrow). H&E stain. Tuberculosis. (e) Lymph node; H&E staining showing granuloma with central caseous necrosis surrounded by histiocytes (macrophages) and mutinucleated giant cells, lymphocytes, and plasma cells. Tuberculosis. (f) Lymph node with acid-fast organisms (stained pink, arrow) inside macrophages. Acid fast staining. *Source:* Images courtesy of Stuart Hunter, Massey University, New Zealand.

tests; sputum culture, acid-fast staining and PCR, and radiography and computed tomography (CT). Throughout the study, the animals that died or were euthanized were subjected to detailed necropsy with histopathology, microbiology, and PCR testing (Jurczynski et al., 2012). The results demonstrated good efficacy for rapid serologic tests, but recommended using a combination of serologic tests, sputum sampling (culture, acid-fast staining and PCR) and CT for captive populations. Although bacterial isolation in culture is the gold standard test, results may take up to eight weeks. Genomic typing is also useful in tracing routes of bacterial spread and pathways for transmission of potentially zoonotic infections. Intradermal skin testing using mycobacterial antigens (*M. bovis* and *M. avium*) have limited efficacy in pinnipeds and are not recommended (Forshaw and Phelps, 1991; Jurczynski et al., 2012).

Differential Diagnoses

In many cases, small granulomas are found incidentally in stranded pinnipeds that died for other reasons or in otherwise healthy fisheries bycatch animals (Hunter et al., 1998; Roe et al., 2019). Histopathology, special stains, culture, and PCR can be used to confirm diagnosis, but similar lesions may also be induced by other bacteria, parasites, or foreign bodies.

Treatment and Management

M. pinnipedii is susceptible to a range of antimicrobials, including rifampicin, isoniazid, streptomycin, ethambutol, and pyrazinamide (Cousins et al., 2003; Kiers et al., 2008). However, given the chronic and often cryptic nature of marine mammal infection and the difficulty in confirming a diagnosis or detecting bacterial shedding, the apparent ease of transmission and the high risk of zoonosis, treatment is not advisable. For animals in captivity, efforts should be aimed at prevention by thorough screening of wild-caught or stranded animals intended for zoo collections. Animals transferred between collections should be subjected to similar screening and quarantine protocols. Mycobacteria are also persistent in the environment and resistant to routine cleaning and disinfection protocols. Finally, cleaning of pens and pools with high pressure cleaning equipment can generate dangerous aerosols.

Mollicutes

Etiology, Host Factors, and Transmission

Mollicutes are a diverse group of small bacteria that lack a cell wall and have a reduced genome. In terrestrial animals and humans, they are commensals or facultative inhabitants of the respiratory and urogenital tracts, sometimes causing respiratory disease or reproductive failure. The most important genera are *Mycoplasma* and *Ureaplasma*. The organisms are shed in body fluids and secretions and are likely transmitted between animals in close contact while hauled out on land or via sexual contact. *Mycoplasma* infection can be transmitted to people through seal bites. *Mycoplasma phocicerebrale* is recognized as the likely cause of "seal finger" in humans, a painful condition characterized by severe cellulitis, and occasionally arthritis (Tryland, 2018).

Clinical and Gross Signs

In 1980, more than 400 harbor seals on the New England coast died of acute pneumonia caused by co-infection with an influenza virus and a novel *Mycoplasma* spp., *M. phocae* (synonymous with *M. phocidae*; Geraci et al., 1984). Pathology in seals infected with both pathogens appeared to be more severe than in individuals infected with influenza virus alone. Two other novel *Mycoplasma* species, *M. phocicerebrale* (formerly, *Mycoplasma phocacerebrale*) and *Mycoplasma phocirhinis* were isolated from harbor seals that died during the 1988 phocine distemper virus (PDV) epidemic, in the North and Baltic seas (Giebel et al., 1991). Detection of mycoplasma in lesions and observed cytotoxicity in vitro (Stadtländer et al., 1994) further supported the hypothesis that mollicute co-infection may exacerbate viral respiratory disease.

In contrast to the potential co-infection role of mycoplasma in harbor seals, *Mycoplasma zalophi*, a novel species isolated from California sea lions, acts as a primary pathogen, causing fatal pneumonia, pleuritis, or septicemia accompanied by suppurative polyarthritis (Haulena et al., 2006). In the same facility, *M. zalophi* was isolated in vitro from subdermal and muscle abscesses, septic joints, and lymph nodes. Lynch et al. (2011b) isolated three *Mycoplasma* spp. (*M. phocae*, *M. zalophi*, and *Mycoplasma* spp. EU714238.1) from nasal swabs of apparently healthy free-ranging Australian fur seals. A fourth species, *Mycoplasma phocicerebrale*, was found in the thymus of an aborted pup and in older aged seals. Isolation of *M. phocicerebrale* from fetal thymus, demonstration of mycoplasma in fetal lung by PCR, and detection of inflammatory lesions consistent with mycoplasma infection on histopathology suggest that these bacteria can potentially cause gestational failure in pinnipeds. Mycoplasmas are commonly isolated from bite wounds on harbor and grey seals (Ayling et al., 2011), so it is no surprise that they may be passed to humans through bites or handling of infected seal tissue.

M. phocicerebrale was isolated from the lungs and livers of harbor porpoises in Europe and *Mycoplasma*species 13CL from the kidney of a Sowerby's beaked whale (*Mesoplodon bidens*) but the pathologic significance is not known (Foster et al., 2011b). Five mycoplasma strains have also been isolated from the oropharynx of southern sea otters (Volokhov et al., 2019). Serological testing via growth inhibition and metabolic inhibition tests employing antiserum to type strains of *M. phocicerebrale*, *Mycoplasma arginini*, *Mycoplasma gateae*, and *Mycoplasma canadense* failed to recognize these novel strains. Based on results from serology and PCR, the southern sea otter strains appear to represent a novel species, *Mycoplasma enhydrae* spp. *nov.*, which was not associated with any specific lesion patterns.

Diagnosis

Mycoplasma culture requires selective media, such as Farrell's or Eaton's mycoplasma medium with added arginine, and incubation at 37°C in a capnophilic atmosphere for up to 14 days (Ayling et al., 2011). They can also be cultured on tryptic soy agar with 5% sheep's blood, chocolate, and MacConkey agar (Haulena et al., 2006). Isolated organisms can be identified using selective growth inhibition tests using a panel of antisera against known mollicutes or by 16S rDNA sequencing (Ayling et al., 2011).

Differential Diagnoses

Many different bacteria and some viral infections can cause lesion patterns similar to those described for *Mycoplasma* and *Ureaplasma* spp. Findings from histopathology should be considered in tandem with results from culture, PCR, or other tests to confirm causal associations between mollicute infection and the observed lesions.

Treatment and Management

Doxycycline and tetracycline are the antibiotics of choice for people with mollicute-infected seal bites (Tryland, 2018). Pinnipeds with abscesses or bite wounds respond well clinically to surgical lancing, flushing, and insertion of drains to treat abscesses, and through-and-through sterile saline joint flushes aimed at treating septic arthritis. Clinical improvement is also noted following treatment with doxycycline and erythromycin.

Fungal Diseases (Dermatophytosis and Systemic Mycosis)

Etiology, Host Factors, and Transmission

At least 28 different fungi have been isolated from 18 marine mammal species, with 37% of cases from free-living stranded animals, and the remaining 63%, from animals in managed care (Burek., 2001; Reidarson et al., 2018). Two different lesion patterns are recognized: Mycoses associated with the pelage and integument (dermatophytes) or claws/nails (onycomycosis), which may cause alopecia, these being more often incidental; and systemic mycoses that are often fatal and, potentially, indicative of underlying immunosuppression. Fungi are ubiquitous in the environment. Many fungi species are saprobes and, under certain circumstances, may become opportunistic pathogens. They gain entry to the body by inhalation, inoculation, or ingestion. Some species of fungi, such as *Candida* spp., are normal flora of the skin or oral cavity, becoming pathogenic only under exceptional circumstances. Many opportunistic fungal pathogens, such as *Histoplasma*, *Cryptococcus*, *Blastomyces* and *Coccidioides* spp. are endemic to specific geographic areas, and are acquired by inhaling infective spores.

Dermatophytosis

Clinical and Gross Signs

Microsporum spp., *Trichophyton* spp., *Fusarium* spp., *Sporothrix schenckii, Trichosporon pullulans, Epidermophyton flocculosum* and *Candida albicans* have been isolated from pinnipeds where the gross lesions were typically discoid foci of alopecia, exposing hyperpigmented, and sometimes erythematous corrugated skin. On histology, there is hyperkeratosis and acanthosis, with fungal hyphae in the keratinized layer of the epidermis and follicles and in the medullae of hair shafts. The lesions are frequently observed at mucocutaneous junctions, nail beds, and axillae. In California sea lions and Steller sea lions such lesions have been associated with *Trichophyton* spp. (Colegrove at al., 2018). *T. equinum* was isolated from alopecic farmed mink (*Mustela vision*; Overy et al., 2015). In preweaned New Zealand sea lion pups, *Fusarium* spp. was isolated from periocular, periaural, sternal, axillary, and perineal foci of dermal alopecia (Duignan, personal communication).

In sirenians, dermal mycosis has been described sporadically in Florida, Antillean, and Amazonian manatees (Owen et al., 2018). The lesions are described as multifocal erosions that progress to white, gray, or reddish-brown plaques, characterized histologically by epidermal hyperplasia and hydropic swelling of acanthocytes. Fungi isolated from these lesions include *Epidermophyton floccosum, Bipolaris hawaiiensis, Cephalosporium, Cercospora* and *Mucor* spp. Additional non-characterized fungi have been observed histologically as with irregularly branching aseptate hyphae with non-parallel walls.

Paracoccidioides brasiliensis is the causative agent of Lobos disease or lobomycosis in cetaceans from warm waters, extending from Florida to South America, and possibly Asia (Vilela and Mendoza, 2018). The characteristic gross lesion is focally extensive to widely disseminated smooth nodular epidermal proliferation that progresses to papules and verrucae which frequently ulcerate. On histology, the dermis is expanded and effaced by lymphohistiocytic to pyogranulomatous inflammation, containing numerous small (6–10 μm) round, thick-walled, periodic acid–Schiff (PAS) and Grocott's methenamine silver (GMS) stain positive yeasts. There is often pseudoepitheliomatous hyperplasia of the epidermis, acanthosis, and parakeratosis, but the expansive dermal lesions may also result in epidermal ulceration that facilitates secondary bacterial infection. The yeasts are typically slow growing and may occur as individual budding cells or chains connected by an isthmus. The cell wall may be pigmented by melanin, which may enhance virulence by protecting the yeasts from oxidation. The lesions are typically slowly progressive and can persist for years.

Diagnosis

For cutaneous lesions, biopsy followed by histopathology (including special stains, such as PAS and GMS) and cell culture or culture of swabs or plucked hair are likely to facilitate diagnosis. Molecular techniques are increasingly used for fungal identification and are especially valuable for cryptic species (Embong et al., 2008; Banos et al., 2018). Long ribosomal amplicons may be used to characterize complex fungal communities from healthy tissues or animals with clinical disease (D'Andreano et al., 2020).

Differential Diagnoses

Bacterial dermatitis and non-infectious causes of alopecia (e.g. endocrinopathies or disorders of molting) should also be considered.

Treatment and Management

Dermatophyte infections are usually treated with topical antifungals, such as enilconazole or ketoconazole, where daily treatment over extended periods is possible. However, for marine mammals, parenteral administration may be more practical. For pinnipeds, terbinafine (2 mg/kg once a day) or lufenuron (60 mg/kg one dose repeated in 15 days) has been used. In odontocetes, voriconazole (1.7 mg/kg orally twice a day for 10 days followed by 1.7 mg/kg once weekly for 5 months) resolved dermal *Fusarium* spp. infection in belugas (Reidarson et al., 2018). Depending on the site of infection, candidiasis is usually treated with topical parenteral antifungals, including itraconazole, fluconazole, voriconazole, nystatin, amphotericin B, and terbinafine. Treatment of Lobos disease using various azole medications has not been successful.

Systemic Mycosis

Clinical and Gross Signs

Zygomycosis is an infection caused by a diverse group of fungi belonging to the orders Mucorales (mucormycosis) and Entomophthorales (entomophthoramycosis). Mucormycosis can be caused by a number of environmental molds including *Mucor*, *Rhizopus*, *Absidia*, *Rhizomucor*, *Aphophysomyces*, and *Saksenaea* spp. The infection may be acquired via inhalation, ingestion, or percutaneous invasion by fungal spores. These fungi have a tropism for blood vessels and are angioinvasive, providing a mechanism for systemic invasion that results in vasculitis, thromboembolism, infarction, ischemia, hemorrhage, and necrosis, especially in the brain, lungs, or kidneys. On histology, suppurative or pyogranulomatous inflammation is often associated with broad ribbon-like thin walled, pauciseptate hyaline hyphae that branch nondichotomously.

Entomopthoramycosis, caused by the genera *Basidiobolous* and *Conidiobolous* spp., occurs sporadically in cetaceans in tropical waters. It usually presents as infection of the skin and subcutis. The fungi occasionally invade blood vessels and spread systemically, similar to mucormycosis. On histology, the hyphae are similar to the mucorales, with broad-branching hyphae and a few septae; infection induces a granulomatous or inflammatory response, with multinucleated giant cells, neutrophils or eosinophils, and Splenore-Höeppli bodies.

Aspergillus spp. are ubiquitous opportunistic fungal pathogens that can cause fatal respiratory or central nervous system infections in cetaceans. Mycotic pneumonia and encephalitis caused by *Aspergillus fumigatus* is often the proximate cause of death in dolphins infected with the immunosuppressive morbillivirus CeMV (Stephens et al., 2014). As with mucormycosis, *Aspergillus* spp. are angioinvasive and disseminate widely. Gross lesions include hemorrhagic grey nodules or cavitation in the lung, kidney or brain. Histopathology reveals masses of septate branching hyphae (Figure 6.29). Infection of the tracheal mucosa can cause segmental granulomatous inflammation and fibrosis with luminal constriction (Delaney et al., 2013). Mycotic otitis associated with *Aspergillus terreus* infection was diagnosed in a stranded harbor porpoise from the eastern North Atlantic. On histology, fungal hyphae are present in the tympanic cavity with pyogranulomatous inflammation and osteolysis of the periotic bone and stapes (Siebert, personal communication).

Coccidioidomycosis is a systemic infection by the dimorphic fungus *Coccidioides* spp., most likely *Coccidioidomycosis immitis*, an endemic soil saprophyte in central and southern California, and a significant and potentially increasing cause of human and animal morbidity and mortality in endemic areas. A second species, *Coccidioidomycosis posadasii*, is endemic to southern California; although *C. posadasii* can also cause coccidioidomycosis in humans and animals, infection has not yet been detected by PCR in marine mammals with disseminated disease. These two closely related fungi are virtually indistinguishable in vitro and on histopathology.

Marine mammals living in or passing through endemic areas are exposed to airborne arthroconidia; fatal infection has been reported most frequently in California sea lions, southern sea otters and, sporadically, in harbor seals, elephant seals, bottlenose dolphins, and harbor porpoises

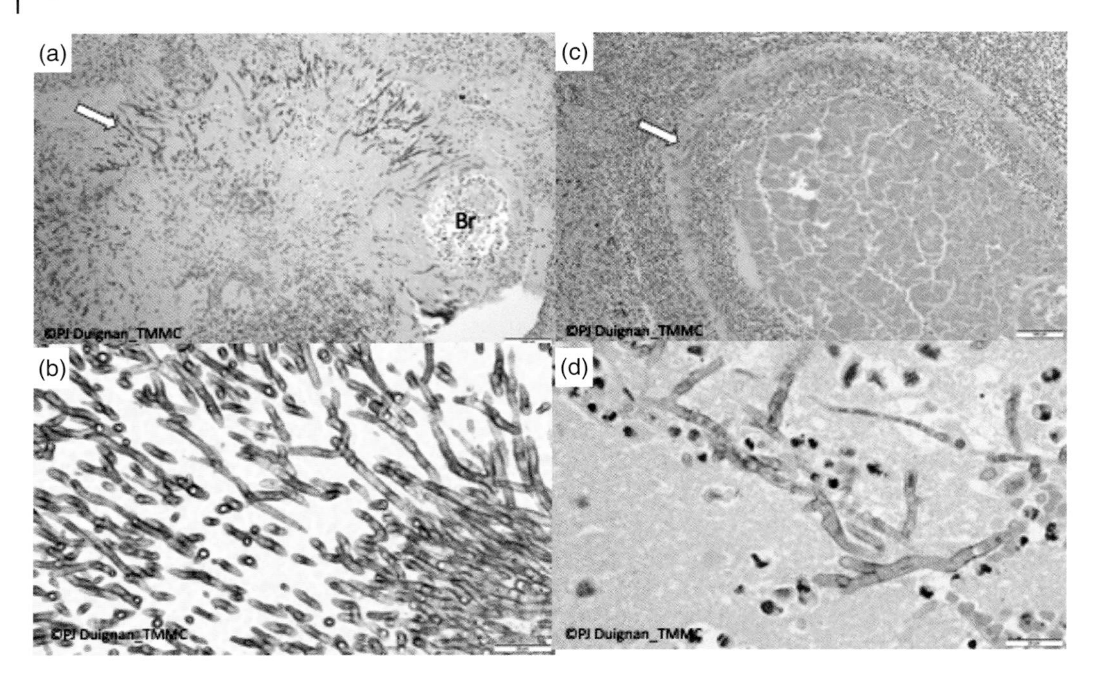

Figure 6.29 Indo-Pacific bottlenose dolphin (Tursiops aduncus). (a) lung, extensive necrosis and granulomatous inflammation with numerous intralesional radiating fungal hyphae (arrow); mycotic invasion of an adjacent bronchiole (Br) is visible at right. (b) Lung from (a), *Aspergillus fumigatus* branching septate hyphae in the parenchyma, Grocott stain. (c) Brain, cerebrum, the wall of an artery (arrow) is heavily infiltrated by interwoven fungal hyphae that are extending into the surrounding neuropil. The latter has been effaced by malacia and extensive inflammatory infiltration. H&E stain. (d) Cerebrum as in (c), showing branching septate hyphae invading the neuropil. There is neuronal necrosis, neutrophil infiltration, and focal hemorrhage. H&E stain. *Source:* Slides from these cases were provided by Dr. N. Stephens, Murdoch University, Western Australia.

(Fauquier et al., 1996; Reidarson et al., 1998; Huckabone et al., 2015). Animals stranding with subacute or chronic pulmonary or disseminated infections are generally emaciated and dyspneic, with severe peripheral lymphadenopathy. At necropsy, pyogranulomatous pleuritis (Figure 6.30a) and pneumonia are often associated with suppurative pleural exudate. Many have pericardial involvement and the resulting suppurative pericardial effusion can cause fatal cor pulmonale (Figure 6.30b). Thoracic and mediastinal lymph nodes may be massively enlarged and firm (Figure 6.30c). Granulomatous inflammation is also frequently found in the meninges, brain, bone, and abdominal viscera. Large thick-walled spherules, often containing numerous endospores are visible on Wright–Giemsa stained wet mounts (Figure 6.30d).

On histology, pyogranulomatous inflammation and necrosis are associated with numerous spherules with a double-contoured refractile wall, enclosing numerous basophilic endospores (Figure 6.30e,f,g,h). Immature spherules range from 10 to 30μm diameter, while mature spherules can be 200 μm in diameter. The fungus produces mycelium in soil, but this stage is rare in living tissue. However, sporulation, mycelial growth, and production of infectious arthroconidia can occur in carcasses at ambient temperature and following exposure to oxygen, posing significant risk of infection to prosectors, laboratory staff, or waste handlers. Following necropsy, waste tissue should be sealed in biohazard bags and held chilled or frozen for incineration; freezing does not kill the fungus (Huckabone et al., 2015). Because the gross lesions are reminiscent of carcinoma,

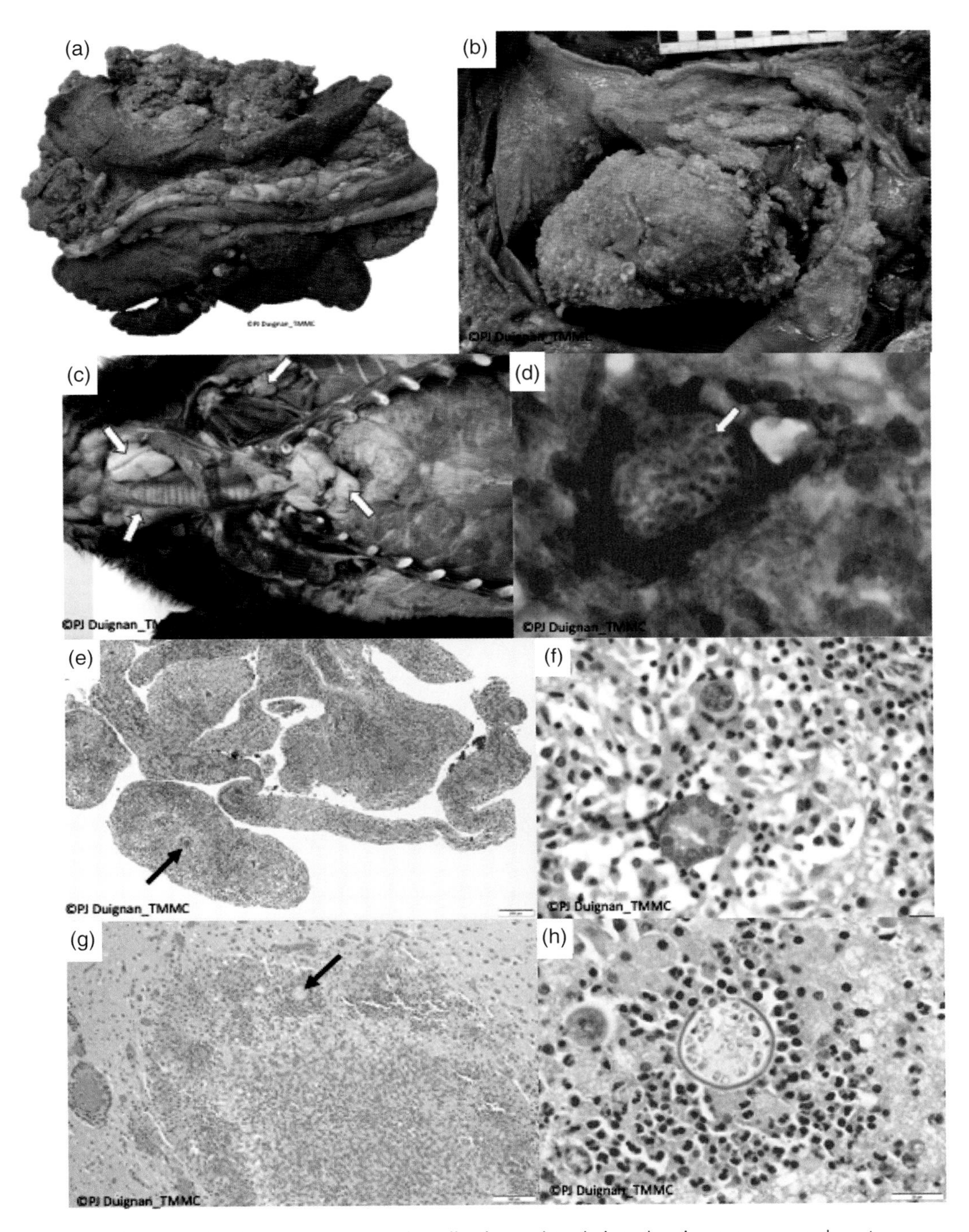

Figure 6.30 (a) California sea lion, lung and mediastinum, dorsal view showing severe granulomatous pleuritis and mediastinitis. Coccidioidomycosis. (b) California sea lion as in (a); the pericardium is markedly thickened and diffusely covered by variably friable to firm tan nodules that also cover the epicardial surface and the visceral and parietal pleura. There is marked hypertrophy of the mediastinal lymph nodes. (c) Southern sea otter, thorax opened to show massively enlarged peripheral and mediastinal lymph nodes (arrows). (d) Southern sea otter, impression smear from a sternal lymph node showing thick-walled *Coccidioides* spp. spherule containing numerous endospores (arrow). Wright–Giemsa stain. (e) California sea lion as in (a) and (b), histopathology of pericardium showing severe granulomatous inflammation with intralesional yeast-like bodies (arrow). H&E stain. (f) California sea lion, pericardium at higher power showing two stages of *Coccidioides immitis* spherule formation, with an immature form above, and a spherule dividing into endospores below. H&E stain. (g) Southern sea otter as in (c), brain with focally extensive malacia and intralesional spherules (arrow). H&E stain. (h) Southern sea otter, *Coccidioides* spp. spherule in the brain surrounded by an intense inflammatory response, H&E stain.

impression smears are useful for diagnosis during necropsy, so that tissues can be handled appropriately. Fungal cultures also pose significant risk to laboratory staff through the production and aerosolization of arthroconidia in vitro; culture of *Coccidioides* spp. should only be attempted by experienced microbiological staff under controlled conditions. Certain ethnic groups, pregnant women, and immune-suppressed people are far more likely to develop severe disseminated infections following *Coccidioides* spp. infection; animal care and necropsy staff should keep this in mind and take precautions when handling suspect cases (Huckabone et al., 2015).

Cryptococcus spp. are yeasts that opportunistically cause pneumonia and lymphadenitis in animals and people. The taxonomy is complex and under review, but three species with pathogenic potential are currently being recognized: *Cryptococcus neoformans, Cryptococcus gatti* and *Cryptococcus albidus*. *C. neoformans* has a worldwide distribution and appears mainly to affect immunocompromised humans, while *C. albidus* is an infrequent cause of dermatitis or systemic disease in humans and terrestrial mammals. *C. albidus* infection is rare in marine mammals, with just one report of granulomatous lymphadenitis in a yearling sea lion that stranded in San Francisco Bay (McLeland et al., 2012). *C. gatti* has a more tropical to subtropical distribution and is more common where there are eucalyptus trees. Recently, it emerged as a pathogen of marine mammals in the northeastern Pacific, when a multispecies outbreak began in 1998, affecting people, companion animals, birds, terrestrial wildlife, harbor and Dall's porpoises, and Pacific white sided dolphins (Stephen et al., 2002). Free-living cetaceans are usually found dead and emaciated, while pinnipeds or cetaceans in managed care may present with respiratory signs and usually die despite treatment (Miller et al., 2002; Rotstein et al., 2010; Rosenberg et al., 2016). Lesions include lymphadenomegaly and granulomatous pneumonia, lymphadenitis, and meningitis. Pulmonary nodules vary from miliary to large confluent, sometimes gelatinous-appearing masses, which are pale yellow, tan, gray, or red, and often have a friable necrotic core. They protrude from the pleural surface and extend deep into the parenchyma. The lesions are often complicated by concurrent bacterial or verminous infection.

Microscopically, acute cases exhibit distension of bronchiolar and alveolar spaces by dense aggregates of encapsulated yeasts, with sparse infiltration by histiocytes and lymphocytes. More chronic cases are characterized by granulomatous inflammation with Langhan's type giant cells, intra- and extracellular yeasts, and perilesional fibrosis. Similar granulomas are common in lymph nodes, brain, kidney, mammary glands, prostate, and adrenal medulla. Vertical transmission has been documented with fetal infection (Norman et al., 2011). Fungal cell walls are best visualized using GMS or Fontana–Masson stain, while the capsules stain red with mucicarmine stain or blue with Alcian blue. Culture and sequencing are used to confirm pathogen identity.

Diagnosis

As for dermatophytes, culture and molecular identification of genus or species are used to diagnose systemic mycoses. For live animals with respiratory disease, bronchoscopy with biopsy or bronchoalveolar lavage followed by cytology and culture can be helpful. Histopathology on biopsy or necropsy tissues with special staining confirm the significance of culture and molecular data (Guarner and Brandt, 2011). As with *Coccidioides* spp., carcass freezing or incineration are advisable to prevent fungal dissemination and minimize human health risks; freezing does not kill *C. gattii* (Huckabone et al., 2015).

Differential Diagnoses

Systemic mycoses often cause focal granulomas that may resemble the response to some bacterial infections, parasites, or metastatic carcinoma. Histopathology and culture can help to differentiate these conditions.

Treatment and Management

Systemic mycoses are often fatal and treatment is variably successful with parenteral antifungals, such as itraconazole, voriconazole, amphotericin B, posaconazole, and fluconazole (Reidarson et al., 2018). Sensitivity testing can guide the best choice of antifungal therapy. For some diseases in free ranging marine mammals, such as coccidioidomycosis or cryptococcosis, affected animals are either found dead or are severely ill at rescue. Diagnosis is made postmortem. Most fungi are poorly transmissible between animals and rarely cause disease outbreaks, but the fungi can become locally endemic if carcasses are improperly handled. Dermatophytes are most likely to spread between haired or fur-bearing pinnipeds. *Paracoccidioides brasiliensis,* the agent of Lobos disease, may also be zoonotic. Systemic mycoses such as aspergillosis are most common in immunocompromised animals, as in the case of those immunosuppressed by prolonged corticosteroid therapy or infected by some immunosuppressive viruses like the CeMV. Patients previously affected by systemic fungal infection that were successfully treated may continue to harbor dormant fungi that can recrudesce, causing clinical disease, if their immune status declines through stress or intercurrent disease.

Viral Diseases

RNA Viruses

Morbillivirus infection

Etiology, Host Factors, and Transmission Over the past three decades, morbilliviruses (family Paramyxoviridae) have emerged as the most pathogenic viruses in marine mammals, with population-level impacts in some odontocetes and phocids (Duignan et al., 2014, 2018a; Van Bressem et al., 2014; Bossart and Duignan, 2019). Sporadic mortality has also been documented in baleen whales and aquatic mustelids. Members of the genus that are known pathogens of aquatic mammals include canine distemper virus, phocine distemper virus (PDV), of which there appears to be one strain, and CeMV (of which there appears to be several strains or clades). Canine distemper virus has caused significant mortality outbreaks in free-living Baikal seals (*Pusa sibirica*) and Caspian seals (*Pusa caspica*). Sporadic mortalities have been diagnosed in northern sea otters, and there is one report from a captive California sea lion (Barrett et al., 2004; White at al., 2018). Harbor seals are particularly susceptible to PDV, based on historic epizootics and immune function studies. Seroconversion can occur in walruses and free-ranging Otariidae, but they are not highly susceptible to clinical disease following PDV infection. CeMV appears to be endemic in pilot whales (*Globicephala* spp.) at least in the North Atlantic, Mediterranean Sea and South Pacific, with a high level of herd immunity in these species and only sporadic mortality. However, CeMV has caused epidemics in other odontocetes, including harbor porpoises, striped dolphins (*Stenella coeruleoalba*), and common dolphins in Europe, bottlenose dolphins along the US Atlantic coast, Guaiana dolphins (*Sotalia guianensis*) in Brazil, and Indo-Pacific bottlenose dolphins and common dolphins in Australia. Sporadic mortality has been documented in various other cetaceans in the North Pacific, North Atlantic, and Mediterranean Sea. While morbilliviruses may be shed in ocular, nasal, oral, anogenital, and mammary gland fluids or secretions, most transmission is likely via aerosol spread to the upper respiratory tract.

Clinical and Gross Signs Initial morbilliviral replication occurs in lymphoid cells; viral entry is mediated by a cell membrane receptor CD150, also called SLAM-F1. Lymphocyte infection facilitates systemic viral spread, but it also causes lymphoid depletion and immunosuppression.

The virus also enters via respiratory epithelial cells, by binding to the PVRL4 receptor. Neurons do not express either of these receptors, so a third mechanism must exist to facilitate cerebral infection. In chronic cases, morbilliviral immunosuppression often results in secondary infections by bacteria, fungi, protozoa (Stephens et al., 2014; Diaz-Delgado et al., 2017); as a result, gross pathology can be highly variable. Animals that die acutely may have interstitial pneumonia with overinflated lungs with prominent rib impressions (Figure 6.31a,b). Phocids with this presentation usually also have marked interlobular emphysema that often extends into the mediastinum, parietal pleura and even the thoracic wall fascia and subcutis. Nail bed and flipper hyperkeratosis are observed in phocids, while buccal and lingual ulcers are described in odontocetes.

On histology, acute cases exhibit interstitial to bronchointerstitial pneumonia, with necrosis of type I pneumocytes and bronchiolar and bronchial epithelium, accompanied by variable interstitial edema or hemorrhage. Later, type II pneumocyte proliferation and syncytial cell formation is the predominant feature, especially in odontocetes (Figure 6.31c,d). In the spleen, thymus, and peripheral lymph nodes, there is profound lymphoid necrosis, follicular depletion, and hyalinosis, and syncytia are often visible within follicles. In the brain, non-suppurative meningoencephalitis is characterized initially by neuronal and glial necrosis, particularly in the cerebrum, which may have a laminar or more random distribution. In the more advanced cases there is neuronophagia, gliosis, gray matter astrocytosis, and myelin depletion in white matter tracts, accompanied by a mononuclear, mainly lymphoplasmacytic, meningeal, and perivascular

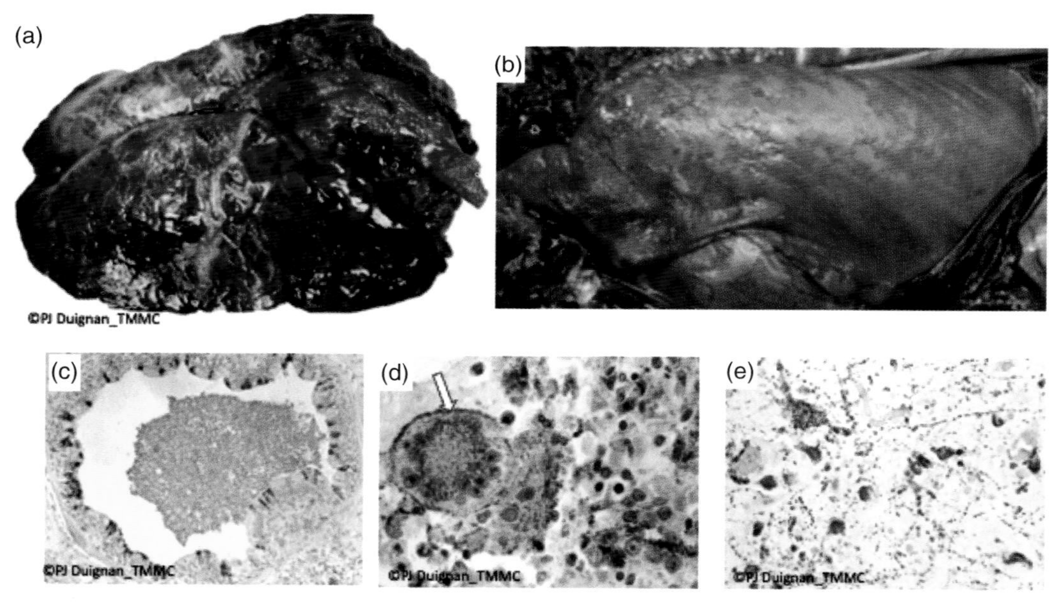

Figure 6.31 (a) Atlantic Harbor seal lung showing diffuse consolidation and congestion with marked interstitial and mediastinal emphysema, phocine distemper virus (PDV) pneumonia. (b) Striped dolphin, lung in situ, interstitial pneumonia, overinflated lung with interstitial to bullous emphysema and rib impressions, cetacean morbillivirus infection. (c) Harbor seal lung, immunohistochemistry, PDV antigen staining (brown) of the bronchiolar epithelial cells. The lumen is partially filled with exudate. (d) Striped dolphin, lung, morbilliviral pneumonia; large syncytial cells are visible in a bronchiole (arrow), with both intracytoplasmic and intranuclear viral antigen staining (brown stain). (e) Harbor seal brain, morbilliviral encephalitis, immunohistochemical staining to show PDV antigen in neuronal cell bodies, axons and glial cells of the cerebrum.

infiltrate. Intracytoplasmic and intranuclear eosinophilic viral inclusions may be detected in epithelial cells of the respiratory, gastrointestinal, and urogenital tracts, including the mammary glands, central nervous system, and lymphoreticular system. These inclusions can be more easily visualized using immunohistochemistry (Figure 6.31d,e). Cetaceans that survive acute or subacute infection may recover sufficient immune function to clear systemic infection, but the virus remains in the brain, where inclusions are rare and syncytia are usually absent; however, neuronal processes will still demonstrate immunostaining. In these cases, defective virus may continue to spread from cell to cell, in a manner similar to humans with measles infection or dogs with CDV, where chronic infection can cause subacute sclerosing panencephalitis or old-dog encephalitis, respectively. In affected dolphins, the lesions are usually in the cortical gray matter, subcortical white matter, and thalamus. There is perivascular mononuclear cuffing, diffuse and focal gliosis, and neuronophagia, but less demyelination. Viral antigen and RNA can be detected, but viable virus is rarely isolated.

Diagnosis Diagnosis is based on histopathology, supplemented by immunohistochemistry and PCR. Virus isolation and characterization is the gold standard. Serology is widely used for epidemiologic studies (Duignan et al., 2014; van Bressem et al., 2014).

Differential Diagnoses For disease outbreaks involving pneumonia and/or encephalitis, other viruses such as influenza or herpesviral infection should be ruled out.

Treatment and Management There is no treatment for clinical disease, but supportive therapy may assist individual cases. A monovalent recombinant CDV vaccine, commercially produced for use in ferrets (Purevax®, Merial Inc., GA) has been used for harbor seals in captivity and for free-living Hawaiian monk seals (Quinley et al., 2013; Baker et al., 2017; Robinson et al., 2018).

Influenza

Etiology, Host Factors, and Transmission There is serological evidence for influenza A virus (IAV, Orthomyxoviridae) infection in several pinniped and cetacean species, as well as sea otters from the North Pacific, Eastern Pacific, North Atlantic, and North Sea (Li et al., 2014; Capuano et al., 2017; Duignan et al., 2018a; Bossart and Duignan, 2019). Disease outbreaks attributed to various influenza subtypes have been documented in free-living harbor seals along the northeastern US Atlantic coast, and from harbor and gray seals in the North Sea (Anthony et al., 2012; Bodewes et al., 2015; Krog et al., 2015; Shin et al., 2019). IAV infects a variety of hosts, including domestic and wild birds, humans, and marine mammals. Influenza B viruses (IBV), in contrast, have only been isolated from humans. On one occasion, the IBV was isolated from a seal. Based on the close genetic relatedness of IAV isolates from marine mammals and wild birds, it has been hypothesized that wild birds are the main source of influenza for marine mammals. The virus may be shed from the respiratory tract as an aerosol and it can also be excreted in feces. Contact between marine mammals and wild birds can occur at haulout sites or when feeding on the same food resources, providing an opportunity for interspecies transmission.

Clinical and Gross Signs Clinical presentation in affected seals includes dyspnea, mucopurulent nasal discharge, and conjunctivitis. Gross and microscopic lesions include acute hemorrhagic interstitial pneumonia with necrotizing bronchitis or bronchiolitis, bronchial gland necrosis, regional hemorrhagic lymphadenopathy, mediastinal, pleural and subcutaneous emphysema, acute conjunctivitis, and suppurative to serosanguinous rhinitis.

Diagnosis Diagnosis is based on histopathology and confirmed by immunohistochemistry using IAV nucleoprotein-specific monoclonal antibody, ELISA serology and reverse transcriptase PCR on lung and upper respiratory tract swabs.

Differential Diagnoses Based on the potential for overlapping clinical signs and gross pathology, morbillivirus and herpesviral infections should be ruled out.

Treatment and Management There is no specific treatment for influenza infection and vaccines have not been used in marine mammals. For marine mammals in captive management, good biosecurity is essential to avoid contact between collection animals and their food and wild birds.

Coronaviruses

Etiology, Host Factors, and Transmission Coronaviruses (CoV) are single-stranded RNA viruses associated with respiratory, gastrointestinal, hepatic, and neurologic disease, in a wide range of vertebrates. Of the four known CoV genera, two (*Alphacoronavirus* and *Gammacoronavirus*) have been associated with outbreaks of respiratory or gastrointestinal disease in captive and free-ranging pinnipeds and cetaceans (Bossart et al., 1990; Nollens et al., 2010; Mihindukulasuriya et al., 2008; Woo et al., 2014; Wang et al., 2020). Alpha HS *CoV* was identified from lung tissue of free-ranging Pacific harbor seals in California. Cetacean coronavirus species include BdCoV HKU22 from captive Indo-Pacific bottlenose dolphins, in Hong Kong, US BdCoV from captive Atlantic bottlenose dolphins in the United States, and BWCoV from a captive beluga whale also in the United States. For some cases, the infection was associated with enteritis or respiratory disease, suggesting that transmission was likely horizontal via the fecal–oral route or by aerosols. Results from the Hong Kong outbreak, where only three of 18 dolphins were found to be infected, would suggest that BdCoV HKU22 is not highly contagious (Woo et al., 2014). No public health risk is known at this time to exist in people exposed to CoV-infected marine mammals.

The novel CoV severe acute respiratory syndrome coronavirus 2 (SARS-CoV-2), the cause of the COVID-19 pandemic, infects hosts through attachment of the viral spike (S) protein receptor binding domain to the angiotensin 1 converting enzyme 2 (ACE2) receptor on host cells. Coronaviruses may adapt to new hosts in part through S mutations that enhance binding affinity for ACE2, a factor that likely allowed SARS-CoV-2 to jump hosts in the first place, while ACE2 is a highly conserved molecule. There are several amino acids known to be important for S protein binding, and mutations in the ACE2 gene that substitute critical amino acids at this site can affect susceptibility to the infection with SARS-CoV-2 (Matahvarajah and Dellaire, 2020).

Using previously published genomes from up to 36 marine mammal species representing cetaceans (baleen whales and odontocetes), pinnipeds (otariids, phocids, walruses), sirenians (West Indian manatees), and fissipeds (polar bears and sea otters) and a modeling approach, it was predicted that cetaceans could be highly susceptible to SARS-CoV-2 infection, pinnipeds less so, followed by polar bears and sea otters (Damas et al., 2020; Matahvarajah et al., 2021). As they have a high number of amino acid substitutions at the ACE2 binding site, both the California sea lion and West Indian manatee are likely to be the most resistant to infection (Mathavarajah et al., 2021). While the risk for human to cetacean transmission is probably highest in captivity, there is also a minimal risk of infection through sewage-contaminated water (Matahvarajah et al., 2021). To date, continuing surveillance of stranded and captive collection marine mammals has found no evidence for SARS-CoV-2 transmission.

Clinical and Gross Signs Lesions associated with suspected coronavirus infection in captive harbor seals included acutely fatal necrotizing enteritis and pulmonary edema (Bossart et al., 1990). For affected harbor seals, CoV antigen was detected by immunofluorescence in intestinal tissue but no virus was isolated. An outbreak of pulmonary congestion, hemorrhage, and consolidation resulted in deaths of 21 free-ranging harbor seals in Northern California (Nollens et al., 2010). Alpha HS CoV was detected in lung from some cases, but causal associations could not be confirmed. The captive-born beluga whale had acute onset generalized respiratory disease and liver failure. Necropsy revealed centrilobular to massive hepatic necrosis and 60–80 nm viral particles were observed on electron microscopy (Mihindukulasuriya et al., 2008). The captive Indo-Pacific bottlenose dolphins had BdCoV detected in routine fecal samples, with no associated morbidity or mortality. Only a small number (3/18) of dolphins were positive for BdCoV and the virus was not detected in California sea lions or harbor seals at the same facility. Seroconversion occurred in the three dolphins from which CoV was isolated (Woo et al., 2014). Clinical signs in the captive Atlantic bottlenose dolphins were acute onset diarrhea, lethargy, and inappetence. Pathogen screening of feces uncovered US BdCoV, but the source of infection was unknown (Wang et al., 2020).

Diagnosis Diagnosis is by respiratory, gastrointestinal, and hepatic symptomatology, pathology (in fatal cases), and etiology confirmation by virus isolation and sequencing.

Differential Diagnoses Differentials include other infectious and parasitic causes of respiratory or gastrointestinal disease or hepatic failure, such as bacteria, other viruses, fungi or harmful algal bloom toxins.

Treatment and Management Case reports for cetaceans and pinnipeds describe either acute onset of clinical signs and sudden death or resolution following a brief period of acute illness without treatment. For the Indo-Pacific bottlenose dolphins, no clinical illness was reported. For marine mammals, particularly cetaceans in long-term captivity, minimizing the risk of human to animal transmission of SARS-CoV-2 would be best practice.

Caliciviruses

Etiology, Host Factors, and Transmission The Caliciviridae encompasses the *Vesivirus*, *Norovirus*, and *Sapovirus* genera, but only vesiviruses are associated with clinical disease or pathology (Duignan et al., 2018a; Bossart and Duignan, 2019). Most marine mammal vesiviruses are strains of vesicular exanthema of swine virus (VESV), including San Miguel sea lion viruses SMSV-1 to SMSV-7, SMSV-9 to 11, SMSV-13 to 17; Steller sea lion vesivirus SLVV-V810 and V1415; walrus calicivirus; cetacean calicivirus (CCV-Tur-1). The pinniped vesiviruses SMSV-8 and SMSV-12 are genetically different from VESV, and they likely represent distinct *Vesivirus* species. Over 40 *Vesivirus* serotypes have been detected in Pacific marine mammals, including California sea lions, northern fur seals, Hawaiian monk seals, Steller sea lions, Pacific walrus (*Odobenus rosmarus divergens*), bottlenose dolphins, gray whales, fin whales (*Balaenoptera physalus*), sei whales (*Balaenoptera borealis*), and sperm whales (*Physeter macrocephalus*). The abundance of caliciviruses in North Pacific marine mammals likely reflects geographically focused research effort, rather than the true global distribution of these viruses.

Clinical and Gross Signs Consistent pathologic findings for otariid *Vesivirus* infections include 1–3 cm diameter epidermal vesicles, usually, on the nonhaired skin of the flippers, which may coalesce and form blisters. Vesicles and ulcers may also involve mucocutaneous junctions of the buccal labia and nares. Viral replication in the stratum spinosum leads to vacuolar degeneration and necrosis, which forms focal intraepidermal vesicles. The vesicles eventually rupture, leaving shallow ulcers that typically heal uneventfully. Although abortion and premature parturition were reported in California sea lions based on virus isolation and serology, there is no evidence for fetal or placental pathology. Caliciviruses are potentially zoonotic, with flu-like symptoms and vesicular skin disease reported after field or laboratory exposure (Tryland, 2018). While noroviruses have not been definitively linked to clinical disease or pathology, porpoise norovirus was shown to replicate in enterocytes. This finding, together with the genetic similarity between porpoise norovirus and oyster-associated fecal-origin noroviruses, raise concern about the zoonotic potential of porpoise norovirus (de Graaf et al., 2017).

Diagnosis Diagnosis is based on the clinical presentation and gross lesions, with molecular techniques (PCR) or virus isolation used for confirmation. Serology is supportive and used for epidemiologic studies.

Differential Diagnoses The presence of clear, fluid-filled vesicles on the nonhaired skin of otariids from the North Pacific is almost pathognomonic for calicivirus infection. In the more chronic stages of infection, the presentation may include dermal ulcers or scar tissue as the vesicles rupture and heal. Other potential differentials include herpesvirus or poxviral infection, bacteria, uremia, or trauma.

Treatment and Management There is no specific cure and, as infection is generally mild and self-limiting, treatment is rarely required.

DNA Viruses

Herpesviruses

Etiology, Host Factors, and Transmission Most herpesviruses identified in aquatic mammals belong to two sub-families, the Alphaherpesvirinae and Gammaherpesvirinae (Duignan et al., 2018a; Bossart and Duignan, 2019). Transmission is likely through direct contact; as for herpesvirus infections in terrestrial mammals, infection is probably lifelong with periods of latency interspersed with clinical recrudescence.

Clinical and Gross Signs Most herpesviruses are associated with relatively minor mucosal or epidermal lesions, but these viruses can occasionally cause fatal systemic or central nervous system infections in pinnipeds and odontocetes. Phocid gammaherpesvirus 1 (GHV1) is a member of the Alphaherpesvirinae, prevalent in Pacific and Atlantic harbor seals and North Atlantic grey seals. Serological surveys show widespread exposure among phocids in both hemispheres. It is associated with epidemic neonatal mortality in harbor seal pups in rehabilitation centers, where it causes hepatic and adrenocortical necrosis; intranuclear inclusions are evident in cells adjacent to necrotic foci. Infected pups can also have oral ulceration, thymic atrophy, and diverse secondary bacterial infections associated with omphalophlebitis, pneumonia and meningoencephalitis. In harbor seal pups under rehabilitation in Europe, mortalities were attributed to interstitial pneumonia and hepatic necrosis.

Otariid GHV1 (also known as otarine herpesvirus 1 or OtGHV1) is a gammaherpesvirus from California sea lions that is directly implicated in the development of urogenital carcinoma, (Gulland et al., 2020; Deming et al., 2021). The virus is endemic and is thought to be transmitted via copulation. Urogenital carcinoma is the primary cause of death for around 20% of subadult and adult sea lions necropsied in Northern California, with up to 26% of all animals in these age classes affected, when nonfatal and microscopic lesions are included (Deming et al., 2018). The virus is always present in sea lions with urogenital carcinoma, being commonly found in tissues of the urogenital tract. Herpesviral oncogenes in a related gammaherpesvirus, human herpesvirus-8, are causally associated with Kaposi's sarcoma. The same oncogenes are also present in OtGHV1 (Deming et al., 2021). Although northern fur seals have a very similar virus, OtGHV4, it lacks oncogenes and it is not associated with neoplasia (Cortés-Hinojosa et al., 2016). Urogenital carcinoma similar to that seen in California sea lions was diagnosed in a South American fur seal from a zoological collection that was likely infected by OtGHV1 in captivity (Dagleish et al., 2013).

In odontocete cetaceans, gammaherpesviruses have been mostly isolated from non-life-threatening skin and genital lesions while a variety of alphaherpesviruses have been associated with skin lesions and also fatal systemic infection and encephalitis (Duignan et al., 2018a; St. Leger et al., 2018; Bossart and Duignan, 2019).

Oral ulcers and plaques with epithelial eosinophilic intranuclear inclusions were observed in northern sea otters that died or were admitted for rehabilitation after the 1989 Exxon Valdez oil spill in Alaska (Tseng et al., 2012). TEM demonstrated the presence of herpesviral virions. A serologic study of otters from the Kodiak archipelago found a high prevalence of exposure to a herpesvirus in live-captured animals. A novel gammaherpesvirus, most closely related to mustelid herpesvirus 1 from badgers, was identified.

Diagnosis Histopathology, immunohistochemistry, TEM, virus isolation, serology, and molecular techniques, are all a useful aid in formulating the diagnosis (Duignan et al., 2018; Bossart and Duignan, 2019; Deming et al., 2021).

Differential Diagnoses Skin and mucosal epithelial lesions may also be caused by caliciviruses, poxviruses, or papillomaviruses, necessitating histopathologic examination of tissues supplemented by molecular techniques. Systemic infection, and in particular encephalitis, has similarities to morbilliviral encephalitis, but other diseases, such as protozoal or bacterial infections, should be considered.

Treatment and Management There are no specific cure or vaccines for herpesviral infections in aquatic mammals.

Papillomaviruses

Etiology, Host Factors, and Transmission There are at least five papillomavirus variants known from aquatic mammals, based on sequencing. Phylogenetically, they are related to papillomaviruses of artiodactylids (Duignan et al., 2018a; Bossart and Duignan, 2019). Like most viruses, they are typically host species specific. The route of transmission is likely horizontal, through mating or other close contact, parturition, or nursing.

Clinical and Gross Signs These viruses are associated with proliferative cutaneous and mucosal lesions in free-ranging and captive cetaceans, manatees, pinnipeds (Figure 6.32a,b), and mustelids. They are generally site-specific in the body, displaying a predilection for the squamous epithelium, causing benign sessile plaques or verrucoid papillomas, or less commonly, malignant neoplasia. Novel papillomaviruses have been identified by molecular, immunohistochemical, and/or classical microscopic techniques in the bottlenose dolphin, orca, sperm whale, West Indian manatee, harbor

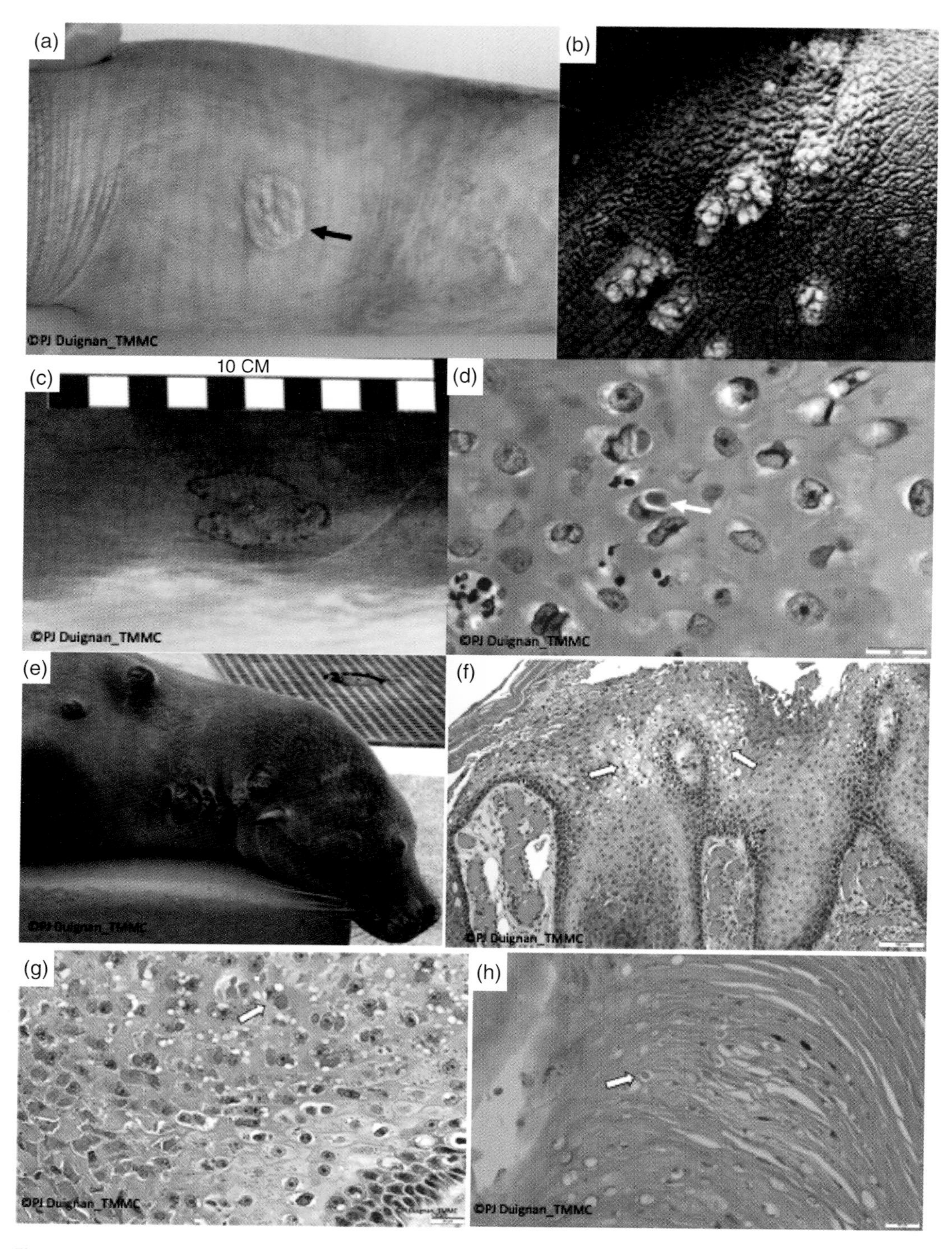

Figure 6.32 (a) Harbor porpoise, penis with raised white firm discoid plaque (arrow) on the base of the penis, Papilloma virus. (b) Manatee, axilla with wart-like exophytic growths. Manatee papilloma virus. *Source:* Photo provided by Dr. G. Bossart, Georgia Aquarium. (c) Harbor porpoise, skin with tattoo-like lesion on the flank, cetacean poxvirus. (d) Harbor porpoise, skin showing large eosinophilic intracytoplasmic inclusions in acanthocytes of the stratum spinosum, cetacean poxvirus. (e) California sea lion, multifocal random raised crusting skin nodules consistent with seal pox. (f) Pacific harbor seal, biopsy of a proliferative skin nodule showing marked parakeratosis, acanthosis and laminar ballooning change (arrows) in the *stratum spinosum*. Consistent with seal pox dermatitis. H&E stain. (g) Pacific harbor seal skin nodule, higher magnification of the *stratum spinosum* showing numerous eosinophilic cytoplasmic inclusions (arrow) consistent with seal pox. H&E stain. (h) Southern sea otter, skin section showing acanthosis and ballooning degeneration of the *stratum spinosum* and numerous cells with eosinophilic cytoplasmic inclusions (arrow). Poxvirus dermatitis. H&E stain.

porpoise, Burmeister's porpoise (*Phocoena spinipinnis*), California sea lion, and southern sea otter. Gastric papillomas associated with papilloma-like virions are also reported in beluga whales. Papillomavirus-associated papillomatosis in Florida manatees was the first viral pathology reported in this species. To date, four novel manatee papillomaviruses (*Trichechus manatus* papillomavirus, TmPV) have been identified, two are cutaneotropic (TmPV1 and TmPV2) and two are mucosotropic (TmPV3 and TmPV4). In manatees, the lesions are variably multifocal, pedunculated, verruciform, or papillary, and white or gray in color. On histology, they are composed of hyperplastic and sometimes dysplastic epithelium. Cells of the stratum granulosum can have vacuolated cytoplasm and pleomorphic nuclei. Inclusion bodies have not been described.

In odontocetes, the mean age for development of papillomas in bottlenose dolphins is 11 years, while for captive dolphins it is 30 years. Lesions are most prevalent on the vaginal, penile, oral, or esophageal mucosa. Papillomas rarely occur on the skin. Papillomas have been observed in harbor porpoises, pilot whales, and killer whales. The gross appearance varies from flat white to tan plaques to proliferative wart-like growths. Histologically, there is hyperplasia of the stratum spinosum on an intact basement membrane supported by a mature fibrovascular core of dermal tissue. Combined herpesvirus and papilloma virus infection in free-ranging and captive odontocetes is associated with genital and oral papillomas and oral squamous cell carcinomas.

Papillomas are a relatively common incidental finding in the oral cavity of young southern sea otters. Next-generation sequencing of viral particles revealed a novel papillomavirus, *Enhydra lutris* papillomavirus 1 (ElPV-1; Fei Fan Ng et al., 2015). The genome of ElPV-1 was obtained. Phylogenetic analysis showed that ElPV-1 is a λ-papillomavirus related to a raccoon papillomavirus (*Procyon lotor* papillomavirus type 1) and a canine oral papillomavirus. Immunohistochemical staining suggested that ElPV-1 is present in intranuclear inclusions and intracytoplasmic keratin granules. Virus-infected cells were scattered throughout the stratum granulosum and stratum spinosum of the gingival and buccal papillomas.

Diagnosis Histopathology, immunohistochemistry using a polyclonal antiserum against bovine papillomavirus 1 and molecular characterization (PCR and sequencing) have been used to confirm diagnosis (Ghim et al., 2014).

Differential Diagnoses Poxviral infection should be ruled out.

Treatment and Management The lesions are generally incidental and of minor clinical significance.

Poxviruses

Etiology, Host Factors, and Transmission Cetacean poxvirus comprises two major lineages: cetacean poxvirus-1 in odontocetes and cetacean poxvirus 2 in Mysticetes (Duignan et al., 2018a; Bossart and Duignan, 2019). They have been documented in southern right whales (*Eubalaenia australis*), humpback whales (*Megaptera novaeangliae*), bowhead whales (*Balaena mysticetus*), harbor and Burmeister's porpoises, and bottlenose, striped, common, dusky (*Lagenorhynchus obscurus*), and Hector's dolphins.

Pinniped parapoxviruses are described for California sea lions, northern fur seals, Pacific harbor seals; ringed (*Pusa hispida*) and spotted seals (*Phoca largha*) from the Arctic; gray and harbor seals from the Atlantic; southern sea lions from South America, Weddell seals from Antarctica; Mediterranean monk seals, and Baikal seals. Parapoxviruses of pinnipeds from the North Pacific and North Atlantic are phylogenetically distinct (Costa et al., 2021). A new species of poxvirus related to an orthopoxvirus was associated with raised, ulcerated, cutaneous lesions in Steller sea lion pups.

A novel poxvirus was described in association with small superficially ulcerated skin lesions in sea otter pups (Tuomi et al., 2014). Bayesian and maximum likelihood phylogenetic analyses found that the virus is divergent from other known poxviruses at a level consistent with a novel genus. These cases were self-limiting and did not appear to be associated with systemic illness.

For all poxviruses, transmission is horizontal. In pinniped pups under rehabilitation, disease outbreaks can occur in crowded pens. Pinniped parapoxvirus is not host specific and can be zoonotic. Cetacean pox is more common in calves and immature animals, but outbreaks and severe infections can occur in older animals under crowded or stressful conditions (van Bressem et al., 2018).

Clinical and Gross Signs Cetacean poxvirus causes "tattoo skin disease," characterized by slightly depressed irregular gray or black dots on the skin that are often arranged in circular or ovoid rings or serpiginous patterns on various parts of the body, but usually on the head, melon, pectoral flippers, dorsal fin, thorax, trunk and flukes (Figure 6.32c). They may persist for months or years and wax and wane, but they are generally benign; severe and extensive infections in juveniles may result in death. Histologic examination of affected skin reveals increased melanocytes in the germinal layer, swelling, and cytoplasmic vacuolation of cells of the stratum intermedium, and hyperplasia and compaction of cells in the stratum externum. Cells of the stratum intermedium have small, variably sized eosinophilic cytoplasmic inclusions that may displace the nucleus (Figure 6.32d). Occasionally, there are intranuclear inclusions. On TEM, the inclusions are typically brick-shaped.

Cutaneous poxvirus lesions of otariids and phocids are proliferative nodules that often ulcerate and are most prevalent on the head at mucocutaneous junctions, but can also be widely distributed on the neck, thorax, or other parts of the body (Figure 6.32eE). Gray or white plaques may occur on the tongue and labia. On histology, there is epidermal and follicular hyperkeratosis and parakeratosis of the stratum spinosum and stratum corneum, often with marked cytoplasmic vacuolation (Figure 6.32f). Keratinocytes of the stratum spinosum may contain low numbers of spherical or irregularly shaped, pale, eosinophilic, intracytoplasmic viral inclusions (Figure 6.32g). A mixed inflammatory cell infiltrate may also be present.

Sea otter cutaneous pox lesions have similar epidermal hyperplasia with ulceration, and rete peg formation projecting into the dermis. Intracytoplasmic inclusions are similar to those in pinnipeds (Figure 6.32h).

Diagnosis The gross appearance of skin lesions and histopathology are characteristic. Electron microscopy and molecular techniques with sequencing can be used for confirmation and phylogenetic studies (Costa et al., 2021).

Differential Diagnoses Papillomaviruses and herpesviruses should be ruled out.

Treatment and Management Outbreaks in pinnipeds under rehabilitation may result in significant proliferative and ulcerative dermatitis, leading to secondary bacterial infection that require antibacterial therapy. Outbreaks should be prevented or managed by good husbandry and sanitary practices. Pinniped parapoxviruses are zoonotic and can cause painful nodular proliferative cutaneous lesions in humans, associated with fever and myalgia (Tryland, 2018). Appropriate personal protective equipment and other precautions should be used when working with stranded and wild pinnipeds. Outbreaks of cetacean pox in managed care dolphins may be severe and prolonged, and can disproportionately affect males (van Bressem et al., 2018). Good husbandry can reduce the risk and magnitude of outbreaks. There is no specific medical therapy or commercially available vaccine.

Adenoviruses

Etiology, Host Factors, and Transmission Aquatic mammal adenoviruses in the genus Mastadenovirus infect cetaceans, pinnipeds, and otters (Duignan et al., 2018a; Bossart and Duignan, 2019). Sea lion adenoviruses (otariid herpesvirus 1, 2) were isolated from California sea lions, while similar adenoviruses were found in liver or feces from South African and South American fur seals, a South American sea lion and a Hawaiian monk seal. They have also been isolated from northern elephant seals (phocid herpesvirus 1), Pacific harbor seal (phocid herpesvirus 2), bottlenose dolphins (Tursiops adenovirus 1), sei whales (*Balaenoptera borealis*), bowhead whales, belugas, harbor porpoises, and polar bears. In otters, canine adenovirus 1 and a novel adenovirus have infected captive Eurasian otters (*Lutra lutra*) and southern sea otters, respectively. Transmission is likely horizontal via feces and other infected body fluids and secretions.

Clinical and Gross Signs Clinical disease is rarely observed or reported. Lesions associated with infection may include acute necrotizing hepatitis, ulcerative keratitis, corneal edema, iridocyclitis, arteritis, and conjunctivitis with endothelial cell infection.

Diagnosis Histopathology may reveal large characteristic intranuclear inclusions in hepatocytes, enterocytes, and endothelial cells. TEM reveals adenovirus-like virions within the nucleus of hepatocytes and endothelial cells.

Differential Diagnoses Other causes of necrotizing hepatitis or conjunctivitis, such as bacterial infections and toxins, must be ruled out.

Treatment and Management There is no specific therapy. There are no vaccines available for aquatic mammals.

Non-Infectious Disease

Neoplasia

Etiology, Host Factors, and Transmission

Newman and Smith (2006) comprehensively reviewed the literature on the occurrence of neoplasia in aquatic mammal taxa from the early 20th to the early 21st century. As with terrestrial wildlife, the prevalence of neoplasia is generally low in aquatic mammals, but benign tumors (e.g. adenomas, leiomyomas, lipomas, and fibrolipomas) have been documented sporadically and opportunistically in both captive and free-ranging animals. Sporadic neoplasia is probably of little importance at the population level. More significant is the high prevalence of malignant neoplasia in some species. Of particular interest are urogenital carcinoma in California sea lions and gastrointestinal adenocarcinomas in beluga whales, in the St. Lawrence River, Canada. Urogenital carcinoma is the most prevalent form of neoplasia in aquatic mammal species. Successive mortality surveys of subadult and adult California sea lions at the Marine Mammal Center in California from 1979 to 1994 (Gulland et al., 1996) and from 1991 to 2000 (Greig et al., 2005) reported a prevalence of 18% (66/370) and 15% (88/568), respectively, for neoplasia cases. One study spanning 2005 to 2015 found little difference in overall prevalence with cancer diagnosed in 14% (263/1917) of necropsied adult sea lions; 90% of those were confirmed to be urogenital carcinoma (Deming et al., 2018). Of sea lions with urogenital carcinoma, 78% had advanced metastatic disease that was diagnosed as the primary cause of death for 95% of these cases. When subclinical cases were included, 26% of subadult and adult sea lions necropsied at the Marine Mammal Center (where standardized histopathology is conducted on the urogenital tract), are diagnosed with either carcinoma in situ or early invasive or metastatic disease (Browning et al., 2015). Because urogenital carcinoma has been prevalent in an easily accessible species for at least four decades, it has become a model for multifactorial carcinogenesis; OtGHV1 infection and organochlorine pollutant contamination are key risk factors (Gulland et al., 2020).

Another gammaherpesvirus, OtGHV3, was found in lymphocytes in a geriatric (24 years) captive male California sea lion which developed acute onset leukemia with multicentric large B cell lymphoma (Venn-Watson et al., 2012). A quantitative PCR assay was developed for the novel virus. By this means, the prevalence and quantity of OtHV3 were then determined among buffy coats from 87 stranded and managed collection sea lions. Stranded sea lions had a higher prevalence of OtHV3 compared with managed collection sea lions (34.9% versus 12.5%), and among the stranded sea lions, yearlings were most likely to be positive (Venn-Watson et al., 2012). The virus is present among free-living sea lions, but little is known about its epidemiology.

A novel gammaherpesvirus, tentatively named miroungine gammaherpesvirus 3 (MirGHV3), was identified in northern elephant seal pups in California with diffuse large B cell lymphoma, but was absent from pups that did not have lymphoma (Martinez et al., 2022). The prevalence of this new virus in the population and whether it is causally linked to the neoplasia is currently unknown. Circular structures that were possibly viral were also present in the cells of a northern fur seal pup with multicentric large cell lymphoma (Stedham et al., 1977). The significance and epidemiology of this possibly new virus are unknown.

Beluga whales in the St. Lawrence seaway are a relict population that is historically subjected to heavy hunting pressure and exposure to some of the most industrially contaminated water in North America. While now protected, population recovery has been slow. Lair et al. (2016) reported on a multi-decade mortality survey (1983–2012) that encompassed necropsy details for 222 of 469 animals found dead over that period. Of these, 39 malignant tumors were diagnosed in 35 of 156 mature adults born in the 1940s and 1950s, but not in any whales born after the year 1971. Neoplasia is rare in free-ranging belugas from other parts of the species' range, suggesting a link with historic environmental contamination of the St. Lawrence seaway by carcinogens (e.g. polychlorinated hydrocarbons), possibly compounded by genetic factors in this small population (Martineau et al., 2002; Lair et al., 2016).

Clinical and Gross Signs

Benign tumors are a common incidental finding at necropsy and are rarely associated with clinical signs. Examples include leiomyomas, chondromas, adrenal phaeochromocytomas, lipomas, or fibromas (Figure 6.33a,b,c; see also Figure 6.49 below).

Malignant and metastatic neoplasms are relatively rare, but they can be associated with significant clinical effects and pathology, depending on the affected organ systems. Leukemia and multicentric lymphoma were recently diagnosed in free-ranging northern elephant seal pups from the central California coast that were admitted for rehabilitation due to malnutrition. Complete blood counts showed a progressive, moderate to marked leukocytosis, characterized by a predominance of large monomorphic mononuclear cells of potentially lymphoid origin, which had flower-shaped

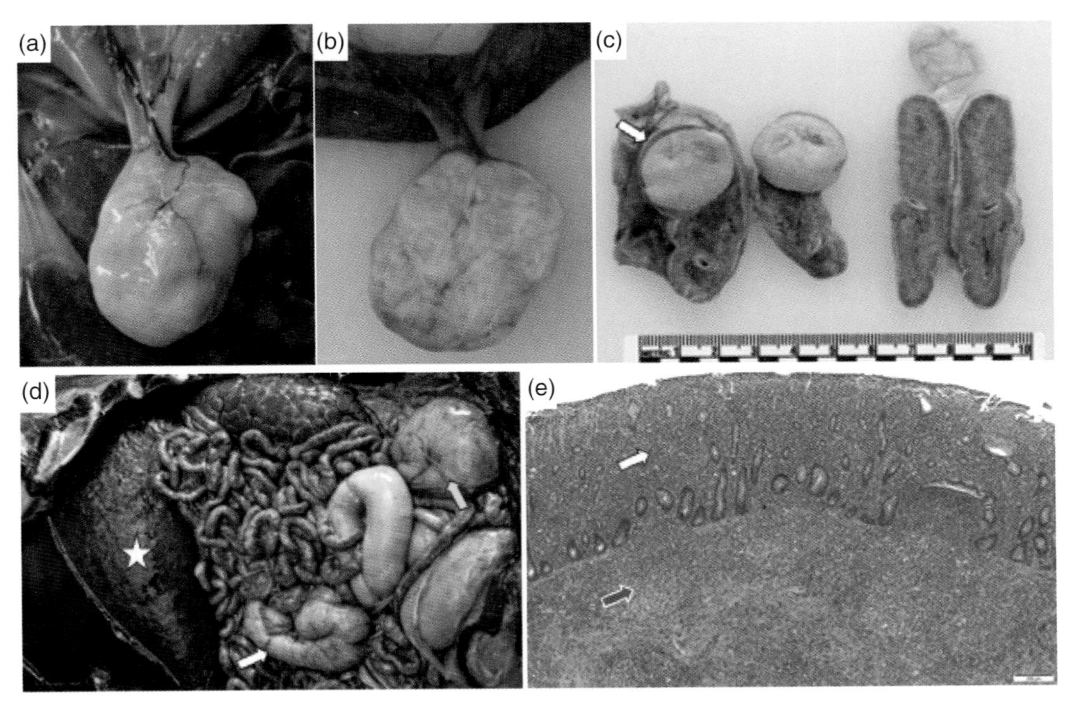

Figure 6.33 (a) California sea lion, jejunal mesentery with pedunculated firm white botryoid mass. (b) California sea lion, sagittal section of the mass showing the internal structure of interwoven fibrous bands separated by adipose tissue, fibrolipoma. (c) California sea lion, the left adrenal gland has a well circumscribed homogenous yellow mass in the medulla surrounded by a thin rim (arrow) of cortical tissue (phaeochromocytoma; for another example see Figure 6.49). (d) Northern elephant seal, abdominal cavity showing splenomegaly (star) and diffuse lymphadenopathy. Deep inguinal lymph node (yellow arrow) and mesenteric lymph node (white arrow). The wall of the small intestine is thickened and corrugated, lymphoma. (e) Ileum, histopathology from the same case, showing marked infiltration of the *lamina propria* (blue arrow) by a uniform population of lymphoblasts that have also effaced most of the mucosa (white arrow). B cell lymphoma, as confirmed by immunohistochemistry, but not shown here. H&E stain.

nuclei (Martinez et al., 2022). At necropsy, there was marked splenomegaly and enlargement of all central and peripheral lymph nodes (Figure 6.33d). On histopathology, the cellular infiltrate was composed of lymphoblasts that variably effaced normal architecture in multiple sites, including skin, intestine, lymph nodes, spleen, tonsils, bone marrow, liver, urinary bladder, and reproductive tract (Figure 6.33e). Immunohistochemical staining of the neoplastic cells was most consistent with a B lymphocyte origin (Pax 5 and CD20 positive with admixed small CD3-positive T lymphocytes and CD204-positive macrophages). PCR and sequencing identified the novel gammaherpesvirus MirGHV3 from affected tissues that was not identified in age-matched controls (Martinez et al., 2022). Another gammaherpesvirus (OtGHV3) was associated with lymphoma in a geriatric captive male sea lion, which died a few days after presenting with acute lymphocytic leukocytosis (Venn-Watson et al., 2012). At necropsy, he had ulceration of the esophagus and stomach. On histopathology, there was multicentric invasion of tissues by neoplastic lymphocytes, as described for the northern elephant seals. The neoplastic cells were diffusely positive for CD20 and negative for CD3, indicating B cell origin. TEM identified herpesvirus particles in esophageal cells.

As another example, a free-ranging river otter was presented to a California veterinary clinic in severe respiratory distress. Radiography revealed multiple intrathoracic masses. Primary pleural

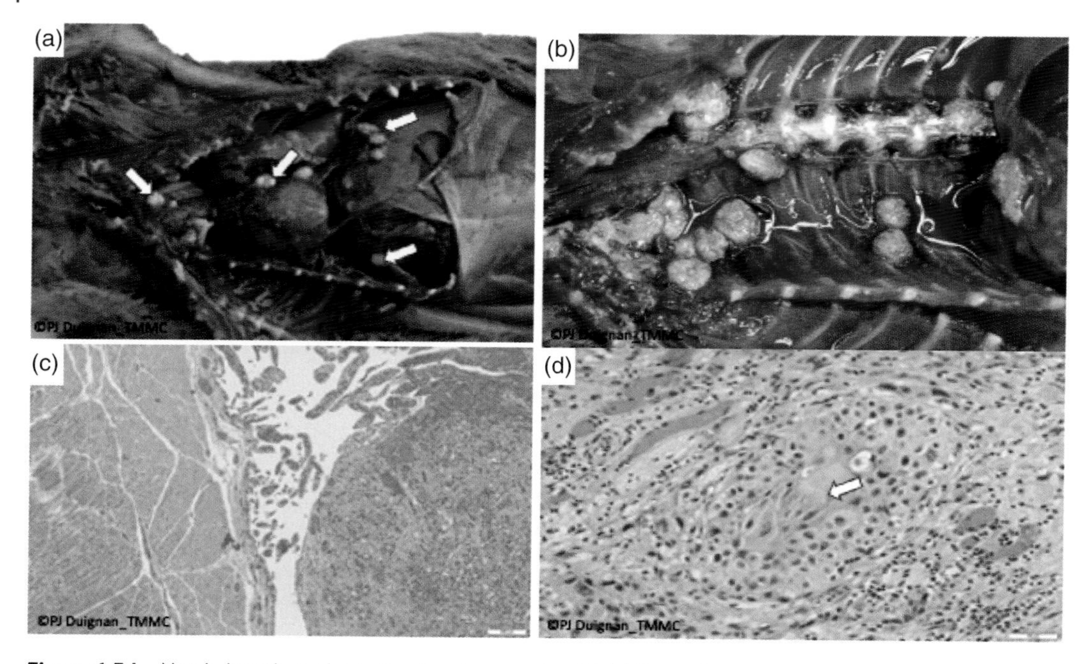

Figure 6.34 North American river otter (*Lontra canadensis*). (a) Thoracic cavity opened to show numerous white or tan firm nodules attached to the pleura and mediastinum and expanding regional lymph nodes. Differentials include neoplasia and granulomatous inflammation. (b) Pluck of (a) removed to show similar nodules attached to the parietal pleura, particularly around the thoracic inlet (left of image). (c) Intercostal muscle (left) and part of a nodule (right), with papillary growth of the parietal pleura extending into the space between. The mass is composed of dense sheets of neoplastic epithelial cells. (d) Histopathology of mass. At higher power, the neoplastic cells exhibit features of squamous cell carcinoma, with keratin production evident as extracellular pink material in the center (arrow).

squamous cell carcinoma was diagnosed on histopathology (van de Velde et al., 2019). In sea otters, an important differential diagnosis is granulomatous pleuritis; the gross neoplastic lesion (Figure 6.34a,b) can be confounded with pyogranulomatous pleuritis caused by the infection with the zoonotic pathogen, *Coccidioides* spp. (Figure 6.30a,b,c,d).

The most significant cancer in marine mammals is urogenital carcinoma in California sea lions from the California coast. It is associated with infection by a gammaherpesvirus, otariid GHV1 and high burdens of persistent organochlorine contaminants (Gulland et al., 2020). California sea lions with advanced urogenital carcinoma usually present with perineal and tarsal edema, and occasionally a prolapsed necrotic vagina or penis, hind limb paresis, decubitus ulceration, or abdominal distension (Figures 6.35 and 6.36).

Urogenital tumors appear to originate in the cervix or proximal vaginal mucosa in females and on the penis or prepuce of males (Figures 6.37, 6.38 and 6.39). Metastasis to regional lymph nodes is common, with the sublumbar chain being the most severely affected, followed by the inguinal, colonic, pancreatic, sternal, bronchial, and mediastinal lymph nodes. Sublumbar lymph nodes become especially enlarged, with loss of normal architecture, a dense sclerotic capsule and often with central coagulative or liquefactive necrosis (Figure 6.37c). These massive tumors obstruct the ureters, leading to hydroureter and hydronephrosis (Figure 6.37b). Lymphatics may also be obstructed by compression or by luminal metastases, causing peripheral edema. Affected animals may present severely azotemic and obtunded, but the gross presentation is highly variable, with

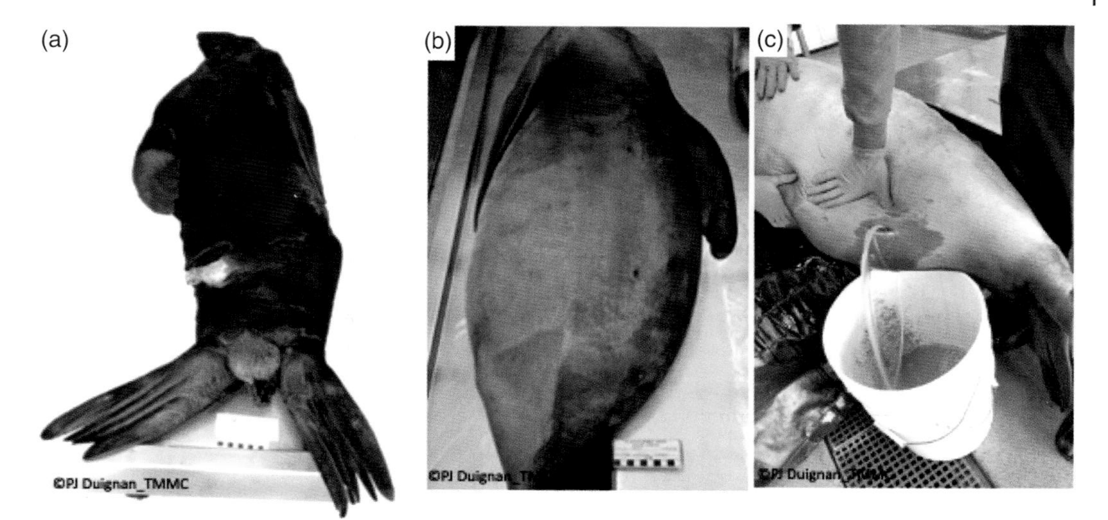

Figure 6.35 California sea lion. (a) Adult male with a prolapsed penis and edematous scrotum and hind flippers suggestive of urogenital carcinoma. Other differentials include balanoposthitis, cystitis, pyelonephritis, peritonitis, spinal/pelvic trauma. (b) Adult female with distended fluid-filled abdomen. Differentials include urogenital carcinoma, cardiomyopathy, hepatopathy, uroabdomen, hemoabdomen, *Coccidioides* spp. infection, and other forms of peritonitis. (c) A different sea lion from (b); abdominal tap produces voluminous yellow translucent transudate.

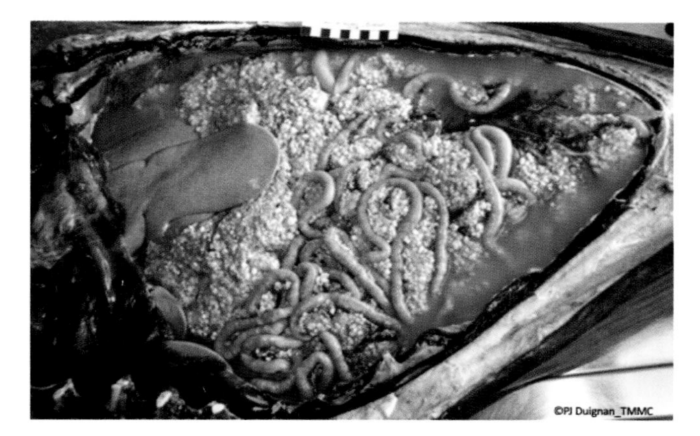

Figure 6.36 California sea lion adult female (as in Figure 6.35c) with the abdomen opened to reveal multifocal white to tan firm nodules multifocally attached to the omentum, mesentery, visceral and parietal peritoneum (carcinomatosis), marked lymphadenomegaly and abundant yellow translucent transudate. Impression smears of nodules showed epithelial cells with few leukocytes, urogenital carcinoma.

some animals having severe abdominal distension and effusion, and carcinomatosis of the serosa, mesentery and omentum (Figures 6.35a,b and 6.36). Other cases may present with discrete to multinodular, white, firm, umbilicated masses on any of the following: gonad, urinary bladder, uterine body and horns, mesometrium, liver, spleen, kidney, adrenals, lungs (Figure 6.40), myocardium, diaphragm, or skeletal muscle.

Vertebral metastases can result in lumbar and sacral fractures (Figure 6.41). On histology, intraepithelial neoplasia may occur multifocally in the cervix, vagina, penis, or prepuce

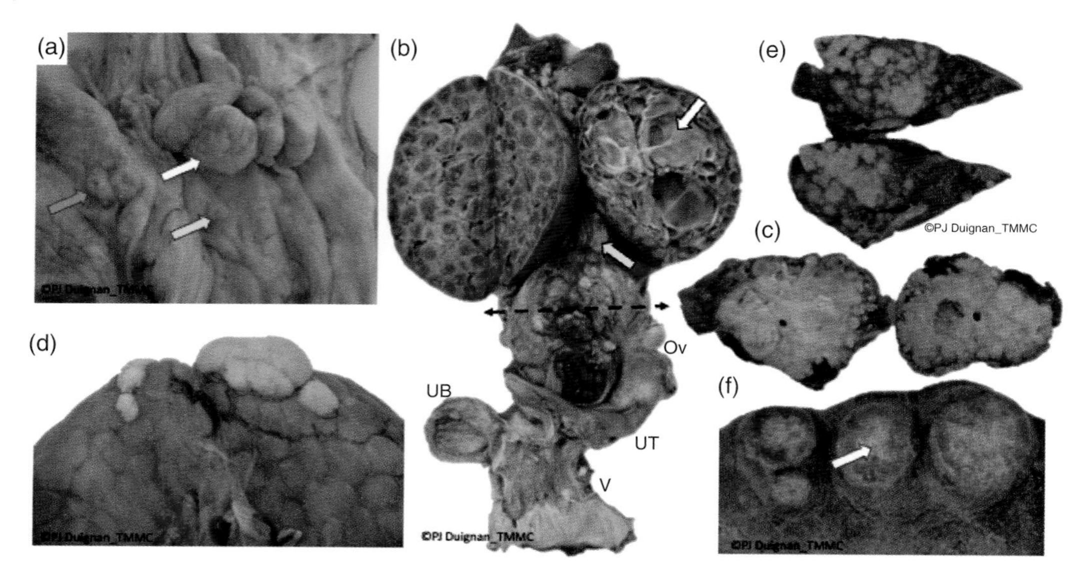

Figure 6.37 California sea lion, adult female. (a) Cervix (white arrow) with proximal vagina (yellow arrow) and urinary bladder (blue arrow), showing an enlarged nodular cervix, thickened nodular vaginal mucosa and multifocal nodules in the trigone of the bladder consistent with urogenital carcinoma. (b) Urogenital tract removed to show multiple cystic spaces in the left kidney (white arrow, hydronephrosis), dilated right ureter (yellow arrow), marked cortical pallor in the left kidney (concurrent leptospiral nephritis). The dashed line indicates the line of section through the sublumbar lymph nodes shown in (c). (c) Sublumbar lymph nodes, cut section showing parenchymal replacement by neoplastic tissue and caseous necrosis. (d) Kidney with nodules of carcinoma implanted on the capsular surface. (e) Liver, cut sections showing invasive carcinoma replacing the normal hepatic parenchyma. (f) Spleen, with four metastatic nodules protruding from the capsular surface. Note the central umbilication characteristic of carcinomas (arrow).

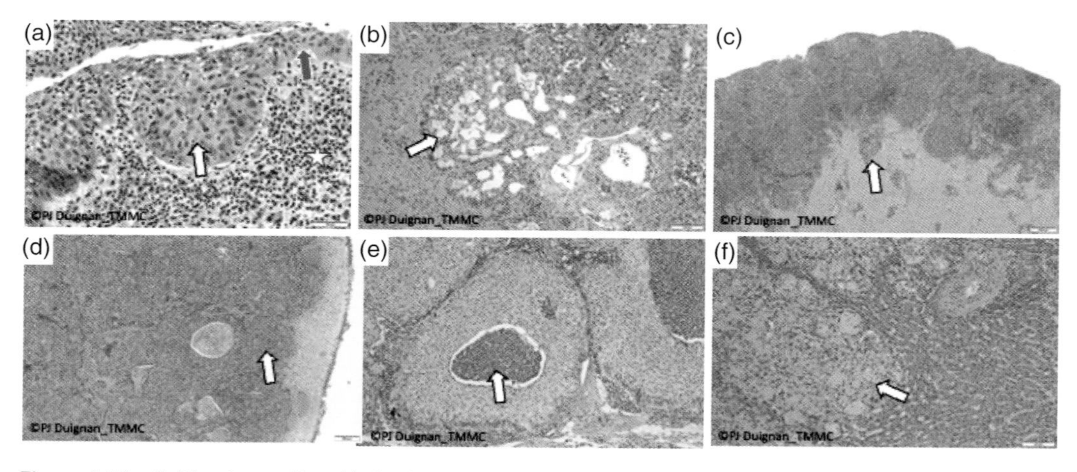

Figure 6.38 California sea lion. (a) Cervix, epithelial dysplasia (blue arrow) and carcinoma *in situ* (white arrow). Note that the basement membrane subtending the epithelium has not been breached by neoplastic epithelial cells. (b) Cervix, urogenital carcinoma showing both a cribriform (arrow) and solid growth pattern. (c) Vagina, massively thickened neoplastic epithelium and carcinoma invading beneath the epithelial basement membrane (arrow). (d) Urinary bladder, carcinoma (basophilic cells, arrow) effacing most of the bladder wall. (e) Inguinal lymph node, carcinoma effacing most of the lymph node architecture with a comedone growth pattern. There is central eosinophilic necrosis (arrow). (f) Liver, the parenchyma is infiltrated and replaced by cords of malignant epithelial cells (arrow).

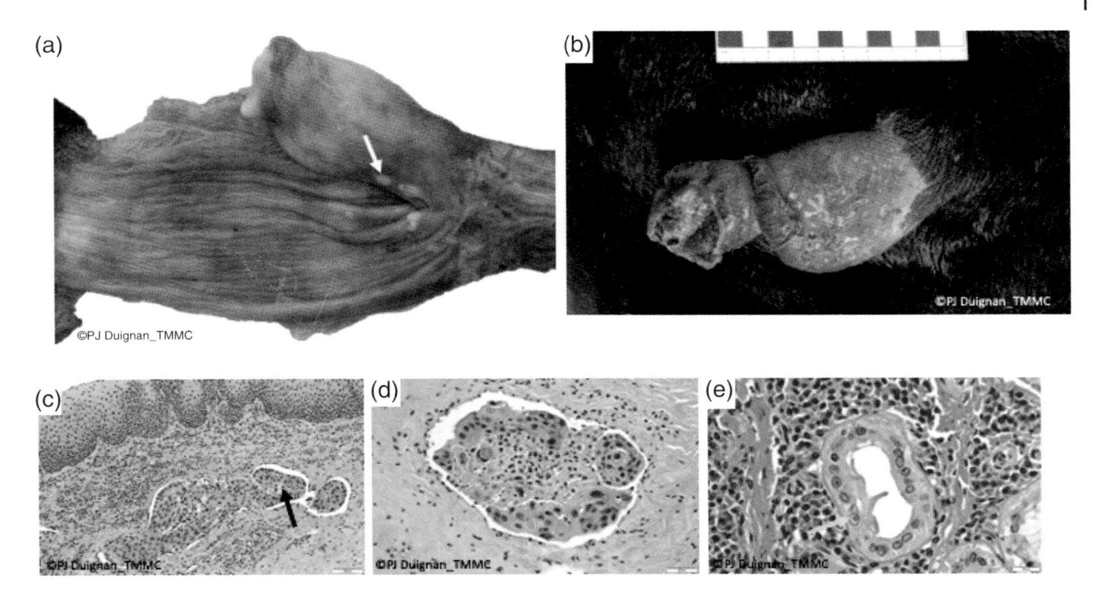

Figure 6.39 California sea lion, adult male. (a) Penis and prepuce with raised pale tan plaques at the base of the penis and proximal prepuce (arrow). (b) Penis, balanoposthitis secondary to urogenital carcinoma. (c) Prepuce histopathology showing multiple carcinoma metastases in submucosal lymphatics (arrow), H&E stain. (d) Prepuce, high magnification view of metastasis composed of highly anaplastic epithelial cells within the lumen of a lymphatic vessel, H&E stain. (e) Prepuce, skin, intranuclear eosinophilic inclusion bodies (arrow), herpesvirus. H&E stain.

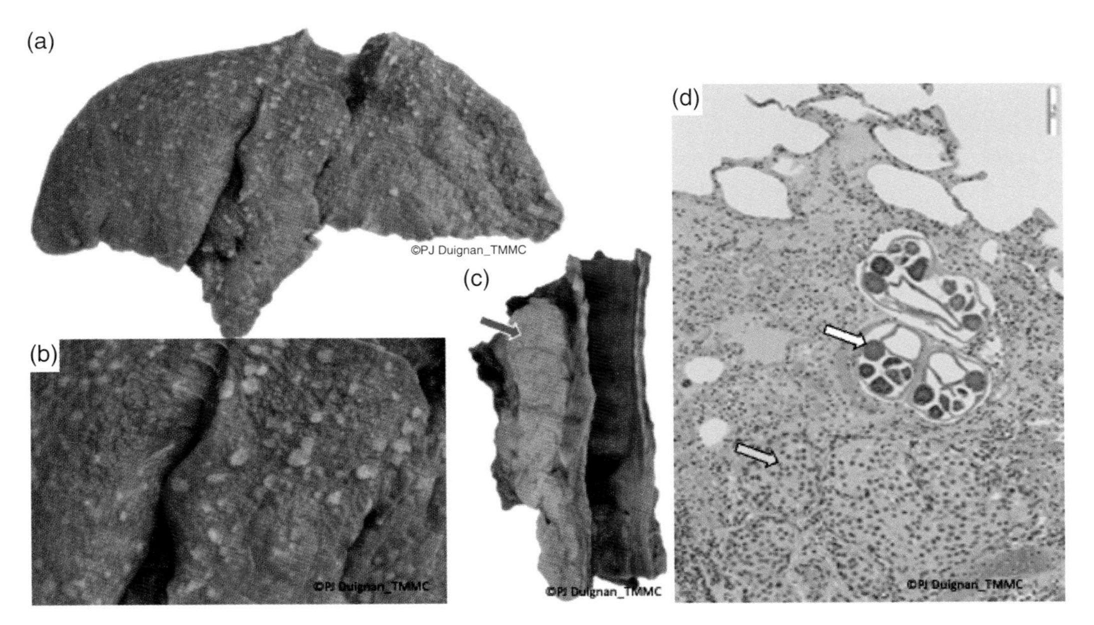

Figure 6.40 California sea lion. (a) Lung, multiple randomly distributed urogenital carcinoma metastases. (b) Lung, close-up of (a) to show the umbilicate structure of the metastases. (c) Bronchus with peribronchial lymph node (arrow) that has been completely effaced by urogenital carcinoma metastases. (d) Lung, histopathology image showing solid nodular carcinoma metastasis (yellow arrow) and a nematode (*Parafilaroides decorus*) within the alveolar parenchyma (white arrow). H&E stain.

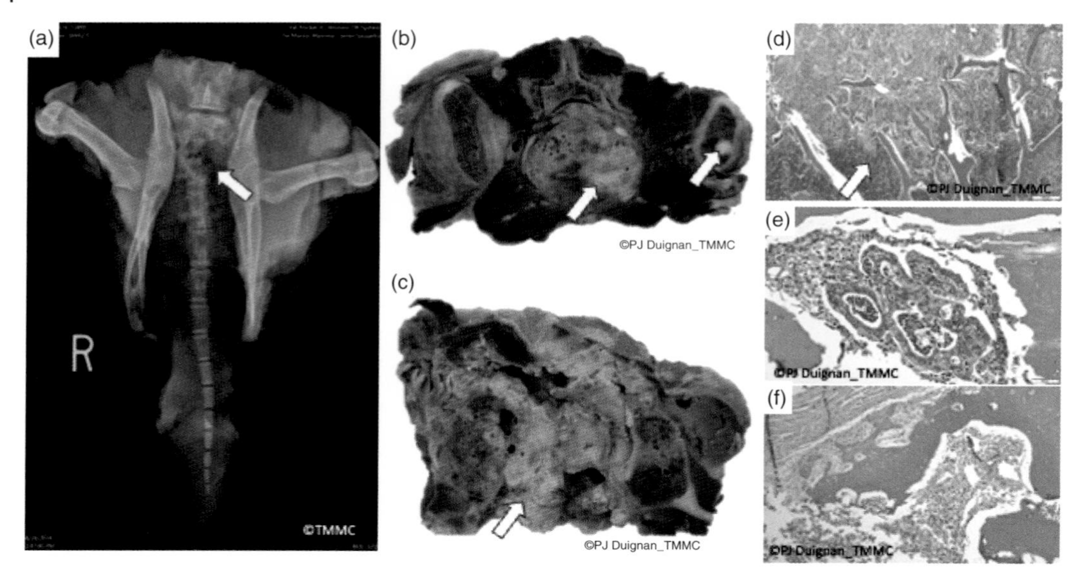

Figure 6.41 California sea lion, subadult female. (a) Pelvic radiograph showing a pathologic fracture of the sacrum with collapse on the left (arrow). (b) Vertebra, section through the first sacral vertebra and ileal wings of the same animal in (a), showing carcinoma (white masses, arrows) infiltrating into the vertebral body and ileum (fixed tissue specimen). (c) Vertebra, section through the sacrum at the site of the pathologic fracture shown in (a); there is extensive invasion and replacement of bone by carcinoma. Fixed tissue specimen. (d) Histopathology of sacral vertebral body showing invading masses of carcinoma (arrow) and loss of bone cortex and trabeculae. H&E stain. (e) Sacrum, higher power of the neoplastic cells in an eroded section of cortical bone. (f) Sacrum, ragged and scalloped fragments of cortical bone at the fracture site. H&E stain.

(Figures 6.38 and 6.39). The affected foci are often extensive and markedly thickened with dysplastic cells, characterized by an increased mitotic rate, and disordered maturation. Although transition zones between relatively normal epithelium and markedly hyperplastic or dysplastic areas are distinctive, early invasion of the lamina propria and submucosa can be more difficult to detect. More advanced invasive lesions show variable morphology with cribriform, squamous, comedone, and basaloid patterns described for metastases (Figure 6.38b,e). Neoplastic cells are polygonal with large nuclei, anisokaryosis, a high mitotic rate, and occasional multinucleated cells. Herpetic eosinophilic intranuclear inclusion bodies are occasionally seen in genital epithelial cells, but these are inconsistent and rare findings in metastases (Figure 6.39eE). Urogenital carcinoma has also been diagnosed in captive California sea lions that were wild-born, and in a captive South American fur seal that was likely in contact with a California sea lions while in captivity (Dagleish et al., 2013).

Gammaherpesvirus-associated lymphoma in sea lions and elephant seal pups in California was first diagnosed on hematology; leukocytosis was characterized by a predominance of large monomorphic mononuclear cells of probable lymphoid origin (Venn-Watson et al., 2012; Martinez et al., 2022). For the elephant seals, flower-shaped nuclei were noted in the neoplastic lymphocytes (Martinez et al., 2022). At necropsy, lymph nodes were generally enlarged and homogenous or nodular on cut section; these lesions were often accompanied by thickening of the gastrointestinal mucosa or skin. Neoplastic infiltration was often associated with ulceration. Histopathologic features consistent with large cell lymphoma were identified to varying degrees of severity in lymph nodes, bone marrow, intestines, liver, tonsils, thyroid, adrenal, spleen, liver, intestines, kidneys, lower urinary tract, and several other organs. Immunohistochemical staining of neoplastic cells was most consistent with B lymphocyte origin, with most cells staining positively for Pax 5, CD20, and CD79a, with admixed smaller numbers of CD3-positive T lymphocytes and CD204-positive macrophages.

Adenocarcinoma of the gastrointestinal tract was the most common tumor (7% of mature animals) for beluga whales of the St. Lawrence River, with salivary gland adenocarcinoma and cholangiocellular carcinomas also detected in this group. The second most common cancer was mammary carcinoma, diagnosed in eight mature females (10% of this age class). There were also two cases of thyroid carcinoma, one lymphoma and two ovarian carcinomas. In total, cancer was diagnosed as the cause of death for 31 belugas or 20% of the mature animal age class, and 14% of the total number of beluga whales necropsied.

Diagnosis

Urogenital carcinoma in sea lions is generally diagnosed antemortem based on the clinical presentation and results of abdominal ultrasound. Females often have marked to severe vulvar edema that may extend to the pelvic flippers, while males may have raised white preputial plaques and a similar edema. Secondary balanoposthitis is common. Lymphoma cases are generally diagnosed by routine hematology and blood smears. Neoplasia in beluga whales is a postmortem diagnosis, based on gross and histopathologic findings.

Differential Diagnoses

Nodules or masses may result from chronic granulomatous inflammation in response to chronic bacterial or mycotic infection, requiring histopathology examination.

Treatment and Management

Medical or surgical intervention is not documented for lymphoma or carcinoma cases.

Toxins

Harmful Algal Blooms

Etiology, Host Factors, and Transmission

Harmful algal blooms composed of planktonic dinoflagellates and cyanobacteria are becoming more frequent in marine, fresh and brackish waters globally, as the climate warms and levels of contamination by nitrogen and phosphorus effluents increase. These blooms have the potential to produce diverse soluble toxins that can exert a range of clinical and pathologic effects on vertebrates, including humans. The most significant dinoflagellate toxins include domoic acid (amnesic shellfish poisoning), brevetoxins (neurotoxic shellfish poisoning), saxitoxin (paralytic shellfish poisoning), okadaic acid (diarrheic shellfish poisoning) and ciguatoxin. Cyanobacteria contain multiple cyanotoxins including microcystins, nodularin, cylindrospermopsin, anatoxins and β-N-methylamino-L-alanine (BMAA). The diatom *Pseudo-nitzschia* spp., the source of domoic acid, has a worldwide distribution including the North Pacific, North Atlantic, Sea of Japan, Gulf of Mexico, and coastal waters of Europe and New Zealand. Toxicosis has been demonstrated or presumed in California sea lions, northern fur seals, southern sea otters, harbor seals, short- and long-beaked common dolphins, bottlenose dolphins, and North Atlantic right whales (Kreuder et al., 2003; Silvagni et al., 2005; Torres de la Riva et al., 2009; Lefebvre et al., 2010; Doucette et al., 2012; McHuron et al., 2013). The toxin is produced during a harmful algal bloom and there can be trophic transfer from algivorous or filter-feeding species, such as anchovies, crustaceans, or mollusks, to marine birds, mammals, and humans. The toxin is distributed in body fluids, can accumulate in fetal tissues and fluids, and may also be transferred via milk to neonates (Rust et al., 2014; Lefebvre et al., 2018).

Saxitoxin is a generic name for at least 50 structurally related algal toxins which occur in temperate waters worldwide, and are produced by the dinoflagellate, *Alexandrium* spp. As with domoic acid, marine mammals are exposed by ingesting prey that have concentrated the toxin. Brevetoxins produced by the dinoflagellate *Karenia brevis* are released by disintegrating cells; liberated toxins can become aerosolized, posing inhalation risk. Brevetoxicosis is most prevalent in waters off the southeastern United States, and can affect manatees, dolphins, fish, sea birds, and humans. Okadaic acid and related dinophysis toxins are produced worldwide by several dinoflagellates and are concentrated in the hepatopancreas and gills of invertebrates such as mollusks. Ciguatoxins are toxic polycyclic polyether neurotoxins produced by dinoflagellates (*Gambierdiscus* spp.), which commonly bioaccumulate in the skin and lipids of tropical reef fish. Microcystins (hepatotoxic shellfish poisoning) are potent cyanotoxins, with over 50 known congeners, produced by certain freshwater and estuarine cyanobacteria, primarily *Microcystis aeruginosa*. Exposure to the cyanotoxin BMAA has been linked to several neurodegenerative diseases in humans, nonhuman primates, and dolphins (Davis et al., 2019). BMAA has been shown to cross the blood–brain barrier, become incorporated into brain proteins and persist in apex predators such as sharks and bottlenose and common dolphins.

Clinical and Gross Signs

Following exposure to domoic acid, pinnipeds, and sea otters with acute toxicosis may exhibit a variety of clinical signs, including neurologic impairment (seizures, disorientation, ataxia, head weaving, pruritis, memory loss, depression or coma), reproductive failure (abortion) or cardiac abnormalities (Brodie et al., 2006; Goldstein et al., 2008; Zabka et al., 2009; Lefebvre et al., 2010; McHuron et al., 2013; Cook et al., 2015; Miller et al., 2021). They may have elevated eosinophils, inappropriate responses on neurologic tests, electroencephalogram (EEG) abnormalities, and in chronic cases, hippocampal atrophy that is detectable by magnetic resonance imaging (MRI; Montie et al., 2010; Gulland et al., 2012). While cetaceans are exposed to domoic acid and high levels have been detected in gastrointestinal tract contents and urine, characteristic neuro- and cardiopathology have not yet been described (Lebebvre et al., 2002).

Domoic acid is an amino acid analog of the excitatory neurotransmitter L-glutamate that binds to alpha-amino-3-hydroxyl-5-methyl-4-isoxazole propionate and kainate receptors in the brain, heart, and other tissues. For marine mammals, domoic acid pathology is best described in California sea lion (Silvagni et al., 2005; Zabka et al., 2009; Buckmaster et al., 2014) and southern sea otter (Miller et al., 2021). Domoic acid-triggered neuronal depolarization results in a cascade of unregulated events, including endogenous glutamate release and activation of voltage-gated calcium channels. The loss of homeostasis and resultant neuronal injury triggered by excessive glutamate receptor activation is termed excitotoxicity. The distribution of glutamate receptors in the brain coincides with findings on histopathology, preferentially affecting regions associated with memory function in California sea lions, humans, and laboratory animal models (Ramsdell, 2010). Brain lesions are centered on the ventral hippocampus and parahippocampal gyrus, may be unilateral or bilateral, and can vary in severity even where bilateral lesions are present (Figures 6.42–6.44). The distribution of lesions within the hippocampal complex can also vary segmentally along the cornu ammonis and dentate gyrus (Silvagni et al., 2005; Goldstein et al., 2009; Miller et al., 2021).

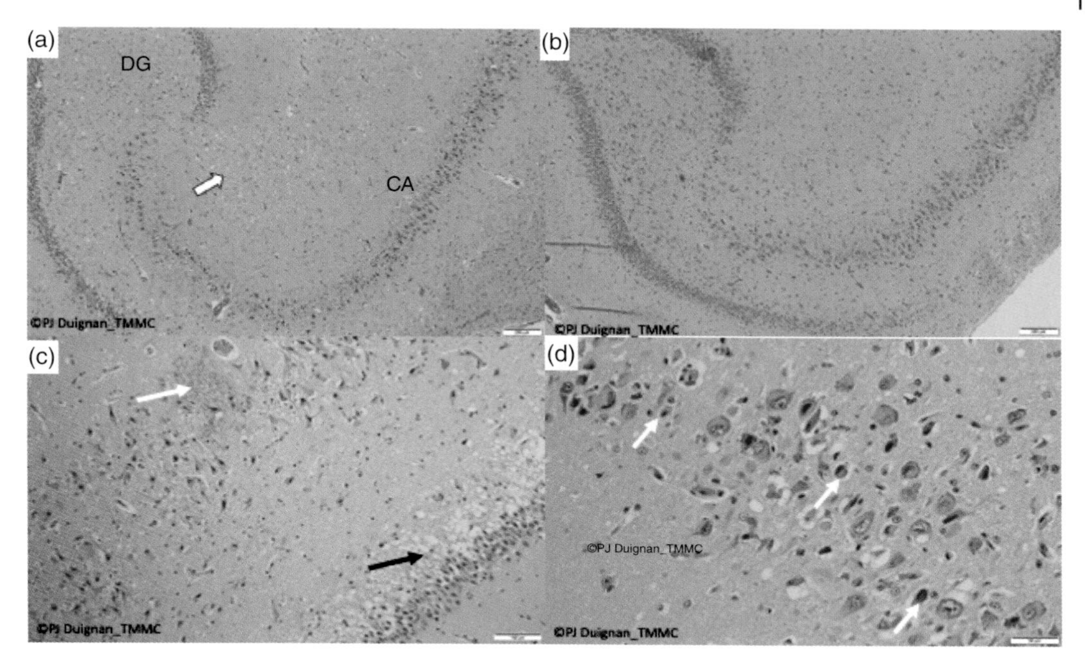

Figure 6.42 Southern sea otter. (a) ventral hippocampus showing the dentate gyrus (DG) to the left and cornu ammonis to the right. Note the reduced density of neurons in the cornu ammonis (CA) and the pallor and vacuolation (arrow) in the neuropil between the dentate gyrus and cornu ammonis. Subacute to chronic domoic acid encephalopathy. (b) Ventral hippocampus from an animal that had toxoplasmosis but not domoic acid intoxication. Compare the neuronal density with (a) and absence of neuropil vacuolation. (c) Hippocampus, high power view, note the focal hemorrhage (white arrow), laminar vacuolation (pallor, black arrow), neuronal necrosis (contracted dark neurons), and focal gliosis (aggregates of smaller cells). Acute to subacute domoic acid encephalopathy. (d) Hippocampus, high magnification view of acute to subacute neuronal necrosis. The necrotic cells are reduced in size and hypereosinophilic (i.e. red and dead, arrows); those that are in the process of dying are shrunken and darker staining, and the few remaining normal neurons are relatively large with pale eosinophilic cytoplasm and large round nuclei. H&E stain.

Where death occurs following acute exposure, neuronal necrosis, and neuropil vacuolation are apparent, affecting the dentate gyrus granular cells, pyramidal neurons of the cornu ammonis, neurons of the amygdala and the pyriform lobe (Figure 6.42). Sea otters with acute, fatal domoic acid toxicosis typically present with neurological signs and severe, diffuse congestion and multifocal microscopic hemorrhages in the brain, spinal cord, cardiovascular system and eyes (Miller et al., 2021).

Areas of most severe depletion of cornu ammonis pyramidal neurons can vary by animal species. In California sea lions (CSL), cells in the cornu ammonis 2 are relatively spared when compared to those in cornu ammonis 1, 3 and 4. If animals die following acute intoxication, gross lesions may be subtle and difficult to detect. Animals that survive acute domoic acid toxicosis may later be admitted to a rehabilitation facility with malnutrition, unusual behavior, intermittent seizures, or apparent blindness. These cases are generally sporadic, single strandings and are usually not temporally linked with algal blooms.

At necropsy, asymmetrical or bilateral hippocampal atrophy are often apparent in coronal sections of fresh or formalin-fixed brain of chronic domoic acid cases, with corresponding expansion of the ventral horn or lateral ventricle (Figure 6.43). Atrophy also affects the parahippocampal

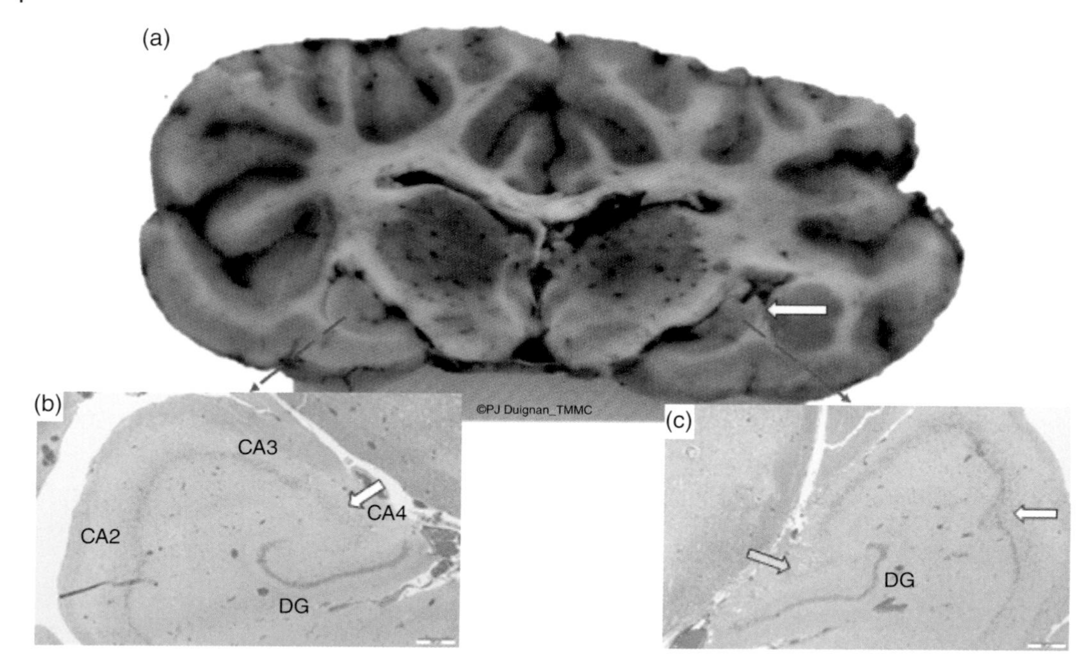

Figure 6.43 Southern sea otter. (a) Brain, chronic domoic acid encephalopathy, fixed brain sliced through the thalamus and ventral hippocampus showing asymmetry of the hippocampus with marked atrophy of the right side (arrow). (b) Left ventral hippocampus of the same otter shown in (a), histopathology section showing mild CA2 distortion and neuronal loss and microvesiculation from CA4. H&E stain. Cornu ammonis (CA), dentate gyrus (DG). (c) Right ventral hippocampus of the same otter in (a) showing marked distortion of CA2 (white arrow) and almost complete loss of CA4 with microvesiculation of the neuropil (yellow arrow). The dentate gyrus is markedly distorted and there is diffuse hippocampal contraction. H&E stain.

gyrus and amygdala, sometimes with marked vacuolation or focally severe tissue cavitation (Figure 6.44). On histology, there is parenchymal loss in the hippocampus and related structures, with mild to severe loss of granular cells in the dentate gyrus and pyramidal neurons of the cornu ammonis, astrocytosis, and oligodendrogliosis, in response to neuronal loss. Mild lymphocytic perivascular cuffing in the parenchyma and focal to diffuse lymphoplasmacytic meningitis may also be present.

Glutamate receptors also occur in the conducting system and other areas of the heart of humans, monkeys, and rats (atrioventricular node, bundle of His and Purkinje fibers, intramural nerve fibers, ganglia cells, and cardiomyocytes); similar receptors are suspected to occur in the heart and conducting system of California sea lions (Zabka et al., 2009). Troponin-I and L-carnitine were not found to be predictive of cardiac damage, suggesting that apoptosis predominates over necrosis in the pathogenesis, and that intermittent arrythmia occurs rather than a continuous functional disturbance (Zabka et al., 2009). Domoic acid cardiomyopathy in pinnipeds is characterized grossly by myocardial flaccidity, pale streaking of the epicardium, which may extend deep into the myocardium, and pericardial effusion (Figure 6.45a). The earliest histological lesion is generally in the septal myocardium, distal to the atrioventricular node, and is characterized by subtle interstitial edema and cytoplasmic vacuolation in Purkinje cells (Figure 6.45b,c). More evolved cases present with myocardial apoptosis or necrosis and loss of necrotized tissue, histiocytic infiltration, fatty replacement, and interstitial fibrosis (Figure 6.45d).

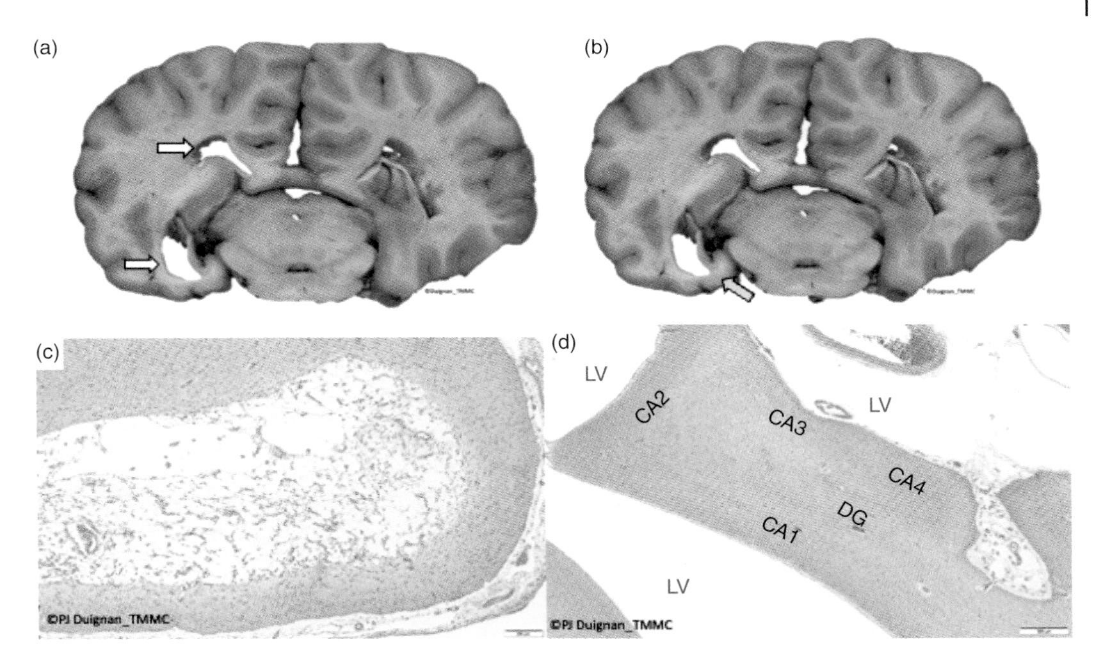

Figure 6.44 Guadalupe fur seal. (a & b) Brain, fixed specimen, serial coronal sections through the midbrain showing apparent distension of the left lateral ventricle (arrows) and severe atrophy and cavitation of the left hippocampus and parahippocampal gyrus (yellow arrow). Chronic domoic acid encephalopathy. (c) Left parahippocampal gyrus showing focally severe malacia (necrosis and tissue loss) resulting in cavitation. H&E stain. (d) Left ventral hippocampus showing marked reduction in size and distortion. There is marked diffuse loss of neurons from cornu ammonis (CA) and dentate gyrus (DG). The relative expansion of the ventral horn of the lateral ventricle (hydrocephalus *ex vacuo*) seen as clear space (LV). H&E stain.

Multiple epidemiologic models confirm that domoic acid toxicosis is a significant risk factor for diagnosis of cardiomyopathy as a primary or contributing cause of death in southern sea otters (Kreuder et al., 2005; Miller et al., 2020). Cardiac lesions in sea otters are progressive with congestion, edema, and generalized pallor seen in acute cases, accompanied by subtle swelling, cytoplasmic vacuolation and hypereosinophilia of cardiomyocytes; small foci of hemorrhage are common in acute cases. In more subacute and chronic cases, the heart is usually grossly enlarged, rounded and pale tan with expanded chambers and variable streaking on the ventricular free wall, papillary muscles, apex and septum (Miller et al., 2021). The histopathology is characterized by multifocal cardiomyocyte necrosis or apoptosis, tissue loss, stromal collapse and fatty or fibrous replacement. These lesions corresponded with the grossly apparent ventricular mottling and streaking. Hyperplastic cardiomyocytes with karyomegaly and/or nuclear rowing (attempted regeneration) occur in some areas. The lesions are often concentrated in the subepicardial and subendocardial ventricular myocardium and the papillary muscles, and they occasionally form discrete, well-demarcated areas of cardiomyocyte loss. Purkinje fiber swelling and cytoplasmic vacuolation are observed as reported for California sea lions (Zabka et al., 2009). Ventricular arterioles (especially in the left ventricular free wall) have progressive mural smooth muscle cell swelling, hypereosinophilia, necrosis or apoptosis, loss, patchy mural hyalinization and thickening, and dystrophic mineralization, accompanied by mild endothelial cell regeneration and hyperplasia.

In pregnant sea lions, domoic acid crosses the placental barrier and causes abruption, leading to abortion. While the main finding in aborted fetuses is cerebral edema, neuronal necrosis can

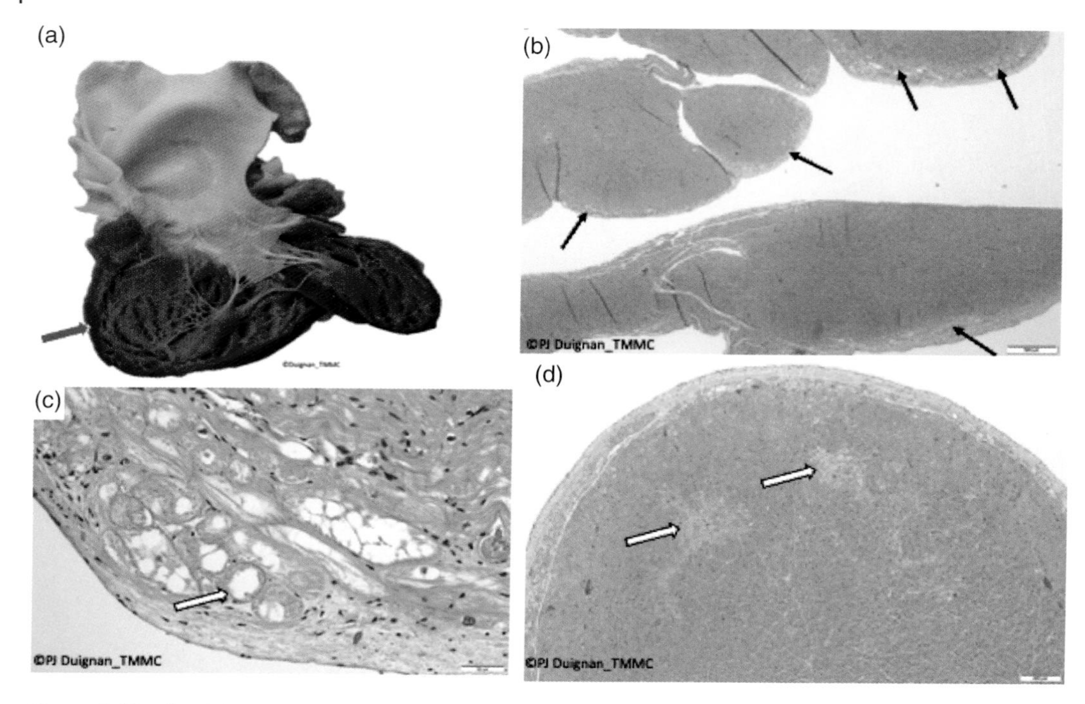

Figure 6.45 Guadalupe fur seal. (a) Heart, domoic acid cardiomyopathy with thinning of the left ventricular wall (arrow) and dilatation of the chamber. (b) Heart, histopathology of the right ventricular free wall (top) and the moderator band (bottom) showing subendocardial vacuolation (arrows). H&E stain. (c) Heart, right ventricular endocardium, showing marked vacuolation of Purkinje cells (arrow). Domoic acid cardiomyopathy, H&E stain. (d) Heart, left ventricle, papillary muscle, showing multifocal myocardial fibrosis (arrow) and myofiber vacuolation. Domoic acid cardiomyopathy, H&E stain.

occur in the laminar cortex, cerebellar Purkinje cells, cingulate to paracingulate gyrus, and all regions of the hippocampal formation (Brodie et al., 2006; Goldstein et al., 2009). Because cerebral hemorrhage was not a feature of domoic acid-induced aborted fetuses, it was proposed that domoic acid-induced seizures in the dam resulted in placental abruption mediated by paroxysmal hypertension that translated to fetal hypertension and brain edema. However, the fetal brain likely expresses glutamate receptors, so a direct mechanism for fetal brain edema may also be a possibility (Costa et al., 2010). Abortion is not an inevitable outcome of intoxication, but even low dose exposure of the dam can result in teratogenesis for the developing fetal brain, due to domoic acid recirculation in fetal fluids, resulting in prolonged domoic acid exposure for fetuses (Lefebvre et al., 2018). Pups may be born apparently unaffected, but as juveniles or subadults, they display aberrant behavior, decreased cognitive ability and a more epileptiform pattern of seizure activity, which can develop with no additional exposure to domoic acid. This syndrome is not associated with detectable central nervous system pathology, via MRI, EEG, and histopathology. Considering the histopathology of brain edema in second to third trimester fetuses exposed to domoic acid, the high vulnerability of fetuses to in utero domoic acid exposure, and the increased excitability of the brain resulting from alterations in neurogenesis, neuromigration and synaptogenesis, fetal exposure to domoic acid may provide a primary explanation for this novel postpartum neurological presentation (Ramsdell and Zabka, 2008; Goldstein et al., 2009).

Saxitoxins are potent sodium channel blockers that bind reversibly to voltage-gated sodium channels on neurons, leading to paralysis. Saxitoxin was one of the first algal bloom toxins linked to marine mammal mortality when a mass stranding of 14 humpback whales occurred in Cape Cod bay. The whales had been actively feeding on mackerel laden with the toxin prior to death (Geraci et al., 1989). As there are no characteristic gross or histologic lesions for saxitoxins in aquatic mammals, diagnosis is based on confirmed exposure and epidemiological correlates.

Brevetoxins are polyether toxins that also bind to voltage-sensitive sodium channels, but to a different site than saxitoxins, causing paralysis. They also have hemolytic properties. Manatees exposed to brevetoxins through ingestion or inhalation show heterophilic and eosinophilic leukocytosis, hemoconcentration, electrolyte abnormalities, and decreased immune responses (Walsh et al., 2015). As with saxitoxins, pathologic changes are nonspecific and include congestion of the respiratory tract and meninges, and variable hemorrhage in the liver, kidneys, gastrointestinal tract, and lungs (Bossart et al., 1998). Brevetoxins demonstrate binding affinity for lymphocytes, macrophages, and microglial cells, and the pathogenesis may involve a cytokine storm or toxic shock (Bossart, 2007). As with saxitoxins, diagnosis is based on biochemical testing of tissues and body fluids, elimination of other causes and epidemiologic factors.

Okadaic acid and related dinophysis toxins are potent inhibitors of specific protein phosphatases, especially serine/threonine phosphatases affecting sodium secretion and solute permeability of the cell membrane. In humans, the symptoms of diarrheic shellfish poisoning include gastrointestinal distress, vomiting, nausea, and diarrhea. Okadaic acid has been detected in manatees and bottlenose dolphins in Florida, sometimes together with brevetoxins (Twiner et al., 2011). Its pathologic significance is yet unknown.

Ciguatoxins are toxic polycyclic polyether neurotoxins; once consumed with the skin of fish, ciguatoxins activate voltage-gated sodium channels, causing synapse depolarization, altered perception of heat and cold, paralysis, and heart failure. The toxins are lipophilic and easily cross the blood–brain barrier, causing central and peripheral nervous signs, that in humans include vomiting, diarrhea, numbness of extremities and lips, reversal of hot/cold sensations, and muscle and joint pain. In aquatic mammals, ciguatoxins was suspected as the cause of death for two Hawaiian monk seals, based on analysis of archived tissue samples (Bottein et al., 2011).

Microcystins act by binding covalently to protein phosphatases, and can cause pansteatitis, hepatic necrosis and nephritis. Microcystin toxicosis was diagnosed as the cause of icterus and massive hepatic necrosis in sea otters in central California, characterized by enlarged friable and hemorrhagic livers; histology revealed hepatocellular necrosis, apoptosis, cytoplasmic vacuolation and hemorrhage (Miller at al., 2010b). Based on laboratory studies, the suspected route of exposure was consumption of contaminated invertebrates that had accumulated the toxin 100-fold over background water levels; multiple marine discharges of microcystin-contaminated fresh water are also documented.

The cyanobacterial neurotoxin BMAA can also bioaccumulate in marine food webs, including in the muscles and fins of sharks. Dietary exposure to this toxin in humans and other primates is associated with development of neurofibrillary tangles and β-amyloid plaques that may be linked to dementia. High BMAA concentrations were found in the brains of stranded bottlenose and common dolphins from the US Atlantic coast; BMAA detection was associated with proliferation of β-amyloid plaques and dystrophic neurites in the auditory cortex, compared to the visual cortex and brainstem (Davis et al., 2019). While the clinical significance of these findings is unknown, cyanotoxin exposure may be an emerging cause of stranding in areas with an increasing frequency of cyanobacterial blooms.

Diagnosis

Very few algal bloom toxins cause pathognomonic lesions as described for domoic acid in pinnipeds and sea otters. For most unusual mortality events, associations between animal mortality and toxic blooms are more often inferred and are based on epidemiologic factors such as temporal association with known toxin-producing algal blooms, clinical signs, presence of toxin in prey species, numbers of animals affected, the variety of predators affected, detection of toxin in body fluids or tissues, and elimination of other potential causes. In some situations, aquatic mammals may be exposed to a cocktail of different toxins that could potentially have synergistic or additive effects (Fire et al., 2011; Fire and van Dolah., 2012). Lethal and sublethal dosages for most of these toxins in aquatic mammals are unknown and are mostly extrapolated from laboratory rodents; these combined factors can make definitive diagnosis challenging for potential algal bloom-associated mortality events.

Differentials

For animals presenting with neurologic clinical signs, differentials include other toxins such as organophosphates, infectious disease (viral, bacterial, protozoal, fungal), cranial trauma, nutritional deficiencies (thiamine), hypernatremia, hyperthermia, metazoan parasites (e.g. *Nasitrema* spp.), or congenital defects. Cardiomyopathy may also be caused by parasitic infection (toxoplasmosis, sarcocystosis), bacterial infection (vegetative endocarditis), or degenerative changes in the myocardium or heart valves (age). Respiratory distress may also be caused by various forms of pneumonia or exposure to other noxious volatiles from the petrochemical industry.

Treatment and Management

Treatment for pinnipeds or sea otters exposed to domoic acid is supportive and includes anticonvulsants, fluid therapy, and anti-inflammatory medication. Seizures can be controlled using benzodiazepines (lorazepam, midazolam, diazepam) or phenobarbital. California sea lions admitted to the Marine Mammal Center are usually treated using phenobarbital (4 mg/kg IM twice a day for two days), lorazepam (0.2 mg/kg IM twice a day for the first two days or longer as needed), subcutaneous fluids and dexamethasone (in the absence of corneal lesions). Alphalipoic acid, an antioxidant that crosses the blood–brain barrier, is also used at 10 mg/kg SC once daily (Field et al., 2018).

For manatees with brevetoxicosis, treatment includes prevention of drowning (using flotation devices) and supportive therapy (fluids, anti-inflammatory drugs, and parenteral antibiotics). Atropine (0.02 mg/kg) and tulathromycin (2.5 mg/kg SQ every seven days for three doses) resulted in successful recovery and release for 93% of cases (Ball et al., 2014). Few if any cetaceans with brevetoxin exposure have survived more than 24 hours under rehabilitation. Oral cholestyramine therapy and supportive care can be used to treat animals with microcystin intoxication (Rankin et al., 2013).

Persistent Organic Pollutants

Etiology, Host Factors, and Transmission

Persistent organic pollutants are anthropogenic chemicals that have been produced on a massive scale since the mid-20th century, with many industrial and agricultural uses including continued use for mosquito control in some parts of the world. They also include chemicals such as dioxins that are produced accidentally as a byproduct of industrial processes or released as a result of combustion (municipal or medical waste incineration or burning of domestic trash). Persistent organic pollutants include polychlorinated biphenyls (multiple congeners), organochlorine pesticides (dieldrin, endrin, heptachlor, hexachlorobenzenes, mirex, toxaphene, polychlorinated dibenzofurans, dichlorodiphenyltrichloroethane (DDT) and its metabolites DDE (1,1-dichloro-2, 2-bis(p-chlorophenyl)ethylene), DDD (dichlorodiphenyldichloroethane), and so on. Although many of these compounds have been banned for decades in some Western countries, residues are still detectable in the blubber of aquatic mammals, often in areas far removed from major industrial and agricultural areas, such as the high Arctic. This is due to environmental persistence, wide dispersal in aquatic environments, and aerosolization. The long lifespan of aquatic mammals and vertical transmission from mother to offspring also contribute to persistence and spread of these anthropogenic pollutants.

Clinical and Gross Signs

Despite numerous publications documenting detection of these chemicals in laboratory animals and free-living wildlife, few studies definitively link chemical detection in tissues or body fluids with clinical illness or gross and microscopic pathology. Lesions or physiological effects in aquatic mammals often attributed to persistent organic pollutants include thymic and splenic lymphoid depletion leading to immune suppression, neoplasia (see section on neoplasia in belugas and California sea lions), dermatitis (squamous metaplasia of sebaceous glands), endocrine disruption, and decreased reproductive success (Beckmen et al., 1997; Martineau et al., 2002; DeGuise et al., 2002).

Diagnosis

Exposure to persistent organic pollutants is determined by measurement of suites of toxins in blubber, other depot fat, liver, kidney or other tissues using biochemical or chromatographic techniques.

Differentials

As for algal bloom toxins, investigation of a mortality event or specific clinicopathologic presentation should encompass all potential epidemiologic variables and eliminate etiologies in a stepwise fashion through microscopic examination and diagnostic testing wherever possible.

Treatment and Management

There is no documented treatment for persistent organic pollutant exposure and because they are ubiquitous in the food web and are able to transfer vertically, avoidance or prevention is difficult.

Heavy Metals

Etiology, Host Factors, and Transmission

Mercury is a toxic non-essential element that can bioaccumulate in marine food webs and is particularly common in areas with current or historic mining practices, such as the Amazon basin and San Francisco bay. Methylmercury is known to cause peripheral and central neuropathies in terrestrial mammals, including humans. While high concentrations have been documented in marine mammal tissues in some parts of the world (e.g. polar bears), there is little evidence for adverse effects (Siebert et al., 1999; Woshner et al., 2001a, b). The proposed tolerance of cetaceans and pinnipeds for mercury may be linked to evolution of detoxification mechanisms involving selenium and proteins (metallothionines and other chelating agents) that bind mercury, zinc, copper, and selenium and sequester them in skin or the liver, where they have minimal apparent effect (O'Hara and Hart 2018).

Clinical and Gross Signs
No significant clinical signs or pathology has been reported.

Diagnosis
Measurement of tissue levels of methylmercury and selenium by liquid chromatography–mass spectrometry.

Differential Diagnoses
Differential diagnoses are not relevant.

Treatment and Management
Treatment is not necessary.

Congenital or Genetic Diseases

Etiology, Host Factors, and Transmission

Congenital defects are rarely reported in free-living aquatic mammals. In wildlife, they may be caused by genetic disorders, maternal and fetal exposure to infectious agents, toxins or nutritional deficiencies, and trauma to developing embryos. The etiology may vary by species and geographic region, necessitating epidemiologic investigation where outbreaks occur. Northern elephant seals are one of the least genetically diverse mammal species on earth (Abadia-Cordoso et al., 2017). One survey of 220 pups that died after rescue found that 5% had one or more congenital defect(s), but a subsequent larger survey found the rate to be approximately 1% (Trupkiewicz et al., 1997; Colegrove et al., 2005).

Clinical and Gross Signs

Defects most commonly affect the brain (hydrocephalus); heart – right ventricular hypoplasia and overriding aorta, atrial (ASD) and ventricular septal defects (VSD), patent ductus arteriosus, pulmonary arterial stenosis; musculoskeletal system (polydactyly, diaphragmatic hernia); kidney (congenital hydronephrosis); lung (dysplasia) and skin (angiomatosis). Clinical signs vary depending on the organ or body system affected and the lesion severity, and may be inapparent, mild or incompatible with life. Many congenital lesions are discovered as incidental findings at necropsy, while others, such as VSD, may be diagnosed antemortem (Dennison et al., 2011a). Harbor seal pups examined at the same hospital had a low (less than 1.5%) frequency of malformations, and this study also determined that the foramen ovale normally closes late in this species (Dennison et al., 2011b). Other defects reported for harbor seals include skeletal malformations (Dennison et al., 2009), hernias (Biancani et al., 2012), intestinal atresia (St. Leger and Nilson, 2014), brain or other neurologic anomalies (McKnight et al., 2005; Harris et al., 2011; Field, 2018), and conjoined twins. A 20-year survey of mortality among northern fur seals on the Pribilof Islands found 33 examples of congenital defects from 2735 necropsied pups, ranging from incidental findings to fatal conditions (Spraker and Lander, 2010).

Among cetaceans, cardiac and skeletal anomalies have been reported. The range of cardiac lesions is similar to that reported from pinnipeds, and includes ASD and VSD, transposition of the great arteries, patent ductus arteriosus, right ventricular hypertrophy, subvalvular pulmonic stenosis with hypoplastic pulmonary artery, and mitral valve and pulmonic or coronary arterial aneurysms (Powell et al., 2009; Scaglione et al., 2013). Malformations of the cranium and axial skeleton are common and include prognathism, double faced monsters, kyphosis and scoliosis, spina bifida, and conjoined twins (van Bressen et al., 2006; deLynn et al., 2011; Groch et al., 2012, Tamburin et al., 2017; St. Leger et al., 2018).

A number of congenital skeletal defects have been described in West Indian manatees, including ectrodactyly of the pectoral flipper, scoliosis, amelia, and open fontanelles (Owen et al., 2018). Defects of internal organs include atresia ani, hernias, and omphalocele.

Focal malformation of the left cerebral temporal lobe was observed in a neonatal sea otter pup that was found stranded alone on the beach and humanely euthanized. On histopathology, free tachyzoites and tissue cysts compatible with *Toxoplasma gondii* were observed in the brain, heart, thymus, liver, lymph nodes and periumbilical adipose. The presence of *T. gondii* within host tissues was associated with lymphoplasmacytic inflammation and tissue necrosis. Brain immunohistochemistry revealed positive staining for tachyzoites and tissue cysts using antiserum raised to *T. gondii*, and parasite DNA was obtained from extracts of brain and muscle by PCR amplification using the diagnostic B1 locus. Transplacental toxoplasmosis was considered a potential cause of the observed brain malformation (Miller et al., 2008).

Recent cases observed at the Marine Mammal Center include kyphosis in an elephant seal and harbor seal pup (Figure 6.46a,b), kyphoscoliosis in a harbor porpoise fetus (Figure 6.46c,d), high

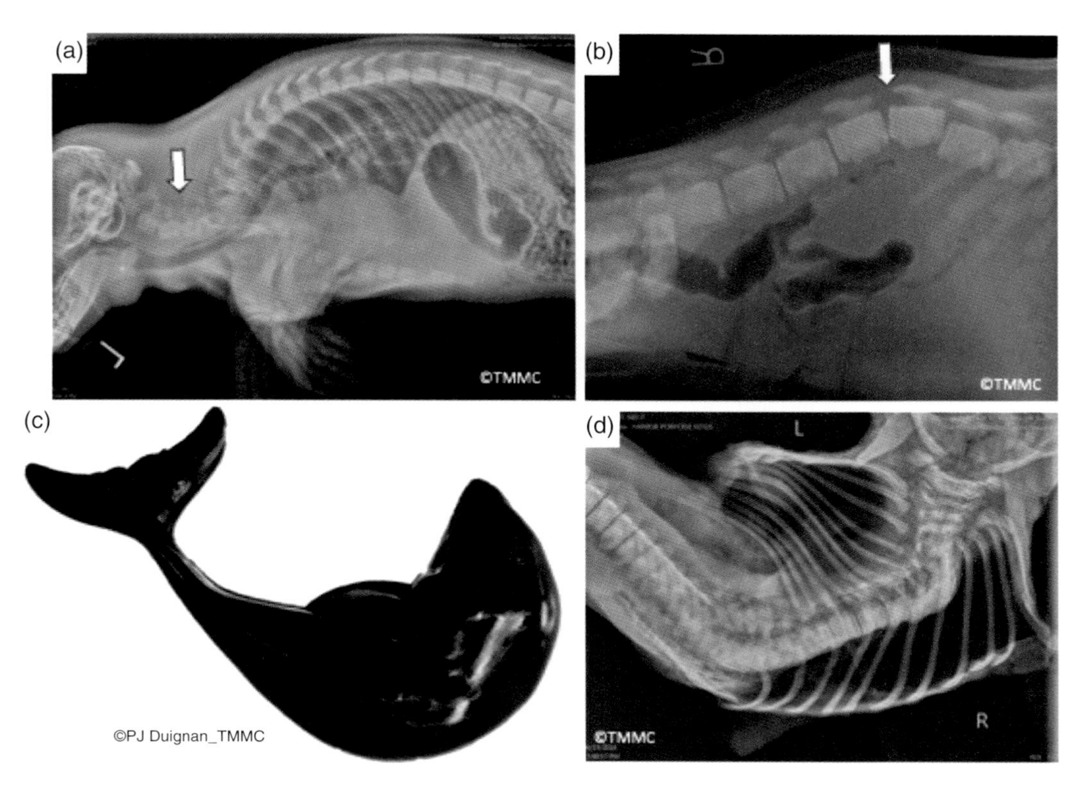

Figure 6.46 (a) Pacific harbor seal, pup, lateral thoracic radiograph showing cervical-thoracic kyphosis (arrow). (b) Northern elephant seal, pup, lateral abdominal radiograph showing lumbar kyphosis between L1 and L3 (arrow). (c) Harbor porpoise (HP), late term fetus, kyphoscoliosis. (d) HP, radiograph of (c), showing craniothoracic and thoracolumbar vertebral deformities.

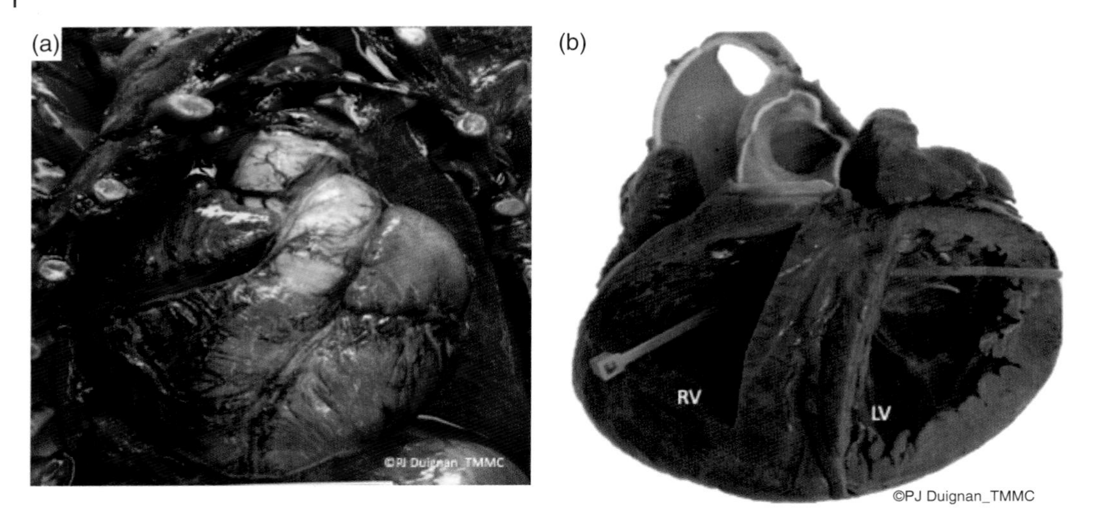

Figure 6.47 Northern elephant seal. (a) Heart with globoid dilated ventricles. (b) Heart as in (a) with ventricles opened to show a high ventricular septal defect between the two chambers. RV, right ventricle; LV, left ventricle.

septal defect in an elephant seal pup with right ventricular hypertrophy (Figure 6.47a,b), subaortic stenosis with distension of the aortic bulb, and left ventricular hypertrophy and dilation in a California sea lion (Figure 6.48), renal and adrenal cysts in a California sea lion (Figure 6.49), bronchial chondral hypoplasia in a harbor seal (Figure 6.50), and cerebellar hypoplasia in a harbor seal (Figure 6.51).

Diagnosis

Based on clinical presentation, age, diagnostic imaging, and necropsy.

Differential Diagnoses

Depending on the lesion location and severity in the affected organ, observed clinical signs may require consideration of infectious disease or trauma as differentials.

Treatment and Management

Treatment is not appropriate for free-living animals. For those in managed care, breeding programs should be reviewed to avoid transmission of potentially heritable defects.

Age-Related or Degenerative Pathology

Etiology, Host Factors, and Transmission

Geriatric disease and degenerative pathology of the cardiovascular system, teeth, bone and joints, and endocrine glands are observed in both free-living marine mammals and those in long-term managed care.

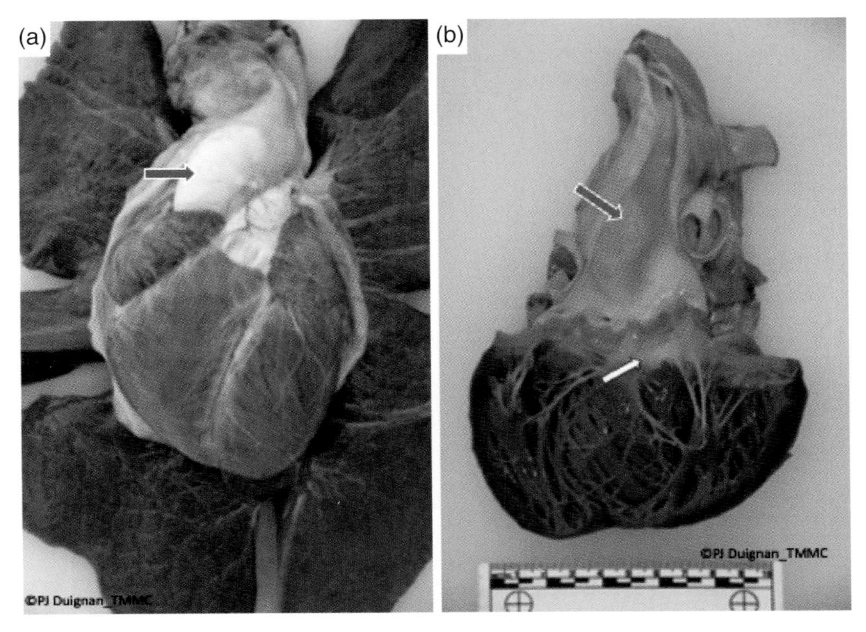

Figure 6.48 California seal lion, juvenile. (a) Heart showing a dilated aortic arch. (b) The left ventricle and aortic arch opened to show a thick band of white fibrous tissue (white arrow) below the aortic valves (causing of outflow stenosis), post-stenotic dilatation of the aorta (caused by turbulent flow) and aortic intimal thickening and corrugation (jet lesions, blue arrow). Upstream from the stenosis there is mild concentric hypertrophy of the left ventricular wall and marked dilatation of the chamber. These lesions are consistent with subaortic stenosis.

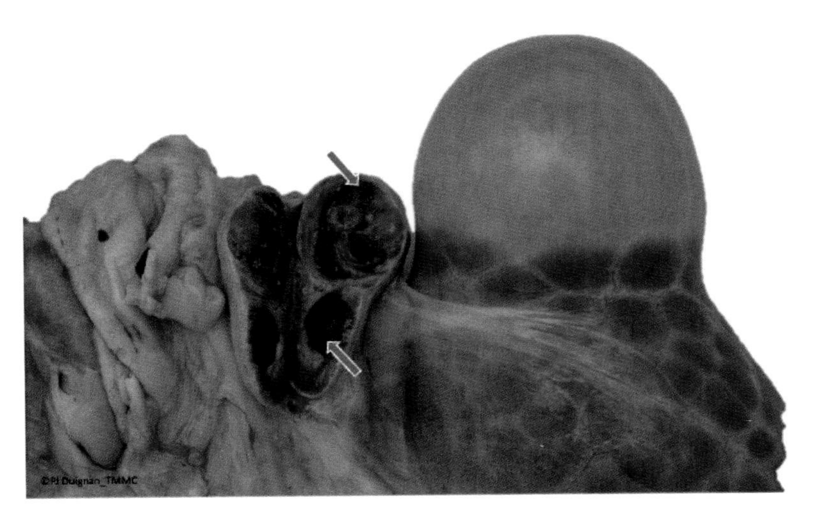

Figure 6.49 California sea lion, adult female, the kidney at right has a large fluid-filled cyst at the cranial pole. The adjacent adrenal gland has tan to brown masses (arrows) effacing most of the medulla (neoplasia; phaeochromocytoma).

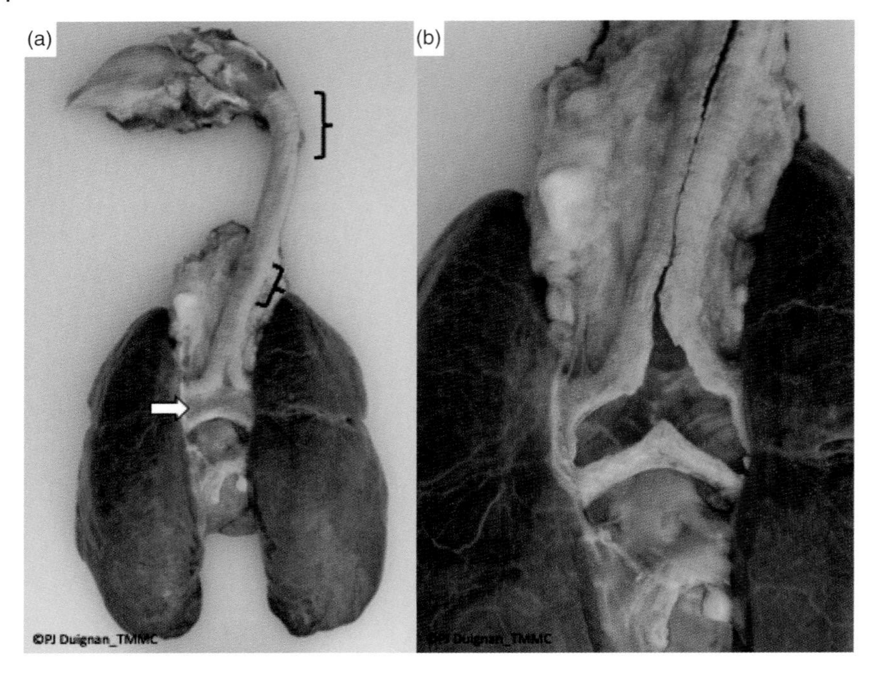

Figure 6.50 Pacific harbor seal, pluck. (a) There is mild stenosis of the trachea immediately caudal to the larynx, and at the thoracic inlet (brackets). At the level of the tracheal bifurcation the cartilage rings are incomplete dorsally (arrow), and this defect continues along both mainstem bronchi. The dorsoventrally flattened and collapsed distal trachea and bronchi are covered dorsally by a thin membrane that acted in a valve-like manner, causing respiratory stridor when the pup was alive. (b) The dorsal membrane has been resected to show the extent of the area that it covered for the mainstem bronchi.

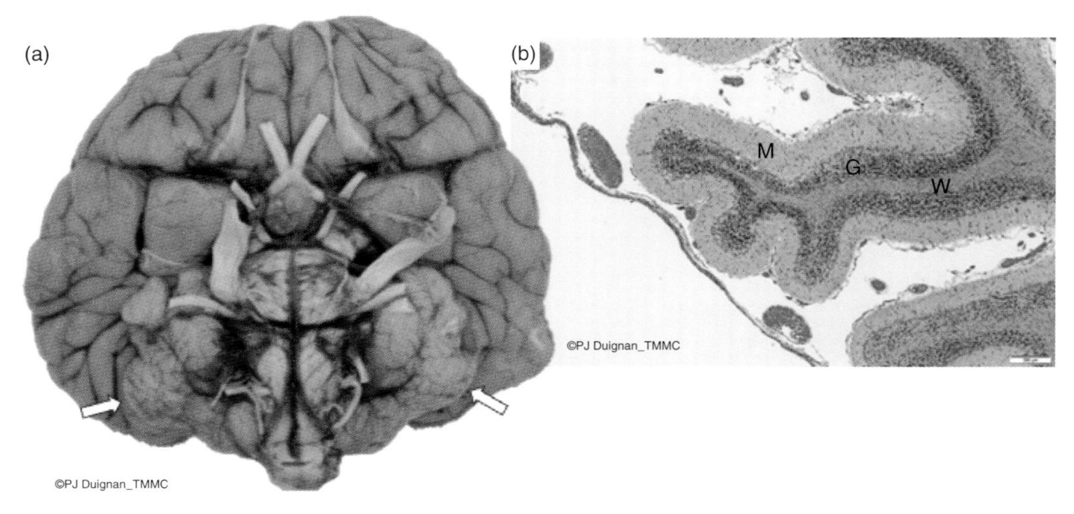

Figure 6.51 Pacific harbor seal. (a) brain ventral aspect, showing lateral cerebellar hemispheres that are approximately 40% smaller than normal (arrows delimit the lateral extremities). The vermis (not shown) was unaffected. Cerebellar hypoplasia. (b) Cerebellum, histopathology of the lateral hemisphere, showing marked hypoplasia of the cerebellar folia, with thinning of both the outer molecular layer (M) and the inner granular layer (G). This is the result of fewer than normal neurons and nuclei in this section. A reduced number of Purkinje cells is visible at the interface between the molecular and granular layers;the Purkinje cells that are present are irregularly spaced. (W, white matter tracts). H&E stain.

Clinical and Gross Signs

Cardiomyopathy and endocardiosis have been described in Florida manatees with histological changes that include cardiomyocyte degeneration, loss of striations, anisokaryosis, and karyomegaly (Bossart et al., 2004; Gerlach et al., 2012, Owen et al., 2012.). In sea otters, degenerative cardiomyopathy also occurs in older animals and endocardiosis of the atrioventricular valves may result in pulmonary or hepatic congestion and chronic fibrosis, depending on which valves are compromised (Figure 6.52).

Numerous other degenerative changes are reported, including periodontal disease, dental attrition, degenerative joint disease, fracture calluses, intervertebral disc disease, and baculum fractures, and digit luxations secondary to intraspecific fighting (Williams et al., 2018). Tooth wear appears to vary between individual otters and may reflect dietary preferences for hard shelled mollusks over softer-bodied prey items (Figure 6.53a). In a study of archival museum crania, approximately half of examined sea otters had significant dental attrition (Winer at al., 2013). In addition, 4% of examined otters had osteoarthritis of the temporomandibular joints, with 30% of these rated as severe (Arzi et al., 2013). However, the clinical significance of this for free-living sea otters is not known.

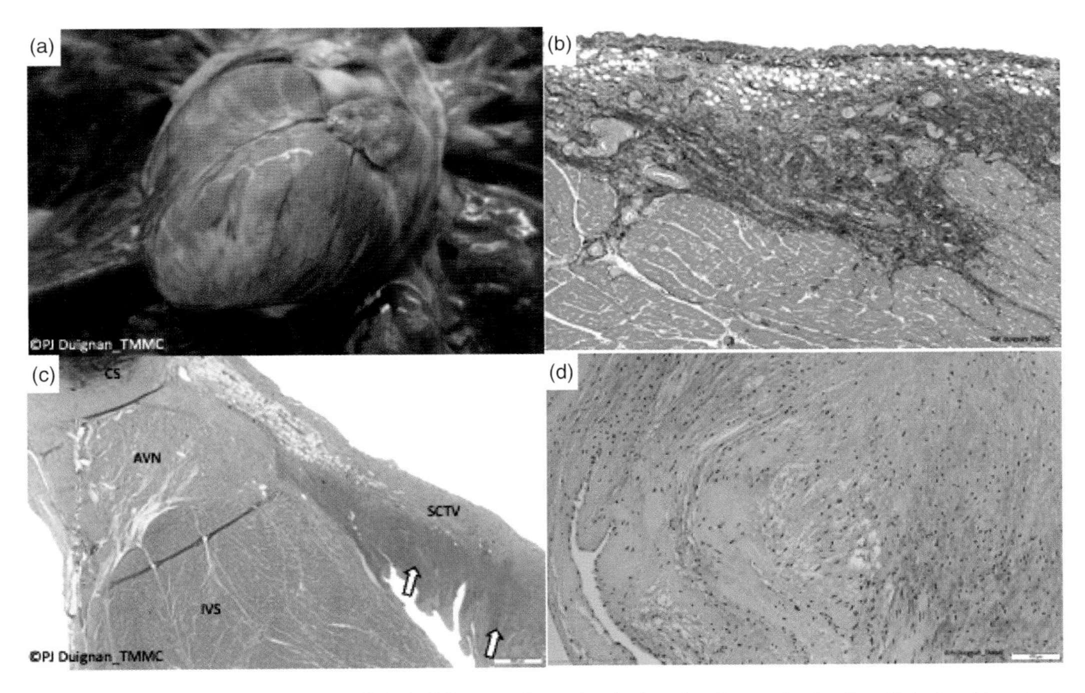

Figure 6.52 Southern sea otter, adult. (a) Heart, enlarged pale heart with marked epicardial streaking over both ventricles. The lungs are diffusely edematous. (b) Heart, histopathology, right ventricular free wall stained to show extensive myocardial fibrosis (blue) extending from the epicardium and in places, traversing the entire ventricular wall. Masson trichrome stain. (c) Heart, section through the right atrium, cardiac skeleton (CS, with cartilage), atrioventricular node, heart base, interventricular septum (IVS) and base of the septal cusp of the tricuspid valve (SCTV) to show marked nodular thickening of the ventricular face of the valve leaflet (endocardiosis), stained pale blue (arrows). (d) Heart, tricuspid valve, high power view showing nodular myxomatous degeneration (valvular endocardiosis) of the septal cusp of the valve that appears as pale blue fibrillar/wispy tissue with few nuclei and areas of vacuolation. H&E staining.

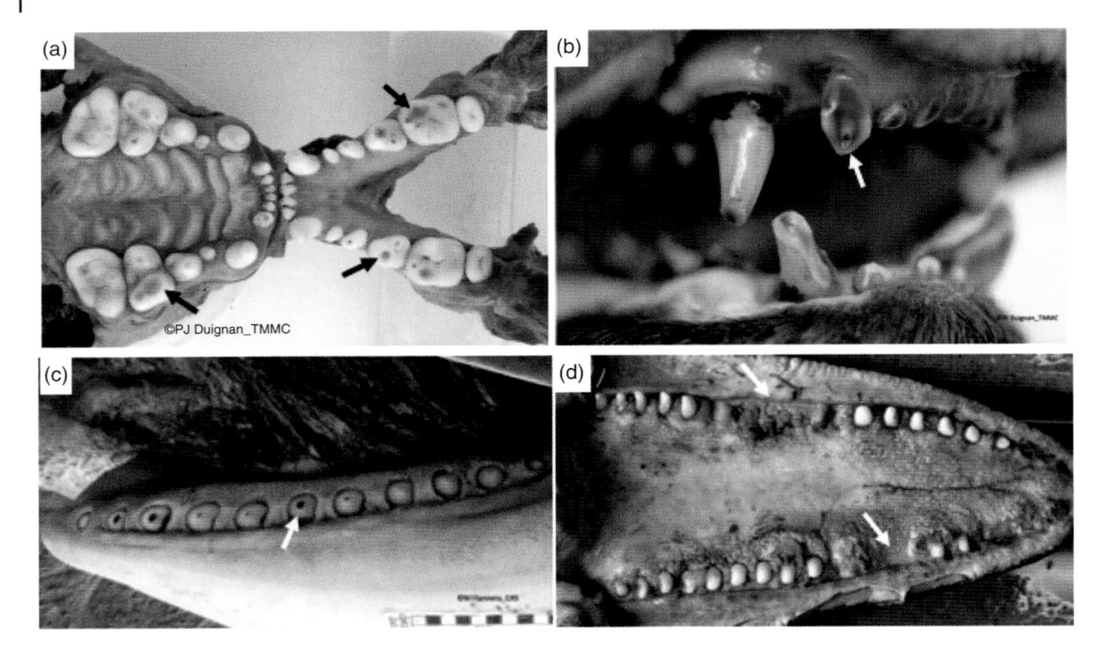

Figure 6.53 (a) Southern sea otter, maxillary and mandibular dental arcades, showing multiple caries-like lesions on the occlusal surfaces (arrows). (b) California sea lion, adult female, showing crown fractures on all four canine teeth and marked abrasion and attrition on the incisors, with exposure of the pulp canal (arrow) on multiple teeth. (c) Killer whale, *Orcinus orca*, subadult male, offshore ecotype. This ecotype of killer whale specializes in eating sharks. Note the extreme dental attrition (arrow) for a subadult animal. Specimen accession number CAS MAM 29219, M. Flannery, California Academy of Sciences, San Francisco, CA. USA. (d) Bottlenose dolphin, adult male, maxilla, showing chronic gingivitis leading to marked dental attrition and loss (arrows).

Dental attrition, fractures, gingivitis, alveolar osteomyelitis, and temporomandibular joint osteoarthritis are relatively common in pinnipeds (Figure 6.53b), (Abbott and Verstraete, 2005; Sinai et al., 2014; Aalderink et al., 2015a, b; Winer et al., 2016a) and polar bears (Winer et al., 2016b). As for sea otters, there appears to be marked individual variation in dental wear based on diet, age, and sex. In a large study of California sea lions, tooth loss, fractures, and dental attrition were more prevalent in males and older animals (Sinai et al., 2014). A similar study of northern elephant seals revealed fewer fractures, but almost half of examined skulls exhibited dental attrition and periodontal lesions in the maxilla or mandible (Abbott and Verstraete, 2005). Odontocetes have dental enamel only at the tip of the tooth crown, and it disappears by attrition with age, increasing their susceptibility to caries-like lesions and dental fractures (Cozzi et al., 2017). Free-living Amazon river dolphins (*Inia geoffrensis*) appear to be particularly susceptible to developing caries-like lesions for unknown reasons (Ness, 1966; Loch et al., 2011). As for pinnipeds, species, age, sex, dietary preference, and learned behavior play a role in determining odontocete dental pathology (Loch et al., 2011; Loch and Simões-Lopes, 2013). Killer whales and false killer whales that selectively prey on elasmobranchs with epidermal denticles are particularly prone to dental abrasion (Figure 6.53c; Ford et al., 2011; Tang et al., 2019). Chronic gingivitis and periodontal disease leading to alveolar osteomyelitis can result in secondary tooth loss in older dolphins (Figure 6.53d).

Degenerative changes have been noted in the endocrine glands of marine mammals. Cystic and adenomatous changes in the thyroids of bottlenose dolphins are regarded as incidental, geriatric changes (St. Leger et al., 2018). Cystic thyroid glands were frequently observed in New Zealand sea lions accidentally caught in fishing nets during the breeding and early lactation season, perhaps suggesting physiological associations (Duignan, personal communication). Similar thyroid changes are rarely observed in stranded adult female California sea lions necropsied at the Marine Mammal Center. In free-living beluga whales, in the St. Lawrence seaway, adenomatous changes correlated with age but again, the clinical significance is unknown (Lair et al., 2016). Adrenal gland hyperplasia, with or without cystic changes, is also common in beluga whales and may increase in prevalence with age; the enlargement can be diffuse or nodular and it generally affects zona fasciculata and zona glomerulosa, and occasionally medulla (Lair et al., 1997).

Diagnosis

Diagnosis is by observation of clinical signs and associated pathology in the context of age.

Differential Diagnoses

Similar pathology may occur as a consequence of chronic inflammation, trauma, diet, or parasitism.

Treatment and Management

For older animals in managed care, good primary care to prevent dental or gingival disease and to manage locomotor issues for animals with degenerative joint disease.

Nutritional and Metabolic Diseases

Etiology, Clinical and Gross Signs, Diagnosis

Malnutrition is a common but variable primary or contributory cause of stranding and death for aquatic mammals (Dailey et al., 2000; Siebert et al., 2001; Kreuder et al., 2003; Greig et al., 2005; Colegrove et al., 2005; Castinel et al., 2007b; Seguel et al., 2013). Malnutrition may result from maternal separation, poor prey availability (e.g. during unusual oceanic events like the El Nino/ Southern oscillation in the Pacific ocean), heavy parasitic burdens or other debilitating disease. Accurate assessment of nutritional status requires knowledge of species biology, migration patterns, breeding, lactation, and molting cycles, as all may influence body condition and may result in significant changes throughout the year.

Hepatic lipidosis is a common finding at necropsy and may be pathologic or physiological, as in young animals, where it reflects the high lipid intake in milk. Lipidosis may occur in stranded animals that are starving and mobilizing their remaining fat reserves or in animals with metabolic derangements caused by intoxication, nutritional deficiencies, or hypoxia.

Urolithiasis is seen in pinnipeds, cetaceans, and river otters. At the Marine Mammal Center, most uroliths tend to be a granular sludge of struvite (magnesium ammonium phosphate) combined with apatite (calcium hydroxyphosphate), located in the renal pelves, ureter, urinary bladder, or urethra (Figure 6.54).

Uroliths can cause obstruction with local urethral mucosal inflammation and hemorrhage. Because there is often bacterial infection (*Klebsiella oxytoca, Escherichia coli* or *Streptococcus phocae*) associated with the uroliths, ascending bacterial infection can lead to cystitis and pyelonephritis (Figure 6.55).

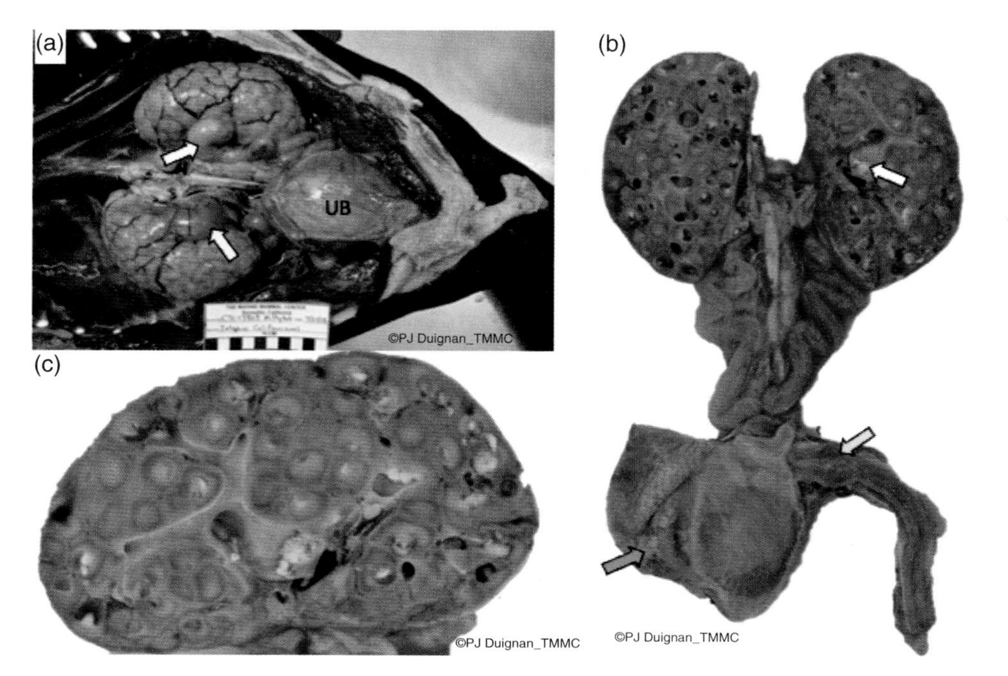

Figure 6.54 California sea lion, subadult male. (a) abdomen opened to show enlarged, pale kidneys, massively distended and tortuous ureters (hydroureter, arrows) and a distended urinary bladder (UB). (b) The urogenital tract has been removed and the kidneys sectioned in the sagittal plane to show dilated, urine-filled pelves (hydronephrosis) and multifocal deposits of white granular material (uroliths, white arrow). The bladder mucosa is thickened and necrotic and is covered by a fibrinous mat (necrotizing fibrinous cystitis, blue arrow); this lesion extends along the entire urethra, which was partially obstructed by uroliths (yellow arrow). (c) Kidney, expanded renal pelves containing yellow/white nephroliths.

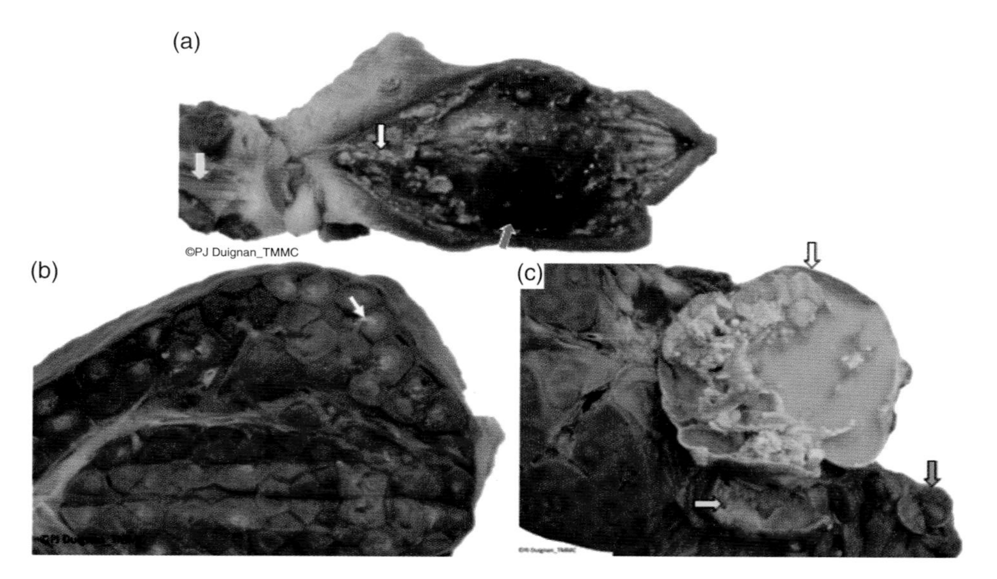

Figure 6.55 Harbor porpoise. (a) Urinary bladder, necrotizing and hemorrhagic cystitis. The trigone is filled with granular debris (white arrow) while the mid and apical mucosa is hemorrhagic (red arrow). The urethra is unaffected (yellow arrow). (b) Kidney from the same animal as (a). Sagittal section to show multiple white concretions (nephroliths) in the renal pelves (arrow). (c) California sea lion, kidneys. The kidney on the left is normal, but the parenchyma of the right kidney (white arrow) has completely atrophied, leaving a connective tissue capsule and some stroma filled with purulent exudate and urine. Below the atrophied kidney, the ureter (yellow arrow) is also dilated and filled with fluid and caseous exudate. Adrenal gland (blue arrow).

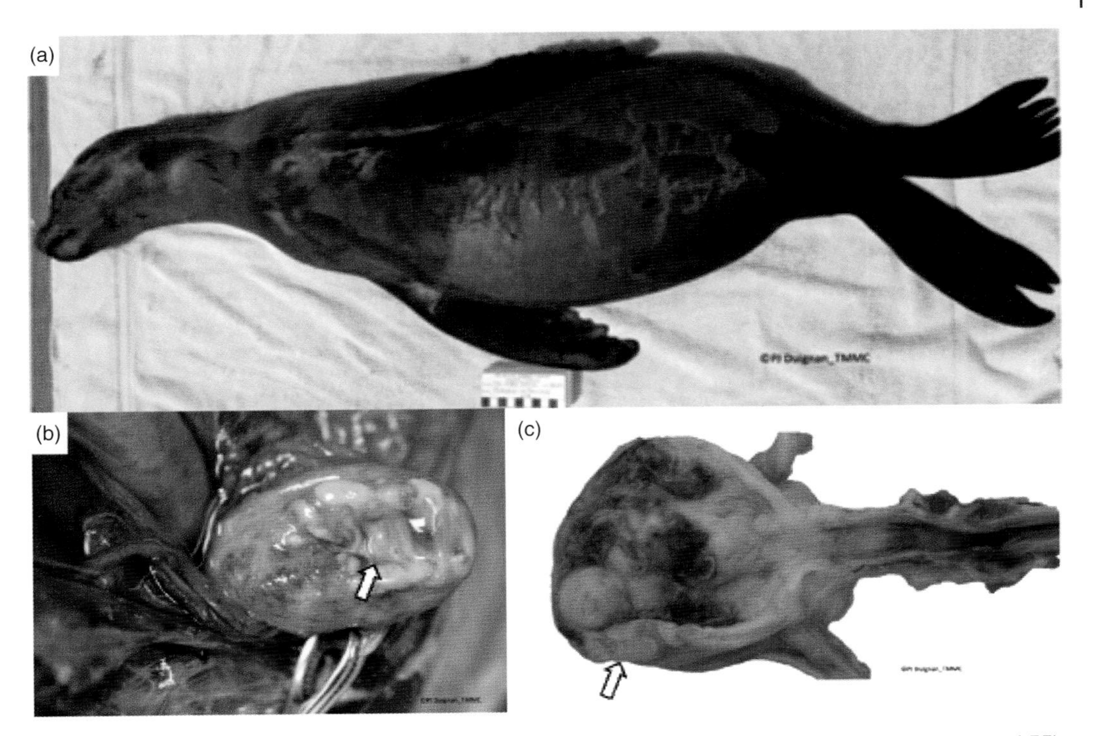

Figure 6.56 California sea lion, adult female. (a) Markedly distended abdomen (compare with Figure 6.33). In this case, the abdomen was filled with urine (uroabdomen). (b) Urinary bladder from (a) in situ showing suppurative transmural necrosis at the apex (arrow). (c) Urinary bladder opened to show necrotizing cystitis affecting the apical half of the organ and transmural necrosis at the point of rupture (arrow).

Complete urethral obstruction or transmural cystitis can result in rupture of the urinary bladder and uroabdomen (uroperitoneum), usually with fatal consequences (Figure 6.56).

Dolphins in managed care can develop uroliths secondary to diets causing urine acidification and high concentrations of excreted purines that can result in supersaturation of sparingly soluble ammonium urate salts (Smith et al., 2014). Advanced cases may present with hematuria and lower tract obstruction, leading to hydroureter, hydronephrosis, cystitis, and renal failure.

Cold stress syndrome is a range of clinical presentations in Florida manatees or dugongs in Australia exposed to water below 20°C, which can result in death (Bossart et al., 2004; Owen et al., 2013). On gross examination, there is emaciation, atrophy of the adipose tissue, an empty upper gastrointestinal tract, and impaction of dry feces in the colon (constipation) due to dehydration. The skin is often hyperkeratotic and fissured, and there may be multifocal ulceration. Secondary bacterial invasion may result in abscesses or pyoderma. On histology, there can be lymphoid depletion and myocardial degeneration, bronchopneumonia, enteritis, and hepatic and pancreatic atrophy, all of which indicate metabolic collapse and immune suppression leading to terminal septicemia or cardiorespiratory failure.

End lactation syndrome in sea otters is characterized by moderate to severe emaciation not attributable to a concurrent, independent disease process, in females dying during late lactation or post-weaning (Figure 6.57) (Chinn et al., 2016). It is a metabolic condition that has been defined for southern sea otters in California, but it could also apply to the northern subspecies; it

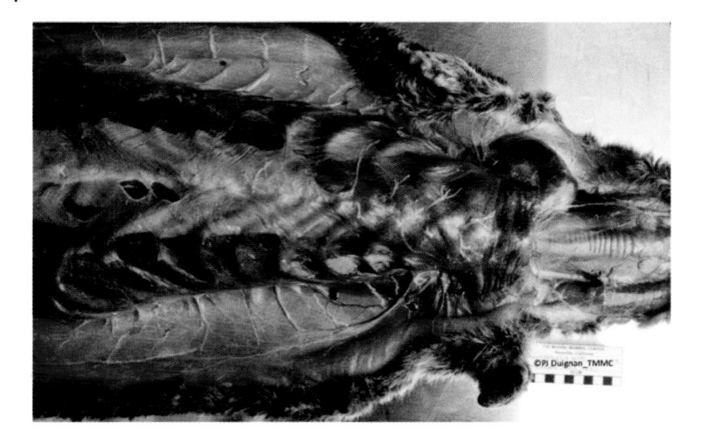

Figure 6.57 Southern sea otter, adult female. The pelt is reflected to show marked generalized atrophy of subcutaneous adipose tissue and generalized atrophy of skeletal muscle. End lactation syndrome.

occurs in relation to the extremely high energetic requirements for sea otters that almost double during pregnancy and lactation. In the above cited study, the researchers tracked a total of 108 adult or aged adult female otters during the period 2005–2012. Over this time, 56% died as a result of end lactation syndrome, with significant risk factors, including the time of year (late spring, the far end of the peak reproductive period for southern sea otters), increased age, and multiparous females. Most animals died during late pup care or immediately post-weaning, with the greatest drop in body condition occurring between early and late pup rearing. The physiology of southern sea otters exacerbates the syndrome in that once sexually mature, females are almost always either pregnant or lactating, with only a brief period during delayed implantation, to recover body condition. Mating is also characterized by aggressive and energetically demanding male behavior.

However, females are not without strategies to optimize reproduction and survival. The first half of the sea otter reproductive cycle (delayed implantation through parturition) appears to be geared toward preloading energy reserves to optimize survival and reproductive success during the extremely metabolically demanding period of pup care that follows. When faced with suboptimal environmental or physiologic conditions, females may reset the timing and energetic demands of reproduction through a prolonged period of delayed implantation, fetal loss, pup abandonment or early weaning. Older females tend to complete pup rearing despite poor nutritional condition, perhaps due to declining reproductive longevity, possibly explaining why end lactation syndrome frequency is highest in older females and those with the most prior pregnancies. Diagnosis of the syndrome requires characterization of the stage of the reproductive cycle, assessment of adipose stores, previous reproductive history (counts of corpora albicantia on ovaries), and environmental conditions.

Treatment and Management

For free-living marine mammals that strand with malnutrition, supportive care with species-appropriate nutrition is sufficient. Urolithiasis is rarely diagnosed antemortem in stranded animals, but for managed care dolphins or pinnipeds, early diagnosis and diet modification are possible.

Miscellaneous Diseases

Amyloidosis

Etiology, Clinical and Gross Signs, Diagnosis

Amyloidosis was first reported in bottlenose dolphins stranded on the Texas coast, in the Gulf of Mexico (Cowan, 1995). In this study, 4 of 21 (19%) necropsied animals were found to have systemic AA amyloid indicative of chronic illness. Amyloid was mostly deposited in the corticomedullary junctions of the kidneys and around blood vessels in the spleen, lungs, myocardium, and acini of the thyroid and salivary glands. Systemic amyloidosis has also been reported for adult Stejneger's beaked whales stranded in the Sea of Japan, with heavy parasite burdens that probably acted as a source of chronic immune stimulation (Tajima et al., 2007, 2015).

In pinnipeds, amyloidosis has been reported in California sea lions with a systemic distribution, primarily involving the kidneys, blood vessels, and thyroid glands (Colegrove et al., 2009). On gross examination, affected kidneys have striking pallor of the cortex and cortico-medullary junction (Figure 6.58). The principal differential diagnosis for this appearance is leptospirosis (compare with Figure 6.22b). However, the histologic lesion is distinct and is characterized by bland pale eosinophilic amorphous deposits in the glomeruli, around blood vessels and in peritubular interstitium of the cortex and corticomedullary junction. Based on biochemistry and immunohistochemistry, the deposited amyloid is type A, and in affected animals, serum amyloid A concentrations are high (;ess than 1200 μg/ml), when compared with results from unaffected sea lions (less than 10 μg/ml).

Treatment and Management

Advanced renal amyloidosis can result in progressive renal failure (azotemia and uremia) for which there is only supportive care for animals in captivity. Most cases are diagnosed postmortem. Associations with chronic illness, such as infectious diseases or parasitism, suggest that good preventive medicine and husbandry reduce the risk of developing amyloidosis.

Gastrointestinal Ulceration

Etiology, Clinical and Gross Signs, Diagnosis

Perforating pyloric and duodenal ulcers in California sea lions are a common cause of sudden death in malnourished yearlings and, occasionally, in older animals. This condition can also be

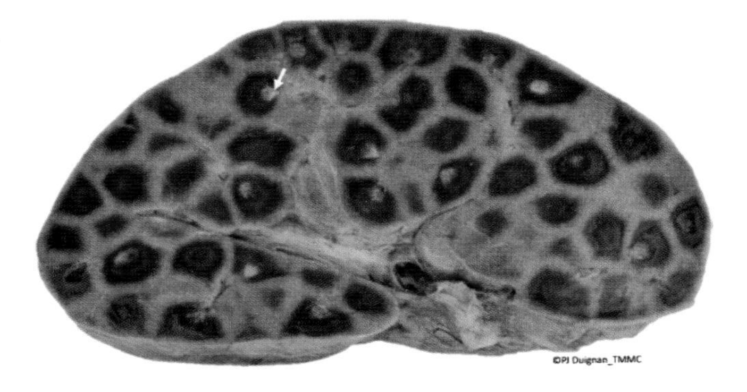

Figure 6.58 California sea lion, male. Enlarged kidney with expanded tan cortices contrasting with the normal color of the medullae. Amyloidosis. Some of the renal pelves are streaked white (mineralization, arrow).

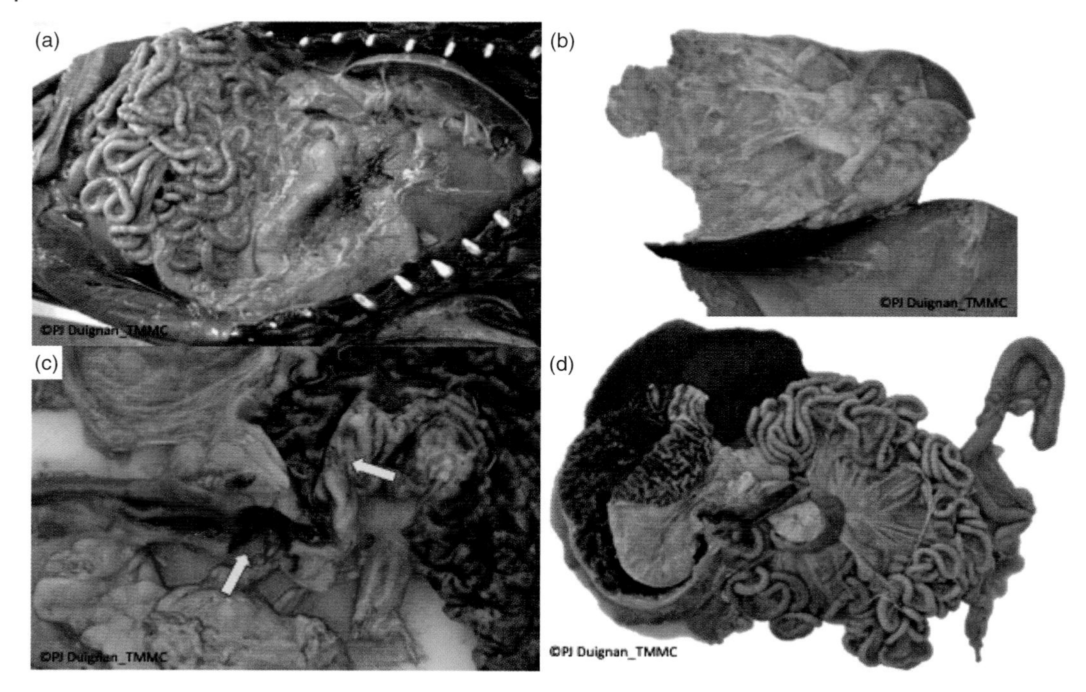

Figure 6.59 California sea lion. (a) Abdominal cavity, fibrinous peritonitis and omentitis. (b) California sea lion as in (a), liver excised, showing thick layer of fibrin loosely attached to the capsule. (c) Stomach of (a), pylorus and proximal duodenum excised and opened to show black coffee-grounds gastric content (digested blood) and perforating pyloric and duodenal ulcers (arrows). (d) Gastrointestinal tract removed and stomach opened along the greater curvature to show the severity of gastric hemorrhage (black fluid is digested blood).

more insidious, resulting in chronic blood loss, melena, anemia, and gradual decline (Figure 6.59). There is no specific association with helminth parasitism or bacterial infection, and histology reveals necrosis and inflammation at the site of perforation. These ulcers may be related to altered gastric emptying in malnourished animals and acid hypersecretion (Zabka et al., 2005). Hemorrhagic gastric ulcers resulting in melena are also common in stranded sea otters, but they are rarely associated with gastric perforation.

Treatment and Management

H2 receptor antagonists (famotidine, ranitidine, and cimetidine) are effective in treating or preventing gastric ulceration in mammals (Scarpignato et al., 1987). In California sea lions at the Marine Mammal Center, famotidine is used for pinnipeds at 0.5 mg/kg IM or PO twice daily; California sea lions have also been treated with cimetidine (5 mg/kg PO) and ranitidine (1.5 mg/kg PO twice daily). Famotidine is also used to treat sea otters (0.5 mg/kg IM or SQ) and odontocete cetaceans (0.5 mg/kg IM every 24 hours twice daily) with gastritis and gastric ulcers.

Cardiomyopathy

Etiology, Clinical and Gross Signs, Diagnosis

Cardiomyopathy of kogiids (pygmy and dwarf sperm whales) was first described from the western Atlantic (Bossart et al., 1985). It is also seen in pygmy sperm whales stranded on the California

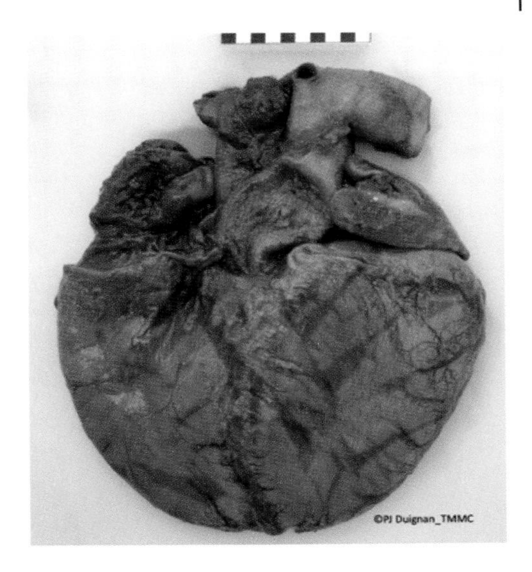

Figure 6.60 Pygmy sperm whale, adult male, heart, cardiomyopathy with large pale flaccid ventricles. Color patterns are an artifact of storage.

coast (Figure 6.60). It is most common in older animals and males. Case review found that the associated myocardial degeneration is progressive, advancing to biventricular dilated cardiomyopathy over time (Bossart et al., 2007). Grossly, the hearts are large and globoid, with a thin, flaccid appearance of the ventricular free walls and interventricular septum. On histology, myocardial degeneration progresses to atrophy. Attempted cardiomyocyte regeneration is characterized by foci of anisokaryosis and nuclear rowing. Interstitial edema is replaced by fibrosis and, occasionally, mononuclear myocarditis. Pulmonary and hepatic congestion occur secondary to cardiac insufficiency.

Cardiomyopathy is the third most common cause of morbidity and mortality in free-ranging southern sea otters, but it is less commonly reported in the northern subspecies (Kreuder et al., 2005; Miller et al., 2020b). Grossly affected otters have an enlarged angular or cubic heart typical of dilated cardiomyopathy, with a mottled orange-brown myocardium (Figure 6.61). On histology, there is myocardial degeneration and replacement fibrosis, often accompanied by a mild lymphocytic to pleocellular infiltrate. Exposure to the algal bloom toxin domoic acid is a significant risk factor for development of dilated cardiomyopathy in otters (Kreuder et al., 2005). In one study, cardiomyopathy was a primary cause of death for 8% (44/560) of examined otters and a primary or contributing cause of death for 41% (229/552; Miller et al., 2020b). Significant risk factors for fatal cardiomyopathy in the same study included being adults or aged adults (11.48 times higher risk) and concurrent diagnosis of probable domoic acid intoxication (4.64 times higher risk), *T. gondii* infection (2.31 times higher risk) or *S. neurona* infection (1.91 times higher risk). This condition in sea otters has many similarities to the cardiomyopathy of domoic acid-exposed California sea lions (see section above on domoic acid toxicosis).

Dermatitis in Northern Elephant Seals

Etiology, Clinical and Gross Signs, Diagnosis

Northern elephant skin disease is a manifestation of chronic ulcerative and pustular dermatitis in molting northern elephant seals, usually yearlings and juveniles (Beckmen et al., 1997). It was a common cause of admission of elephant seals to California rehabilitation centers in the 1980s and

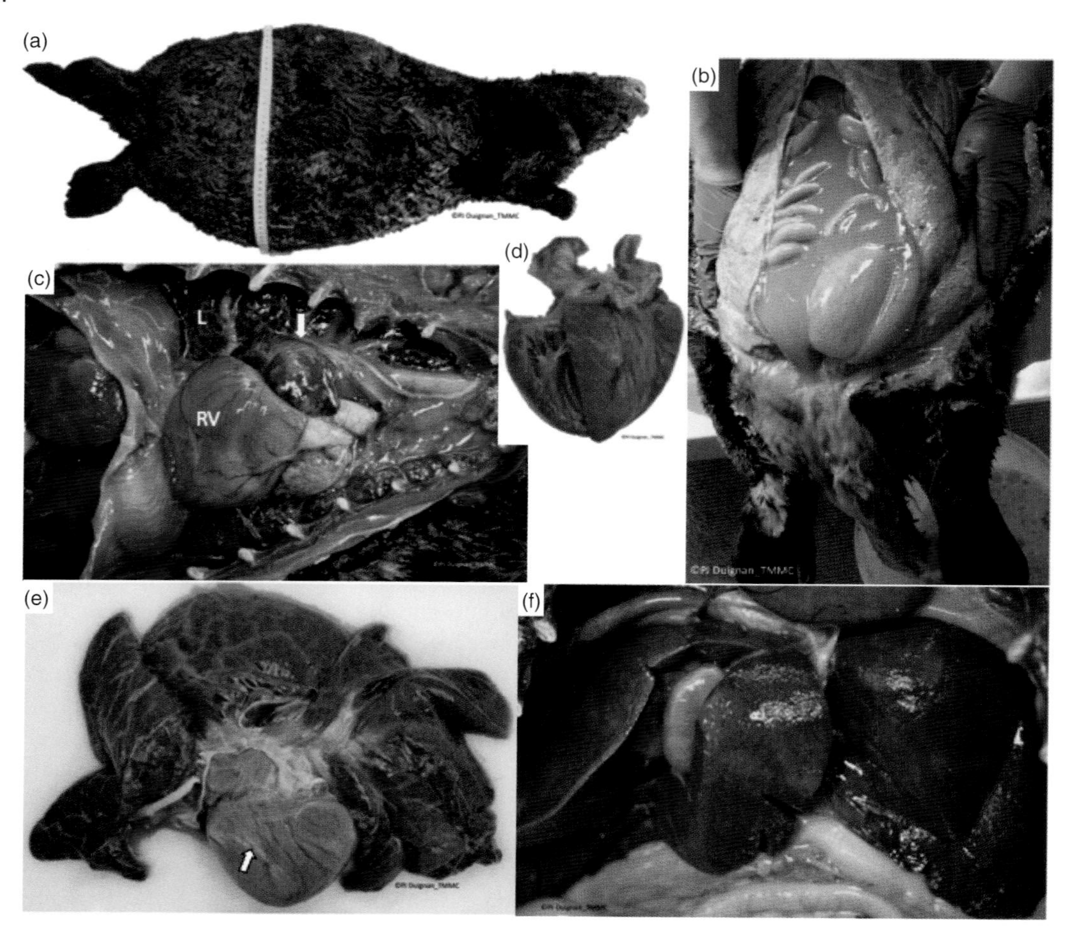

Figure 6.61 Southern sea otter, adult female. (a) Markedly distended abdomen. Main differentials in this case would be cardiomyopathy with heart failure leading to ascites, hepatopathy, dystocia, septic peritonitis and coccidioidomycosis. (b) Abdomen opened to release a large volume of opaque pink ascites. (c) Heart in situ, the heart is enlarged and angular or cubic with markedly dilated right atrium (arrow) and ventricle (RV). The lungs (L) are diffusely edematous and the liver is congested. (d) The excised heart is diffusely pale with white streaks in the ventricular myocardium. (e) The pluck excised to show the dilated pale heart with white epicardial streaking (arrow). The lungs are diffusely congested and edematous with marked distension of interlobular septae. (f) The liver is enlarged, rounded and dark, with a rough cobblestone surface (Morocco leather texture). The green/yellow structure is the distended gall bladder.

1990s, but it has only been seen sporadically since then. The gross appearance varied markedly, from focal alopecia and hyperpigmentation with multifocal ulceration to locally extensive epidermal necrosis. The animals are usually severely dehydrated and emaciated. Microscopically, there is hyperkeratosis, ulceration, squamous metaplasia of sebaceous ducts and atrophy of the glands, and surface proliferation of different microorganisms, including bacteria, fungi, and algae (Figure 6.62). Hematology and serum chemistry are indicative of stress, and in some cases septicemia. Beckmen at al. (1997) discounted hypothyroidism, vitamin A deficiency, genetic predisposition, and specific pathogens in the etiology of this condition. However, serum concentrations of PCBs (e.g. DDT and DDE) were elevated relative to age-matched controls. This group of lipophilic

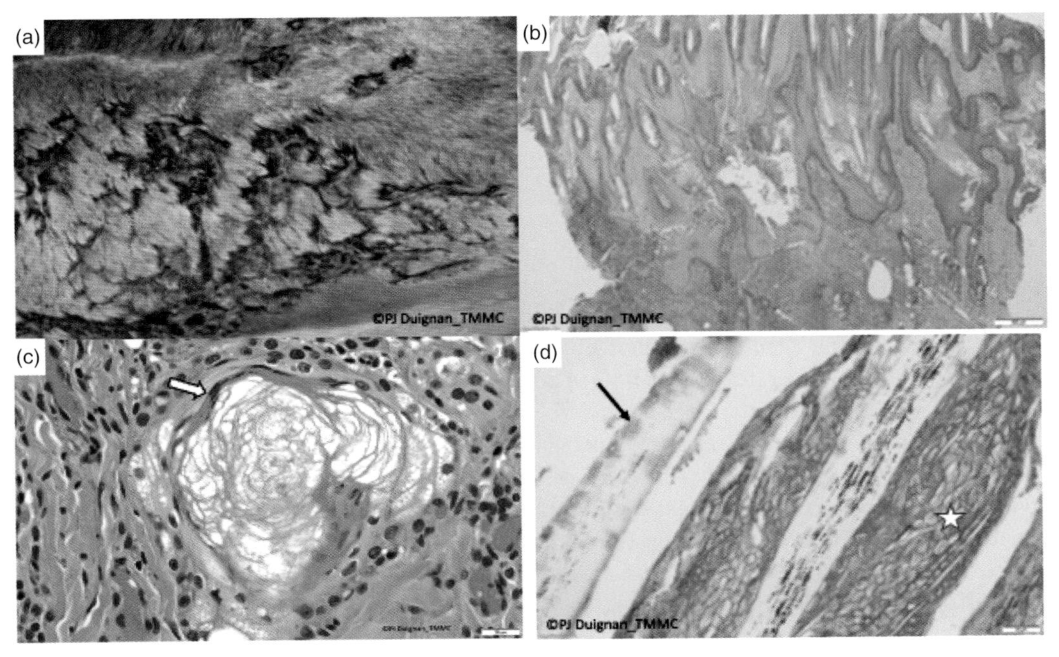

Figure 6.62 Northern elephant seal, yearling. (a) Skin on the flank showing multifocal deep ulcers and fissures with superficial suppurative exudate. Northern elephant seal skin disease. (b) Skin, histopathology, low power view showing hyperkeratosis, acanthosis, follicular keratitis, squamous metaplasia of sebaceous ducts and marked superficial dermatitis. H&E stain. (c) Skin, higher magnification view of a sebaceous gland characterized by atrophy and squamous metaplasia (arrow). H&E stain. (d) Skin, two adjacent hair shafts shown at high magnification; dense mats of periodic acid–Schiff positive fungal hyphae encircle one hair shaft (star) while the cortex of the other shaft has a scalloped appearance, associated with bacterial colonization (arrow).

persistent organic pollutants can concentrate in marine food webs and interfere with thyroid hormone homeostasis. While the hyperplastic changes seen on microscopy are nonspecific, squamous metaplasia of sebaceous ducts was observed. Transformation of sebaceous glands into sebaceous cysts is pathognomonic in people and other mammals with confirmed exposure to polyhalogenated aromatic hydrocarbons. Although these results are not definitive, they suggest a potential role for polyhalogenated aromatic hydrocarbon exposure.

Treatment and Management

Severe cases of northern elephant seal skin disease usually have a variety of bacteria associated with the skin ulceration; antimicrobial therapy may be warranted, together with fluid therapy and parenteral nutrition.

Alopecia in Pinnipeds and Polar Bears

Etiology, Clinical and Gross Signs, Diagnosis

Alopecia (focal hair thinning and loss) has been observed in several species of free-living marine mammals including northern elephant seals (see above), Australian fur seals, southern sea lions, gray seals, ringed seals, Pacific walrus, and polar bears (Beckmen et al., 1997; Lynch et al., 2011c; Pistorius and Baylis, 2011; Atwood et al., 2015; Pugliares-Bonner et al., 2018). Alopecia has also been observed in California sea lions, Guadalupe fur seals, northern fur seals, harbor seals, and a ribbon seal (Duignan et al., 2018b). In some studies, alopecia has been associated with elevated concentrations of PCBs (Beckmen et al. 1997), while in others, it has been attributed to nutrient deficiencies (Trites and Donnelly, 2003), ectoparasites (Dailey, 2001; McHuron et al., 2013; Javeed et al., 2021), or fungi (Guillot et al., 1998). However, in many cases the causative agent remains unknown.

Alopecia is of concern for marine mammals, such as fur seals and polar bears, which depend on a thick fur coat and blubber for insulation, but probably less so for phocids or walruses, which rely more exclusively on blubber. Polar bears experience marked temperature differences between Arctic water and air as they travel and forage on sea ice. Individuals with alopecia may have difficulty maintaining adequate thermoregulation and require additional energy to maintain a constant core body temperature. The elevated energy demands on alopecic animals could have an adverse effect on body condition and survival.

Since 1989, a syndrome has been recognized in Australian fur seals on islands off the southeast of the continent that manifests as bilaterally symmetrical alopecia. It occurs predominantly in juveniles, and it has a strong sex bias toward females (Lynch et al., 2011c). It also occurs in adult females but has never been seen in postpubescent males. The prevalence is highest in one colony (approximately 30,000 fur seals) in the northwestern Bass Strait, where a distinct seasonal pattern is noted; cases peak in spring and summer, with up to 50% of juvenile females affected. Thermal images indicated that alopecic and normal areas of the dorsal thorax had a mean difference of 6.6°C, and affected animals were in significantly poorer body condition than unaffected animals. While the etiology remains elusive, the condition occurs in fur seals at specific locations, but not at rookeries greater than 300 km distant, suggesting involvement of an unknown factor that is intrinsic to the environment of the NW Bass Straits.

Since the late 1990s, focally symmetrical alopecia of the head, neck, and shoulders has been reported for polar bears of the southern Beaufort sea (Atwood et al., 2015). Since polar bears rely on a thick blubber layer and a dense hair coat for insulation, this finding raised concerns of increased energy demands and potential for mortality. The lesions were characterized by guard hair loss and thinning of the underfur, with exudation and crusting of the skin surface; affected bears were thinner than controls without alopecia. Males were more likely to be affected than females and affected animals had reduced body weight. However, it is not known whether the reduced weight was due to increased energetic demands or an underlying disease process. To date, the etiology of alopecia in this species is unknown.

Since mid-2011, overlapping spatially and temporally with the polar bear alopecia events, increased sightings of alopecia in northern phocids (ringed, spotted, bearded and ribbon seals) and walrus has been recorded. An unusual mortality event was declared in December 2011, and it continued through 2016. A second unusual mortality event was declared during 2018– 020 (NOAA Fisheries, 2022). Affected seals were sometimes found dead, but more often they were reported by subsistence hunters in Alaska or Arctic Canada. There were two primary gross presentations in ice seals. In the first, the animals were in excellent body condition, with no indication of disease other than hair loss. The second presentation involved systemic illness, with ulcerative dermatitis, and often, signs of septicemia. Extensive diagnostic and environmental testing failed to identify a common etiology or pathogenesis. In 2017, a ribbon seal with extensive alopecia, but otherwise in good body condition, stranded in central California (Figure 6.63a,b,d,e,f). It matched the first type case definition described above for the unusual mortality event in ice seals; histological findings in the skin were also similar, with superficial scalloping of the remaining hair shafts (trichilemmal keratolysis) associated with a halophilic bacterium, that may be a commensal and not a primary

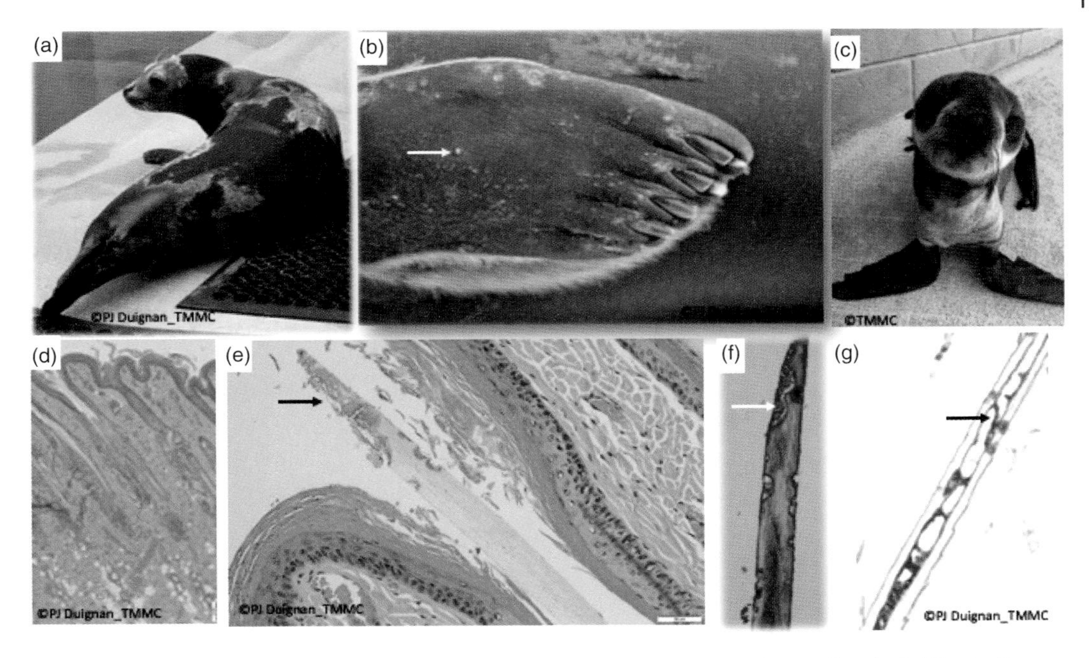

Figure 6.63 (a) Ribbon seal (*Histriophoca fasciata*) Arctic phocid extralimital stranding in California. Note the extensive alopecia (as indicated by black skin). (b) Ribbon seal, pectoral flipper close-up to show alopecia and comedones (skin nodules, arrow). (c) Northern fur seal, *Callorhinus ursinus*, pup with extensive loss of dark brown guard hairs, revealing the tan underfur. (d) Ribbon seal skin biopsy from area of alopecia, showing no significant inflammation or follicular atrophy. H&E staining. (e) High power view of a follicular ostium showing a fractured hair shaft with a scalloped cortical surface associated with adherent bacteria or possible fungi (arrow). H&E staining. (f) Ribbon seal hair shaft stained with Gram stain, showing clusters of bacteria in the excavated cortex (arrow). (g) Fur seal hair showing fungus-like hyphal structures in the cortex of the hair (arrow). periodic acid–Schiff staining.

pathogen (Duignan et al., 2018b). In this case, the etiology was suggestive of a telogen defluxion, as described in humans or terrestrial mammals subjected to an acute stressor or systemic illness. Similar guard hair degradation has been observed in stranded northern fur seals and Guadalupe fur seals at the Marine Mammal Center (Figure 6.63c,g).

Treatment and Management

The etiology of alopecia in phocids, fur seals, and polar bears is still under investigation; no defined treatment or management protocols are currently in effect.

Freshwater Skin Disease

Etiology, Host Factors, and Transmission

Freshwater skin disease is a syndrome observed in coastal or estuarine cetaceans exposed to a sudden, profound and prolonged drop in salinity (from greater than 30 ppt to less than 5 ppt), usually following fresh water influx from flooding or storm events (Duignan et al., 2020). It may also occur in cetaceans that swim up-river of their own volition or become trapped in fresh water following a hurricane, cyclone, or a similar event (Gulland et al., 2008; Mullin et al., 2015). This is an emerging condition that is likely linked to climate change.

Clinical and Gross Signs

In the acute stages, freshwater skin disease is characterized by a change of color with dull white to pale patches occurring extensively over the epidermis. If the animal remains in hyposaline water, this progresses to cell rupture, ulceration, and invasion by opportunistic pathogens (Figure 6.64a,b,c). The compromised epidermis at any stage may be overgrown by algal mats, resulting in green to orange discoloration (Figure 6.64d). Acute changes on histology include swelling or ballooning of cells in the stratum spinosum (reversible hydropic degeneration; Figure 6.64e). Rake marks (epidermal tooth marks from conspecifics) may act as points of entry for the hyposaline water. For many dolphins, secondary pathogen invasion leads to pustular dermatitis with deep ulceration and may progress to systemic infection and death (Figure 6.64f). In addition to dermatitis and secondary infection, serum electrolyte imbalances may occur, including decreased osmolarity and reduced sodium and chloride, associated with overhydration due to increased transcutaneous water absorption and solute loss (Ewing et al., 2017; McClain et al., 2020). Corneal opacity (edema) has also been observed in dolphins residing in hyposaline waters for prolonged periods or in dolphins rescued from freshwater habitats (Deming et al., 2020).

Diagnosis

Diagnosis is based on the clinical presentation, clinical history, and lesions, in combination with the ambient conditions where the affected animals were found.

Differentials

Ultraviolet (UV) exposure, dermatitis, or systemic infection in immunocompromised animals (e.g. morbillivirus infection) should be considered.

Treatment and Management

Where possible, return out-of-habitat cetaceans to normal osmolarity seawater and provide supportive care for animals with advanced lesions.

Ultraviolet Irradiation (Sunburn)

Etiology, Host Factors, and Transmission

Sunburn can occur in stranded cetaceans and animals housed in pools without shade cover.

Clinical and Gross Signs

As with terrestrial mammals, the first indication is epidermal edema, followed by superficial epidermal sloughing and ulceration, as the basal layers of the epidermis are killed by UV irradiation. Degeneration of cells in the stratum spinosum includes individual cell contraction and dissociation (Martinez-Levasseur et al., 2011). The effects of UV irradiation are exacerbated by dehydration and skin desiccation, resulting in degeneration, fragmentation, and lifting of external layers of the stratum spinosum. In severe cases, the entire epidermis can slough, exposing congested, hemorrhagic, and edematous dermis. Remarkably, if the insult is removed, the animal can make a full recovery by epidermal migration with minimal scar formation.

Diagnosis

The stranding history or husbandry conditions should be considered, together with the gross appearance of the lesions.

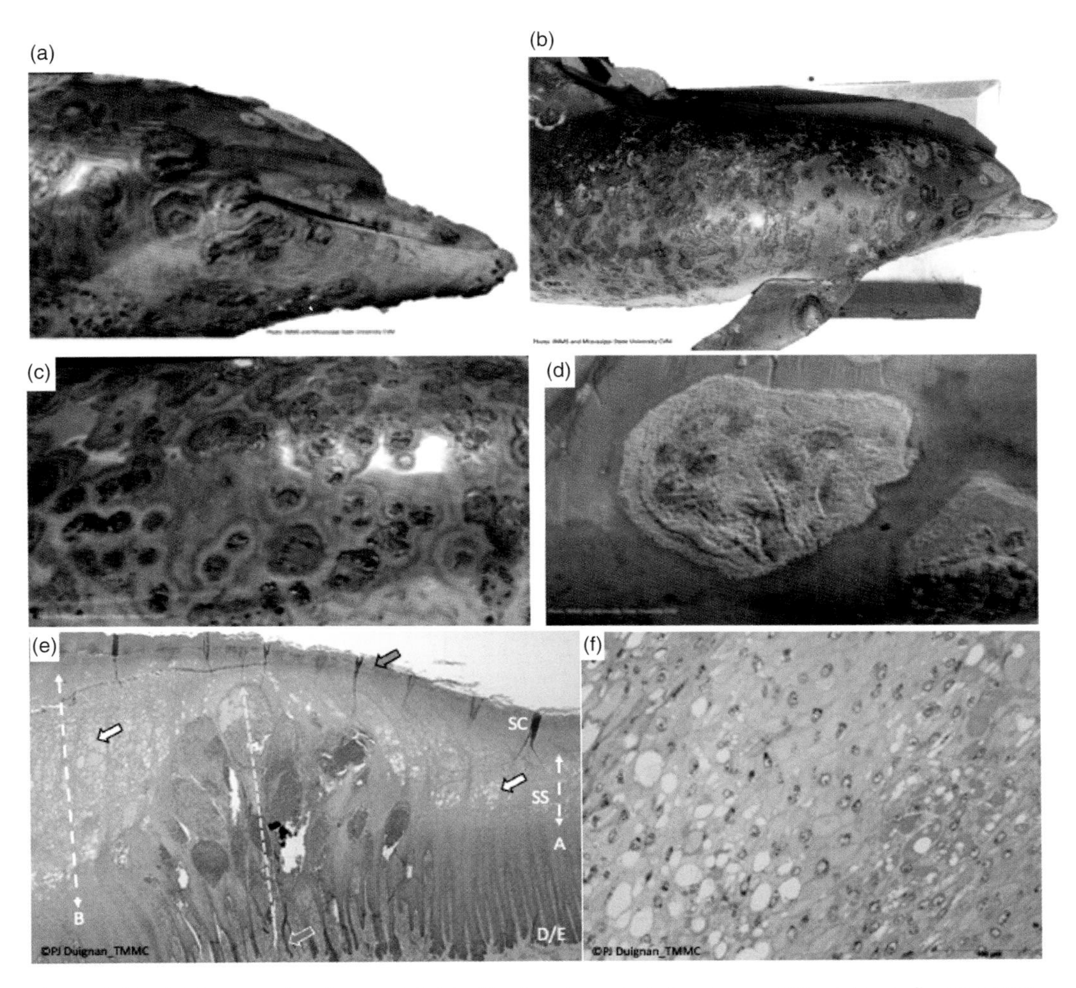

Figure 6.64 (a) Common bottlenose dolphin (*Tursiops truncatus*) showing multifocal to confluent target-like ovoid ulcers and plaques on the head and rostrum. Freshwater skin disease. (b) This view of the same dolphin shows that the lesions cover over 70% of the epidermis, including the dorsal fin and pectoral flipper. (c) Close-up of the target-like discrete to confluent, ulcers on the flank, surrounded by a central zone of pallor and a dark outer margin. (d) Raised plaques composed of bacterial, fungal and algal mats (yellow, green and orange discoloration). (e) Indo-Pacific bottlenose dolphin (*Tursiops aduncus*), full depth of the epidermis from the interdigitating dermal–epidermal junction (D/E) through the stratum spinosum (SS) to the outer stratum corneum (SC). Centrally, there is neutrophilic inflammation surrounding vessels of the superficial dermis (red arrow) with expansion of pustules up through the SS (dashed yellow arrow) to eventually rupture through the SC and result in an ulcer. To each side of the section, there is marked expansion of the SS, as a result of hydropic change. Note the difference between A on the right, where the hydropic change is mild by comparison with the left side B, where hydropic change has progressed to cell rupture and vesiculation of the epidermis. The SC is diffusely thickened and colonized by bacteria, algae and other opportunistic microorganisms (blue arrow). (F) *Stratum spinosum*, higher power view showing early hydropic swelling of acanthocytes exposed to low salinity water. Affected cells are enlarged, with diffusely pale cytoplasm. Source: (a–d) Dr. T. Morgan, Mississippi State University, USA; (e, f) Dr. N. Stephens, Murdoch University, Western Australia.

Differential Diagnoses

Rule out fresh-water exposure for marine dolphins.

Treatment and Management

Cetaceans have remarkable ability to heal skin lesions but may benefit from antimicrobial therapy to manage secondary infections. For stranded animals grounded between tides, covering exposed skin with wet towels can help protect the skin from UV light, desiccation, and wind. Topical UV-protectant creams can also be used on the exposed skin.

Angiomatosis

Etiology, Host Factors, and Transmission

Angiomatosis is a vascular condition of unknown etiology, reported in stranded dolphins from the Gulf of Mexico, Southern California, and the Canary Islands (Turnbull and Cowan, 1999; Diaz-Delgado et al., 2012; St. Leger et al., 2018).

Clinical and Gross Signs

UV irradiation is characterized by a proliferation of small blood vessels focally, multifocally, or diffusely throughout the lungs, with no inflammation, exudation, or alveolar hemorrhage (Figure 6.65). Changes may also be observed in adjacent lymph nodes. Angiomatosis my reduce alveolar air space and compromise breathing, but there is no clinical evidence to confirm this finding.

Diagnosis

UV irradiation is usually found incidentally in stranded dolphins and is diagnosed by histopathology.

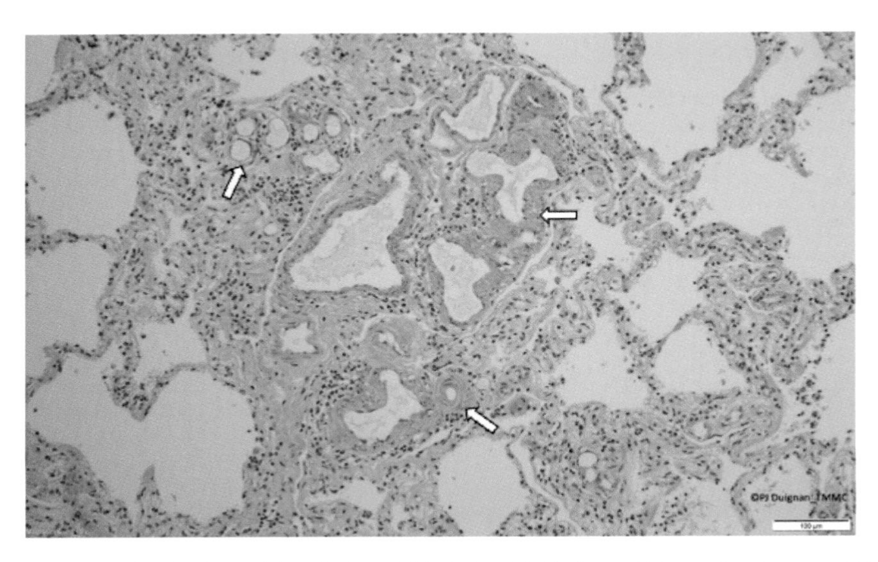

Figure 6.65 Northern right whale dolphin (*Lissodelphis borealis*) lung, showing a proliferation of small thick-walled tortuous blood vessels (arrows) acting as a space-occupying lesion and replacing functional respiratory parenchyma. Angiomatosis.

Differentials
Hemangioma or hemangiosarcoma.

Treatment and Management
There is no reported treatment and there is no indication that treatment or preventive measures are required.

Trauma

Predation and Interspecific Aggression

Sea otters are noted for their feisty nature; aggressive interactions may be directed toward other species, such as harbor seals, or may occur as part of normal breeding behavior. After mating, female southern sea otters frequently have a lacerated nasal planum that may remain ulcerated for an extended period, and eventually heal by scar formation (Figure 6.66). This condition is less common in female northern sea otters.

Pinniped species with marked sexual dimorphism and mating systems based on males holding a breeding territory or defending a group of females can result in frequent injury or mortality of females due to male aggression. At one breeding site for New Zealand sea lions, 14% of adult female mortality was attributed to attempted copulation, with death resulting from drowning, suffocation in sand, cranial or spinal fractures, hemoabdomen, or bite wounds (Lenting et al., 2019). Similar trauma and mortality among females was reported for northern elephant seals and Hawaiian monk seals (LeBoeuf and Mesnick, 1991; Atkinson et al., 1994). Pinnipeds may also be predators of other marine mammals. Sea lions of most species, and particularly subadult and adult males, are noted for infanticide and cannibalism, and for preying upon adult female fur seals or their pups (Gentry and Johnson, 1981; Harcourt, 1993; Bradshaw et al., 1998; Wilkinson et al., 2000; Womble and Conlon, 2010). Walrus, while highly social at haul sites, are also aggressive and can inflict deep tusk injuries and blunt trauma from crushing their conspecifics. They are also known predators of smaller phocids, such as ringed seals (Duignan et al., 1994). Intraspecific predation

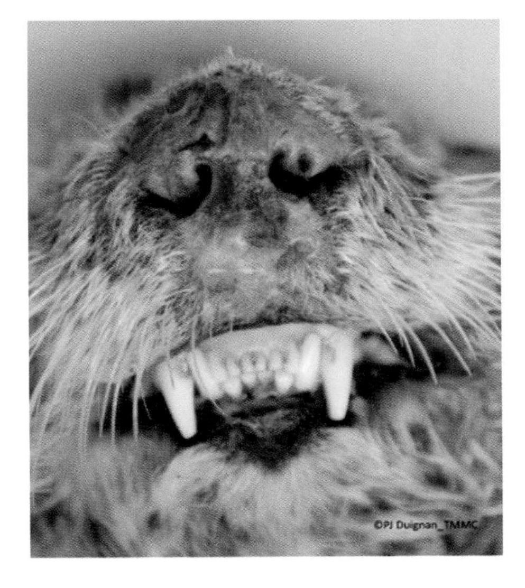

Figure 6.66 Southern sea otter, adult female, showing extensive deep ulceration of the nasal planum, with suppurative inflammation. Conspecific bite trauma from a male sea otter during copulation.

and cannibalism are also well documented among polar bears (Amstrup et al., 2006). For many years, on beaches around the North Sea, harbor seals and juvenile gray seals were found dead with unusual deep spiral lacerations running from the head to the thorax and abdomen. The regularity of the lesions suggested mechanical injury, such as boat propellor strike. Around the same time, harbor porpoises were also found with bite wounds and tissue removed. Eventually, fieldwork and forensic pathology revealed that the culprits were adult gray seals (Jauniaux et al., 2014; Leopold et al., 2015; Stringell et al., 2015; Brownlow et al., 2016).

Harbor porpoises and other small odontocetes, such as the calves of Rissos's dolphins, are also the victims of interspecific aggression by bottlenose dolphins; lack of meat or blubber consumption suggests that predation is not the motive (Patterson et al., 1998; Barnett et al., 2009; Cotter et al., 2012; Wilkin et al., 2012). The behavior, often dubbed "porpicide," was first documented on the Scottish east coast, but it is also very common on the California coast, where diagnosis is based on gross findings that include skin rakes (bite marks) with an interdental distance of approximately 10 mm (equivalent to that of subadult male *Tursiops truncatus*), (Figure 6.67a), extensive subcuticular and muscular contusions (Figure 6.67b) and skeletal fractures that can involve the mandibles, cranium, ribs, and spinal column (Figure 6.67c,d). Absence of fresh rake marks reduces the likelihood of *Tursiops* aggression (Chantra et al., 2017; Halaska et al., 2018). Bottlenose dolphins appear to be the main aggressors but are probably not the only species to behave in this manner. Larrat and others (2012) reported evidence that Atlantic white-sided dolphins also kill harbor porpoise calves. The reason for interspecific aggression without predation is not known. However,

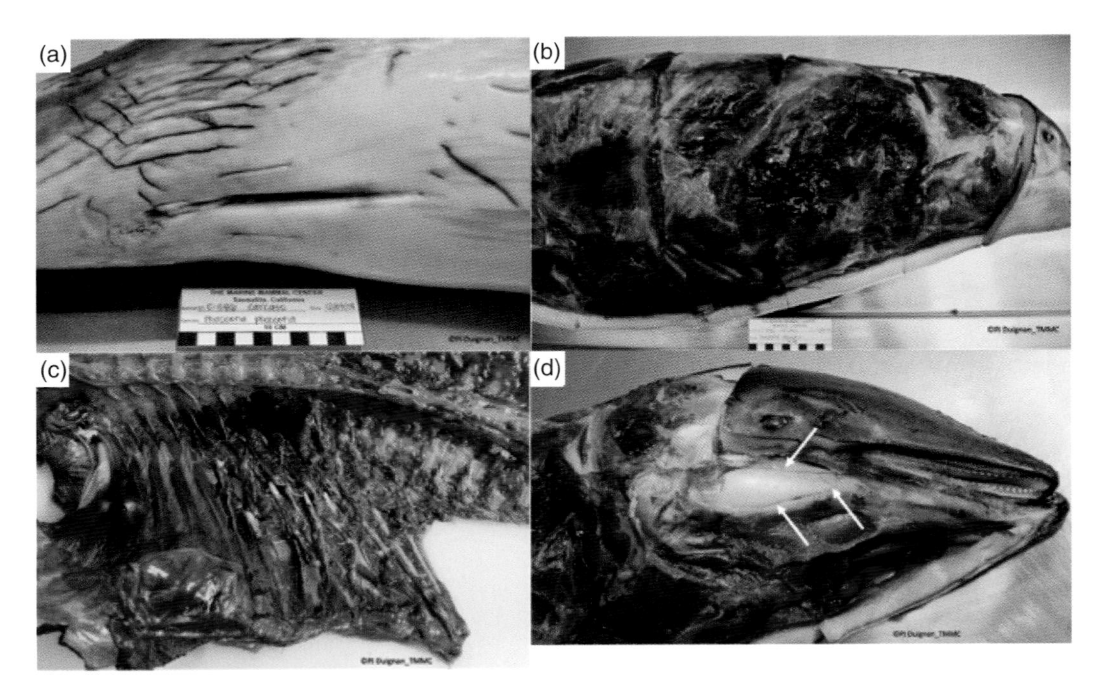

Figure 6.67 Harbor porpoise, juvenile female. (a) Deep rake marks spaced approximately 1 cm apart, along the flank and peduncle. Bottlenose dolphin-inflicted trauma. (b) The blubber is flensed off the thorax and abdomen to show extensive contusion of the subtending subcutis and skeletal muscles, consistent with blunt force trauma inflicted by a bottlenose dolphin. (c) Multiple comminuted and compound rib fractures and subpleural and diffuse intercostal hemorrhage. (d) Comminuted fractures of the right ramus of the mandible (arrows).

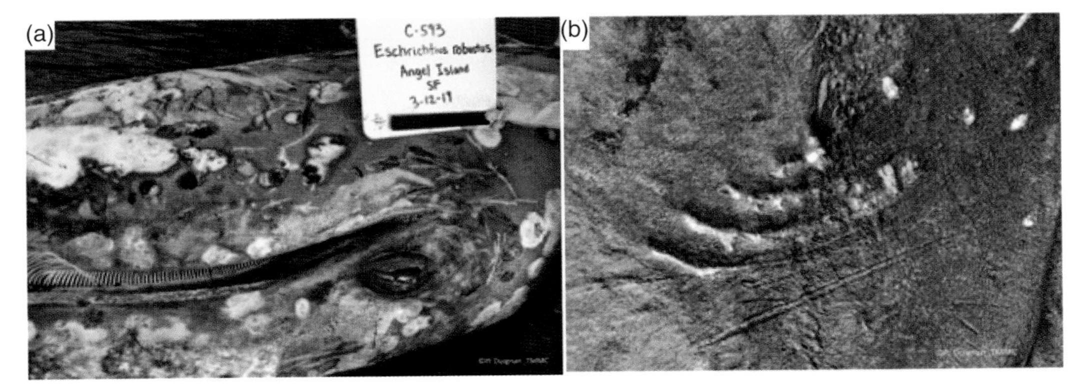

Figure 6.68 Gray whale, yearling. (a) punctate and linear mandibular lacerations consistent with prior attempted killer whale predation. (b) Tail fluke from the same whale, showing four distinct suspect killer whale tooth lacerations.

bottlenose dolphins are known to carry out infanticide; extension of this behavior to harbor porpoises is one potential hypothesis for porpicide (Patterson et al., 1998; Cotter et al., 2012).

A more conventional predation interaction between cetacean species is the interaction between the mammal-predating ecotype of killer whales and their prey. Killer whales have been documented to prey upon baleen whales, small odontocetes, pinnipeds, and sea otters, from polar to tropical waters globally (Baird et al., 2006; Barrett-Lennard et al., 2011; Pitman et al., 2015; Visser et al., 2010; Weller et al., 2018; Willoughby et al., 2020). Animals that survive the predation attempt may be left with bite-wound scars (rake marks) on the pectoral flippers, flukes, or mandibles (Figure 6.68).

Sharks are formidable marine mammal predators, but many animals survive the initial attack and escape predation. However, these bites can ultimately prove fatal through blood loss and shock, sepsis or stranding, and humane euthanasia (Figure 6.69). At both ends of the current southern sea otter range, shark predation is a significant obstacle for recolonization of the remaining California coast by sea otters. For example, in central California, along a stretch of coast extending from the elephant seal rookery of Año Nuevo to Monterey Bay, great white sharks (*Carcharodon carcharias*) are an important cause of sea otter death (Kreuder et al., 2003; Miller et al., 2020b). All sea otter victims appear to have been bitten, but not consumed. Based on wound healing and bacterial invasion, more than half (53%; 84/161) of southern sea otters with shark bite survived the initial trauma but succumbed to secondary infections days to weeks later (Miller et al., 2020b). Significant risk factors for death due to white shark bite included subadult age class, excellent or good nutritional condition at stranding, stranding during fall or winter, and stranding within the highest risk zones for white shark bite at the northern and southern ends of the southern sea otter range (Miller et al., 2020b).

An unusual form of predation on cetaceans has been documented for southern right whale calves attacked by kelp gulls (*Larus dominicanus*), which eat the skin from the whale's backs (McAloose et al., 2016). The predatory behavior has resulted in calf deaths from secondary infection, as well as altered behavior by the calves to avoid the birds, resulting in increased energetic demands.

When prey species turn the tables on their would-be aquatic mammal predators, the result can be serious injuries or death. There are numerous examples in the literature of stranded animals presenting with injuries inflicted by elasmobranch spines embedded in their head, face, or

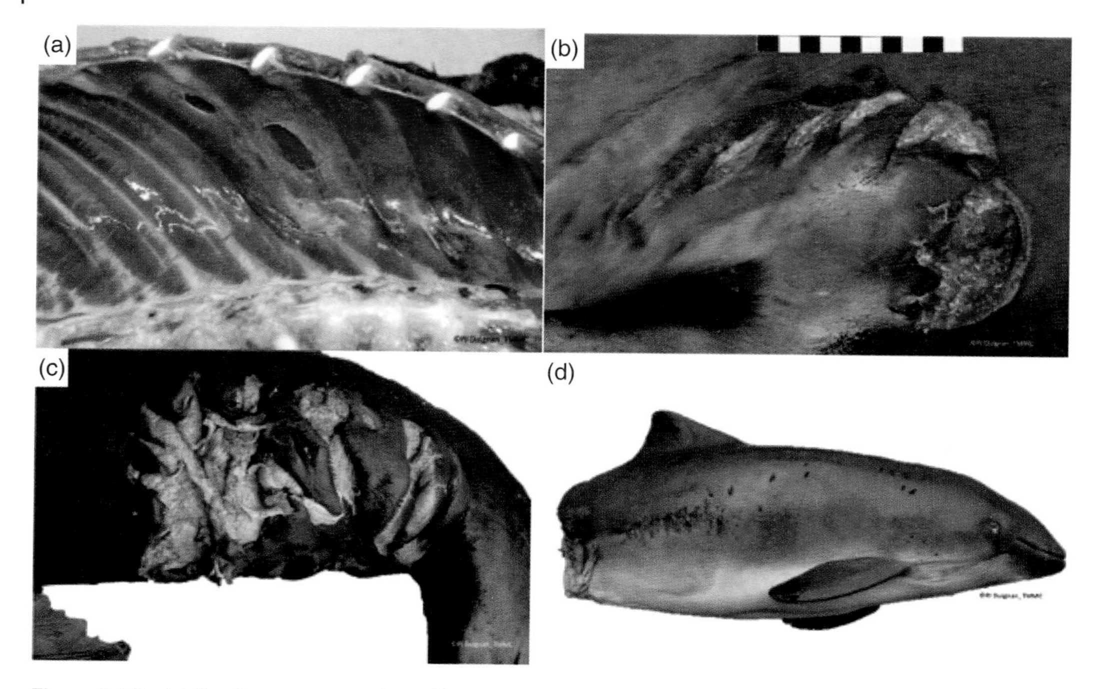

Figure 6.69 (a) Southern sea otter, juvenile male. Right thoracic wall showing two lacerations through the intercostal muscle and parietal pleura associated with shark bite. Pneumothorax was the cause of death. (b) California sea lion, adult female, arc of deep triangular lacerations over the shoulder of the right pectoral flipper. Probable great white shark, *Carcharodon carcharias*, attack. (c) California sea lion, adult male, great white shark bite on the abdomen. (d) Harbor porpoise, peduncle amputation. Probable great white shark attack.

gastrointestinal tract, some causing fatal hemorrhage or injury to vital organs (Figure 6.70; Walsh et al., 1988; Duignan et al., 2000; Akmajian et al., 2012). Sometimes, the predator tries to swallow a prey animal that is simply too big to swallow; in dolphins, the epiglottis (goose beak) can be displaced, causing asphyxiation (St. Leger et al., 2018; Elliser et al., 2020), or as Stephens et al. (2017) reported, the prey, in this case an octopus, fought back, resulting in the same outcome for the dolphin.

Human Interaction

Human interaction is a growing cause of morbidity and mortality for marine mammals globally, and it takes many forms, including direct killing by gunshot and explosive devices ("seal bombs"; Figure 6.71a,b); deep lacerations and amputations caused by propellors or entangled cables or fishing gear (Figure 6.71c,d); and emaciation from chronically entangled marine debris.

Large baleen whales appear to be particularly susceptible to blunt and sharp force trauma from container ships or other large vessels (Figure 6.72). Entrapment underwater and asphyxiation in gill nets or other fishing equipment, also known as peracute underwater entrapment; decompression sickness (the bends) from a sudden change in dive depth, either as a result of net entrapment and abrupt ascent, or rapid ascent in response to sonar from naval or oil and gas vessels; barotrauma or blast trauma from underwater explosions or sonar, are all potential causes of mortality for cetaceans and pinnipeds, but they require highly detailed and specific forensic necropsy.

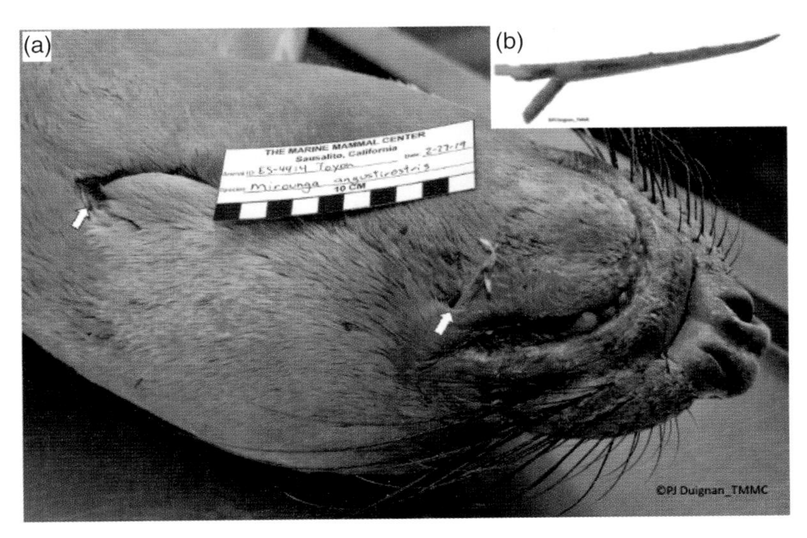

Figure 6.70 (a) Northern elephant seal, weaned pup, multiple fistulous tracks draining from skin of the mandible (arrows), one of which has a protruding sting ray barb. (b) The barb was embedded 6 cm into the soft tissue of the mandible, resulting in local necrosis and a suppurative inflammation.

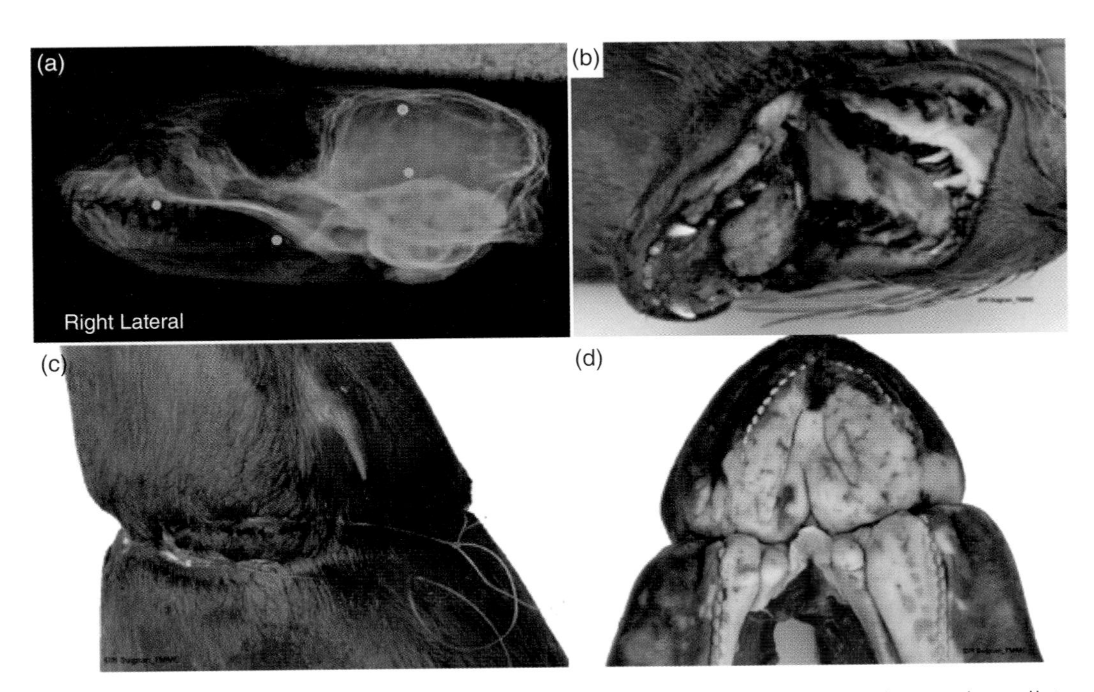

Figure 6.71 Human interaction trauma. (a) Pacific harbor seal, cranial radiograph showing gunshot pellets. (b) California sea lion, adult female, bilateral mandibular fracture. Trauma caused either by entanglement or an explosive deterrent (seal bomb). (c) California sea lion, monofilament netting encircling the neck and deeply embedded into the tissues. Commercial gill net fishery interaction. (d) Harbor porpoise, fishing line encircling the mandibles and deeply incised into the soft tissue.

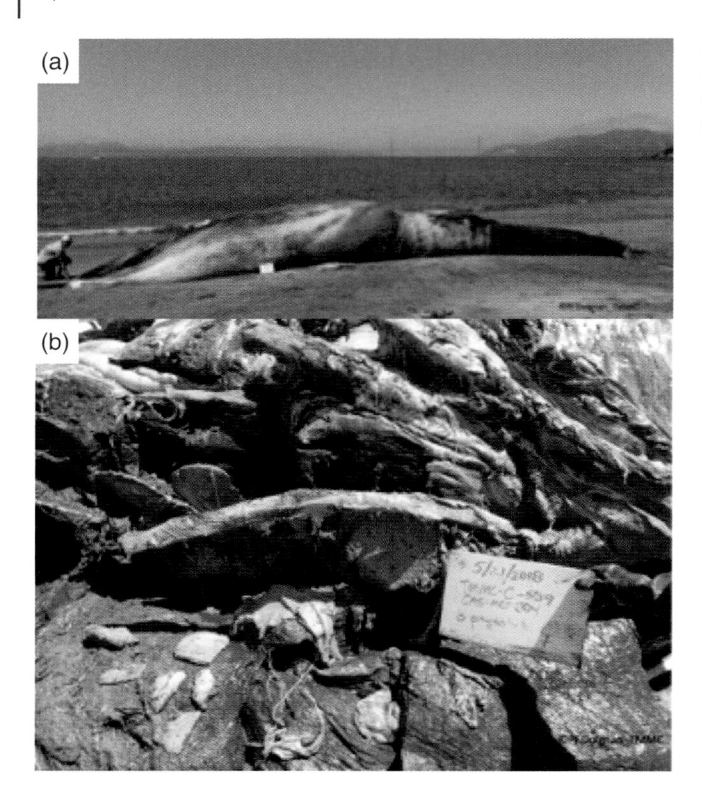

Figure 6.72 (a & b) Fin whale (*Balaenoptera borealis*) struck by a container ship with multiple vertebral and rib fractures.

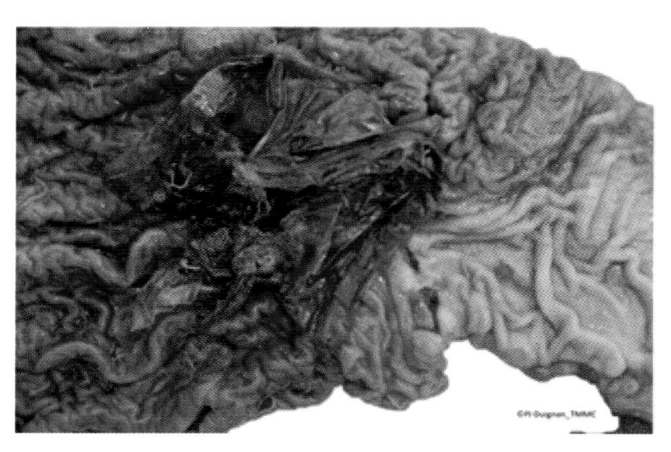

Figure 6.73 California sea lion, stomach opened to show multiple gastric ulcers, several nematodes and a plastic bag.

The pathology associated with each of these forms of adverse human interaction and methods for diagnosis have been described in some detail elsewhere (Arbelo et al., 2013; Bernaldo de Quirós et al., 2011, 2018, 2019; Moore et al., 2013; Raverty et al., 2018; St. Leger et al., 2018; Owen et al., 2018).

Another form of adverse human impact on aquatic animals is accidental ingestion of plastics (macro- or microplastics), or other floating debris (Figure 6.73). Social media is replete with images of stranded whale stomachs filled with plastic debris. However, the global impact and significance of this problem is poorly understood, and better scientific documentation is required. The species that appear most vulnerable to plastic debris ingestion from the water column would be baleen whales, such as humpback whales, that engage in lunge feeding. Benthic-feeding gray whales are also at risk of ingesting debris on the sea floor, while species that suction feed on cephalopods or cnidaria, such as beaked whales or sperm whales, may also ingest floating plastic waste. Plastics have the potential to cause gastrointestinal obstruction, ulceration, perforation, peritonitis, and death. In addition, degradation of certain plastics may release potentially toxic chemicals, such as PCBs that, when absorbed, may cause immune response or endocrine modulating effects, along with plasticizers, pigments, flame retardants, or heavy metals.

Acknowledgments

Marine mammal necropsies and sampling are conducted at the Marine Mammal Center, under National Oceanic and Atmospheric Administration permit 18786-04. The author thanks the necropsy and clinical staff at the Marine Mammal Center for assistance with cases shown in this chapter. New Zealand field research team, particularly Dr. Ian Wilkinson, Department of Conservation, and Dr. Aurelie Castinel. Narwhal field research team and, in particular, Dr. Sandie Black, University of Calgary, Dr. Steve Ferguson, Department of Fisheries and Oceans, Canada, and the late Jack Orr, DFO.

Bibliography

Aalderink MT, Nguyen HP, Kass PH, et al. 2015a. Dental and temporomandibular joint pathology of the Eastern Pacific harbour seal (*Phoca vitulina richardsi*). *J Comp Pathol* 152(4), 335–344.

Aalderink MT, Nguyen, HP, Kass, PH, et al. 2015b. Dental and temporomandibular joint pathology of the northern fur seal (*Callorhinus ursinus*). *J Comp Pathol* 152(4):325–334.

Abadía-Cardoso A, Freimer NB, Deiner, K Garza JC. 2017. Molecular population genetics of the northern elephant seal *Mirounga angustirostris*. *J Heredity* 108(6):618–627.

Abbott C, Verstraete FJM. 2005. The dental pathology of northern elephant seals (*Mirounga angustirostris*). *J Comp Pathol* 132(2–3):169–178.

Acevedo-Whitehouse K, Spraker TR, Lyons E, et al. 2006. Contrasting effects of heterozygosity on survival and hookworm resistance in California sea lion pups. *Mol Ecol* 15(7):1973–1982.

Acevedo-Whitehouse K, Petetti L, Duignan P, Castinel A. 2009. Hookworm infection, anaemia and genetic variability of the New Zealand sea lion. *Proc R Soc B* 276(1672):3523–3529.

Acevedo-Whitehouse K, Gulland FM, Bowen L. 2018. MHC class II DRB diversity predicts antigen recognition and is associated with disease severity in California sea lions naturally infected with *Leptospira interrogans*. *Infect Genet Evol* 57:158–165.

Akmajian AM, Lambourn DM, Lance MM, et al. 2012. Mortality Related to spotted ratfish (*Hydrolagus colliei*) in Pacific harbor seals (*Phoca vitulina*) in Washington State. *J Wildl Dis* 48(4):1057–1062.

Amstrup SC, Stirling I, Smith TS, et al. 2006. Recent observations of intraspecific predation and cannibalism among polar bears in the southern Beaufort Sea. *Polar Biol* 29(11):997–1002.

Anthony SJ, St Leger JA, Pugliares K, et al. 2012. Emergence of fatal avian influenza in New England harbor seals. *MBio* 3(4):e00166–12.

Arbelo M, de los Monteros AE, Herráez P, et al. 2013. Pathology and causes of death of stranded cetaceans in the Canary Islands (1999—2005). *Dis Aquat Organ* 103(2):87–99.

Arzi B, Winer JN, Kass PH, Verstraete FJM. 2013. Osteoarthritis of the temporomandibular joint in southern sea otters (*Enhydra lutris nereis*) *J Comp Pathol* 149(4):486–494.

Atkinson S, Becker BL, Johanos TC, et al. 1994. Reproductive morphology and status of female Hawaiian monk seals (*Monachus schauinslandi*) fatally injured by adult male seals. *Reproduction* 100(1):225–230.

Atwood T, Peacock E, Burek-Huntington K, et al. 2015. Prevalence and spatio-temporal variation of an alopecia syndrome in polar bears (*Ursus maritimus*) of the southern Beaufort Sea. *J Wildl Dis* 51(1):48–59.

Ayling RD, Bashiruddin S, Davison NJ, et al. 2011. The occurrence of *Mycoplasma phocicerebrale*, *Mycoplasma phocidae*, and *Mycoplasma phocirhinis* in grey and common seals (*Halichoerus grypus* and *Phoca vitulina*) in the United Kingdom. *J Wildl Dis* 47(2)\;471–475.

Aznar FJ, Agustí C, Littlewood DTJ, et al. 2007. Insight into the role of cetaceans in the life cycle of the tetraphyllideans (Platyhelminthes: Cestoda). *Int J Parasitol* 37(2):243–255.

Baker JD, Harting AL, Barbieri MM, et al. 2017. Modeling a morbillivirus outbreak in Hawaiian monk seals (*Neomonachus schauinslandi*) to aid in the design of mitigation programs *J Wildl Dis* 53(4):736–748.

Baird RW, McSweeney DJ, Bane C, et al. 2006. Killer whales in Hawaiian waters: information on population identity and feeding habits. *Pacific Sci* 60(4):523–530.

Balbuena JA, Simpkin A. 2014. Role of *Crassicauda* sp in natural mortality of pantropical spotted dolphins *Stenella attenuata*: a reassessment. *Dis Aquat Organ* 108(1):83–89.

Ball R, Walsh C, Flewelling L, et al. 2014. Clinical pathology, serum brevetoxin, and clinical signs of Florida Manatees (*Trichechus manatus latirostris*) during the brevetoxin-related mortality event in Southwest Florida. *International Association for Aquatic Animal Medicine 2014 Proceedings Online* https://www.vin.com/apputil/content/defaultadv1.aspx?id=6251877&pid=11397 (accessed 7 October 2022).

Banos S, Lentendu G, Kopf A, et al. 2018. A comprehensive fungi-specific 18S rRNA gene sequence primer toolkit suited for diverse research issues and sequencing platforms. *BMC Microbiol* 18(1):1–15.

Barnett J, Davison N, Deaville R, et al. 2009. Postmortem evidence of interactions of bottlenose dolphins (*Tursiops truncatus*) with other dolphin species in south-west England. *Vet Rec* 165(15):441–444.

Barrett T, Wohlsein P, Bidewell CA, Rowell SF. 2004. Canine distemper virus in a Californian sea lion (*Zalophus californianus*). *Vet Rec* 154:334–336.

Barrett-Lennard LG, Matkin CO, Durban JW, et al. 2011. Predation on gray whales and prolonged feeding on submerged carcasses by transient killer whales at Unimak Island, Alaska. *Mar Ecol Prog Ser* 421:229–241.

Bartlett G, Miller W, Dominik C, et al. 2016. Prevalence, pathology and potential risk factors associated with *Streptococcus phocae* infection in southern sea otters (*Enhydra lutris nereis*) (2004–2010). *J Wildl Dis* 52:1–9.

Bastida R, Loureiro J, Quse V, et al. 1999. Tuberculosis in a wild subantarctic fur seal from Argentina. *J Wildl Dis* 35(4):796–798.

Beck C, Forrester DJ. 1988. Helminths of the Florida manatee, *Trichechus manatus latirostris*, with a discussion and summary of the parasites of sirenians. *J Parasitol* 74(4:628–637.

Beckmen KB, Lowenstine LJ, Newman J, et al. 1997. Clinical and pathological characterization of northern elephant seal skin disease. *J Wildl Dis* 33(3):438–449.

Bergeron E, Measures LN, Huot J. 1997. Lungworm (*Otostrongylus circumlitus*) infections in ringed seals (*Phoca hispida*) from eastern Arctic Canada. *Can J Fish Aquat Sci* 54(10):2443–2448.

Bernardelli A, Bastida R, Loureiro J, et al. 1996. Tuberculosis in sea lions and fur seals from the south-western Atlantic coast. *Rev Sci Tech* 15:985–1005.

Bernaldo De Quirós Y, González-Díaz Ó, Saavedra P, et al. 2011. Methodology for in situ gas sampling, transport and laboratory analysis of gases from stranded cetaceans. *Sci Rep* 1:193.

Bernaldo de Quirós Y, Hartwick M, Rotstein DS, et al. 2018. Discrimination between bycatch and other causes of cetacean and pinniped stranding. *Dis Aquat Organ* 127(2):83–95.

Bernaldo De Quirós Y, Fernandez A, Baird RW, et al. 2019. Advances in research on the impacts of anti-submarine sonar on beaked whales. *Proc R Soc B* 286(1895):20182533.

Biancani B, Field CL, Dennison S, et al. 2012. Hiatal hernia in a harbor seal (*Phoca vitulina*) pup. *J Zoo Wildl Med* 43(2):355–359.

Birkenheuer AJ, Harms CA, Neel J, et al. 2006. The identification of a genetically unique piroplasma in North American river otters (*Lontra canadensis*). *Parasitology* 134(5):631–635.

Blair D. 1981. The monostome flukes (Digenea: Families Opisthotrematidae Poche and Rhodbiopoeidae Poche) parasitic in sirenians (Mammalia: Sirenia). *Aust J Zool Suppl Ser* 29(81):1–54.

Boardman WS, Shephard L, Bastian I, et al. 2014. *Mycobacterium pinnipedii* tuberculosis in a free-ranging Australian fur seal (*Arctocephalus pusillus doriferus*) in South Australia. *J Zoo Wildl Med* 45(4):970–972.

Bodewes R, Bestebroer TM, van der Vries E, et al. 2015. Avian influenza A (H10N7) virus-associated mass deaths among harbor seals. *Emerg Infect Dis* 21(4):720–722.

Bonar CJ, Wagner RA. 2003. A third report of "golf ball disease" in an Amazon River dolphin (*Inia geoffrensis*) associated with *Streptococcus iniae*. *J Zoo Wildl Med* 34(3):296–301.

Bonar CJ, Boede EO, Hartmann MG, et al. 2007. A retrospective study of pathologic findings in the Amazon and Orinoco river dolphin (Inia geoffrensis) in captivity *J Zoo Wildl Med* 38(2):177–191.

Bossart GD. 2007. Emerging diseases in marine mammals: from dolphins to manatees. *Microbe* 2(11):544–549.

Bossart GD, Schwartz P. 1990. Acute necrotizing enteritis associated with suspected coronavirus infection in three harbor seals (*Phoca vitulina*). *J Zoo Wildl Med* 21:84–87.

Bossart GD, Duignan PJ. 2019. Emerging viruses in marine mammals. *CABI Rev* 13(052): doi: https://doi.org/10.1079/PAVSNNR201813052.

Bossart GD, Odell DK, Altman NH. 1985. Cardiomyopathy in stranded pygmy and dwarf sperm whales. *J Am Vet Med Assoc* 187(11):1137–1140.

Bossart GD, Baden DG, Ewing RY, et al. 1998. Brevetoxicosis in manatees (*Trichechus manatus latirostris*) from the 1996 epizootic: gross, histologic, and immunohistochemical features. *Toxicol Pathol* 26(2):276–282.

Bossart GD, Meisner RA, Rommel SA, et al. 2004. Pathologic findings in Florida manatees (*Trichechus manatus latirostris*). *Aquat Mammals* 30(3):434–440.

Bossart GD, Hensley G, Goldstein JD, Kroell K. 2007. Cardiomyopathy and myocardial degeneration in stranded pygmy (*Kogia breviceps*) and dwarf (*Kogia sima*) sperm whales. *Aquat Mammals* 33(2):214–222.

Bottein MYD, Kashinsky L, Wang Z, et al. 2011. Identification of ciguatoxins in Hawaiian monk seals *Monachus schauinslandi* from the northwestern and main Hawaiian Islands. *Environ Sci Technol* 45(12):5403–5409.

Bradshaw CJ, Lalas C, McConkey S. 1998. New Zealand sea lion predation on New Zealand fur seals. *N Z J Marine Freshwater Res* 32(1):101–104.

Brodie EC, Gulland FM, Greig DJ, et al. 2006. Domoic acid causes reproductive failure in California sea lions (*Zalophus californianus*). *Marine Mammal Sci* 22(3):700–707.

Browning HM, Gulland FM, Hammond JA, et al. 2015. Common cancer in a wild animal: the California sea lion (*Zalophus californianus*) as an emerging model for carcinogenesis. *Phil Trans R Soc B* 370(1673):20140228.

Brownlow A, Onoufriou J, Bishop A, et al. 2016. Corkscrew seals: grey seal (*Halichoerus grypus*) infanticide and cannibalism may indicate the cause of spiral lacerations in seals. *PloS One* 11(6): e0156464.

Buck JD, Shepard LL, Bubucis PM, et al. 1989. Microbiological characteristics of white whale (*Delphinapterus leucas*) from capture through extended captivity. *Can J Fish Aquat Sci* 46(11):1914–1921.

Buck JD. 1991. Recovery of *Vibrio metschnikovii* from market seafood. *J Food Saf* 12(1):73–78.

Buckle K, Roe WD, Howe L, et al. 2017. Brucellosis in endangered Hector's Dolphins (*Cephalorhynchus hectori*). *Vet Pathol* 54(5):838–845.

Buckmaster PS, Wen X, Toyoda I, et al. 2014. Hippocampal neuropathology of domoic acid–induced epilepsy in California sea lions (*Zalophus californianus*). *J Comp Neurol* 522(7):1691–1706.

Buergelt CD, Bonde RK, Beck CA, O'Shea TJ. 1984. Pathologic findings in manatees in Florida. *J Am Vet Med Assoc* 185(11):1331–1334.

Burek KA. 2001. Mycotic diseases. In: Williams E, Barker I, eds. *Infectious Diseases of Wild Mammals*, 3rd edn., 514–531. Ames, IA: Iowa State University Press.

Burgess TL, Johnson CK, Burdin A, et al. 2017. Brucella infection in Asian sea otters (*Enhydra lutris lutris*) on Bering Island, *Russia. J Wildl Dis* 53(4):864–868.

Canales R, Sanchez-Okrucky R, Bustamante L, et al. 2020. Melioidosis in a bottlenose dolphin (*Tursiops truncatus*) after a hurricane in the Caribbean islands. *J Zoo Wildl Med* 51(2):443–447.

Carlson-Bremer DP, Gulland FM, Johnson CK, et al. 2012. Diagnosis and treatment of *Sarcocystis neurona*-induced myositis in a free-ranging California sea lion. *J Am Vet Med Assoc* 240(3):324–328.

Capuano AM, Miller M, Stallknecht DE, et al. 2017. Serologic detection of subtype–specific antibodies to influenza A viruses in southern sea otters (*Enhydra lutris nereis*). *J Wildl Dis* 53(4):906–910.

Castinel A, Grinberg A, Pattison R, et al. 2006. Characterization of Klebsiella pneumoniae isolates from New Zealand sea lion (*Phocarctos hookeri*) pups during and after the epidemics on Enderby Island, Auckland Islands, *Vet Microbiol* 122:178–184.

Castinel A, Duignan PJ, Lyons ET, et al. 2007a. Epidemiology of hookworm (*Uncinaria* spp) infection in New Zealand (Hooker's) sea lion (*Phocarctos hookeri*) pups on Enderby Island, Auckland Islands (New Zealand) during the breeding seasons from 1999/2000 to 2004/2005. *Parasitol Res* 101(1):53–62.

Castinel A, Duignan PJ, Pomroy WE, et al. 2007b. Neonatal mortality in New Zealand sea lions (*Phocarctos hookeri*) at Sandy Bay, Enderby Island, Auckland Islands from 1998 to 2005. *J Wildl Dis* 43(3):461–474.

Chang EK, Miller MA, Shahin K, et al. 2021. Genetics and pathology associated with Klebsiella pneumoniae isolates from North American Pacific Coastal marine mammals. *Vet Microbiol* 265: 109307.

Chantra R, Simeone C, Duignan P, et al. 2017. Understanding harbor porpoise trauma cases in northern California through necropsy and dolphin sighting data. Poster Presentation: The Southern California Marine Mammal Workshop, Long Beach, CA January 27–28, 2017.

Chinn SM, Miller MA, Tinker MT, et al. 2016. The high cost of motherhood: End–lactation syndrome in southern sea otters (Enhydra lutris nereis) on the Central California Coast, USA. *J Wildl Dis* 52 (2):307–318.

Chilvers BL, Duignan PJ, Robertson BC, et al. 2009. Effects of hookworms (*Uncinaria* sp) on the early growth and survival of New Zealand sea lion (*Phocarctos hookeri*) pups. *Polar Biol* 32(2):295–302.

Choi YK, Kang MS, Sohn HR, Kim DY. 2003. Disseminated ciliated protozoan infection in a Pacific dolphin (*Tursiops gilli*). *Vet Rec* 153(23):714–715.

Colegrove KM, Greig DJ, Gulland FM. 2005. Causes of live strandings of northern elephant seals (*Mirounga angustirostris*) and Pacific harbor seals (*Phoca vitulina*) along the central California coast, 1992–2001. *Aquat Mammals* 31(1):1–10.

Colegrove KM, Gulland FMD, Harr K, et al. 2009. Pathological features of amyloidosis in stranded California sea lions (*Zalophus californianus*). *J Comp Pathol* 140(2–3):105–112.

Colegrove KM, St Leger JA, Raverty S, et al. 2010. Salmonella Newport omphaloarteritis in a stranded killer whale (*Orcinus orca*) neonate. *J Wildl Dis* 46(4):1300–1304.

Colegrove KM, Venn-Watson S, Litz J, et al. 2016. Fetal distress and in utero pneumonia in perinatal dolphins during the Northern Gulf of Mexico unusual mortality event. *Dis Aquat Organ* 119(1):1–16.

Colegrove KM, Burek-Huntington KA, Roe W. 2018. Pinnipediae. In: Terio KA, McAloose D, St Leger J, eds. *Pathology of Wildlife and Zoo Animals*, 569–592. London: Academic Press.

Cook PF, Reichmuth C, Rouse AA, et al. 2015. Algal toxin impairs sea lion memory and hippocampal connectivity, with implications for strandings. *Science* 350(6267):1545–1547.

Cortés-Hinojosa G, Gulland FM, DeLong R, et al. 2016. A novel gammaherpesvirus in northern fur seals (*Callorhinus ursinus*) is closely related to the California sea lion (*Zalophus californianus*) carcinoma-associated otarine herpesvirus-1. *J Wildl Dis* 52(1):88–95.

Costa LG, Giordano G, Faustman EM. 2010. Domoic acid as a developmental neurotoxin. *Neurotoxicology* 31(5):409–423.

Costa H, Klein J, Breines EM, et al. 2021. A comparison of parapoxviruses in North American pinnipeds. *Front Vet Sci* 8: 653094.

Cotter MP, Maldini D, Jefferson TA. 2012. "Porpicide" in California: killing of harbor porpoises (*Phocoena phocoena*) by coastal bottlenose dolphins (*Tursiops truncatus*). *Marine Mammal Sci* 28(1):E1–E15.

Cousins DV, Bastida B, Cataldi A, et al. 2003. Tuberculosis in seals caused by a novel member of the *Mycobacterium tuberculosis* complex: *Mycobacterium tuberculosis* subsp pinnipedae subsp nov. *Int J Syst Evol Microbiol* 53:1305–1314.

Cowan DF. 1995. Amyloidosis in the bottlenose dolphin (*Tursiops truncatus*). *Vet Pathol* 32:311–314.

Cozzi B, Huggenberger S, Oelschläger HA. 2016. *Anatomy of Dolphins: Insights into body structure and function*, 339–368. San Diego, CA: Academic Press.

Dagleish MP, Barley J, Howie FE, et al. 2007. Isolation of Brucella species from a diseased atlanto-occipital joint of an Atlantic white-sided dolphin (*Lagenorhynchus acutus*). *Vet Rec* 160:876–878.

Dagleish MP, Barley J, Finlayson J, et al. 2008. *Brucella ceti* associated pathology in the testicle of a harbour porpoise (*Phocoena phocoena*). *J Comp Pathol* 139(1):54–59.

Dagleish MP, Barrows M, Maley M, et al. 2013. The first report of otarine herpesvirus-1-associated urogenital carcinoma in a South American fur seal (*Arctocephalus australis*). *J Comp Pathol* 149(1):119–125.

Dailey M. 2001. Parasitic diseases. In: Dierauf LA, Gulland FMD, eds. *CRC Handbook of Marine Mammal Medicine*, 2nd edn., 357–382. Boca Raton, FL: CRC Press.

Dailey M, Stroud R. 1978. Parasites and associated pathology observed in cetaceans stranded along the Oregon coast. *J Wildl Dis* 14(4):503–511.

Dailey M, Walsh M, Odell D, Campbell T. 1991. Evidence of prenatal infection in the bottlenose dolphin (*Tursiops truncates*) with the lungworm *Halocercus lagenorhynchi* (Nematoda: Pseudaliidae). *J Wildl Dis* 27(1):164–165.

Dailey M, Ellin R, Parás A. 2005. First report of parasites from pinnipeds in the Galapagos Islands, Ecuador, with a description of a new species of Philophthalmus (Digenea: Philophthalmidae). *J Parasitol* 91(3):614–617.

Dailey MD. 1970. The transmission of *Parafilaroides decorus* (Nematoda: Metastrongyloidea) in the California sea lion (*Zalophus californianus*). *Proc Helminth Soc Washington* 37(2):215–222.

Dailey MD, Walker WA. 1978. Parasitism as a factor (?) in single strandings of southern California cetaceans. *J Parasitol* 64(4):593–596.

Dailey MD, Vogelbein W, Forrester DJ. 1988. *Moniligerum blairi* ng, n sp and *Nudacotyle undicola* n sp (Trematoda: Digenea) from the West Indian Manatee, *Trichechus manatus L. Syst Parasitol* 11(2):159–163.

Dailey MD, Gulland FM, Lowenstine LJ, et al. 2000. Prey, parasites and pathology associated with the mortality of a juvenile gray whale (*Escherichia robustus*) stranded along the northern California coast. *Dis Aquat Organ* 42(2):111–117.

Dailey MD, Haulena M, Lawrence J. 2002. First report of a parasitic copepod (*Penella balaenoptererae*) infestation on a pinniped. *J Zoo Wildl Med* 33(1):62–65.

Damas J, Hughes GM, Keough KC, et al. 2020. Broad host range of SARS-CoV-2 predicted by comparative and structural analysis of ACE2 in vertebrates. *Proc Natl Acad of Sci* 117(36):22311–22322.

D'Andreano S, Cuscó A, Francino O. 2020. Rapid and real-time identification of fungi up to species level with long amplicon nanopore sequencing from clinical samples. *Biol Methods Protocols* 6(1):bpaa026.

Davis DA, Mondo K, Stern E, et al. 2019. Cyanobacterial neurotoxin BMAA and brain pathology in stranded dolphins *PLoS One* 14(3):e0213346.

Davison NJ, Simpson VR, Chappell S, et al. 2010. Prevalence of a host-adapted group B *Salmonella enterica* in harbour porpoises (*Phocoena phocoena*) from the south-west coast of England. *Vet Rec* 167(5):173–176.

Degollada E, Domingo M, Alonso JM, et al. 1996. Nocardiosis in a striped dolphin (*Stenella coeruleoalba*). Proceedings 3rd ECS Workshop on Cetacean Pathology: Lung Pathology. *ECS Special Issue* 37:16–18.

Degollada E, Andre M, Arbelo M, Fernandez A. 2002. Incidence, pathology and involvement of Nasitrema species in odontocete strandings in the Canary Islands. *Vet Rec* 150(3):81–81.

De Graaf AS, Shaughnessy PD, McCully RM, Verster AJ. 1980. Occurrence of *Taenia solium* in a Cape fur seal (*Arctocephalus pusillus*). *Onderstepoort J Vet Res* 47:119–120.

De Guise S, Beckmen KB, Holladay SD. 2002. Contaminants and marine mammal immunotoxicology and pathology. In: Vos JG, Bossart G, Fournier M, O'Shea T, eds. *Toxicology of Marine Mammals*, 50–66. Boca Raton, FL: CRC Press.

Delaney MA, Terio KA, Colegrove KM, et al. 2013. Occlusive fungal tracheitis in 4 captive bottlenose dolphins (*Tursiops truncatus*). *Vet Pathol* 50(1):172–176.

Delaney MA, Colegrove KM, Spraker TR, et al. 2014. Isolation of Leptospira from a phocid: acute renal failure and mortality from leptospirosis in rehabilitated northern elephant seals (*Mirounga angustirostris*), California, USA. *J Wildl Dis* 50(3):621–627.

DeLynn R, Lovewell G, Wells RS, Early G. 2011. Congenital scoliosis of a bottlenose dolphin. *J Wildl Dis* 47(4):979–983.

Deming AC, Colegrove KM, Duignan PJ, et al. 2018. Prevalence of urogenital carcinoma in stranded California sea lions (*Zalophus californianus*) from 2005–2015. *J Wildl Dis* 54(3):581–586.

Deming AC, Wingers NL, Moore DP, et al. 2020. Health impacts and recovery from prolonged freshwater exposure in a common bottlenose dolphin (*Tursiops truncatus*). *Front Vet Sci* 7:235.

Deming AC, Wellehan JFX, Colegrove KM, et al. 2021. Unlocking the roles of a genital herpesvirus, Otarine Herpesvirus-1, in California sea lion cervical carcinoma. *Animals (Basel)* 11:491.

Dennison SE, Forrest LJ, Fleetwood ML, Gulland FM. 2009. Concurrent occipital bone malformation and atlantoaxial subluxation in a neonatal harbor seal (*Phoca vitulina*). *J Zoo Wildl Med* 40(2):385–388.

Dennison SE, Van Bonn W, Boor M, et al. 2011a. Antemortem diagnosis of a ventricular septal defect in a California sea lion *Zalophus californianus*. *Dis Aquat Organ* 94(1):83–88.

Dennison SE, Boor M, Fauquier D, et al. 2011b. Foramen ovale and ductus arteriosus patency in neonatal harbor seal (*Phoca vitulina*) pups in rehabilitation. *Aquat Mammals* 37(2):161–166.

Dent CES, Miller MA, Batac F, et al. 2019. Pathology and epidemiology of nasopulmonary acariasis (*Halarachne* sp) in southern sea otters (*Enhydra lutris nereis*). *Int J Parasitol* 9:60–67.

Díaz-Delgado J, Arbelo M, Sacchini S, et al. 2012. Pulmonary angiomatosis and hemangioma in common dolphins (*Delphinus delphis*) stranded in Canary Islands. *J Vet Med Sci* 74(8):1063–1066.

Díaz-Delgado J, Fernández A, Xuriach A, et al. 2016. Verminous arteritis due to *Crassicauda* sp in Cuvier's beaked whales (*Ziphius cavirostris*). *Vet Pathol* 53(6):1233–1240.

Díaz-Delgado J, Sierra E, Vela AI, et al. 2017. Coinfection by *Streptococcus phocae* and cetacean morbillivirus in a short-beaked common dolphin *Delphinus delphis*. *Dis Aquat Organ* 124(3):247–252.

Di Renzo L, Di Francesco G, Profico C, et al. 2017. *Vibrio parahaemolyticus*- and *V alginolyticus*-associated meningo-encephalitis in a bottlenose dolphin (*Tursiops truncatus*) from the Adriatic coast of Italy. *Res Vet Sci* 115:363–365.

Doucette GJ, Mikulski CM, King KL, et al. 2012. Endangered North Atlantic right whales (*Eubalaena glacialis*) experience repeated, concurrent exposure to multiple environmental neurotoxins produced by marine algae. *Environ Res* 112:67–76.

Dróżdż J. 1987. Oocysts of six new *Coccidiomorpha* species from pinnipeds of King George Island (South Shetlands, Antarctica). *Acta Protozool* 26:263–266.

Dubey JP, Murata FHA, Cerqueira-Cézar CK, et al. 2021. Epidemiologic and public health significance of *Toxoplasma gondii* infections in bears (*Ursus* spp): a 50 year review Including recent genetic evidence. *J Parasitol* 107(3):519–528.

Duignan PJ. 1999. Pathology and disease investigations. In: Baker A, ed. *Unusual Mortality of the New Zealand Sea Lion, Phocarctos hookeri, Auckland Islands, January–February 1998*. Wellington, New Zealand: Department of Conservation.

Duignan PJ. 2000. Diseases of cetaceans and pinnipeds. In: *Post Graduate Foundation in Veterinary Science. Marine Wildlife Proceedings* 335, 419–462. Sydney, Australia: University of Sydney.

Duignan PJ, Saliki JT, St Aubin DJ, et al. 1994. Neutralizing antibodies to phocine distemper virus in Atlantic walrus (*Odobenus rosmarus rosmarus*) from Arctic Canada. *J Wildl Dis* 30:90–94.

Duignan PJ, Norman RJ de B, Pomroy W, et al. 1999. Renal crassicaudiasis in Cuvier's Beaked whales: Incidental finding or cause of adult mortality? Proceedings of the New Zealand Society for Parasitology Inc. *N Z J Zool* 28:225–226.

Duignan PJ, Hunter JEB, Visser IN, et al. 2000. Sting ray spines: a potential cause of killer whale mortality in New Zealand. *Aquat Mammals* 26:143–147.

Duignan PJ, Van Bressem MF, Baker JD, et al. 2014. Phocine distemper virus: current knowledge and future directions. *Viruses* 6:5093–5134.

Duignan PJ, Van Bressem MF, Kennedy-Stoskopf S. 2018a. Viruses of marine mammals. In: Gulland FMD, Dierauf LA, Whitman KL, eds. *CRC Handbook of Marine Mammal Medicine*, 3rd edn., 331–366. Boca Raton, FL: CRC Press.

Duignan PJ, McClain AM, Peters-Kennedy J, et al. 2018b. Alopecia in an extra-limital ribbon seal (*Histriophoca fasciata*) stranded in central California: similarities and differences to the Alaskan Northern Pinniped UME Alopecia and Dermatitis Syndrome. International Association for Aquatic Animal Medicine 2018 Proceedings Online. https://www.vin.com/apputil/content/defaultadv1.aspx?pId=20778&id=8505000 (accessed 7 October 2022).

Duignan PJ, Whitmer ER, McClain AM, et al. 2019. Descriptive epidemiology and pathology of the 2018 leptospirosis epidemic in California sea lions (*Zalophus californianus*). Presented at the World Marine Mammal Conference, Barcelona, Spain 8–12 December 2019.

Duignan PJ, Stephens NS, Robb K. 2020. Fresh water skin disease in dolphins: a case definition based on pathology and environmental factors in Australia. *Sci Rep* 10(1):1–17.

Duncan C, Kersh GJ, Spraker T, et al. 2012. *Coxiella burnetii* in northern fur seal (*Callorhinus ursinus*) placentas from St Paul Island, *Alaska. Vector Borne Zoonotic Dis* 12(3):192–195.

Duncan C, Dickerson B, Pabilonia K, et al. 2014b. Prevalence of *Coxiella burnetii* and *Brucella* spp in tissues from subsistence harvested northern fur seals (*Callorhinus ursinus*) of St Paul Island, *Alaska, Acta Vet Scand* 56(1):67.

Duncan C, Gill VA, Worman K, et al. 2015. *Coxiella burnetii* exposure in northern sea otters *Enhydra lutris kenyoni*. *Dis Aquat Organ* 114(1):83–87.

Duncan CG, Tiller R, Mathis D, et al. 2014a. *Brucella placentitis* and seroprevalence in northern fur seals (*Callorhinus ursinus*) of the Pribilof Islands, Alaska. *J Vet Diagn Invest* 26(4):507–512.

Dunn JL, Buck JD, Robeck TR. 2001. Bacterial diseases of cetaceans and pinnipeds. In: Dierauf LA, Gulland FMD, eds. *CRC Handbook of Marine Mammal Medicine*, 2nd edn., 309–336. Boca Raton, FL: CRC Press.

Elliser CR, Calambokidis J, D'Alessandro DN, et al. 2020. Prey-related asphyxiation in harbor porpoises (*Phocoena phocoena*) along the US West Coast: importance of American shad (*Alosa sapidissima*) on adult female harbor porpoise mortality. *Oceans* 1:94–108.

Embong Z, Hitam WHW, Yean CY, et al. 2008. Specific detection of fungal pathogens by 18S rRNA gene PCR in microbial keratitis. *BMC Ophthalmol* 8(1):1–8.

Estes J, Hatfield BB, Ralls K, Ames J. (2003) Causes of mortality in California sea otters during periods of population growth and decline. *Marine Mammal Sci* 19(1):198–216.

Ewing RY, Mase-Guthrie B, McFee W, et al. 2017. Evaluation of serum for pathophysiological effects of prolonged low salinity water exposure in displaced bottlenose dolphins (*Tursiops truncatus*). *Front Vet Sci* 4:80.

Faulkner J, Measures LN, Whoriskey FG. 1998. Stenurus minor (Metastrongyloidea: Pseudaliidae) infections of the cranial sinuses of the harbour porpoise, *Phocoena phocoena. Can J Zoo* 76(7):1209–1216.

Fauquier DA, Gulland FMD, Trupkiewicz JG, et al. 1996. Coccidioidomycosis in free-living California sea lions (*Zalophus californianus*) in central California. *J Wildl Dis* 32(4):707–710.

Fauquier D, Gulland F, Haulena M, et al. 2004. Meningoencephalitis in two stranded California sea lions (*Zalophus californianus*) caused by aberrant trematode migration. *J Wildl Dis* 40(4):816–819.

Fauquier DA, Kinsel MJ, Dailey MD, et al. 2009. Prevalence and pathology of lungworm infection in bottlenose dolphins *Tursiops truncatus* from southwest Florida. *Dis Aquat Organ* 88(1):85–90.

Fenwick SG, Duignan PJ, Nicol CM, et al. 2004. A comparison of Salmonella serotypes isolated from New Zealand sea lions and feral pigs on the Auckland Islands by pulsed-field gel electrophoresis. *J Wildl Dis* 40:566–570.

Fidalgo SG, Wang Q, Riley TV. 2000. Comparison of methods for detection of *Erysipelothrix* spp and their distribution in some Australasian seafoods. *Appl Environ Microbiol* 66(5):2066–2070.

Field CL. 2018. The brain game: diagnosis of neurologic disease in stranded Pacific harbor seal (*Phoca vitulina richardsi*) pups. Presented at the International Association of Aquatic Animal Medicine Conference, Long Beach, CA 19th–23nd May, 2018.

Field CL, Gulland FMD, Johnson SP, et al. 2018. Seal and sea lion medicine. In: Gulland FMD, Dierauf LA, Whitman KL, eds. *CRC Handbook of Marine Mammal Medicine*, 3rd ed., 909–934. Boca Raton, FL: CRC Press.

Fire SE, Wang Z, Byrd M, et al. 2011. Co-occurrence of multiple classes of harmful algal toxins in bottlenose dolphins (*Tursiops truncatus*) stranding during an unusual mortality event in Texas, USA. *Harmful Algae* 10(3):330–336.

Fire SE, Van Dolah FM. 2012. Marine biotoxins. In: Aguirre AA, Ostfeld RS, Daszak P, eds. *New Directions in Conservation Medicine: Applied cases of ecological health*, 374–389. New York, NY: Oxford University Press.

Forbes LB. 2000. The occurrence and ecology of Trichinella in marine mammals. *Vet Parasitol* 93(3–4):321–334.

Forbes LB, Nielsen O, Measures L, Ewalt DR. 2000. Brucellosis in ringed seals and harp seals from Canada. *J Wildl Dis* 36(3):595–598.

Ford JK, Ellis GM, Matkin CO, et al. 2011. Shark predation and tooth wear in a population of northeastern Pacific killer whales. *Aquat Biol* 11(3):213–224.

Forshaw D, Phelps GR. 1991. Tuberculosis in a captive colony of pinnipeds. *J Wildl Dis* 27(2):288–295.

Foster G, Jahans KL, Reid RJ, Ross HM. 1996. Isolation of Brucella species from cetaceans, seals, and an otter. *Vet Rec* 138:583–586.

Foster G, Ross HM, Patterson IAP, et al. 1998. *Actinobacillus scotiae* sp nov, a new member of the family Pasteurellaceae Pohl (1979) 1981 isolated from porpoises (*Phocoena phocoena*). *Int J Syst Evol Microbiol* 48(3):929–933.

Foster G, Patterson IAP, Munro DS. 1999. Monophasic group B Salmonella species infecting harbour porpoises (*Phocoena phocoena*) inhabiting Scottish coastal waters. *Vet Microbiol* 65(3):227–231.

Foster G, MacMillan AP, Godfroid J, et al. 2002. A review of *Brucella* sp infection of sea mammals with particular emphasis on isolates from Scotland. *Vet Microbiol* 90(1–4):563–580.

Foster G, Holmes B, Steigerwalt et al. 2004. *Campylobacter insulaenigrae* sp nov, isolated from marine mammals. *Int J Syst Evol Microbiol* 54(6):2369–2373.

Foster G, Osterman BS, Godfroid J, et al. 2007. *Brucella ceti* sp nov and *Brucella pinnipedialis* sp nov for Brucella strains with cetaceans and seals as their preferred hosts. *Int J Syst Evol Microbiol* 57(11):2688–2693.

Foster G, Higgins R, Leclair D, et al. 2011a. Proposal of *Bisgaardia hudsonensis* gen nov, sp nov and an additional genomospecies, isolated from seals, as new members of the family Pasteurellaceae. *Int J Syst Evol Microbiol* 61(12):3016–3022.

Foster, G, McAuliffe, L, Dagleish, MP, Barley, J, Howie, F, Nicholas, RA and Ayling, RD (2011b) Mycoplasma species isolated from harbor porpoises (Phocoena phocoena) and a Sowerby's beaked whale (Mesoplodon bidens) stranded in Scottish waters *J Wildl Dis* 47(1):206–211.

Fujioka RS, Greco SB, Cates MB, Schroeder JP. 1988. *Vibrio damsela* from wounds in bottlenose dolphins *Tursiops truncates*. *Dis Aquat Organ* 4(1):1–8.

Fulde M, Valentin-Weigand P. 2013. Epidemiology and pathogenicity of zoonotic streptococci. *Curr Top Microbiol Immunol* 386:49–81.

Garner MM, Lambourn DM, Jeffries SJ, et al. 1997. Evidence of Brucella infection in Parafilaroides lungworms in a Pacific harbor seal (*Phoca vitulina richardsi*). *J Vet Diagn Invest* 9(3):298–303.

Garner HM, Barr BC, Packham AE, et al. 1997. Fatal hepatic sarcocystosis in two polar bears (*Ursus maritimus*). *J Parasitol* 83(3):523–526.

Gehring EA, Mergl JC, Cornell LH. 2013. *Nocardia paucivorans* in a juvenile beluga whale (*Delphinapterus leucas*). International Association of Aquatic Animal Medicine Conference Proceedings. https://www.vin.com/apputil/content/defaultadv1.aspx?id=5768640&pid=11375& (accessed 9 October 2022).

Gentry RL, Johnson JH. 1981. Predation by sea lions on northern fur seal neonates. *Mammalia* 45(4):423–430.

Geraci JR, Aubin DJS. 1987. Effects of parasites on marine mammals. *Int J Parasitol* 17(2):407–414.

Geraci JR, Dailey MD, Aubin DS. 1978. Parasitic mastitis in the Atlantic white-sided dolphin, *Lagenorhynchus acutus*, as a probable factor in herd productivity. *J Fish Board Can* 35(10):1350–1355.

Geraci JR, Fortin JF, Aubin DS, Hicks BD. 1981. The seal louse, *Echinophthirius horridus*: an intermediate host of the seal heartworm, *Dipetalonema spirocauda* (Nematoda). *Can J Zool* 59(7):1457–1459.

Geraci JR, Aubin DJS, Barker IK, et al. 1984. Susceptibility of grey (*Halichoerus* grypus) and harp (*Phoca groenlandica*) seals to the influenza virus and mycoplasma of epizootic pneumonia of harbor seals (*Phoca vitulina*). *Can J Fish Aquat Sci* 41(1):151–156.

Geraci JR, Anderson DM, Timperi RJ, et al. 1989. Humpback whales (*Megaptera novaeangliae*) fatally poisoned by dinoflagellate toxin. *Can J Fish Aquat Sci* 46(11):1895–1898.

Gerber JA, Roletto J, Morgan LE, et al. 1993. Findings in pinnipeds stranded along the central and northern California coast, 1984–1990. *J Wildl Dis* 29(3):423–433.

Gerlach TJ, Wit MD, Landolfi JA. 2012. Diaphragmatic hernia and right-sided heart enlargement in a Florida manatee (*Trichechus manatus latirostris*). *J Wildl Dis* 48(4):1102–1104.

Ghim SJ, Joh J, Mignucci-Giannoni AA, et al. 2014. Genital papillomatosis associated with two novel mucosotropic papillomaviruses from a Florida manatee (*Trichechus manatus latirostris*). *Aquat Mammals* 40(2):195–200.

Giebel J, Meier J, Binder A, et al. 1991. *Mycoplasma phocarhinis* sp nov and *Mycoplasma phocacerebrale* sp nov, two new species from harbor seals (*Phoca vitulina* L). *Int J Syst Evol Microbiol* 41(1):39–44.

Gilmartin WG, Vainik PM, Neill VM. 1979. Salmonellae in feral pinnipeds off the southern California coast. *J Wildl Dis* 15(4):511–514.

Godfroid J, Saegerman C, Wellemans V, et al. 2002. How to substantiate eradication of bovine brucellosis when aspecific serological reactions occur in the course of brucellosis testing. *Vet Microbiol* 90(1–4):461–477.

Goertz CE, Walton R, Rouse N, et al. 2013. *Vibrio parahaemolyticus*, a climate change indicator in Alaska marine mammals. International Association of Aquatic Animal Medicine Conference Proceedings. https://www.vin.com/apputil/content/defaultadv1.aspx?pId=11375&meta=Generic&catId=35416&id=5768586&ind=41&objTypeID=17 (accessed 9 October 2022).

Goldstein T, Mazet JAK, Zabka TS, et al. 2008. Novel symptomatology and changing epidemiology of domoic acid toxicosis in California sea lions (*Zalophus californianus*): an increasing risk to marine mammal health. *Proc R Soc B* 275(1632):267–276.

Goldstein T, Zabka TS, DeLong RL, et al. 2009. The role of domoic acid in abortion and premature parturition of California sea lions (*Zalophus californianus*) on San Miguel Island, California. *J Wildl Dis* 45(1):91–108.

González-Barrientos R, Morales JA, Hernández-Mora G, et al. 2010. Pathology of striped dolphins (*Stenella coeruleoalba*) infected with *Brucella ceti*. *J Comp Pathol* 142(4):347–352.

Gosselin JF, Measures LN, Huot J. 1998. Lungworm (Nematoda: Metastrongyloidea) infections in Canadian phocids. *Can J Fish Aquat Sci* 55(4):825–834.

Greig DJ, Gulland FM, Kreuder C. 2005. A decade of live California sea lion (*Zalophus californianus*) strandings along the central California coast: causes and trends, 1991–2000. *Aquat Mammals* 31(1):11–22.

Greig DJ, Gulland FM, Smith WA, et al. 2014. Surveillance for zoonotic and selected pathogens in harbor seals *Phoca vitulina* from central California. *Dis Aquat Organ* 111(2):93–106.

Groch KR, Marcondes MC, Colosio AC, and Catão-Dias JL. 2012. Skeletal abnormalities in humpback whales *Megaptera novaeangliae* stranded in the Brazilian breeding ground. *Dis Aquat Organ* 101(2):145–158.

Guarner J, Brandt ME. 2011. Histopathologic diagnosis of fungal infections in the 21st century. *Clin Microbiol Rev* 24(2):247–280.

Guillot J, Petit T, Degorce-Rubiales F, et al. 1998. Dermatitis caused by *Malassezia pachydermatis* in a California sea lion (*Zalophus californianus*). *Vet Rec* 142:311–312.

Gulland F, Hall A, Ylitalo G, et al. 2020. Persistent contaminants and herpesvirus OtHV1 are positively associated with cancer in wild California sea lions (*Zalophus californianus*). *Front Mar Sci* 7:602565.

Gulland FM, Nutter FB, Dixon K, et al. 2008. Health assessment, antibiotic treatment, and behavioral responses to herding efforts of a cow–calf pair of humpback whales (*Megaptera novaeangliae*) in the Sacramento River Delta, California. *Aquat Mammals* 34(2):182–192.

Gulland FM, Hall AJ, Greig DJ, et al. 2012. Evaluation of circulating eosinophil count and adrenal gland function in California sea lions naturally exposed to domoic acid. *J Am Vet Med Assoc* 241(7):943–949.

Gulland FMD, Trupkiewicz JG, Spraker TR, Lowenstine LJ. 1996. Metastatic carcinoma of probable transitional cell origin in 66 free-living California sea lions (*Zalophus californianus*), 1979 to 1994. *J Wildl Dis* 32(2):250–258.

Gulland FMD, Beckmen K, Burek K, et al. 1997. Nematode (*Otostrongylus circumlitus*) infestation of northern elephant seals (*Mirounga angustirostris*) stranded along the central California coast. *Mar Mammal Sci* 13(3):446–458.

Guzmán-Verri C, Gonzalez-Barrios R, Hernandez G, et al. 2012. *Brucella ceti* and brucellosis in cetaceans. *Front Cell Infect Microbiol* 2:1–22.

Halaska BL, Johnson SP, DeRango EL, Duignan PJ. 2018. First evidence of interspecies interaction between a Risso's dolphin and coastal bottlenose dolphin in the San Francisco Bay area. International Association of Aquatic Animal Medicine Conference, Long Beach, CA, 19–23 May, 2018. https://www.vin.com/apputil/content/defaultadv1.aspx?pId=20778&meta=Generic&catId=113367&id=8504894&ind=112&objTypeID=17 (accessed 9 October 2022).

Hanni KD, Mazet JA, Gulland FM, et al. 2003. Clinical pathology and assessment of pathogen exposure in southern and Alaskan sea otters. *J Wildl Dis* 39(4):837–850.

Hansen MJ, Bertelsen MF, Delaney MA, et al. 2013. *Otariodibacter oris* and Bisgaardia genomospecies 1 isolated from infections in pinnipeds. *J Wildl Dis* 49(3):661–665.

Harris HS, Facemire P, Greig DJ, et al. 2011. Congenital neuroglial heterotopia in a neonatal harbor seal (*Phoca vitulina richardsi*) with evidence of recent exposure to polycyclic aromatic hydrocarbons. *J Wildl Dis* 47(1):246–254.

Harcourt R. 1993. Individual variation in predation on fur seals by southern sea lions (*Otaria byronia*) in Peru. *Can J Zool* 71(9):1908–1911.

Haulena M, Gulland FM, Lawrence JA, et al. 2006. Lesions associated with a novel *Mycoplasma* sp in California sea lions (*Zalophus californianus*) undergoing rehabilitation. *J Wildl Dis* 42(1):40–45.

Hays R, Measures LN, Huot J. 1998. Euphausiids as intermediate hosts of Anisakis simplex in the St Lawrence estuary. *Can J Zool* 76(7):1226–1235.

Heckmann RA, Jensen LA, Warnock RG, Coleman B. 1987. Parasites of the bowhead whale, *Balaena mysticetus. Great Basin Natur* 47(3):355–372.

Hermosilla C, Silva LM, Kleinertz S, et al. 2016. Endoparasite survey of free-swimming baleen whales (*Balaenoptera musculus, B physalus, B borealis*) and sperm whales (*Physeter macrocephalus*) using non/minimally invasive methods. *Parasitol Res* 115(2):889–896.

Houde M, Measures LN, Huot J. 2003. Experimental transmission of *Pharurus pallasii* (Nematoda: Metastrongyloidea), a lungworm of the cranial sinuses of the beluga whale (*Delphinapterus leucas*), to fish. *Can J Zool* 81(3):364–370.

Hsu CK, Melby Jr EC, Altman NH. 1974. *Eimeria phocae* sp n from the harbor seal (*Phoca vitulina concolor*). *J Parasitol* 60(3):399–402.

Huckabone SE, Gulland FM, Johnson SM, et al. 2015. Coccidioidomycosis and other systemic mycoses of marine mammals stranding along the central California, USA coast: 1998–2012. *J Wildl Dis* 51(2):295–308.

Huggins JL, Raverty SA, Norman SA, et al. 2015. Increased harbor porpoise mortality in the Pacific Northwest, USA: understanding when higher levels may be normal. *Dis Aquat Organ* 115(2):93–102.

Hughes SN, Greig DJ, Miller WA, et al. 2013. Dynamics of *Vibrio* with virulence genes detected in Pacific harbor seals (*Phoca vitulina richardsi*) off California: implications for marine mammal health. *Microb Ecol* 65(4):982–994.

Hunter JEB, Duignan PJ, Dupont C, et al. 1998. First report of potentially zoonotic tuberculosis in fur seals in New Zealand. *N Z Med J* 111:130–131.

Jabbar A, Beveridge I, Bryant MS. 2015. Morphological and molecular observations on the status of *Crassicauda magna*, a parasite of the subcutaneous tissues of the pygmy sperm whale, with a re-evaluation of the systematic relationships of the genus *Crassicauda*. *Parasitol Res* 114(3):835–841.

Jaime-Andrade G, Avila-Figueroa D, Lozano-Kasten J, et al. 1997. Acute Chagas' cardiopathy in a polar bear (*Ursus maritimus*) in Guadalajara, Mexico. *Rev Soc Bras Med Trop* 30(4):337–340.

Jang S, Wheeler L, Carey RB, et al. 2010. Pleuritis and suppurative pneumonia associated with a hypermucoviscosity phenotype of *Klebsiella pneumoniae* in California sea lions (*Zalophus californianus*). *Vet Microbiol* 141(1–2):174–177.

Jauniaux T, Petitjean D, Brenez C, et al. 2002. Post-mortem findings and causes of death of harbour porpoises (*Phocoena phocoena*) stranded from 1990 to 2000 along the coastlines of Belgium and Northern France. *J Comp Pathol* 126(4):243–253.

Jauniaux T, Garigliany MM, Loos P, et al. 2014. Bite injuries of grey seals (*Halichoerus grypus*) on harbour porpoises (*Phocoena phocoena*). *PloS One* 9(12): e108993.

Javeed N, Foley J, Oliver-Guimera A, et al. 2021. Demodectic mange in threatened southern sea otters (*Enhydra lutris nereis*). *Vet Dermatol* 32(3):211–e55.

Jensen SK, Nymo IH, Forcada J, et al. 2013. Brucella antibody seroprevalence in Antarctic seals (*Arctocephalus gazella*, *Leptonychotes weddellii* and *Mirounga leonina*). *Dis Aquat Organ* 105(3):175–181.

Jepson PD, Baker JR, Kuiken T, et al. 2000. Pulmonary pathology of harbour porpoises (*Phocoena phocoena*) stranded in England and Wales between 1990 and 1996. *Vet Rec* 146(25):721–728.

Jurczynski K, Lyashchenko KP, Scharpegge J, et al. 2012. Use of multiple diagnostic tests to detect *Mycobacterium pinnipedii* infections in a large group of South American sea lions (*Otaria flavescens*). *Aquat Mammals* 38(1):43–55.

Kane EA, Olson PA, Gerrodette T, Fiedler PC. 2008. Prevalence of the commensal barnacle *Xenobalanus globicipitis* on cetacean species in the eastern tropical Pacific Ocean, and a review of global occurrence. *Fish Bull* 106(4):395–404.

Kaye S, Johnson S, Rios C, Fletcher DJ. 2017. Plasmatic coagulation and fibrinolysis in healthy and Otostrongylus-affected Northern elephant seals (*Mirounga angustirostris*). *Vet Clin Pathol* 46(4):589–596.

Keenan-Bateman TF, McLellan WA, Harms CA, et al. 2016. Prevalence and anatomic site of *Crassicauda* sp infection, and its use in species identification, in kogiid whales from the mid-Atlantic United States. *Mar Mammal Sci* 32(3):868–883.

Keenan-Bateman TF, McLellan WA, Costidis AM, et al. 2018. Habitat use pattern of the giant parasitic nematode *Crassicauda magna* within the pygmy sperm whale *Kogia breviceps*. *Dis Aquat Organ* 127 (3):163–175.

Kersh GJ, Lambourn DM, Self JS, et al. 2010. *Coxiella burnetii* infection of a Steller sea lion (*Eumetopias jubatus*) found in Washington State. *J Clin Microbiol* 48(9):3428–3431.

Kersh GJ, Lambourn DM, Raverty SA, et al. 2012. *Coxiella burnetii* infection of marine mammals in the Pacific Northwest, 1997–2010. *J Wildl Dis* 48(1):201–206.

Kiers A, Klarenbeek A, Mendelts B, et al. 2008. Transmission of *Mycobacterium pinnipedii* to humans in a zoo with marine mammals. *Int J Tuberculosis Lung Dis* 12(12):1469–1473.

Kikuchi S. 1993. *Bolbosoma capitatum* (Acanthocephala) from false killer whales, *Pseudorca crassidens*, and its pathogenicity. *Japan J Parasitol* 42:398–408.

Kinoshita R. 2008. Melioidosis in marine mammals. In: Miller ME, Fowler RE, eds., 299–307. *Zoo and Wild Animal Medicine*. Philadelphia, PA: Elsevier Health Sciences.

Kinsel MJ, Boehm JR, Harris B, Murnane RD. 1997. Fatal *Erysipelothrix rhusiopathiae* septicemia in a captive Pacific white-sided dolphin (*Lagenorhyncus obliquidens*). *J Zoo Wildl Med* 28(4):494–497.

Knowles S, Lynch D, Thomas N. 2020. Leptospirosis in Northern Sea Otters (*Enhydra lutris kenyoni*) from Washington, USA. *J Wildl Dis*, 56(2):466–471.

Kreuder C, Miller MA, Jessup DA, et al. 2003. Patterns of mortality in southern sea otters (*Enhydra lutris nereis*) from 1998–2001. *J Wildl Dis* 39(3):495–509.

Kreuder C, Miller MA, Lowenstine LJ, et al. 2005. Evaluation of cardiac lesions and risk factors associated with myocarditis and dilated cardiomyopathy in southern sea otters (*Enhydra lutris nereis*). *Am J Vet Res* 66(2):289–299.

Krog JS, Hansen MS, Holm E, et al. 2015. Influenza A (H10N7) virus in dead harbor seals, *Denmark. Emerg Infect Dis* 21(4):684–687.

Kuzmina TA, Spraker TR, Kudlai O, et al. 2018. Metazoan parasites of California sea lions (*Zalophus californianus*): a new data and review. *Int J Parasitol* 7(3):326–334.

Lacave G, Cui Y, Salbany A, et al. 2019. Erysipelas vaccination protocols in dolphins *Tursiops truncatus* evaluated by antibody responses over twenty continuous years. *Dis Aquat Organ* 134(3):237–255.

Lainson R, Naiff RD, Best RC,Shaw, JJ. 1983. *Eimeria trichechi* n sp from the Amazonian manatee, *Trichechus inunguis* (Mammalia: Sirenia). *Syst Parasitol* 5(4):287–289.

Lair S, Beland P, De Guise S, Martineau D. 1997. Adrenal hyperplastic and degenerative changes in beluga whales. *J Wildl Dis* 33(3):430–437.

Lair S, Measures LN, Martineau D. 2016. Pathologic findings and trends in mortality in the beluga (*Delphinapterus leucas*) population of the St Lawrence Estuary, Quebec, Canada, from 1983 to 2012. *Vet Pathol* 53(1):22–36.

Lambertsen RH. 1986. Disease of the common fin whale (*Balaenoptera physalus*): crassicaudiosis of the urinary system. *J Mammal* 67(2):353–366.

Lambertsen RH. 1997. Natural disease problems of the sperm whale. *Biologie* 67(Suppl):105–112.

Lambourn DM, Garner M, Ewalt D, et al. 2013. *Brucella pinnipedialis* infections in Pacific harbor seals (*Phoca vitulina richardsi*) from Washington State, USA. *J Wildl Dis* 49(4):802–815.

Lapointe JM, Duignan PJ, Marsh AE, et al. 1998. Meningoencephalitis due to a Sarcocystis neurona-like protozoan in Pacific harbor seals (*Phoca vitulina richardsi*). *J Parasitol* 84(6):1184–1189.
Lapointe JM, Gulland FMD, Haines D, et al. 1999. Placentitis due to *Coxiella burnetii* in a Pacific harbor seal (*Phoca vitulina richardsi*). *J Vet Diagn Invest* 11:541–543.
Larrat S, Lair S. 2012. Rake marks on a harbor porpoise (*Phocoena phocoena*) calf suggestive of a fatal interaction with an Atlantic white-sided dolphin (*Lagenorhynchus acutus*). *Aquat Mammals* 38(1):86–91.
Lawson PA, Falsen E, Foster G, et al. 2001. *Arcanobacterium pluranimalium* sp nov, isolated from porpoise and deer. *Int J Syst Evol Microbiol* 51(1):55–59.
Lawson PA, Foster G, Falsen E, Collins MD. 2005. *Streptococcus marimammalium* sp nov, isolated from seals. *Int J Syst Evol Microbiol* 55(1):271–274.
Le Boeuf BJ, Mesnick S. 1991. Sexual behavior of male northern elephant seals: I Lethal injuries to adult females. *Behaviour* 116(1–2):143–162.
Lefebvre KA, Bargu S, Kieckhefer T, Silver MW. 2002. From sanddabs to blue whales: the pervasiveness of domoic acid. *Toxicon* 40(7):971–977.
Lefebvre KA, Robertson A, Frame ER, et al. 2010. Clinical signs and histopathology associated with domoic acid poisoning in northern fur seals (*Callorhinus ursinus*) and comparison of toxin detection methods. *Harmful Algae* 9(4):374–383.
Lefebvre KA, Hendrix A, Halaska B, et al. 2018. Domoic acid in California sea lion fetal fluids indicates continuous exposure to a neuroteratogen poses risks to mammals. *Harmful Algae* 79:53–57.
Lehnert K, Raga JA, Siebert U. 2005. Macroparasites in stranded and bycaught harbour porpoises from German and Norwegian waters. *Dis Aquat Organ* 64(3):265–269.
Lehnert K, Raga JA, Siebert U. 2007a. Parasites in harbour seals (*Phoca vitulina*) from the German Wadden Sea between two phocine distemper virus epidemics. *Helgoland Mar Res* 61(4):239–245.
Lehnert K, Fonfara S, Wohlsein P, Siebert U. 2007b. Whale lice (*Isocyamus delphinii*) on a harbour porpoise (*Phocoena phocoena*) from German waters. *Vet Rec* 161:526–528.
Lehnert K, von Samson-Himmelstjerna G, Schaudien D, et al. 2010. Transmission of lungworms of harbour porpoises and harbour seals: molecular tools determine potential vertebrate intermediate hosts. *Int J Parasitol* 40(7):845–853.
Lehnert K, Seibel H, Hasselmeier I, et al. 2014. Increase in parasite burden and associated pathology in harbour porpoises (*Phocoena phocoena*) in West Greenland. *Polar Biol* 37(3):321–331.
Lehnert K, Schwanke E, Hahn K, et al. 2016. Heartworm (*Acanthocheilonema spirocauda*) and seal louse (*Echinophthirius horridus*) infections in harbour seals (*Phoca vitulina*) from the North and Baltic Seas. *J Sea Res* 113:65–72.
Lehnert K, IJsseldijk LL, Uy ML, et al. 2021. Whale lice (*Isocyamus deltobranchium* and *Isocyamus delphinii*; Cyamidae) prevalence in odontocetes off the German and Dutch coasts: morphological and molecular characterization and health implications. *Int J Parasitol* 15:22–30.
Leidenberger S, Harding K, Härkönen T. 2007. Phocid seals, seal lice and heartworms: a terrestrial host–parasite system conveyed to the marine environment. *Dis Aquat Organ* 77(3):235–253.
Lempereur L, Delobelle M, Doom M, et al. 2017. *Crassicauda boopis* in a fin whale (*Balaenoptera physalus*) ship-struck in the eastern North Atlantic Ocean. *Parasitol Open* 3:E9. doi:10.1017/pao.2017.10.
Lenting B, Gartrell B, Kokosinska A, et al. 2019. Causes of adult mortality in two populations of New Zealand sea lions (*Phocarctos hookeri*). *Anim Vet Sci* 7:10057.
Leonardi MS, Palma RL. 2013. Review of the systematics, biology, and ecology of lice from pinnipeds and river otters (Insecta: Phthiraptera: Anoplura: Echinophthiriidae). *Zootaxa* 3630(3):445–466.
Leopold MF, Begeman L, van Bleijswijk JD, et al. 2015. Exposing the grey seal as a major predator of harbour porpoises. *Proc R Soc B* 282(1798):20142429.

Li Z, Ip HS, Trost JF, et al. 2014. Serologic evidence of influenza a(h1n1) PDM09 virus infection in northern sea otters. *Emerg Infect Dis* 20(5):915–917.

Lindsay SA, Gray R. 2021. A novel presentation of tuberculosis with intestinal perforation in a free-ranging Australian sea lion (*Neophoca cinerea*). *J Wildl Dis* 57(1):220–224.

Linn LM, Gardner J, Warrilow D, et al. 2001. Arbovirus of marine mammals: a new alphavirus isolated from the elephant seal louse, *Lepidophthirus macrorhini. J Virol* 75(9):4103–4109.

Liong E, Hammond DD, Vedros N. 1985. *Pseudomonas pseudomallei* infection in a dolphin (*Tursiops gilli*): a case study. *Aquat Mammals* 1:20–22.

Littnan CL, Stewart BS, Yochem PK, Braun R. 2006. Survey for selected pathogens and evaluation of disease risk factors for endangered Hawaiian monk seals in the main Hawaiian Islands. *EcoHealth* 3(4):232–244.

Loch C, Grando LJ, Kieser JA, Simões-Lopes PC. 2011. Dental pathology in dolphins (Cetacea: Delphinidae) from the southern coast of Brazil. *Dis Aquat Organ* 94(3):225–234.

Loch C, Simoes-Lopes PC. 2013. Dental wear in dolphins (Cetacea: Delphinidae) from southern Brazil. *Arch Oral Biol* 58(2):134–141.

Lyons ET, DeLong RL, Spraker TR, et al. 2005. Seasonal prevalence and intensity of hookworms (*Uncinaria* spp) in California sea lion (*Zalophus californianus*) pups born in 2002 on San Miguel Island, *California. Parasitol Res* 96(2):127–132.

Lyons ET, DeLong RL, Nadler SA, et al. 2011. Investigations of peritoneal and intestinal infections of adult hookworms (*Uncinaria* spp) in northern fur seal (*Callorhinus ursinus*) and California sea lion (*Zalophus californianus*) pups on San Miguel Island, California (2003). *Parasitol Res* 109(3):581–589.

Lynch M, Duignan PJ, Taylor T, et al. 2011a. Epizootiology of Brucella infection in Australian fur seals. *J Wildl Dis* 47(2):352–363.

Lynch M, Taylor TK, Duignan PJ, et al. 2011b. Mycoplasmas in Australian fur seals: identification and association with abortion. *J Vet Diagn Invest* 23(6):1123–1130.

Lynch M, Kirkwood R, Mitchell A, et al. 2011c. Prevalence and significance of an alopecia syndrome in Australian fur seals (*Arctocephalus pusillus doriferus*). *J Mammal* 92(2):342–351.

Ma H, Overstreet RM, Sniezek JH, et al. 2006. Two new species of symbiotic ciliates from the respiratory tract of cetaceans with establishment of the new genus Planilamina n gen (Dysteriida, Kyaroikeidae). *J Eukaryot Microbiol* 53(6):407–419.

Mackereth GF, Webb KM, O'keefe JS, et al. 2005. Serological survey of pre-weaned New Zealand fur seals (*Arctocephalus forsteri*) for brucellosis and leptospirosis. *N Z Vet J* 53(6):428–432.

Marcer F, Negrisolo E, Franzo G, et al. 2019. Morphological and molecular characterization of adults and larvae of *Crassicauda* spp (Nematoda: Spirurida) from Mediterranean fin whales *Balaenoptera physalus* (Linnaeus, 1758). *Int J Parasitol* 9:258–265.

Marcus AD, Higgins DP, Gray R. 2014. Epidemiology of hookworm (*Uncinaria sanguinis*) infection in free-ranging Australian sea lion (*Neophoca cinerea*) pups. *Parasitol Res* 113(9):3341–3353.

Marcus AD, Higgins DP, Gray R. 2015. Health assessment of free-ranging endangered Australian sea lion (*Neophoca cinerea*) pups: effect of haematophagous parasites on haematological parameters. *Comp Biochem Physiol A* 184:132–143.

Martineau D, Lemberger K, Dallaire A, et al. 2002. Cancer in wildlife, a case study: beluga from the St Lawrence estuary, Québec, *Canada. Environ Health Perspect* 110(3):285–292.

Martinez ME, Stacy NI, Wellehan JFX, et al. 2022. Diffuse large B cell lymphoma and a novel gammaherpesvirus in northern elephant seals (*Mirounga angustirostris*). *Dis Aquat Organ* 149:59–70.

Martinez-Levasseur LM, Gendron D, Knell RJ, et al. 2011. Acute sun damage and photoprotective responses in whales. *Proc R Soc B* 278(1711):1581–1586.

Mathavarajah S, Dellaire G. 2020. Lions, tigers, and kittens too: ACE2 and susceptibility to COVID-19. *Evol Med Publ Health* 2020(1):109–113.

Mathavarajah S, Stoddart AK, Gagnon GA, Dellaire G. 2021. Pandemic danger to the deep: the risk of marine mammals contracting SARS-CoV-2 from wastewater. *Sci Total Environ* 760:143346.

Mavrot F, Orsel K, Hutchins W, et al. 2020. Novel insights into serodiagnosis and epidemiology of Erysipelothrix rhusiopathiae, a newly recognized pathogen in muskoxen (*Ovibos moschatus*). *PloS One* 15(4):pe0231724.

Mayer KA, Dailey MD, Miller MA. 2003. Helminth parasites of the southern sea otter *Enhydra lutris nereis* in central California: abundance, distribution, and pathology. *Dis Aquat Organ* 53(1):77–88.

McAloose D, Rago MV, Di Martino M, et al. 2016. Post-mortem findings in southern right whales *Eubalaena australis* at Península Valdés, Argentina, 2003–2012. *Dis Aquat Organ* 119(1):17–36.

McClain AM, Daniels R, Gomez FM, et al. 2020. Physiological effects of low salinity exposure on bottlenose dolphins (Tursiops truncatus) *J Zool Botanic Gardens* 1(1):61–75.

McClelland G. 1993. *Eimeria phocae* (Apicomplexa: Eimeriidae) in harbour seals *Phoca vitulina* from Sable Island, Canada. *Dis Aquat Organ* 17:1–8.

McClelland G. 2002. The trouble with sealworms (*Pseudoterranova decipiens* species complex, Nematoda): a review. *Parasitology* 124(7):183–203.

McDonald WL, Jamaludin R, Mackereth G, et al. 2006. Characterization of a *Brucella* sp strain as a marine-mammal type despite isolation from a patient with spinal osteomyelitis in New Zealand. *J Clin Microbiol* 44(12):4363–4370.

McHuron E, Miller MA, Gardiner CH, Harvey JT. 2013A. *Pelodera strongyloides* infection in Pacific harbor seals (*Phoca vitulina richardii*) from California. *J Zoo Wildl Med* 44:799–802.

McHuron EA, Greig DJ, Colegrove KM, et al. 2013B. Domoic acid exposure and associated clinical signs and histopathology in Pacific harbor seals (*Phoca vitulina richardii*). *Harmful Algae* 23:28–33.

McIlhattan TJ, Martin JW, Wagner RJ, Iversen JO. 1971. Isolation of Leptospira pomona from a naturally infected California sea lion, Sonoma County, California. *J Wildl Dis* 7(3):195–197.

McKnight CA, Reynolds TL, Haulena M, et al. 2005. Congenital hemicerebral anomaly in a stranded Pacific harbor seal (*Phoca vitulina richardsi*). *J Wildl Dis* 41(3):654–658.

Mcleland S, Duncan C, Spraker T, et al. 2012. *Cryptococcus albidus* infection in a California sea lion (*Zalophus californianus*). *J Wildl Dis* 48(4):1030–1034.

Measures L. 2018. Helminths and parasitic arthropods. In: Gulland FMD, Dierauf LA, Whitman KL, eds. *CRC Handbook of Marine Mammal Medicine*, 3rd ed., 471–500. Boca Raton, FL: CRC Press.

Measures LN, Béland P, Martineau D, Guise SD. 1995. Helminths of an endangered population of belugas, *Delphinapterus leucas*, in the St Lawrence estuary, Canada. *Can J Zool* 73(8):1402–1409.

Migaki G, van Dyke DON, Hubbard RC. 1971. Some histopathological lesions caused by helminths in marine mammals. *J Wildl Dis* 7(4):281–289.

Mihindukulasuriya KA, Wu G, St Leger J, et al. 2008. Identification of a novel coronavirus from a beluga whale by using a panviral microarray. *J Virol* 82(10):5084–5088.

Miller M, Shapiro K, Murray MJ, et al. 2018. Protozoan parasites of marine mammals. In: Gulland FMD, Dierauf LA, Whitman KL, eds. *CRC Handbook of Marine Mammal Medicine*, 3rd ed., 429–465. Boca Raton, FL: CRC Press.

Miller MA, Gardner IA, Kreuder C, et al. 2002. Coastal freshwater runoff is a risk factor for *Toxoplasma gondii* infection of southern sea otters (*Enhydra lutris nereis*). *Int J Parasitol* 32(8):997–1006.

Miller MA, Conrad PA, James ER, et al. 2008. Transplacental toxoplasmosis in a southern sea otter (*Enhydra lutris nereis*). *Vet Parasitol* 153:12–18.

Miller MA, Byrne BA, Jang SS, et al. 2010a. Enteric bacterial pathogen detection in southern sea otters (Enhydra lutris nereis) is associated with coastal urbanization and freshwater runoff. *Vet Res* 41(1):1–13.

Miller MA, Kudela RM, Mekebri A, et al. 2010b. Evidence for a novel marine harmful algal bloom: Cyanotoxin (microcystin) transfer from land to sea otters. *PLoS One* 5(9):e12576.

Miller MA, Burgess TL, Dodd EM, et al. 2017. Isolation and characterization of marine brucellae from a southern sea otter (*Enhydra lutris nereis*), California, USA. *J Wildl Dis* 53(2):215–224.

Miller MA, Duignan PJ, Dodd E, et al. 2020a. Emergence of a zoonotic pathogen in a coastal marine sentinel: *Capillaria hepatica* (syn *Calodium hepaticum*) associated hepatitis in southern sea otters (*Enhydra lutris nereis*). *Front Mar Sci* 7:335.

Miller MA, Moriarty ME, Henkel L, et al. 2020b. Predators, disease, and environmental change in the nearshore ecosystem: mortality in southern sea otters (*Enhydra lutris nereis*) from 1998–2012. *Front Mar Sci* 7:582.

Miller MA, Moriarty ME, Duignan PJ, et al. 2021. Clinical signs and pathology associated with domoic acid toxicosis in southern sea otters (*Enhydra lutris nereis*). *Front Mar Sci* 8: https://doiorg/103389/fmars2021585501.

Miller WG, Adams LG, Ficht TA, et al. 1999. Brucella-induced abortions and infection in bottlenose dolphins (*Tursiops truncatus*). *J Zoo Wildl Med* 30(1):100–110.

Miller WG, Padhye AA, van Bonn W, et al. 2002. Cryptococcosis in a bottlenose dolphin (*Tursiops truncatus*) caused by *Cryptococcus neoformans* var gattii. *J Clin Microbiol* 40(2):721–724.

Minor C, Kersh GJ, Gelatt T, et al. 2013. *Coxiella burnetii* in northern fur seals and Steller sea lions of Alaska. *J Wildl Dis* 49(2):441–446.

Montie EW, Wheeler E, Pussini N, et al. 2010. Magnetic resonance imaging quality and volumes of brain structures from live and postmortem imaging of California sea lions with clinical signs of domoic acid toxicosis. *Dis Aquat Organ* 91(3):243–256.

Moore MJ, van der Hoop J, Barco SG, et al. 2013. Criteria and case definitions for serious injury and death of pinnipeds and cetaceans caused by anthropogenic trauma. *Dis Aquat Organ* 103(3):229–264.

Morell M, Lehnert K, IJsseldijk LL, et al. 2017. Parasites in the inner ear of harbour porpoise: cases from the North and Baltic Seas. *Dis Aquat Organ* 127(1):57–63.

Morimitsu T, Nagai T, Ide M, et al. 1987. Mass stranding of Odontoceti caused by parasitogenic eighth cranial neuropathy. *J Wildl Dis* 23(4):586–590.

Morimitsu T, Kawano H, Torihara K, et al. 1992. Histopathology of eighth cranial nerve of mass stranded dolphins at Goto Islands, *Japan. J Wildl Dis* 28(4):656–658.

Mullin K, Barry KP, Sinclair C, et al. 2015. *Common Bottlenose Dolphins (Tursiops truncatus) in Lake Pontchartrain, Louisiana, 2007 to mid-2014.* NOAA Technical Memorandum NMFS-SEFSC-673. Pascagoula, MS: National Oceanic and Atmospheric Administration.

Nadler SA, Lyons ET, Pagan C, et al. 2013.) Molecular systematics of pinniped hookworms (Nematoda: Uncinaria): species delimitation, host associations and host-induced morphometric variation. *Int J Parasitol* 43(14):1119–1132.

Neimanis AS, Moraeus C, Bergman A, et al. 2016. Emergence of the zoonotic biliary trematode *Pseudamphistomum truncatum* in grey seals (*Halichoerus grypus*) in the Baltic Sea. *PLoS One* 11(10):e0164782.

Ness AR. 1966. Dental caries in the platanistid whale *Inia geoffrensis*. *J Comp Pathol* 76:271–279.

Newman SJ, Smith SA. 2006. Marine mammal neoplasia: a review. *Vet Pathol* 43(6):865–880.

Ng TFF, Miller MA, Kondov NO, et al. 2015. Oral papillomatosis caused by *Enhydra lutris* papillomavirus 1 (ElPV-1) in southern sea otters (*Enhydra lutris nereis*) in California, USA. *J Wildl Dis* 51(2):446–453.

Nielsen O, Stewart RE, Nielsen K, et al. 2001. Serologic survey of *Brucella* spp antibodies in some marine mammals of North America. *J Wildl Dis* 37(1):89–100.

Nielsen O, Nielsen K, Braun R, Kelly L. 2005. A comparison of four serologic assays in screening for Brucella exposure in Hawaiian monk seals. *J Wildl Dis* 41(1):126–133.

Nielsen KA, Owen HC, Mills PC, et al. 2013. Bacteria isolated from dugongs (*Dugong dugon*) submitted for postmortem examination in *Queensland, Australia, 2000–2011 J Zoo Wildl Med* 44(1):35–41.

NOAA Fisheries. 2022. 2018–2022 Ice seal unusual mortality event in Alaska. https://www.fisheriesnoaagov/alaska/marine-life-distress/2018-2022-ice-seal-unusual-mortality-event-alaska (accessed 10 September 2022).

Nollens HH, Wellehan JF, Archer L, et al. 2010. Detection of a respiratory coronavirus from tissues archived during a pneumonia epizootic in free-ranging Pacific harbor seals *Phoca vitulina richardsii*. *Dis Aquat Organ* 90(2):113–120.

Nollens HH, Giménez-Lirola LG, Robeck TR, et al. 2016. Evaluation of anti-Erysipelothrix rhusiopathiae IgG response in bottlenose dolphins *Tursiops truncatus* to a commercial pig vaccine. *Dis Aquat Organ* 121(3):249–256.

Norman SA, Raverty S, McLellan B, et al. 2005. Multidisciplinary investigation of harbor porpoises (*Phocoena phocoena*) stranded in Washington State from 2 May–2 June 2003 coinciding with the mid-range sonar exercises of the USS SHOUP. NOAA Technical Memorandum NMFS–NWR–34. Washington, DC: NOAA Northwest Fisheries, US Department of Commerce, National Oceanic and Atmospheric Administration, National Marine Fisheries Service.

Norman SA, Raverty S, Zabek E, et al. 2011. Maternal–fetal transmission of *Cryptococcus gattii* in harbor porpoise. *Emerg Infect Dis* 17(2):304.

Nutting WB, Dailey MD. 1980. Demodicosis (Acari: Demodicidae) in the California sea lion, *Zalophus californianus. J Med Entomol* 17(4):344–347.

Nymo IH, Tryland M, Godfroid J. 2011. A review of *Brucella* infection in marine mammals, with special emphasis on *Brucella pinnipedialis* in the hooded seal (*Cystophora cristata*). *Vet Res* 42(1):93.

O'Hara TM, Holcomb D, Elzer P, et al. 2010. Brucella species survey in polar bears (*Ursus maritimus*) of northern Alaska. *J Wildl Dis* 46(3):687–694.

O'Hara TM, Hart L. 2018. Environmental toxicology. In: Gulland FMD, Dierauf LA, Whitman KL, eds. *CRC Handbook of Marine Mammal Medicine*, 3rd ed., 297–317. Boca Raton, FL: CRC Press

Ohishi K, Zenitani R, Bando T, et al. 2003. Pathological and serological evidence of Brucella infection in baleen whales (Mysticeti) in the western North Pacific. *Comp Immunol Microbiol Infect Dis* 26(2):125–136.

Olsen OW, Lyons ET. 1962. Life cycle of the hookworm, *Uncinaria lucasi* Stiles, of northern fur seals, *Callorhinus ursinus*, on the Pribilof Islands in the Bering Sea. *J Parasitol* 48(2):42–43.

Onderka DK. 1989. Prevalence and pathology of nematode infections in the lungs of ringed seals (*Phoca hispida*) of the western arctic of Canada. *J Wildl Dis* 25(2):218–224.

Opriessnig T, Shen HG, Bender JS, et al. 2013. *Erysipelothrix rhusiopathiae* isolates recovered from fish, a harbour seal (*Phoca vitulina*) and the marine environment are capable of inducing characteristic cutaneous lesions in pigs. *J Comp Pathol* 148(4):365–372.

O'Shea TJ, Homer BL, Greiner EC, Layton AW. 1991. *Nasitrema* sp associated encephalitis in a striped dolphin (*Stenella coeruleoalba*) stranded in the Gulf of Mexico. *J Wildl Dis* 27(4):706–709.

Overy DP, Marron-Lopez F, Muckle A, et al. 2015. Dermatophytosis in farmed mink (*Mustela vison*) caused by *Trichophyton equinum*. *J Vet Diagn Invest* 27(5):621–626.

Owen H, Gillespie A, Wilkie I. 2012. Postmortem findings from dugong (*Dugong dugon*) submissions to the University of Queensland: 1997–2010. *J Wildl Dis* 48(4):962–970.

Owen H, Flint M, de Wit M. 2018. Sirenia. In: Terio KA, McAloose D, St Leger J, eds. *Pathology of Wildlife and Zoo Animals*, 593–606. London, UK: Academic Press.

Owen HC, Flint M, Limpus CJ, et al. 2013. Evidence of sirenian cold stress syndrome in dugongs *Dugong dugon* from southeast Queensland, Australia. *Dis Aquat Organ* 103(1):1–7.

Palmgren H, McCafferty D, Aspan A, et al. 2000. Salmonella in sub-Antarctica: low heterogeneity in Salmonella serotypes in South Georgian seals and birds. *Epidemiol Infect* 125(2):257–262.

Parsons ECM, Jefferson TA. 2000. Post-mortem investigations on stranded dolphins and porpoises from Hong Kong waters. *J Wildl Dis* 36(2):342–356.

Pascual S, Abollo E, Lopez A. 2000. Elemental analysis of cetacean skull lesions associated with nematode infections. *Dis Aquat Organ* 42(1):71–75.

Patterson IAP, Reid RJ, Wilson B, et al. 1998. Evidence for infanticide in bottlenose dolphins: an explanation for violent interactions with harbour porpoises? *Proc R Soc Lond B* 265(1402):1167–1170.

Pereira EM, Müller G, Secchi E, et al. 2013. Digenetic trematodes in South American sea lions from southern Brazilian waters. *J Parasitol* 99(5):910–913.

Pesapane R, Dodd E, Javeed N, et al. 2018. Molecular characterization and prevalence of *Halarachne halichoeri* in threatened southern sea otters (*Enhydra lutris nereis*). *Int J Parasitol* 7(3):386–390.

Peterson JC, Hoggard W. 1996. First sperm whale (*Physeter macrocephalus*) record in Mississippi. *Gulf Caribb Res* 9(3):215–217.

Pistorius PA, Baylis AMM. 2011. A bald encounter: hairless southern sea lion at the Falkland Islands. *Polar Biol* 34(1):145–147.

Pitman RL, Totterdell JA, Fearnbach H, et al. 2015. Whale killers: prevalence and ecological implications of killer whale predation on humpback whale calves off Western Australia. *Mar Mammal Sci* 31:629–657.

Poester F, Nielsen K, Ernesto Samartino L, Ling Yu W. 2010. Diagnosis of brucellosis. *Open Vet Sci J* 4(1):46–60.

Polo F, Figueras MJ, Inza I, et al. 1999. Prevalence of Salmonella serotypes in environmental waters and their relationships with indicator organisms. *Antonie van Leeuwenhoek* 75(4):285–292.

Powell JW, Archibald RT, Cross CA, et al. 2009. Multiple congenital cardiac abnormalities in an Atlantic bottlenose dolphin (*Tursiops truncatus*). *J Wildl Dis* 45(3):839–842.

Poynton SL, Whitaker BR, Heinrich AB. 2001. A novel trypanoplasm-like flagellate *Jarrellia atramenti* ng, n sp (Kinetoplastida: Bodonidae) and ciliates from the blowhole of a stranded pygmy sperm whale *Kogia breviceps* (Physeteridae): morphology, life cycle and potential pathogenicity. *Dis Aquat Organ* 44(3):191–201.

Prager KC, Greig DJ, Alt DP, et al. 2013. Asymptomatic and chronic carriage of *Leptospira interrogans* serovar Pomona in California sea lions (*Zalophus californianus*). *Vet Microbiol* 164(1–2):177–183.

Pugliares-Bonner K, McKenna K, Sette L, et al. 2018. Prevalence of alopecia in gray seals *Halichoerus grypus atlantica* in Massachusetts, USA, 2004–2013. *Dis Aquat Organ* 131(3):167–176.

Quinley N, Mazet JA, Rivera R, Schmitt, et al. 2013. Serologic response of harbor seals (*Phoca vitulina*) to vaccination with a recombinant canine distemper vaccine. *J Wildl Dis* 49(3):579–586.

Raga JA, Balbuena JA. 1990. A new species of the genus Crassicauda Leiper et Atkinson, 1914 (Nematoda: Spiruroidea) from the penis of *Globicephala melas* (Traill, 1809) (Cetacea: Globicephalidae) in the western Mediterranean Sea. *Ann Parasitol Hum Comp* 65(5–6):255–261.

Ramsdell JS. 2010. Neurological disease rises from ocean to bring model for human epilepsy to life. *Toxins* 2(7):1646–1675.

Ramsdell JS, Zabka TS. 2008. In utero domoic acid toxicity: a fetal basis to adult disease in the California sea lion (*Zalophus californianus*). *Mar Drugs* 6(2):262–290.

Rankin KA, Alroy KA, Kudela RM, et al. 2013. Treatment of cyanobacterial (microcystin) toxicosis using oral cholestyramine: case report of a dog from Montana. *Toxins* 5: 1051–1063.

Raverty S, Duignan PJ, Jepson P, Morel M. 2018. Necropsy procedures and sampling for marine mammal gross necropsy. In: Gulland FMD, Dierauf LA, Whitman KL, eds. *CRC Handbook of Marine Mammal Medicine*, 3rd ed., 249–266. Boca Raton, FL: CRC Press.

Ready ZC, Whitmer ER, Wright SE, et al. 2021. Clinical and microbiological characterization of lymph node abscessation in pup and yearling California sea lions (*Zalophus californianus*) undergoing rehabilitation. *J Zoo Wildl Med* 52(4):1149–1158.

Reif JS, Kliks MM, Aguirre AA, et al. 2006. Gastrointestinal helminths in the Hawaiian monk seal (*Monachus schauinslandi*): associations with body size, hematology, and serum chemistry. *Aquat Mammals* 32(2):157–167.

Reidarson TH, Griner LA, Pappagianis D, McBain J. 1998. Coccidioidomycosis in a bottlenose dolphin. *J Wildl Dis* 34(3):629–631.

Reidarson TH, García-Párraga D, Wiederhold NP. 2018. Marine mammal mycoses. In: Gulland FMD, Dierauf LA, Whitman KL, eds. *CRC Handbook of Marine Mammal Medicine*, 3rd ed., 389–424. Boca Raton, FL: CRC Press.

Robinson SJ, Barbieri MM, Murphy S, et al. 2018. Model recommendations meet management reality: implementation and evaluation of a network-informed vaccination effort for endangered Hawaiian monk seals. *Proc R Soc Lond B* 285(1870):20171899.

Roe W, Rogers L, Gartrell B, et al. 2010. Serological evaluation of New Zealand sea lions for exposure to Brucella and Leptospira spp. *J Wildl Dis* 46(6):1295–1299.

Roe WD, Rogers L, Pinpimai K, et al. 2015. Septicaemia and meningitis caused by infection of New Zealand sea lion pups with a hypermucoviscous strain of *Klebsiella pneumoniae*. *Vet Microbiol* 176(3–4):301–308.

Roe WD, Lenting B, Kokosinska A, et al. 2019. Pathology and molecular epidemiology of *Mycobacterium pinnipedii* tuberculosis in native New Zealand seals, sea lions and dolphins. *PLoS One* 14(2):e0212363.

Rosenberg JF, Haulena M, Hoang LM, et al. 2016. *Cryptococcus gattii* type VGIIa infection in harbor seals (*Phoca vitulina*) in British Columbia, *Canada*. *J Wildl Dis* 52(3):677–681.

Rotstein DS, West K, Levine G, et al. 2010. *Cryptococcus gattii* VGI in a spinner dolphin (*Stenella longirostris*) from Hawaii. *J Zoo Wildl Med* 41(1):181–183.

Rust L, Gulland F, Frame E, Lefebvre K. 2014. Domoic acid in milk of free-living California marine mammals indicates lactational exposure occurs. *Mar Mammal Sci* 30(3):1272–1278.

St Leger JA, Begeman L, Fleetwood M, et al. 2009) Comparative pathology of nocardiosis in marine mammals. *Vet Pathol* 46(2):299–308.

St Leger JA, Nilson EM. 2014. Intestinal atresia in a harbor seal (*Phoca vitulina*) and a review of congenital conditions of the species. *Aquat Mammals* 40(2):207–213.

St Leger JA, Raverty S, Mena A. 2018. Cetacea. In: Terio KA, McAloose D, St Leger J, eds. *Pathology of Wildlife and Zoo Animals*, 533–568. London, UK: Academic Press.

Scaglione FE, Bollo E, Pregel P, et al. 2013. Heart pathologies in dolphins stranded along the northwestern Italian coast. *Dis Aquat Organ* 107(1):31–36.

Scarpignato C, Tramacere R, Zappia L. 1987. Antisecretory and antiulcer effect of the H2-receptor antagonist famotidine in the rat: comparison with ranitidine. *Br J Pharmacol* 92(1):153–159.

Schell DM, Rowntree VJ, Pfeiffer CJ. 2000. Stable-isotope and electron-microscopic evidence that cyamids (Crustacea: Amphipoda) feed on whale skin. *Can J Zool* 78(5):721–727.

Scholz T, Kuchta R. 2016. Fish-borne, zoonotic cestodes (Diphyllobothrium and relatives) in cold climates: a never-ending story of neglected and (re)-emergent parasites. *Food Waterborne Parasitol* 4:23–38.

Schulman FY, Lipscomb TP. 1999. Dermatitis with invasive ciliated protozoa in dolphins that died during the 1987–1988 Atlantic bottlenose dolphin morbilliviral epizootic. *Vet Pathol* 36(2):171–174.

Seguel M, Paves H, Paredes E, Schlatter R. 2013. Causes of mortality in South American fur seal pups (*Arctocephalus australis gracilis*) at Guafo Island, southern Chile (2004–2008). *Mar Mammal Sci* 29(1):36–47.

Seguel M, Munoz F, Navarrete MJ, et al. 2017a. Hookworm infection in South American fur seal (*Arctocephalus australis*) pups: pathology and factors associated with host tissue damage and mortality. *Vet Pathol* 54(2):288–297.

Seguel M, Gottdenker NL, Colegrove K, et al. 2017b. Hypervirulent *Klebsiella pneumoniae* in California sea lions (*Zalophus californianus*): pathologic findings in natural infections. *Vet Pathol* 54(5):846–850.

Seguel M, Nadler S, Field C, Duignan P. 2018. Vasculitis and thrombosis due to the sea lion lungworm, *Parafilaroides decorus*, in a Guadalupe fur seal (*Arctocephalus philippii townsendi*). *J Wildl Dis* 54(3):638–641.

Seguel M, Gutiérrez J, Hernández C, et al. 2018. Respiratory mites (*Orthohalarachne diminuata*) and β-hemolytic Streptococci-associated bronchopneumonia outbreak in South American Fur seal pups (*Arctocephalus australis*). *J Wildl Dis* 54(2):380–385.

Seguel M, Colegrove KM, Field C, et al. 2019. Polyphasic rhabdomyositis in California sea lions (*Zalophus californianus*): pathology and potential causes. *Vet Pathol* 56(4):619–629.

Shin DL, Siebert U, Lakemeyer J, et al. 2019. Highly pathogenic avian influenza A (H5N8) virus in gray seals, *Baltic Sea. Emerg Infect Dis* 25(12):2295–2298.

Shon AS, Bajwa RP, Russo TA. 2013. Hypervirulent (hypermucoviscous) *Klebsiella pneumoniae*: a new and dangerous breed. *Virulence* 4(2):107–118.

Schulman FY, Lipscomb TP. 1999. Dermatitis with invasive ciliated protozoa in dolphins that died during the 1987–1988 Atlantic bottlenose dolphin morbilliviral epizootic. *Vet Pathol* 36(2):171–174.

Shockling Dent CE, Miller MA, Batac F, et al. 2019. Pathology and epidemiology of nasopulmonary acariasis (*Halarachne* sp) in southern sea otters (*Enhydra lutris nereis*). *Int J Parasitol Parasites Wildl* 9:60–67.

Siebert U, Joiris C, Olsbeek L, et al. 1999. Potential relation between mercury concentrations and necropsy findings in cetaceans from German waters of the North and Baltic Seas. *Mar Pollut Bull* 38(4):285–295.

Siebert U, Wünschmann A, Weiss R, et al. 2001. Post-mortem findings in harbour porpoises (*Phocoena phocoena*) from the German North and Baltic Seas. *J Comp Pathol* 124(2–3):102–114.

Silvagni PA, Lowenstine LJ, Spraker T, et al. 2005. Pathology of domoic acid toxicity in California sea lions (*Zalophus californianus*). *Vet Pathol* 42(2):184–191.

Sinai NL, Dadaian RH, Kass PH, Verstraete FJM. 2014. Dental pathology of the California sea lion (*Zalophus californianus*). *J Comp Pathol* 151(1):113–121.

Smith CR, Poindexter JR, Meegan JM, et al. 2014. Pathophysiological and physicochemical basis of ammonium urate stone formation in dolphins. *J Urol* 192(1):260–266.

So SY, Chau PY, Leung YK, Lam. WK 1984. First report of septicaemic melioidosis in Hong Kong. *Trans R Soc Trop Med Hyg* 78(4):456–459.

Sohn AH, Probert WS, Glaser CA, et al. 2003. Human neurobrucellosis with intracerebral granuloma caused by a marine mammal *Brucella* spp. *Emerg Infect Dis* 9(4):485–488.

Soto E, Abdelrazek S, Basbas C, et al. 2020. Environmental Persistence and disinfectant susceptibility of *Klebsiella pneumoniae* recovered from marine mammals. *Vet Microbiol* 241: 108554.

Spraker TR, DeLon, RL, Lyons ET, Melin SR. 2007. Hookworm enteritis with bacteremia in California sea lion pups on San Miguel Island. *J Wildl Dis* 43(2):179–188.

Spraker TR, Lander ME. 2010. Causes of mortality in northern fur seals (*Callorhinus ursinus*), St Paul Island, Pribilof Islands, Alaska, 1986–2006. *J Wildl Dis* 46(2):450–473.

Stadtländer CTH, Madoff S. 1994. Characterization of cytopathogenicity of aquarium seal mycoplasmas and seal finger mycoplasmas by light and scanning electron microscopy. *Zentralbl Bakteriol* 280(4):458–467.

Steadham MA, Casey HW. 1977. Lymphosarcoma in an infant northern fur seal (*Callorhinus ursinus*). *J Wildl Dis* 13(2):176–179.

Stephen C, Lester S, Black W et al. 2002. Multispecies outbreak of cryptococcosis on southern Vancouver Island, British Columbia. *Can Vet J* 43(10):792–794.

Stephens N, Duignan PJ, Wang J, et al. 2014. Cetacean morbillivirus in coastal Indo-Pacific bottlenose dolphins, Western Australia. *Emerg Infect Dis* 20(4):666–670.

Stephens N, Duignan PJ, Symons J, et al. 2017. Death by octopus (*Macroctopus maorum*): laryngeal luxation and asphyxiation in an Indo-Pacific dolphin (*Tursiops aduncus*). *Mar Mammal Sci* 33(4):1204–1213.

Stoddard RA, Gulland FM, Atwill ER, et al. 2005. Salmonella and Campylobacter spp in northern elephant seals, California. *Emerg Infect Dis* 11(12):1967–1969.

Stoddard RA, Miller WG, Foley JE, et al. 2007. *Campylobacter insulaenigrae* isolates from northern elephant seals (*Mirounga angustirostris*) in California. *Appl Environ Microbiol* 73(6):1729–1735.

Stratton M, Duignan PJ, Forester N, et al. 2001. Prevalence of potentially pathogenic bacteria in New Zealand sea lions (*Phocarctos hookeri*). Presented at the 14th Biennial Conference on the Biology of Marine Mammals, Vancouver.

Stringell T, Hill D, Rees D, et al. 2015. Predation of harbour porpoises (*Phocoena phocoena*) by grey seals (*Halichoerus grypus*) in Wales. *Aquat Mammals* 41(2):188–191.

Sweeney JC, Ridgway SH. 1975. Common diseases of small cetaceans. *J Am Vet Med Assoc* 167(7):533–540.

Sweeney JC, Reddy ML, Lipscomb TP, et al. 1999. *Handbook of Cetacean Cytology*. San Diego, CA: Dolphin Quest.

Tachibana M, Watanabe K, Kim S, et al. 2006. Antibodies to *Brucella* spp in Pacific bottlenose dolphins from the Solomon Islands. *J Wildl Dis* 42(2):412–414.

Tajima Y, Shimada A, Yamada TK, Cowan DF. 2007. Amyloidosis in two Stejneger's beaked whales (*Mesoplodon stejnegeri*) stranded at the Sea of Japan. *J Zoo Wildl Med* 38:108–113.

Tajima Y, Maeda K, Yamada TK. 2015. Pathological findings and probable causes of the death of Stejneger's beaked whales (*Mesoplodon stejnegeri*) stranded in Japan from 1999 and 2011. *J Vet Med Sci* 77(1):45–51.

Tamburin E, Carone E, Lopez IG, Magaña FG. 2017. First report of gray whale (*Eschrichtius robustus*, Lilljeborg, 1861) conjoined twin calves in the Eastern Pacific Ocean. *Turk J Zool* 41(5):951–954.

Tang KN, Winer JN, McKlveen T, et al. 2019. Computed tomography of the mandibles of a stranded offshore killer whale (*Orcinus orca*). *J Comp Pathol* 168:35–40.

Taurisano ND, Butler BP, Stone D, et al. 2018. *Streptococcus phocae* in marine mammals of northeastern pacific and arctic Canada: a retrospective analysis of 85 postmortem investigations. *J Wildl Dis* 54(1):101–111.

Thepthai C, Smithtikarn S, Suksuwan M, et al. 2005. Serodiagnosis of melioidosis by a competitive enzyme–linked immunosorbent assay using a lipopolysaccharide–specific monoclonal antibody. *Asian Pacific J Allergy Immunol* 23(2–3):12 –132.

Thompson PJ, Cousins DV, Gow BL, et al. 1993. Seals, seal trainers, and mycobacterial infection. *Am J Respir Crit Care Med* 147(1):164–167.

Thornton SM, Nolan S, Gulland FM. 1998. Bacterial isolates from California sea lions (*Zalophus californianus*), harbor seals (*Phoca vitulina*), and northern elephant seals (*Mirounga angustirostris*) admitted to a rehabilitation center along the central California coast, 1994–1995. *J Zoo Wildl Med* 29(2):171–176.

Tomaselli M, Ytrehus B, Opriessnig T, et al. 2022. Contagious ecthyma dermatitis as a portal of entry for *Erysipelothrix rhusiopathiae* in muskoxen (*Ovibos moschatus*) of the Canadian Arctic. *J Wildl Dis* 58(1):228–231.

Toplu N, Aydoğan A, Oguzoglu TC. 2007. Visceral leishmaniosis and parapoxvirus infection in a Mediterranean monk seal (*Monachus monachus*). *J Comp Pathol* 136(4):283–287.

Torres De La Riva GT, Johnson CK, Gulland FM, et al. 2009. Association of an unusual marine mammal mortality event with Pseudo-nitzschia spp blooms along the southern California coastline. *J Wildl Dis* 45(1):109–121.

Trites AW, Donnelly CP. 2003. The decline of Steller sea lions Eumetopias jubatus in Alaska: a review of the nutritional stress hypothesis. *Mammal Rev* 33(1):3–28.

Trupkiewicz JG, Gulland FMD, Lowenstine LJ. 1997. Congenital defects in northern elephant seals stranded along the central California coast. *J Wildl Dis* 33(2):220–225.

Tryland M. 2018. Zoonoses and public health. In: Gulland FMD, Dierauf LA, Whitman KL, eds. *CRC Handbook of Marine Mammal Medicine*, 3rd ed., 47–62. Boca Raton, FL: CRC Press.

Tryland M, Derocher AE, Wiig Ø, Godfroid J. 2001. *Brucella* sp antibodies in polar bears from Svalbard and the Barents Sea. *J Wildl Dis* 37(3):523–531.

Tryland M, Sørensen KK, Godfroid J. 2005. Prevalence of *Brucella pinnipediae* in healthy hooded seals (*Cystophora cristata*) from the North Atlantic Ocean and ringed seals (*Phoca hispida*) from Svalbard. *Vet Microbiol* 105(2):103–111.

Tryland M, Nymo IH, Nielsen O, et al. 2012. Serum chemistry and antibodies against pathogens in Antarctic fur seals, Weddell seals, crabeater seals, and Ross seals. *J Wildl Dis* 48(3):632–645.

Tryland M, Larsen AK, Nymo IH. 2018. Bacterial infections and diseases. In: Gulland FMD, Dierauf LA, Whitman KL, eds. *CRC Handbook of Marine Mammal Medicine*, 3rd ed., 367–388. Boca Raton, FL: CRC Press.

Tseng M, Fleetwood M, Reed A, et al. 2012. Mustelid herpesvirus-2, a novel herpes infection in northern sea otters (*Enhydra lutris kenyoni*). *J Wildl Dis* 48(1):181–185.

Tuomi PA, Murray MJ, Garner MM, et al. 2014. Novel poxvirus infection in northern and southern sea otters (*Enhydra lutris kenyoni* and *Enhydra lutris neiris*), Alaska and California, USA. *J Wildl Dis*, 50(3):607–615.

Turnbull BS, Cowan DF. 1999. Angiomatosis, a newly recognized disease in Atlantic bottlenose dolphins (*Tursiops truncatus*) from the Gulf of Mexico. *Vet Pathol* 36(1):28–34.

Twiner MJ, Fire S, Schwacke L, et al. 2011. Concurrent exposure of bottlenose dolphins (*Tursiops truncatus*) to multiple algal toxins in Sarasota Bay, Florida, USA. *PLoS One* 6(3):e17394.

Upton SJ, Odell DK, Bossart GD, Walsh MT. 1989. Description of the oocysts of two new species of Eimeria (Apicomplexa: Eimeridae) from the Florida manatee, Trichechus manatus (Sirenia: Trichechidae). *J Protozool* 36(1):87–90.

Van Bolhuis GH, Philippa JDW, Osterhaus ADME, et al. 2007. Fatal enterocolitis in harbour seals (*Phoca vitulina*) caused by infection with *Eimeria phocae*. *Vet Rec* 160(9):297–300.

Van Bressem MF, Van Waerebeek K, Montes D, et al. 2006. Diseases, lesions, and malformations in the long-beaked common dolphin Delphinus capensis from the Southeast Pacific. *Dis Aquat Organ* 68(2):149–165.

Van Bressem MF, Van Waerebeek K, Flach L, et al. 2008. *Skin Diseases in Cetaceans*. SC/60/DW8. Santiago, Chile: International Whaling Commission.

Van Bressem MF, Duignan PJ, Baynard A, et al 2014. Cetacean morbillivirus: current knowledge and future directions. *Viruses* 6:5145–5181.

Van Bressem MF, Van Waerebeek K, Duignan PJ. 2018. Epidemiology of tattoo skin disease in captive common bottlenose dolphins (*Tursiops truncatus*): are males more vulnerable than females? *J Appl Anim Welfare Sci* 21(4):305–315.

Van Bressem MF, Duignan PJ, Raga JA, et al. 2020. *Crassicauda* spp cranial lesions in Indian Ocean humpback dolphins and Indo-Pacific bottlenose dolphins from South Africa: conservation implications. *Dis Aquat Organ* 139:93–103.

Van de Velde N, Demetrik DJ, Duignan PJ. 2019. Primary pleural squamous cell carcinoma in a free-ranging River otter (*Lontra canadensis*). *J Wildl Dis* 53(3): 728–732.

Venn-Watson S, Benham C, Gulland FM, et al. 2012. Clinical relevance of novel otarine herpesvirus-3 in California sea lions (*Zalophus californianus*): lymphoma, esophageal ulcers, and strandings. *Vet Res* 43(1):1–9.

Vilela R, Mendoza L. 2018. *Paracoccidioidomycosis ceti* (lacaziosis/lobomycosis) in dolphins. In: Seyedmousavi S, de Hoog GS, Guillot J, Verweij PE, eds. *Emerging and Epizootic Fungal Infections in Animals*, 177–196. Cham, Switzerland: Springer.

Visser IN, Zaeschmar J, Halliday J, et al. 2010. First record of predation on false killer whales (*Pseudorca crassidens*) by killer whales (*Orcinus orca*). *Aquat Mammals* 36:195–204.

Weller DW, Bradford AL, Lang AR, et al. 2018. Prevalence of killer whale tooth rake marks on gray whales off Sakhalin Island, *Russia. Aquat Mammals* 44(6):643–652.

Willoughby AL, Ferguson MC, Stimmelmayr R, et al. 2020. Bowhead whale (*Balaena mysticetus*) and killer whale (*Orcinus orca*) co-occurrence in the US Pacific Arctic, 2009–2018: evidence from bowhead whale carcasses. *Polar Biol* 43:1669–1679.

Volokhov DV, Batac F, Gao Y, et al. 2019. *Mycoplasma enhydrae* sp nov isolated from southern sea otters (*Enhydra lutris nereis*). *Int J Syst Evol Microbiol* 69(2):363–370.

Walsh MT, Beusse D, Bossart GD, et al. 1988. Ray encounters as a mortality factor in Atlantic bottlenose dolphins (*Tursiops truncatus*). *Mar Mammal Sci* 4(2):154–162.

Walsh CJ, Butawan M, Yordy J, et al. 2015. Sublethal red tide toxin exposure in free-ranging manatees (*Trichechus manatus*) affects the immune system through reduced lymphocyte proliferation responses, inflammation, and oxidative stress. *Aquat Toxicol* 161:73–84.

Wang L, Maddox C, Terio K, et al. 2020. Detection and characterization of new coronavirus in bottlenose dolphin, United States, 2019. *Emerg Infect Dis* 26(7):1610 –1612.

Welsh T, Burek-Huntington K, Savage K, et al. 2014. Sarcocystis canis associated hepatitis in a Steller sea lion (*Eumetopias jubatus*) from Alaska. *J Wildl Dis* 50(2):405–408.

Wessels M, Barnett J, Bexton S, et al. 2019. A novel pulmonary vasculitis in grey seals (*Halichoerus grypus*) associated with *Otostrongylus circumlitus* infection. Presented at the World Marine Mammal Conference, Barcelona, December 2019.

Whitaker DM, Reichley SR, Griffin MJ, et al. 2018. Hypermucoviscous *Klebsiella pneumoniae* isolates from stranded and wild-caught marine mammals of the US Pacific coast: prevalence, phenotype, and genotype. *J Wildl Dis* 54(4):659–670.

White CL, Lankau EW, Lynch D, et al. 2018. Mortality trends in northern sea otters (*Enhydra lutris kenyoni*) collected from the coasts of Washington and Oregon, USA (2002–15). *J Wildl Dis* 54(2):238–247.

Whitmer E, Borremans B, Duignan PJ, et al. 2021. Classification and regression tree (CART) analysis for predicting prognosis in wildlife rehabilitation: a case study of leptospirosis in California sea lions (*Zalophus californianus*). *J Zoo Wildl Med* 52(1):38–48.

Whoriskey ST, Duignan PJ, McClain AM, et al. 2021. Clinical signs, treatment and outcome for California sea lions (*Zalophus californianus*) with sarcocystis-associated polyphasic rhabdomyositis. *J Am Vet Med Assoc* 259(10):1196–1205.

Wilkin SM, Cordaro J, Gulland FM, et al. 2012. An unusual mortality event of harbor porpoises (*Phocoena phocoena*) off central California: increase in blunt trauma rather than an epizootic. *Aquat Mammals* 38 (3):301–310.

Wilkinson IS, Childerhouse SJ, Duignan PJ, Gulland FMD. 2000. Infanticide and cannibalism in the New Zealand sea lion, *Phocarctos hookeri. Mar Mammal Sci* 16(2):494–500.

Wilkinson IS Duignan PJ Grinberg A, et al. 2006. Klebsiella pneumoniae epidemics: possible impact on New Zealand sea lion recruitment. In: Trites A, Atkinson S, DeMaster D, et al., eds. *Sea Lions of the World*, 385–406. Fairbanks, AK: Alaska Sea Grant College Program, University of Alaska.

Williams BH, Huntington KB, Mille M. 2018. Mustelids. In: Terio KA, McAloose D, St Leger J, eds. *Pathology of Wildlife and Zoo Animals*, 287–304. London, UK: Academic Press.

Williams KM, Fessler MK, Bloomfield RA, et al. 2020. A novel quantitative real-time PCR diagnostic assay for fecal and nasal swab detection of an otariid lungworm, *Parafilaroides decorus. Int J Parasitol Parasites Wildl* 12:85–92.

Winer JN, Liong SM, Verstraete FJM. 2013. The dental pathology of southern sea otters (*Enhydra lutris nereis*). *J Comp Pathol* 149(2–3):346–355.

Winer JN, Arzi B, Leale DM, et al. 2016a. Dental and temporomandibular joint pathology of the walrus (*Odobenus rosmarus*). *J Comp Pathol* 155(2–3):242–253.

Winer JN, Arzi B, Leale DM, et al. 2016b. Dental and temporomandibular joint pathology of the polar bear (*Ursus maritimus*). *J Comp Pathol* 155(2–3):231–241.

Womble JN, Conlon S, 2010. Observation of Steller sea lion (*Eumetopias jubatus*) predation on a harbor seal (*Phoca vitulina richardsi*) in the Glacier Bay region of Southeastern Alaska. *Aquat Mammals* 36(2):129–137.

Woo PCY, Lau SKP, Lam CSF, et al. 2014. Discovery of a novel bottlenose dolphin coronavirus reveals a distinct species of marine mammal cornonavirus in Gammacoronavirus. *J Virol* 88:1318–1331.

Woodard JC, Zam SG, Caldwell DK, Caldwell MC. 1969. Some parasitic diseases of dolphins. *Pathol Vet* 6(3):257–272.

Woshner VM, O'Hara TM, Bratton GR, Beasley VR. 2001a. Concentrations and interactions of selected essential and non-essential elements in ringed seals and polar bears of Arctic Alaska. *J Wildl Dis* 37(4):711–721.

Woshner VM, O'Hara TM, Bratton GR, et al. 2001b. Concentrations and interactions of selected essential and non-essential elements in bowhead and beluga whales of Arctic Alaska. *J Wildl Dis* 37(4):693–710.

Wu Q, McFee WE, Goldstein T, et al. 2014. Real-time PCR assays for detection of *Brucella* spp and the identification of genotype ST27 in bottlenose dolphins (*Tursiops truncatus*). *J Microbiol Methods* 100:99–104.

Yang S, Zabka TS, Baumgartner W, et al. 2018. Characterization of arterial vasculopathy in juvenile northern elephant seals, associated with *Otostrongylus circumlitus* infection. Presented at the American College of Veterinary Pathology, Annual Conference, Washington, DC, November 3rd–7th, 2018.

Zabka TS, Lowenstine LJ, Gulland FMD. 2005. Normal gastrointestinal anatomy and perforating ulcerative gastroduodenitis in California sea lions (*Zalophus californianus*). International Association of Aquatic Animal Medicine Conference Proceedings. https://www.vin.com/apputil/content/defaultadv1.aspx?pId=11195&meta=generic&catId=30723&id=3980675&ind=36&objTypeID=17 (accesed 10 October 2022).

Zabka TS, Goldstein T, Cross C, et al. 2009. Characterization of a degenerative cardiomyopathy associated with domoic acid toxicity in California sea lions (*Zalophus californianus*). *Vet Pathol* 46(1):105–119.

Zarnke RL, Saliki JT, Macmillan AP, et al. 2006. Serologic survey for *Brucella* spp, phocid herpesvirus-1, phocid herpesvirus-2, and phocine distemper virus in harbor seals from Alaska, 1976–1999. *J Wildl Dis* 42(2):290–300.

Zhang ER, Duignan PJ, Seguel M, et al. 2019. Sarcocystis neurona type II and type VI is associated with recently described polyphasic rhabdomyositis in stranded California sea lions. Presented at the World Marine Mammal Conference, Barcelona, Spain Dec, 8th–12th, 2019.

Zuerner RL, Alt DP. 2009. Variable nucleotide tandem-repeat analysis revealing a unique group of Leptospira interrogans serovar Pomona isolates associated with California sea lions. *J Clin Microbiol* 47(4):1202–1205.

Appendix 6.1

Clinical Signs of Mammals

Clinicopathologic presentation	Differential etiologic diagnoses
Sudden death	Trauma, asphyxiation, intoxication (e.g. domoic acid, saxitoxin, microcystins, brevetoxin), cardiac failure (cardiomyopathy, cardiac infarction, cor pulmonale), cerebral hemorrhage (secondary to trematodiasis or mycotic arteritis), gastrointestinal perforation (parasitic, foreign body, stress), fatal congenital defect
Poor growth	Vitamin deficiency, stress, insufficient nutritional intake, premature parturition or maternal separation, heavy parasitism, congenital defect (e.g. cardiac, musculoskeletal)
Uncoordinated locomotion, nervousness, obtunded	Generalized infectious disease (virus, bacteria), central nervous system disease (viral, protozoal, bacterial, neurotoxin e.g. domoic acid, saxitoxin), myopathy/ myositis (vitamin E deficiency, infection e.g. *Sarcocystis neurona* rhabdomyositis, trichinosis), trauma, nutritional deficiency (e.g. thiamine, vitamin E), cerebral edema (freshwater exposure, systemic disease e.g. leptospirosis)
Abortion	Viral infection (morbilliviruses), bacteria (*Leptospira* spp., *Brucella* spp., *Coxiella* spp., *Mycoplasma*/*Ureaplasma* spp.), protozoa (*Toxoplasma* spp., *Sarcocystis* spp.), algal bloom toxins (domoic acid), nutritional deficiency, trauma, endocrine-disrupting toxins (persistent organic pollutants)
Skin:	
Hemorrhage/ petechiae/ ecchymosis	Bacterial septicemia (eg. *Erysipelas* sp.), trauma, uremia (e.g. leptospirosis)
Ulcers/necrosis/ inflammation	Viruses (morbillivirus, caliciviruses, herpesviruses), bacteria (leptospiral uremia, septicemia, mycosis), fungi (candidiasis)
Vesicles	Viruses (Caliciviruses), thermal or chemical injury
Hyperplasia/nodules	Viruses (poxviruses, papilloma viruses, morbilliviruses), bacteria (dermatophilosis), fungi (*Paracoccidioides brasiliensis* or Lobos disease, various dermatophytes), ectoparasites (mites, lice, copepods)
Alopecia	Physiologic or metabolic (abnormal molt), fungi (dermatophytosis), ectoparasites (sucking lice, demodicosis), nutritional deficiency, idiopathic
Upper respiratory:	
Nasal discharge	Serous, mucoid, mucopurulent – nasal or sinus parasites (respiratory mites, trematodes, nematodes), bacterial infection (*Streptococcus* spp., *Arcanobacterium* spp., *Mycoplasma* spp. etc.), fungi (various opportunists e.g. *Aspergillus* spp.), viral infection (morbilliviruses, influenza A, herpesviruses)
Epistaxis	Trauma, parasites (respiratory mites, nematodes e.g. *Otostrongylus circumlitus*, mycoses e.g. aspergillosis), pulmonary or gastric hemorrhage (e.g. ulcers)
Obstruction (rales)	Foreign body (e.g. fish hook, fish bones or other prey), laryngeal luxation (dolphins), laryngeal paralysis (strophy of laryngeal muscles e.g. *Sarcocystis neurona* associated rhabdomyositis)

(*Continued*)

Clinicopathologic presentation	Differential etiologic diagnoses
Lung:	
Pneumonia	Bacteria (numerous), viruses (e.g. morbillivirus, influenza A virus), parasites (e.g. metastrongyle nematodes, respiratory mites), fungi (systemic mycoses), toxins (harmful algal blooms, oil and gas hydrocarbons)
Hemorrhage	infarction (e.g. otostrongyliasis), septicemia, trauma
Nodules	Granulomas (e.g. parasites, *Mycobacteria*, fungi), abscesses, neoplasia (primary or metastatic)
Edema	Asphyxiation, congestive heart failure
Thorax and mediastinum:	
Pneumothorax	Trauma (pulmonary rupture or body wall perforation), barotrauma (forced/rapid ascent)
Hemothorax	Trauma (blunt force or perforating), pulmonary infarction (e.g. otostrongyliasis in phocids), neoplasia
Effusion (inflammatory)	Bacteria (e.g. pyogenic *Streptococci*, *Nocardia* spp., *Klebsiella pneumoniae*), fungi (systemic mycoses)
Hydrothorax	congestive heart failure, endocardiosis/mitral endocarditis, cardiomyopathy, asphyxiation, neoplasia (lymphatic obstruction)
Emphysema	Viral pneumonia (morbillivirus, influenza A), bacterial or parasitic pneumonia
Nodules	Granulomas (parasitic, bacterial, mycotic), neoplasia (e.g. carcinoma, mesothelioma), abscesses
Pleuritis	Bacteria (e.g. *Klebsiella pneumoniae*, *Nocardia* spp.), fungi (*Coccidioides immitis*, *Cryptococcus gatti*)
Mouth/pharynx/esophagus:	
Vesicles	Virus
Nodules	Granuloma (bacterial, parasitic), neoplasia (e.g. tonsillar squamous cell carcinoma, leiomyoma), abscess
Distension/impaction	Megaesophagus (*Sarcocystis neurona* rhabdomyositis), obstruction (foreign body e.g. fishing gear), congenital defect (e.g. hiatal hernia, pyloric stenosis)
Teeth: Abrasion, fractures, laxity, attrition	Related to diet, learned behaviors, trauma, gingivitis.
Eye:	
Corneal ulcers	Fungus, bacterial septicemia, trauma, hyposalinity, ultraviolet light
Conjunctivitis	Bacteria, fungi, virus (e.g. influenza A), mollicutes, trauma
Endocrine:	
Thyroid enlargement	Congenital hyperplastic goiter (captive dolphins), cysts (incidental in older cetaceans and pinnipeds), adenomas (age related)
Adrenal enlargement	Cortical, medullar or extracapsular hyperplasia common in older delphinids, neoplasia (pheochromocytoma, carcinoma metastases), abscesses
Adrenal cortical atrophy	In dolphins associated with petroleum exposure

Clinicopathologic presentation	Differential etiologic diagnoses
Brain:	Seizures, depression, altered behavior and ambulation, central blindness
Suppurative meningitis	Various bacteria
Nonsuppurative meningitis	(protozoal e.g. *Toxoplasma* spp., *Sarcocystis* spp., *Neospora* spp., or viral e.g. morbillivirus, herpesvirus)
Intoxication	(HAB toxins eg., domoic acid, saxitoxin)
Infarct	Systemic mycosis (e.g. *Aspergillus fumigatus*), bacteria, aberrant parasites (e.g. Trematoda: *Nasitrema* spp.)
Muscle:	
Atrophy	Emaciation, denervation, trauma, chronic myositis (e.g. *Sarcocystis neurona* rhabdomyositis), myopathy (capture, compartment syndrome)
Hemorrhage	Trauma, septicemia
Nodules/swelling	Parasite granulomas (cestodes, nematodes), abscess, neoplasia
Skeletal deformity:	
Spinal	Congenital defect (scoliosis, kyphosis, spina bifida), metabolic bone disease, fracture and callus, neoplasia
Cranial	Congenital defects, parasitic osteolysis (e.g. *Crassicauda* spp.)
Degenerative arthritis, spondylitis, spondylosis	secondary to inflammatory arthritis, old age, trauma
Abdomen:	
Ascites	Cardiomyopathy, hepatopathy, neoplasia (lymphatic obstruction), malnutrition
Effusion (inflammatory)	Peritonitis (bacterial, parasitic), perforation, hepatitis, pancreatitis, septicemia, abscess rupture, carcinomatosis, systemic mycosis (e.g. coccidioidomycosis)
Uroabdomen	Ascending urogenital infection, urolithiasis, urinary bladder rupture, balanoposthitis
Hemoabdomen	Trauma, gastric or duodenal perforation, neoplasia
Nodules	Granulomas (parasites e.g. cestodes, nematodes, trematodes), neoplasia (e.g. carcinomas, leiomyoma, mesothelioma), fluid-filled cysts (cestodes, congenital cysts of the urogenital tract)
Kidney:	
Diffuse swelling/ pallor	Inflammation (bacterial e.g. leptospirosis), amyloidosis, neoplasia (e.g. lymphoma).
Cystic change	Congenital defect, hydronephrosis
Necrosis	Bacterial or parasitic infection (e.g. *Crassicauda* spp.), neoplasia
Granulomas/nodules	Bacteria, fungi, parasites (e.g. cestodes or nematodes), neoplasia (e.g. urogenital carcinoma), hypoplasia, dysplasia
Hemorrhage/ congestion	Bacterial infection (mixed ascending, leptospirosis), septicemia, infarction
Spleen and lymph nodes:	
Diffuse splenomegaly	Bacterial septicemia, neoplasia (e.g. lymphosarcoma), congestion (barbiturate euthanasia)

(*Continued*)

Clinicopathologic presentation	Differential etiologic diagnoses
Splenic nodules	granulomas (bacterial, fungal, parasitic), hematoma, hyperplasia, neoplasia (e.g. metastases)
Multiple accessory spleens	Normal anatomic variation
Peripheral lymphadenopathy	Systemic bacterial or mycotic infection (e.g. coccidioidomycosis), tuberculosis (southern hemisphere otariids), neoplasia (lymphosarcoma)
Liver:	
Necrosis	Virus (e.g. herpesvirus, adenovirus), bacteria, toxins (e.g. microcystin), hypoxia (congestive heart failure)
Nodules	Granulomas (parasitic, bacterial, mycotic), neoplasia, encysted parasites, biliary ectasia (e.g. trematodes), hyperplasia
Enlarged, tan/ yellow, friable	Fat accumulation – excessive nutrition or cachexia, toxicosis, neonate (milk fat)
Shrunken, firm, dark	Atrophy (cachexia), hemosiderosis, fibrosis
Stomach:	
Ulcers	Parasites (nematodes, trematodes), bacteria, uremia, stress, neoplasia
Nodules	Neoplasia (leiomyoma, carcinoma, lymphosarcoma), granulomas (parasites)
Hemorrhage	Gastritis (bacterial, parasitic), perforation (stress ulcers), foreign body (rocks, fishing hooks, sting ray spines, etc.)
Impaction	Pyloric obstruction (foreign body, torsion)
Intestines:	
Hemorrhage	Bacteria (eg. Salmonella spp., Clostridium spp., E. coli), parasites (eg. Unsinaria spp. hookworms), protozoa (eg. Eimeria spp.), perforating ulcers (eg. stress, bacteria), foreign bodies (eg., fishing gear, sting ray spines)
Ulcers	Stress, bacterial or mycotic infection
Nodules	parasitic granulomas or cysts, abscesses, leiomyomas, adenocarcinoma
Reproductive:	
Nodules	
Dystocia	Obesity, nutrition, dehydration, primipara, abnormal eggs, improper temperatures, improper cage/environment, oviduct infection/torsion/ compression, ectopic egg, oviduct prolapse, nutritional hyperparathyroidism (T), hypovitaminosis A (T), hypocalcemia
Enlarged ovary/uterus	
Fetal demise	
Heart:	
Murmur	Vegetative valvular endocarditis, mitral endocardiosis, congenital or ontogenetic defects, cardiomyopathies
Electrocardiogram anomalies	Infarction, conduction defects (domoic acid intoxication)
White streaks	Myocarditis (protozoal eg. sarcocystosis, toxoplasmosis or bacterial e.g. streptococcal), myopathy (nutritional, toxic e.g. domoic acid)
Hemorrhage	Thrombosis and infarction
Nodules	Abscesses, neoplasia (e.g. carcinoma metastases)
Increased radiographic profile	Dilated cardiomyopathy, pericarditis, pericardial effusion

Part II

Epidemiology and Animal Health Economics

Introduction

Aquatic animal diseases have become important obstacles facing national and international aquaculture sustainability and growth. These diseases also impact efforts to replenish natural populations. Epidemiology is an important aspect of aquatic veterinary medicine. In many clinical cases you will need to carry out further diagnostic tests, decide on whether to treat or cull during a disease outbreak, design a surveillance system, consider the presence or absence of pathological organisms to implement and focus biosecurity, or set up a trial to prove efficacy of a new treatment. Epidemiological methods will help you make the right decision.

Using epidemiological tools can appear daunting and certainly requires understanding if these techniques are to be fully exploited. You need to understand and write mathematical notation, understand frequentist and Bayesian probabilities, have knowledge of different probability distributions, remember formulae and how to write them in to a spreadsheet. Then there is a concern over how good the data are and if you have enough. Couple this with the need in some cases for special computer programs and it is no wonder the average practitioner is deterred from using many of these techniques on a daily basis. There are several simple methodologies, and even those requiring computer spreadsheets, once set up, can provide better insight and can be used repeatedly.

The aim of this part of the book is to provide examples to help you understand why and how you could use these methodologies, with examples you can set up on your own computer/tablet/phone. In most cases, you need very few data points (3–5), although the more data, and/or the more accurate your data, the closer to "reality" any outcome is likely to be. Remember, much of this information is based on probabilities, likelihoods, and odds, and is a prediction of a potential future through modelling that potential future. All can be updated in the light of new evidence. However, the authors hope to demonstrate that even in a "data poor" environment, with a little thought, these techniques can be extremely effective.

How to use these chapters? The focus is on providing various equations for probabilities, helping you to become more proficient in entering equations into spreadsheets, and including summary information of why you would use these techniques, with some potential pitfalls. At best, we hope that the information can make you a better thinker and help to promote better clinical outcomes. The text provides a basic understanding of techniques, and is not exhaustive. If you are completely new to veterinary epidemiology, then you should refer to a standard veterinary epidemiology text.

Pathology and Epidemiology of Aquatic Animal Diseases for Practitioners, First Edition.
Edited by Laura Urdes, Chris Walster, and Julius Tepper.

There are six chapters in this section:

- Epidemiology keyword refresher.
- Probabilities and probability distributions – brief descriptions.
- Data Sources – using and assessing.
- Diagnostics – sampling and diagnostic testing.
- Biosecurity – the use of risk assessment, surveillance, outbreak investigation, modelling disease outbreaks.
- Animal health economics – production functions, whether to treat or not, cost benefit analysis.

7

Epidemiology Keyword Refresher

Chris Walster and Leo Foyle

Biosecurity

There are a number of definitions of biosecurity, but essentially it is the application of practices that aim to prevent or reduce the ability of relevant infectious agents to gain entry to, or spread within, a defined unit. Biosecurity impacts on human health (e.g. zoonoses, foodborne illness), animal health, animal welfare (e.g. stress through increased handling, improved health), the environment (e.g. waste discharges), biodiversity (e.g. introduction of alien species or aquatic nuisance species) and production economics (e.g. decreased disease helping to increase production). In this chapter, we focus on processes and procedures involved in the prevention, control, and eradication of infectious diseases. An alternative term that can be used is *biological risk management*.

A central component of biosecurity is defining the epidemiological unit. It could be a zone – national or regional – or a single tank. Biosecurity is sometimes described as "porous." Just because there is a biosecurity plan in place, it does not mean that infectious organisms will not spread. Hence, the term "biological risk management" perhaps more accurately reflects the approach required. Biosecurity plans also need to include a containment strategies and contingency plans, should an infectious organism relevant to the plan enter the epidemiological unit.

Design Prevalence

Disease prevalence (P*), also known as minimum expected prevalence or maximum acceptable prevalence, is the disease prevalence level set to calculate disease prevalence in a population. The null hypothesis states that disease is present at or greater than P*. This hypothesis can be rejected if sufficient samples from the population are negative. In most cases, for disease freedom, a P* of less than 2% is used, the usual World Organisation for Animal Health (WOAH) level, but it can be varied depending on the type of disease or what your trading partner requires.

Pathology and Epidemiology of Aquatic Animal Diseases for Practitioners, First Edition.
Edited by Laura Urdes, Chris Walster, and Julius Tepper.

Epidemiology

Epidemiology is the study of the occurrence and distribution of diseases in populations and the factors that influence disease occurrence. It asks who has what, when, where, why, and how. Epidemiology is:

- Being a disease detective
- Knowing how much disease there is
- Identifying risk factors for diseases
- Suggesting hypotheses for new causal mechanisms
- Working to find the best means to minimize risks and control diseases
- Making observations on representative samples of populations and generalizing relationships identified to apply to the whole population. These relationships are usually identified based on statistical association between, for example, a risk factor and a disease, but this does not imply cause and effect.

Many epidemiological principles apply to biosecurity, such as risk analysis, surveillance, outbreak investigation, sampling, and diagnostic testing. Observations made can be summarized by statistics and hypotheses tested. Using epidemiology tools assist in the development, implementation and ongoing activities of any biosecurity plan including requirements of auditing and certifying.

Epidemiological Unit

With infectious disease, epidemiological units are the basic unit relevant to disease control. They can be anything that can be spatially defined or is a contiguous area in which an infectious or contagious disease can be transmitted and maintained between individuals of a population. Meaningful systems can be implemented to prevent introduction, control, or eradication of disease. Thus, an epidemiological unit can be defined geographically as a country, region, watershed, or offshore island, or as a farm or single fish tank.

Incidence

Incidence is the number of new cases in a known population over a specified period, the total animal time at risk. An individual animal spends a certain amount of time at risk (animal time at risk). Over a period, there are a certain number of new cases. Incidence can be expressed as a proportion of non-diseased animals becoming diseased over a period of time (cumulative incidence), or as a measure of how rapidly non-diseased animals become diseased over time (the incidence rate). It can be expressed simply but it is usually expressed related to the population at risk in units such as cases per animal per week or year.

Likelihood ratios

The *likelihood ratio of a positive test* (LR+) is the ratio of the likelihood of a positive test in an animal that truly has the disease to the likelihood of a positive test in an animal that does not have the disease. The *likelihood ratio of a negative test* (LR–) is the ratio of the likelihood of a negative test in

Table 7.1 Liklihood ratios.

	The animal is:	
Test result	**Diseased (case)**	**Not diseased (control)**
Positive	P_{true} (a)	P_{false} (b)
Negative	N_{false} I	N_{true} (d)

I, incidence; N, negative; P, positive; Se, is sensitivity; Sp is specificity.

an animal that truly has the disease to the likelihood of a negative test in animal that does not have the disease (Table 7.1).

$$LR+ = \left(P_{true}/P_{true} + N_{false}\right) \div \left(P_{false}/P_{false} + N_{true}\right) \text{ or } \left(a/a + c\right)/\left(b/b + d\right) \text{or } Se \div \left(1 - Sp\right)$$

$$LR- = \left(N_{false}/P_{true} + N_{false}\right) \div \left(N_{true}/P_{false} + N_{true}\right) \text{ or } \left(c/a + c\right)/\left(a/b + a\right) \text{ or } \left(1 - Se\right) \div Sp$$

The likelihood ratio combines information about the sensitivity and specificity. It tells you how much a positive or negative result changes the likelihood that an animal would have the disease. It is not affected by the prevalence.

Likelihood ratios are actually odds which are different to probabilities. For example, a probability of 25% corresponds to odds of 1 : 3. To convert between probability and odds:

$$\text{Odds} = \text{probability}/\left(1 - \text{probability}\right)$$

$$\text{Probability} = \text{odds}/\left(1 + \text{odds}\right)$$

Monitoring

Monitoring is often used interchangeably with surveillance, when in fact they are two separate but related concepts. Monitoring is the routine collection, and often transmission, of observations and information on productivity and disease within a defined population (e.g. farm, area, country). Much monitoring information is done on the farm, particularly information relating to production records.

Odds Ratio

"Odds" are a ratio of probabilities: the ratio of the probability of an even occurring to the probability of it not occurring. Where we cannot sample from the whole population at risk but require a way to compare the effect of a risk factor then the odds ratio (OR) is used. There is still a need for "cases" and "controls" but we only need to test these individuals. In a 2 × 2 table, the odds of being a case in the exposed group is a/b, the odds of being a case in the non-exposed group is c/d (Table 7.2). The ratio of these odds is the *odds ratioI,* ad/bc (sometimes called the cross-product ratio):

$$\text{Odds ratio} = \left(a/b\right)/\left(c/d\right) = \left(ad\right)/\left(bc\right)$$

Table 7.2 Odds ratios.

	The animal is:	
	Diseased (case)	**Not diseased (control)**
Exposed	a	b
Non-exposed	c	d

Table 7.3 Predictive values.

	The animal is:	
	Diseased (case)	**Not diseased (control)**
Test result positive	P_{true} (a)	P_{false} (b)
Test result negative	N_{false} I	N_{true} (d)

Predictive values

The inferences that can be drawn from a test result are given by the positive (PPV) and negative predictive values (NPV). Sensitivity (Se) and specificity (Sp) are called the test characteristics that we need to know, but we also need to know the likelihood that the animal is diseased (i.e. disease prevalence), and the diagnostic criteria/signs (which affect the pretest probability – how certain we are that the animal has the disease) to interpret the result correctly (Table 7.3).

PPV is the proportion of positive tests that are truly positive, and NPV is the proportion of negative tests that are truly negative changes. Both depend on the prevalence of the disease in question. Se and Sp are characteristics of a test, and are not affected by the prevalence.

$$Se = P_{true} / P_{true} + N_{false} \text{ or } a/(a+c)$$

$$Sp = N_{true} / P_{false} + N_{true} \text{ or } d/(b+d)$$

$$PPV = P_{true} / (P_{true} + P_{false}) \text{ or } a/(a+b)$$

$$NPV = N_{true} / (N_{false} + N_{true}) \text{ or } d/(c+d)$$

Prevalence

Prevalence is the number of cases or attributes of interest in a known population at a designated period. If time is not specified, it is usually called point prevalence. It is the ratio of the number of cases/total population at risk, and is unlikely to be constant due to changes in the number of cases or variations in the population at risk. It is unitless and is often quoted between 0 and 1.0, although it can be expressed as a percentage (i.e. if the number of cases at a given time in a population of 100 at risk is 10, the prevalence is 0.1 or 10%). Prevalence is a useful measure if we are interested in the number of existing cases to measure the effectiveness of a disease control measure/surveillance and is essential for evaluating diagnostic tests.

Probability (Frequentist)

Probability is a measure between 0 and 1.0. It can be thought of as the frequency of an event relative to the total number of events that occur. Probability drawn from a single study can be called frequentist. If p is the probability that something happens, then $1–p$ is the probability that it will not. If two outcomes are independent, then the probability that both occur is the product $(p_a \times p_b)$ of their probabilities. The probability that either one or the other occurs is the sum of their probabilities minus the product:

$$\left(\left(p_a + p_b\right) - \left(p_a \times p_b\right)\right)$$

Finally, if two outcomes are mutually exclusive then the probability of one or the other is the sum of the two probabilities $(p_a + p_b)$.

Probability (Bayesian)

Bayesian statistics considers use of probability distributions to describe the uncertainty of events. The Bayesian approach starts with a prior probability regarding the event, based on previous knowledge, and then updates that probability based on new evidence or test results, yielding a posterior probability. While not always explicit, a likelihood function can be applied between the prior and posterior.

Probability Notation

Independent Probabilities

If two events A and B are independent, then the probability (P) of event A occurring at the same time as or immediately followed by event B is the product of these two probabilities, which can be written as:

$$\mathrm{P}(\mathrm{A} \cap \mathrm{B}) = \mathrm{P}(\mathrm{A}) \times \mathrm{P}(\mathrm{B})$$

Conditional Probabilities

If an animal is test negative (T^-) then what is the probability that it is disease positive (D^+)? This can be expressed as $P(D^+|T^-)$, which is the probability that an animal is disease positive given that it is test negative. This is a conditional probability and is the same as 1–NPV. To calculate 1–NPV, we first need to calculate the NPV:

$$\mathrm{NPV} = \mathrm{P}(\mathrm{D}- \mid \mathrm{T}-) = \frac{Sp(1-p)}{p(1-Se)+(1-p)Sp}$$

where p = prevalence of infection; Se = test sensitivity; Sp = test specificity.

Table 7.4 Relative risk.

	The animal is:	
	Diseased (case)	**Not diseased (control)**
Exposed	a	b
Non-exposed	c	d

Relative Risk

The relative risk (RR) is the risk of developing disease (or an event) relative to the exposure. It is a ratio of the incidence of disease in the exposed group to the incidence of disease in the unexposed group. Using the 2 × 2 table (Table 7.4), we can calculate that the risk in the exposed group as a/(a+b) and the risk in the non-exposed group is c/(c+d). Therefore, the relative risk (RR) is a(c+d)/c (a+b). A RR of 3 indicates that the incidence of disease in exposed individuals is 3 times that of unexposed individuals. A RR less than 1.0 indicates a negative association (protective?), while RR = 1.0 indicates no statistical association.

Sensitivity

Sensitivity (Se) is the ability of a test to detect disease in a diseased animal (+ve, +ve) based on the "true status of the animal" or more commonly based on a "gold standard" test (which may be imperfect). Se is a proportion and is not affected by the prevalence.

Specificity

Specificity (Sp) is the ability of the test to detect the absence of disease in a healthy animal (–ve, –ve) based on the "true status of the animal" or more commonly based on a "gold standard" test (which may be imperfect). Sp is a proportion and is not affected by the prevalence.

Surveillance

Surveillance is the collection, recording and analysis of data and can be thought of as monitoring with analysis and the intent to take action. Predetermined goals and thresholds must be set and the action that will be taken to control disease must be decided. Additionally, the information recorded can be communicated to other interested parties if necessary.

Probabilities and Probability Distributions

Independent Probabilities

If two events A & B are independent, then the probability (P) of event A occurring at the same time as, or immediately followed by event B is the product of these two probabilities which can be written:

$$P(A \cap B) = P(A) \times P(B)$$

When tossing a coin, the probability of obtaining a head (H), followed by a tail (T), followed by a head (H) is:

$$P(H \cap T \cap H) = P(H) \times P(T) \times P(H) = 0.5 \times 0.5 \times 0.5 = 0.125 = 12.5\%$$

If we have a disease prevalence of 40% then the probability of choosing an infected fish at random can be expressed as $P(D^+) = 0.4$. The probability of selecting 10 infected fish at random is:

$$= P(D^+ \cap D^+ \cap D^+ \cap D^+ \cap D^+ \cap D^+ \cap D^+ \cap D^+ \cap D^+ \cap D^+)$$

$$= P(D^+) \times P(D^+) \times P(D^+) \times P(D^+) \times P(D^+) \times P(D^+) \times P(D^+) \times P(D^+) \times P(D^+) \times P(D^+)$$

$$= 0.4 \times 0.4 \times 0.4 \times 0.4 \times 0.4 \times 0.4 \times 0.4 \times 0.4 \times 0.4 \times 0.4 \times 0.4$$

$$= 0.4^{10} = 0.000105 = 0.0105\%$$

- The probability that all n fish in a group are infected is $P(D^+)n$
- The probability that none of the n fish in a group is infected is $(1–P(D^+))n$
- The probability that at least one of the n fish is infected is $1–(1–P(D^+))n$

Conditional Probabilities

The probability that B will occur given A has already occurred is called a conditional probability and can be written:

$$P(B \mid A)$$

- If A and B are independent, then $P(B|A) = P(B)$ and $P(A|B) = P(A)$ and the probability of A followed by B is: $P(A \cap B) = P(A) \times P(B)$
- If the occurrence of B is dependent on A, then the probability of A followed by B is: $P(A \cap B) = P(A) \times P(B|A)$

Using the fish example above, we test one of the fish and want to know the probability that it is test positive (T^+) given that it is infected (D^+) which can be written $P(T^+|D^+)$ and is the test sensitivity (**Se**). Using a test with a sensitivity of 0.9 and assuming that the probability that a fish is infected then:

$$P(D^+ \cap T^+) = P(D^+) \times P(T^+ \mid D^+) = 0.4 \times 0.9 = 0.36$$

(note that $P(D^+)$ is the disease prevalence p)

The probability that there is at least one test positive and infected fish amongst a group of size n selected at random is:

$$P((D^+ \cap T^+) \geq 1) = 1 - (1 - P(D^+) \times P(T^+ \mid D^+))^n = 1 - ((1-p) \times Se)n$$

Mutually Exclusive Probabilities

If two or more events cannot happen together then they are mutually exclusive. Suppose that we have a tank containing fish species A, B and C. If species A is 50% of the tank population, species B is 15%, and species C is 35% then the probability of selecting either species A or species C is:

$$P(A \cup C) = P(A) + P(C) = 0.5 + 0.35 = 0.85 = 85\%$$

Independent Events That Can Occur Simultaneously

If our tank of fish is now infected with two diseases, disease Y with probability of 0.2 and disease Z with probability of 0.8 and we assume they can independently infect our three species of fish, what is the probability of having both Y and Z diseases:

$$P(Y \cap Z) = P(Y) \times P(Z) = 0.2 \times 0.8 = 0.16$$

We now want to know the probability of selecting a fish at random that will have either disease Y or disease Z. Since some fish have both diseases, we need to subtract this probability:

$$P(Y \cup Z) = P(Y) + P(Z) - P(Y \cap Z) = 0.2 + 0.8 - 0.16 = 0.84$$

Probability Distributions

A *variable* can be any characteristic whose value varies for different objects or subjects. It is a random variable if it can take different values as a result of a random process. Random variables are divided into:

1) Discrete variables that can take on only a limited number of values (e.g. number of infected animals or number of test positive animals) and its corresponding distribution will also be discrete (e.g. a bar graph):
   a) Litter size is a discrete variable and by observing different litter sizes we could determine their relative frequency and plot the results on a bar graph. This relative frequency is the actual probability of occurrence, and this probability is referred to as the *probability mass (function)* with all the individual probabilities adding up to one.
   b) To calculate the probability of a litter size less than or equal to a certain value, we calculate the *cumulative probability (function)* by adding the respective probabilities for each value up to and including our certain variable.
   c) To calculate the mean of the distribution, we multiply the litter size by its respective probability divided by the number of litters. This is essentially a *weighted average*.
   d) Some discrete variables can be treated as continuous where the gap between allowable values is considered to be insignificant (e.g. bacterial cell counts or fecal egg counts).
2) Continuous variables are random variables that can take on any value within a given range (e.g. bodyweight – the scale can be divided into smaller and smaller units) and its distribution will also be continuous (e.g. a histogram).
   a) The cumulative probability can be calculated as in point 1b.
   b) Instead of defining a continuous distribution directly from the data you could use a mathematical function, such as the normal distribution function which is defined by two parameters, the mean μ, and standard deviation σ.
   c) A normal distribution is unimodal, symmetrical about the mean (the mean, median, and mode are all equal) and 95% of the distribution lies within $\pm$ 1.96 standard deviations of the mean while 99% lies within $\pm$ 3 standard deviations from the mean.
   d) The relative frequency of a continuous variable refers to an interval rather than an exact value.
3) For a continuous variable, probability is correctly referred to as *probability density* and the area under the curve must add up to one.

Some examples of distributions are shown in Box 7.1. The formula used in the examples in Box 7.1 are all deterministic – that is, the formula is not random. The same input/s will provide the same output/s (result/s). To change the result, you need to change the input.

Box 7.1 Some Examples of Distributions

Discrete distributions:

- Binomial
- Discrete
- Hypergeometric
- Negative binomial
- Poisson

Continuous distributions:

- Beta
- Normal
- Gamma
- Lognormal
- Triangular
- Pert
- Uniform

For example, to understand or visualize the definitions of cumulative and probability mass function then, for example, run the binomial process example: enter the number of successes (x) and the numbers from 1 to 20, record the results in columns, and graph the results (using either a column or line graph) for the cumulative or probability mass function. The cumulative graph will result in something that looks like an S-shaped line between 0 and 1. We can then sum the probability that the number of successes will be less than or equal to X number of successes. The probability graph will look like a distribution curve and is the probability of occurrence.

Distributions Used to Model a Binomial Process

A binomial experiment or process has five characteristics:

1) It consists of n identical trials.
2) The outcome of any trial is either a success or a failure.
3) The probability of a success p is constant.
4) The trials are independent.
5) The interest is in x, the number of successes observed in n trials, for $x = 0, 1, 2, \ldots n$.

It is characterized by two parameters, the number of trials n, and the probability p, that each trial is successful. The outcome is expressed as the number of successes x. Once two of the values n, p, or x is known the third one can be estimated from the following distributions:

Binomial Distribution

Binomial distribution is used to model the number of successes x; for example, the probability of selecting (x) diseased animals when selecting (n) animals from an infected population:

$$x = \text{binomial}\left(n, p\right)$$

Syntax for Excel

Number_s	The number of successes in trials (the value of x you wish to evaluate).
Trials	The number of independent trials (n).
Probability_s	The probability of success on each trial (p).
Cumulative	A logical value (e.g. 1 = true, 0 = false) that determines the form of the function. If cumulative is TRUE, then BINOM. DIST returns the cumulative distribution function (≈ area under the distribution curve), which is the probability that there are at most number_s successes; if FALSE, it returns the probability mass function, which is the probability that there are number_s successes.

Beta Distribution

Beta distribution is used to model the probability of success p (e.g. estimating the sensitivity of a test):

$$p = \text{beta}(\alpha_1, \alpha_2) = \text{beta}(x+1, n-x+1)$$

α_1 and α_2 are parameters that define the shape of the distribution. Since its domain is restricted to ≥ 0 and ≤ 1 it provides a convenient way of modelling uncertainty about the parameter p in a binomial process. Some useful applications of the beta distribution are shown in Table 7.5.

Example

A total of 9 of 10 animals known to be infected were positive to a serological test so we can estimate the sensitivity of the test as 90% (i.e. the probability that the test is positive given the animal is infected ($P(T^+|D^+)$). However, the sample size is small, so how confident are we that this is a reasonable estimate? By replacing α_1 with $(x + 1)$ where x is the number of successes and α_2 with $(n - x + 1)$ where n is the number of trials, we can model this uncertainty.

Syntax for Excel

X	The value between A(alpha) and B(beta) at which (you want) to evaluate the function.
Alpha (α_1)	A parameter of the distribution ($x + 1$).
Beta (α_2)	A parameter of the distribution ($n - x + 1$).
Cumulative	A logical value that determines the form of the function. If cumulative is TRUE, BETA. DIST returns the cumulative distribution function; if FALSE, it returns the probability density function.
A	Optional. A lower bound to the interval of x.
B	Optional. An upper bound to the interval of x.

Table 7.5 Some applications of the beta distribution.

Application	Number (n)	Number (x)
Test sensitivity	Diseased animals	Diseased animals that test positive
Test specificity	Non-diseased animals	Non-diseased animals that test negative
	Animals	Diseased animals
Estimating a probability when there are no "successes"[a]	Animals sampled	Zero

[a] For example, estimating prevalence when none of the animals sampled is found to be infected.

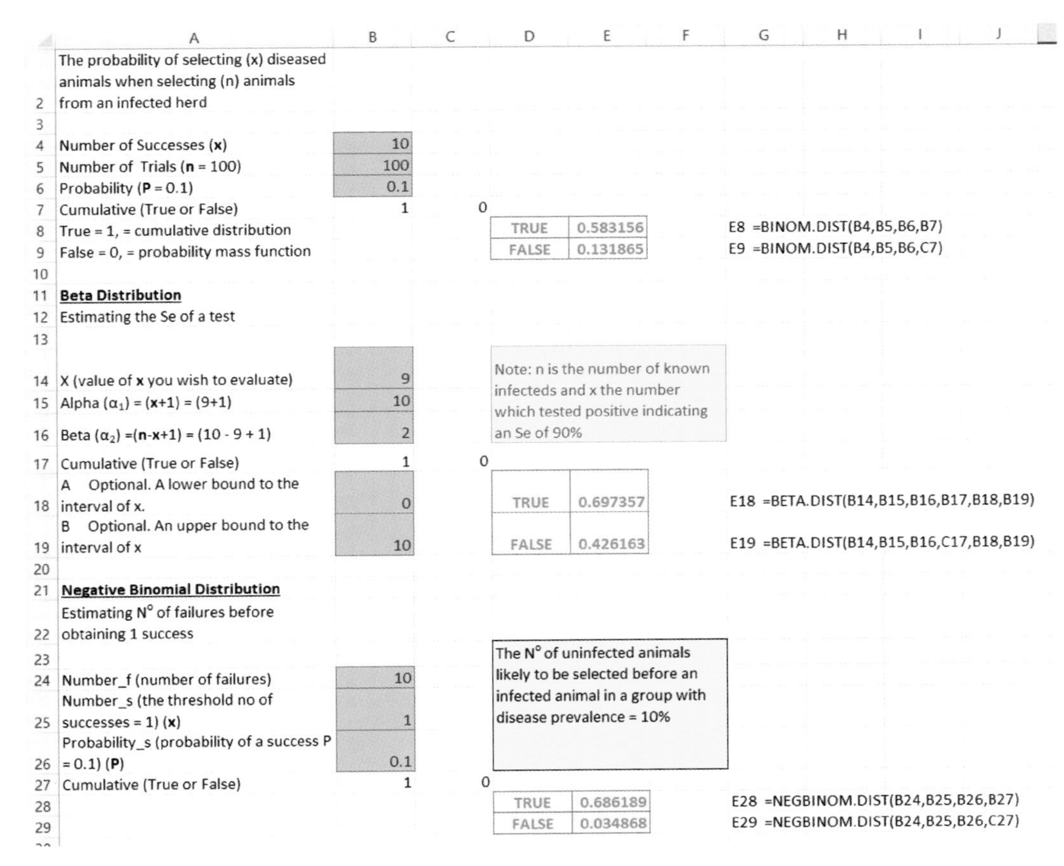

Figure 7.1 Beta distributions.

Negative Binomial Distribution

Negative binomial distribution is used to model the number of trials *n*, undertaken before *x* successes have occurred (Figure 7.1):

$$n = x + \text{negative binomial}(x, p)$$

The outcome is expressed as the number of failures there will be before *x* successes have occurred. The distribution is used to estimate the number of trials *n* required before *x* successes have occurred by adding the number of successes *x* and the number of failures, Negbin(*x*, p).

Example

How many animals could we select from an infected population with a disease prevalence of 10%, before including an infected animal in the group? The formula is:

$$\text{Negbin}(1, \text{O.I})$$

since we are interested in the number of uninfected animals ("failures") before obtaining the first infected one. If we were interested in the number of animals needed to include one infected animal the formula would be:

$$1 + \text{Negbin}(1, \text{O.1})$$

Syntax for Excel

Number_f	The number of failures (e.g. test negative).
Number_s	The threshold number of successes. X
Probability_s	The probability of a success. P
Cumulative	A logical value that determines the form of the function. If cumulative is TRUE, NEGBINOM. DIST returns the cumulative distribution function; if FALSE, it returns the probability density function.

Distributions Used to Model a Poisson Process

A Poisson process has four characteristics:

1) It models the number of events x, that occur in an interval t, of space or time.
2) It is characterized by one parameter lambda (λ), the average number of events per unit interval of space or time.
3) There is a constant and continuous probability of an event occurring per unit interval.
4) The number of events that occur in any one interval is independent of the number that occur in any other interval. It does not matter how far apart the events are in space or time.

The interval t can be measured in space (e.g. per liter, kilogram, kilometer) or time (e.g. second, hour, day, year) and the mean number of events per unit interval λ can also be expressed as $1/\beta$ where β is the mean interval between events. The Poisson process can be modelled using three distributions:

- Poisson
- Gamma (a)
- Gamma (b)

Poisson Distribution

A Poisson distribution is used to model the number of events x in an interval of time t:

$$x = \text{Poisson}\left(\lambda \times t\right) or\ x = \text{Poisson}\left(\frac{t}{\beta}\right)$$

It provides a good approximation for estimating the number of events in an interval such as the number of outbreaks of a disease per year (Figure 7.2).

Example Estimate the number of disease outbreaks (x) expected in the next six months given that historical information suggests an outbreak occurs on average every 24 months. The mean interval between events β is 24 (months), λ is 1/24 (0.04) outbreaks per month and $t = 6$ (months):

$$x = \text{Poisson}\left(\frac{t}{\beta}\right) = \text{Poisson}\left(\frac{6}{24}\right)$$

Syntax for Excel

X	The number of events (in time (t) you want to evaluate).
Mean	The expected numeric value $\left(=\left(\frac{t}{\beta}\right)\right)$.

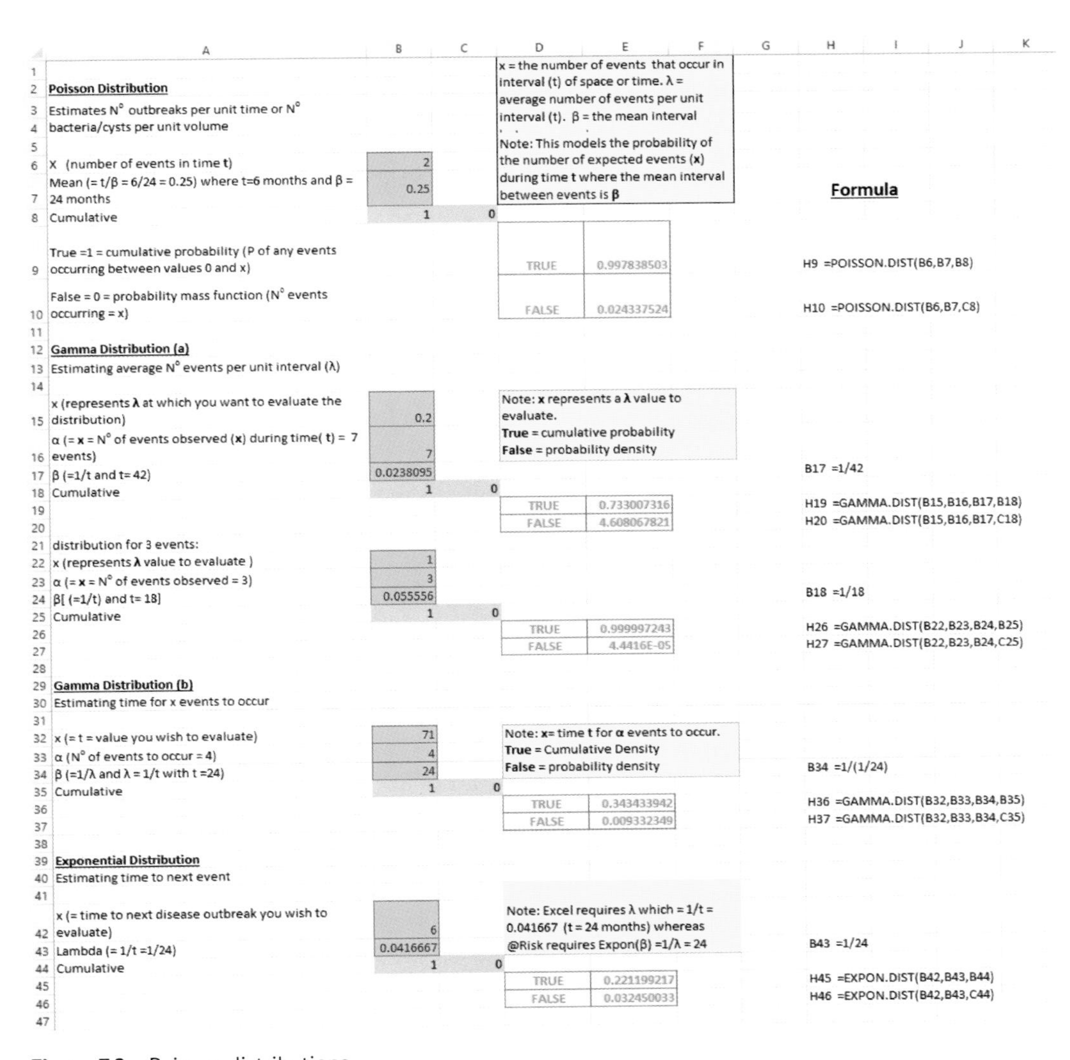

Figure 7.2 Poisson distributions.

Cumulative — A logical value that determines the form of the probability distribution returned. If cumulative is TRUE, POISSON. DIST returns the cumulative Poisson probability that the number of random events occurring will be between zero and x inclusive; if FALSE, it returns the Poisson probability mass function that the number of events occurring will be exactly x.

Gamma Distribution (a)

Gamma distribution (a) is used to model a distribution of λ (the average (or mean) number of events per unit interval):

$$\lambda = \text{Gamma}\left(x, \frac{1}{t}\right)$$

Example Suppose that we observe three disease outbreaks over a period of 18 months, we could estimate that the mean number of outbreaks per month is 0.17 (3/18), presuming that the outbreaks satisfy the Poisson characteristics. Gamma distribution can be used to model the uncertainty surrounding λ (0.17). If we extend the observed period to 42 months and find there are seven outbreaks, we would be increasingly confident that the "true" mean number of outbreaks per month is 0.17.

Syntax for Excel

X	The value at which you want to evaluate the distribution (= λ at which you want to evaluate the distribution).
Alpha	A parameter to the distribution (= number of events observed (x) during time (t)).
Beta	A parameter to the distribution ($=1/t = \lambda$). If beta = 1, GAMMA. DIST returns the standard gamma distribution.
Cumulative	A logical value that determines the form of the function. If cumulative is TRUE, GAMMA. DIST returns the cumulative distribution function; if FALSE, it returns the probability density function.

Gamma Distribution (b)

Gamma distribution (b) is the distribution of the time until the next x events have occurred:

$$t_x = \text{Gamma}\left(x, \frac{1}{\lambda}\right) = \text{gamma}(x, \beta)$$

Syntax for Excel:

X	The value at which you want to evaluate the distribution (= time for x events to occur).
Alpha	A parameter to the distribution (= number of events to occur).
Beta	A parameter to the distribution ($=1/\lambda$ and $\lambda = 1/t$). If beta = 1, GAMMA. DIST returns the standard gamma distribution.
Cumulative	A logical value that determines the form of the function. If cumulative is TRUE, GAMMA. DIST returns the cumulative distribution function; if FALSE, it returns the probability density function.

Exponential Distribution

Exponential distribution is used to model a distribution of the time until the next event has occurred:

$$t_{\text{next}} = \text{Expon}\left(\frac{1}{\lambda}\right) = \text{gamma}\left(1, \frac{1}{\lambda}\right) = \text{Expon}(\beta) = \text{gamma}(1, \beta)$$

The Expon(β) is equivalent to a gamma(x, β) where the number of events x is equal to one. If we estimate that the mean interval between outbreaks of a particular disease is 24 months ($\beta = 24$), we could define a distribution for the length of time it is likely to take before we can expect the next outbreak.

Syntax for Excel

X	The value of the function (the time you wish to evaluate).
Lambda	The parameter value ($1/t$ where $t = \beta$).
Cumulative	logical value that indicates which form of the exponential function to provide. If cumulative is TRUE, EXPONDIST returns the cumulative distribution function; if FALSE, it returns the probability density function.

Hypergeometric Distribution

$$x = \text{hypergeom}\left(n,\ D,\ M\right)$$

A hypergeometric process is characterized by three parameters:

1) The sample size n
2) The number of individuals with the characteristic of interest D (e.g. infected).
3) The population size M.

The outcome is expressed as number of successes x in the sample (Figure 7.3). The probability of success in a hypergeometric process changes each time an individual is selected and removed from the population. It is effectively modelling sampling without replacement.

Example There are five infected animals ($D = 5$) in a batch of 100 animals ($M = 100$) and D/M is initially 0.05. If the first animal selected is infected, then $D/M = 4/99 = 0.04$. However, if it is uninfected then $D/M = 5/99 = 0.051$. As a result, the probability measured by D/M changes depending on whether the previous animal was infected or not (i.e. P is no longer independent of the outcome of the previous trial). This contrasts with the binomial process, where the probability of success P remains constant, and the result of each trial is independent. The binomial process is effectively modelling sampling with replacement. If sample size n is small (less than one tenth the

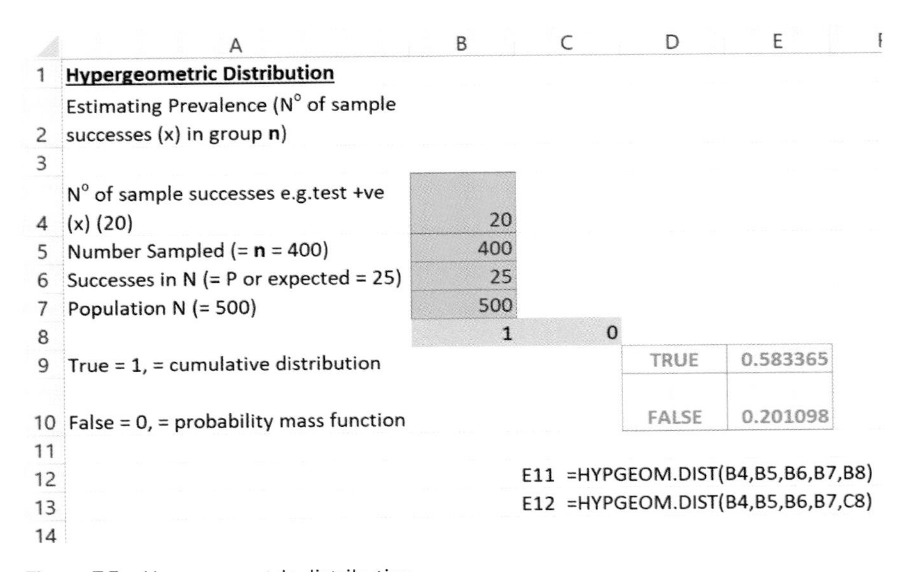

	A	B	C	D	E
1	Hypergeometric Distribution				
2	Estimating Prevalence (N° of sample successes (x) in group **n**)				
3					
4	N° of sample successes e.g.test +ve (x) (20)	20			
5	Number Sampled (= **n** = 400)	400			
6	Successes in N (= P or expected = 25)	25			
7	Population N (= 500)	500			
8		1	0		
9	True = 1, = cumulative distribution			TRUE	0.583365
10	False = 0, = probability mass function			FALSE	0.201098
11					
12				E11 =HYPGEOM.DIST(B4,B5,B6,B7,B8)	
13				E12 =HYPGEOM.DIST(B4,B5,B6,B7,C8)	
14					

Figure 7.3 Hypergeometric distribution.

population size M), the binomial distribution closely approximates the hypergeometric distribution but as the ratio of M/n falls below 10 there is an increasing disparity between the two distributions. As the ratio approaches 1, the binomial distribution predicts a probability of having more infected animals in the group selected than can exist in the whole batch.

Syntax for Excel

Sample_s	The number of successes in the sample (x).
Number_sample	The size of the sample (n).
Population_s	The number of successes in the population.
Number_pop	The population size (N).
Cumulative	A logical value that determines the form of the function. If cumulative is TRUE, then HYPGEOM. DIST returns the cumulative distribution function; if FALSE, it returns the probability mass function.

Lognormal Distribution

Lognormal distribution is used to model disease incubation periods for example (Figure 7.4):

$$\text{Lognorm}(\mu, \sigma)$$

$$\text{Tlognorm}(\mu, \sigma, \text{minimum}, \text{maximum})$$

The parameters, μ and σ are the actual mean and standard deviation of the lognormal distribution. It often provides a good representation for data that extend from zero and are positively skewed (e.g. have a longer right hand tail) such as population sizes, carcass weights and disease incubation periods. The lognormal distribution extends from zero to plus infinity so it may need to be truncated (constrained) to avoid implausible values.

Example Model the incubation period for a particular disease as Lognorm(5,3). If this disease had a minimum and maximum incubation period of 2 and 14 days, respectively, there is a reasonable chance that some random samples drawn from the distribution would fall outside this range. As a result, we may need to truncate the distribution so that sensible values are sampled.

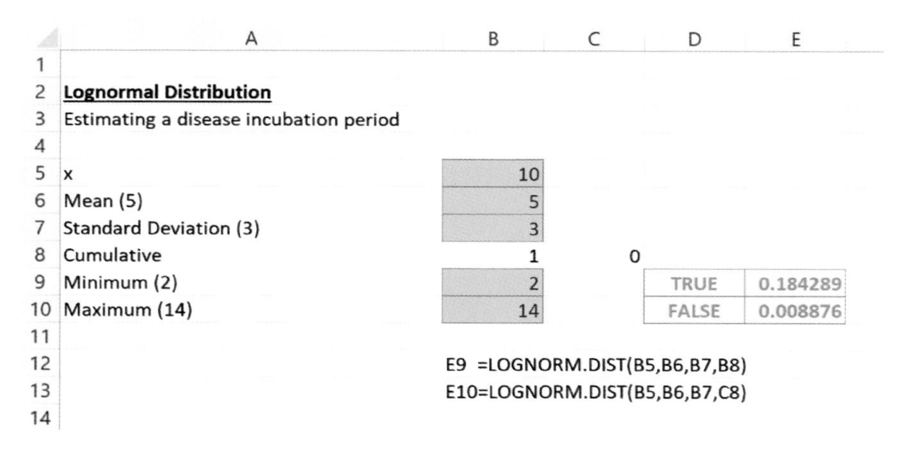

	A	B	C	D	E
1					
2	Lognormal Distribution				
3	Estimating a disease incubation period				
4					
5	x	10			
6	Mean (5)	5			
7	Standard Deviation (3)	3			
8	Cumulative	1	0		
9	Minimum (2)	2		TRUE	0.184289
10	Maximum (14)	14		FALSE	0.008876
11					
12		E9 =LOGNORM.DIST(B5,B6,B7,B8)			
13		E10=LOGNORM.DIST(B5,B6,B7,C8)			
14					

Figure 7.4 Lognormal distribution.

Syntax for Excel

X	The value at which to evaluate the function.
Mean	The mean of ln(x).
Standard_dev	The standard deviation of ln(x).
Cumulative	A logical value that determines the form of the function. If cumulative is TRUE, LOGNORM. DIST returns the cumulative distribution function; if FALSE, it returns the probability density function.

Normal Distribution

The normal distribution (μ, σ) is symmetrical about its mean, with 99.9% of its values lying within ± 3 standard deviation of the mean (Figure 7.5). Many naturally occurring variables such as weight, physiological characteristics, pH of tissues and fluids and milk and egg production are normally distributed. Others are normally distributed following some transformation of the data, for example a log transformation of a set of data on the incubation period of a disease.

Syntax for Excel

X	The value for which you want the distribution.
Mean	The arithmetic mean of the distribution.
Standard_dev	The standard deviation of the distribution.
Cumulative	A logical value that determines the form of the function. If cumulative is TRUE, NORM. DIST returns the cumulative distribution function; if FALSE, it returns the probability mass function

Pert Distribution

Pert(minimum, most likely, maximum):

$$\text{Pert}(a, b, c) = \text{beta}(\alpha_1, \alpha_2) \times (c - a) + a$$

$$\mu(\text{mean}) = \frac{a + 4b + c}{6}$$

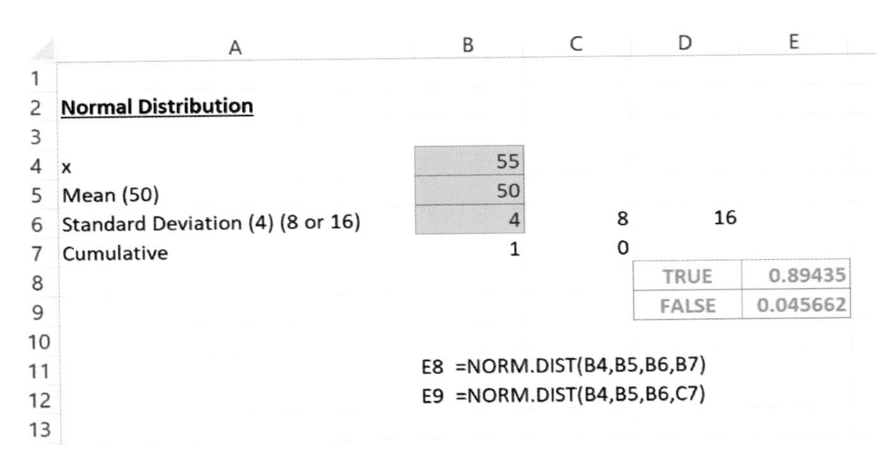

Figure 7.5 Normal distribution.

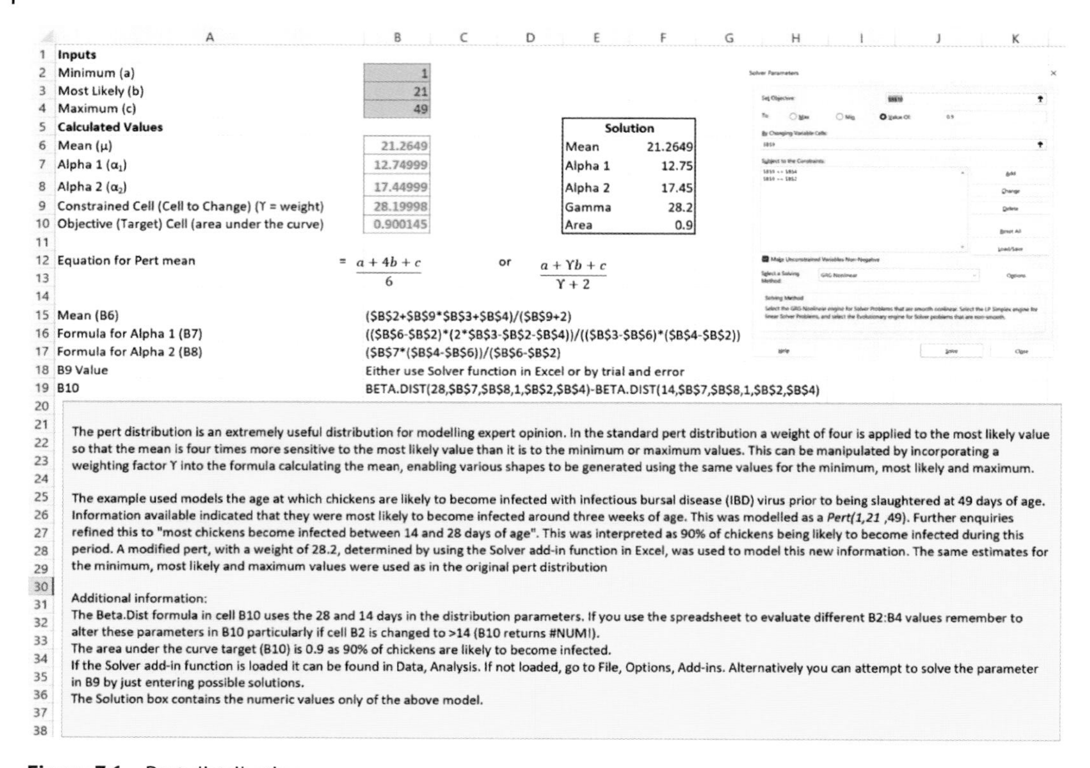

	A	B	C	D	E
1	**Inputs**				
2	Minimum (a)	1			
3	Most Likely (b)	21			
4	Maximum (c)	49			
5	**Calculated Values**				
6	Mean (μ)	21.2649			
7	Alpha 1 (α_1)	12.74999			
8	Alpha 2 (α_2)	17.44999			
9	Constrained Cell (Cell to Change) (ϒ = weight)	28.19998			
10	Objective (Target) Cell (area under the curve)	0.900145			
12	Equation for Pert mean	$= \frac{a+4b+c}{6}$		or	$\frac{a+\Upsilon b+c}{\Upsilon+2}$
15	Mean (B6)	($B$2+$B$9*$B$3+$B$4)/($B$9+2)			
16	Formula for Alpha 1 (B7)	(($B$6-$B$2)*(2*$B$3-$B$2-$B$4))/(($B$3-$B$6)*($B$4-$B$2))			
17	Formula for Alpha 2 (B8)	($B$7*($B$4-$B$6))/($B$6-$B$2)			
18	B9 Value	Either use Solver function in Excel or by trial and error			
19	B10	BETA.DIST(28,$B$7,$B$8,1,$B$2,$B$4)-BETA.DIST(14,$B$7,$B$8,1,$B$2,$B$4)			

Solution	
Mean	21.2649
Alpha 1	12.75
Alpha 2	17.45
Gamma	28.2
Area	0.9

The pert distribution is an extremely useful distribution for modelling expert opinion. In the standard pert distribution a weight of four is applied to the most likely value so that the mean is four times more sensitive to the most likely value than it is to the minimum or maximum values. This can be manipulated by incorporating a weighting factor ϒ into the formula calculating the mean, enabling various shapes to be generated using the same values for the minimum, most likely and maximum.

The example used models the age at which chickens are likely to become infected with infectious bursal disease (IBD) virus prior to being slaughtered at 49 days of age. Information available indicated that they were most likely to become infected around three weeks of age. This was modelled as a *Pert(1,21 ,49)*. Further enquiries refined this to "most chickens become infected between 14 and 28 days of age". This was interpreted as 90% of chickens being likely to become infected during this period. A modified pert, with a weight of 28.2, determined by using the Solver add-in function in Excel, was used to model this new information. The same estimates for the minimum, most likely and maximum values were used as in the original pert distribution

Additional information:
The Beta.Dist formula in cell B10 uses the 28 and 14 days in the distribution parameters. If you use the spreadsheet to evaluate different B2:B4 values remember to alter these parameters in B10 particularly if cell B2 is changed to >14 (B10 returns #NUM!).
The area under the curve target (B10) is 0.9 as 90% of chickens are likely to become infected.
If the Solver add-in function is loaded it can be found in Data, Analysis. If not loaded, go to File, Options, Add-ins. Alternatively you can attempt to solve the parameter in B9 by just entering possible solutions.
The Solution box contains the numeric values only of the above model.

Figure 7.6 Pert distribution

The pert distribution is a modification of the beta distribution, which models minimum, most likely, and maximum estimates (Figure 7.6). It provides a more natural shape than the triangular distribution and is not as influenced by the extreme (minimum and maximum) values. It is very good for modelling expert opinion. In the standard pert distribution, a weight of four is applied to the most likely value so that the mean is four times more sensitive to it than the other two. This weighting can be manipulated by incorporating a weighting factor ϒ into the formula to enable different shapes to be generated using the same minimum, most likely and maximum values.

$$\mathrm{M} = \frac{a + \Upsilon b + c}{\Upsilon + 2}$$

There is no pert function in Excel.

Using and Assessing Data Sources

Figure 7.7 looks informative at first sight but what data does it provide? It is clearly a sample of a larger population but there is no indication of the size of the whole population. It could be presumed or hoped that the animals were selected at random, but there is no evidence of whether the sample is representative. There is information missing to be able to assess the validity and precision of the results. To address this uncertainty, we could gather more data to give greater confidence that the result (e.g. sample mean) – is "correct" but this would take time and increase costs.

	A	B	C	D
1	Weight in Kg	Value or	Excel Function	Brief Description
2		Formula	Used	
3	50	10	COUNT	Sample Size (n)
4	54	0.05	α	(=95% CI) Required for Confidence T (=100 x (1- α) = 95%)
5	46	48.500	AVERAGE	Mean (Strictly sample average x̄ whereas μ = population mean)
6	47	4.577	STDEV.S	SD (σ̂) based on a sample (would use STDEV.P (σ) if a population)
7	44	3.274	CONFIDENCE T	Returns the CI (confidence interval)for a pop mean using students t value
8	52	51.774		Upper 95% CL (confidence limit)
9	47	45.226		Lower 95% CL
10	56	1.447	SQRT	Standard Error of the mean
11	41	2.262		t value with (n-1) df
12	48			
13			Excel Formula	
14		B1	=COUNT(A4:A13)	B6 =B6+B8
15		B2	= numerical value	B7 =B6-B8
16		B3	=AVERAGE(A4:A13)	B8 =B7/SQRT(B4)
17		B4	=STDEV.S(A4:A13)	B9 =B8/B11
18		B5	=CONFIDENCE.T(B5,B7,B4)	

Figure 7.7 Basic statistics.

We could also look for analogies in other reports indicating a similar mean, increasing our confidence to use our data as a basis for any decision.

Both above approaches are reasonable, but is there a way to improve confidence without collecting more data and avoiding the increased costs? A stochastic modelling approach may achieve this end. This approach estimates probability distributions of possible outcomes by taking random variation of one or more inputs into account. It can be done by sampling a hypothetical sampling distribution of the mean and the standard deviation and running a Monte Carlo simulation. When the graphs of the results produced are compared it can be seen there is little difference between the two distributions (Figure 7.8). The means are identical, and although there is some inflation in the variance of the mixed model, as shown in the tails of the distribution, the difference is minor. In this case, it would be reasonable to ignore the uncertainty in bodyweight based on a random sample of 10. The Figure 7.8 illustrates the graphs produced using classical statistics. This is a four-step process:

1) Collection of initial data and analysis
2) Derive a sampling distribution for the mean and standard deviation
3) Assessing the uncertainty by comparing models. A first order model is produced where the sampling distributions for the mean and standard deviation are set to their expected values, and compared to a mixed model where uncertain and variable components are modelled together
4) Compare the simulation graphs.

We could also use parametric and non-parametric bootstrap methods. Figure 7.8 is an example that occurs in many animal health situations– the problem of limited data. As authors, we should always fully record how the data were produced, from what, and for what purpose. As a consumer of data, there is always a need to check whether the data look correct (missing data, unexpected outliers) and have been analyzed correctly, particularly where that analysis is through statistics (if a paper identifies a statistician, then the statistical analysis should be correct). Through modelling and an understanding of statistics it is possible, even in data poor environments, to reduce uncertainty and confirm that the data are useable.

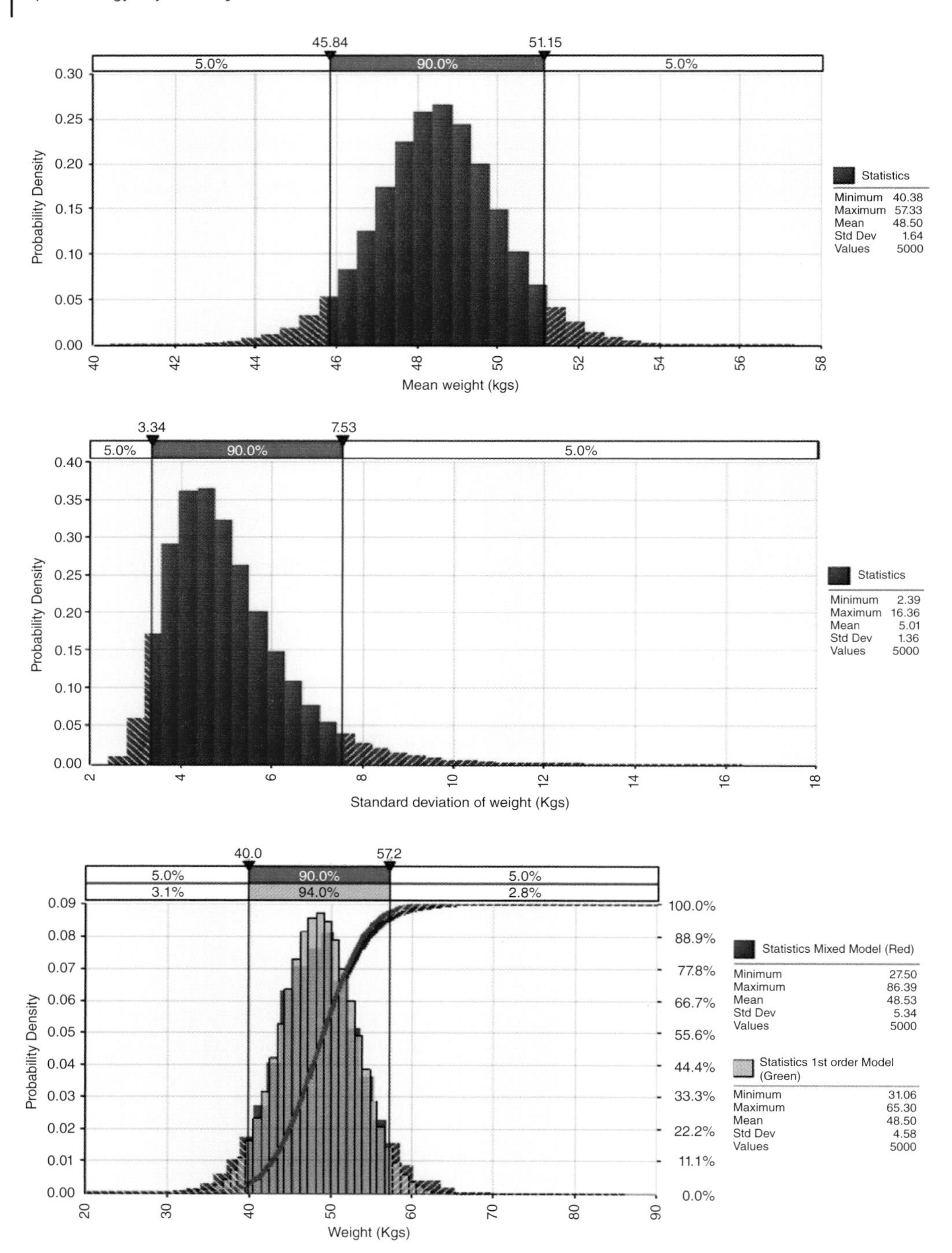

Figure 7.8 Modelling uncertainty.

If access to a statistician is difficult, or third-party add-ins that allow Excel to perform stochastic modelling are unavailable, it is possible to carry out Monte Carlo simulations in standard Excel. Producing meaningful figures to describe it, however, is difficult. A framework that could be used would be based on the following, but it still does not get around any problem of poor quality or lack of data.

Before providing a brief description of the various studies we first need to consider the following terms:

- *Precision* can be thought of as how consistently an effect has been assessed in a series of measures. By increasing the sample size, the precision increases, but it can be decreased, if at the same time the "noise" in the system is increased. This noise may be removed by accounting for, for example, sex or age, or any other variable that might affect the result.
- *Validity* in a test or technique is a measure of the test doing what it is supposed to do, and can be thought of as lack of systematic error or bias. While palpation is a reasonably valid method of diagnosing a fracture, a more accurate diagnosis is achieved by using a technique such as radiography, which has a higher validity.
- *Confounding* is when a causal variable is not only associated with the outcome of interest but also another putative causal variable (e.g. sex, age, disease duration). This confounding variable is non-random, and is typically a risk factor for the disease in question. Confounding is of particular relevance in case–control studies where subjects are chosen based on presence or absence of disease and where subjects may share many risk factors, some statistically significant but not causal.
- *Selection bias* is where we fail to ensure the sample is representative of the whole population of interest. This can be caused by failing to account for disease clustering (e.g. using a specific locality or facility such as a fish processing plant as a representative of the entire population of fish at sea), failure in the randomization process, ignoring the disease status of the sample.
- *Misclassification* leads to cases and controls being confused, possibly as a result of the sensitivity and specificity of diagnostic criteria.
- *Recall bias* is a particular problem in retrospective studies, where the "subject" is required to remember or recollect events linked to a disease.
- *Generalizability* to other situations beyond the actual study.

There are many other forms of bias. See Thrusfield (2018) for more detail.

Descriptive Epidemiology

Descriptive epidemiology can be described as information on the presence or absence of the disease within an epidemiological unit, country or the world. It includes data on the prevalence, the results of any surveillance carried out either by the competent authority or the facility, which can be either passive or active, and the generation of case reports.

Knowing the prevalence of a disease is important when it comes to interpreting a diagnostic test and also the disease's potential relevance to any biosecurity plan. Evidence for prevalence may be available from the competent authority, from production records (disease present or not after at least two production cycles) or it needs to be generated from sampling carried out within the epidemiological unit. Surveillance may be carried out by the competent authority on known diseases with serious economic consequences or as a public good (see Chapter 10). For an epidemiological unit, surveillance is the monitoring for disease presence and the actions that presence instigates. Case reports can be a quick way of alerting others to the possible presence of an emerging or re-emerging disease. While descriptive epidemiology provides useful information for the practitioner and the epidemiological unit, it may or may not be generalizable (externally valid).

Analytic Epidemiology

Cross-sectional studies

These look at a population or sub-population at an instance in time and result in prevalence ratios.

Cohort Studies

Cross-sectional studies follow a group of animals who have a similar experience (e.g. smolts in a similar environment) and are usually prospective. They typically compare an exposed with a nonexposed cohort over a period of time. Animals can be removed from the study due to death, sale, disease, or being no longer at risk. The results are expressed as risk of disease, relative risk (exposed, non-exposed), and the incidence rate. One drawback is that the cohort may experience varying risk during the period of study.

Case–Control Studies

It is necessary to identify two groups (cases and controls) and to provide an accurate and consistent case definition. The study compares case and controls for certain risk factors. The results are expressed as odds. The odds of being a case given exposure, the odds of being a case given non-exposure and the odds ratio of exposed versus non-exposed.

Selection of cases requires a clear case definition and must be from a population of interest. Controls must be selected from the same population. They must be selected independently of exposure and be eligible to be a case if they become "diseased". It is acceptable to have more than one control per case.

Ecologic Studies

An ecologic study is a unit of observation in a population or community. Disease rates and exposures are measured in a variety of populations and any relationship is examined.

Randomized Controlled Trials

Randomized controlled trials (RCTs) test whether a "treatment" has an effect. The population must all be considered as "cases" and is typically split into two groups: treated and non-treated. Selection for each group must be at random. Groups can be single blinded, where the subject does not know whether they have received the treatment, which helps to account for any placebo effect. Double-blinded RCTs are where neither the subject nor the operator knows whether they have received the treatment, which helps to account for any operator effect. Triple blinded RCTS are where the subject, the operator, and the statistician are unaware of which treatment has been received.

Expert Opinion

Expert opinion, while useful, is subject to bias and is rather hard to define, as it could either be a consensus opinion provided by a group of people, or an individual who has reviewed the scientific literature; or it could be a group of people who have reviewed the available expert opinion. This all seems rather tautological and maybe easier to provide the clear example of the WOAH *Aquatic Animal Health Code and Manual*, where the information contained, mainly on listed diseases, is reviewed every couple of years or when there is a significant change, by a panel of recognized experts. The Code and Manual are a good starting point for any biosecurity plan.

Further Reading

Kirkeby C, Brookes VJ, Ward MP, et al. A practical introduction to mechanistic modeling of disease. *Front. Vet. Sci.* 2021; 7: 546651.

Mancy R, Brock PM, Kao RR. An Integrated Framework for Process-Driven Model Construction in Disease Ecology and Animal Health. Front. Vet. Sci. 2017; 4:155.

Petrie A, Watson P. *Statistics for Veterinary and Animal Science*, 3rd edn. Hoboken, NJ: Wiley; 2013.

Sergeant E, Perkins N. *Epidemiology for Field Veterinarians: An introduction*. Wallingford, UK: CABI; 2015.

Thrusfield M, Christley R. *Veterinary Epidemiology*, 4th ed. Hoboken, NJ: Wiley; 2018.

Wei Y, Sha F, Zhao Y, et al. Better modelling of infectious diseases: lessons from COVID-19 in China. *BMJ* 2021; 375 :n2365.

8

Diagnostics: Sampling and Diagnostic Testing

Chris Walster and Leo Foyle

Diagnosis is a Bayesian process (Bours, 2021; Mandel, 2014). As you are dealing with probabilities, it can be far from certain. This uncertainty partially stems from Koch's postulates not being applicable to all the diseases we recognize today (Evans, 1976), and there rarely being a "gold standard" test available. In infectious and non-infectious disease, clinicians start with a pretest probability, which is usually the disease prevalence in the population of the animal/s being cared for. A clinical examination or diagnostic test is then carried out, and from this, you obtain a post-test probability is obtained. At some point, the clinician will have whittled down their list of differential diagnoses and feel confident that they have the diagnosis.

We tend to think of a "test" as being a laboratory test to confirm a diagnosis and rarely think that a clinical examination, or even taking a history, is actually a test, which can be measured using the exact same measurements such as sensitivity (Se), specificity (Sp) and positive predictive value (PPV). While your brain seems pretty good at doing these things during the consultation process (certainly for experienced clinicians), it is not actually very good at getting them right. When measured, clinicians are unexpectedly poor at coming up with the right probabilities, let alone the negative predictive value (NPV). A famous statistician in the UK admitted that despite 40 years of teaching statistics, when presented with a probability problem, he often needed five minutes to sit down and think about it. Some of what is presented in the rest of this chapter might appear daunting, so sit down and think about it, if it is a spreadsheet, set it up, and try altering the data. See what happens and if that does not work, turn the results into a graph so you can visualize it.

Test Characteristics

Se, Sp, positive likelihood ratio (LR+) and negative likelihood ratio (LR–) are fixed properties and do not change with prevalence. However, the PPV, which is the proportion of positive tests that are truly positive, and the NPV, which is the proportion of negative tests that are truly negative do (Caraguel et al., 2015; Parikh et al., 2008, 2009; Coulthard, 2006). This is best demonstrated by an example interpretation of a test result, although it is an unlikely scenario in clinical practice because of the numbers of animals tested. As well as the Se and Sp of the test, you need to know the prevalence or your best guestimate. As an example, a disease with high morbidity and mortality is unlikely to be present if no deaths or clinical signs are noticed, so it would be safe to assume

Pathology and Epidemiology of Aquatic Animal Diseases for Practitioners, First Edition.
Edited by Laura Urdes, Chris Walster, and Julius Tepper.

a very low prevalence. However, with a disease of low morbidity and mortality it would be more prudent to assume a higher prevalence. We wish to know what a test result actually means. In this example, the test has an Se of 80% and an Sp of 95%:

$$LR+ = Se \div (1 - Sp) = 0.80 \div (1 - 0.95) = 16$$
$$LR- = (1 - Se) \div Sp = (1 - 0.80) \div 0.95 = 0.21$$

The prevalence of the disease is 1 in 100 (1%) and we have tested 1000 animals (Table 8.1). Remember that converting to odds is odds = probability/(1-probability) and from odds to probability is probability = odds/(1+ odds):

- Pretest odds for a positive result is known/presumed disease positive (prevalence) divided by known/presumed disease negative = 0.01/0.99 = 0.0101
- Pretest odds for a negative result is 0.99/0.01 = 99
- For a positive result post-test odds = pretest odds × likelihood ratio = 0.0101 × 16 = 0.162
- For a negative result post-test odds = pretest odds × likelihood ratio = 99 × 0.21 = 20.79
- Post-test probability for a positive result = 0.162/(1 + 0.162) = 13.9%
- Post-test probability for a negative result = 20.79/(1 + 20.79) = 95.4%
- The proportion of positive tests that are truly positive (PPV) = a/(a + b) = 8/58 = 14%
- The proportion of negative tests that are truly negative (NPV) = d/(c + d) = 940/942 = 99.8%

Thus, we can be fairly confident that a negative test result is accurate, but we are still very uncertain what a positive test result actually means. If we now make the prevalence of the disease 50 in 100 (50%) and we test 1000 animals (Table 8.2).

- For a positive result post-test odds = pretest odds × likelihood ratio = 1 × 16 = 16 = 94.1%
- For a negative result post-test odds = pretest odds × likelihood ratio = 1 × 0.21 = 0.21 = 82.6%

Table 8.1 The "truth."

Test results	Disease positive	Disease negative	Total
Positive	8[1] (a)	50 (b)	58
Negative	2 I	940 [2] (d)	942
Total	10	990	1000

[1] the number truly positive = 0.80 (Se) × 10 (10 being the number we know to be positive at 1% of 1000).
[2] the number truly negative = 0.95 (Sp) × 990 (990 being the number we know to be negative at 99% of 1000).

Table 8.2 The "truth."

Test results	Disease positive	Negative	Total
Positive	400 (a)	25 (b)	425
Negative	100 I	475 (d)	575
Total	500	500	1000

	A	B	C	D	E	F	G	H	I
1	Calculating LR. Odds and probabilties								
2			Cell Formula without =						
3	LR+	16.0000	G9/(1-G10)				The "truth"		
4	LR-	0.2105	(1-G9)/G10				Disease Positive	Disease Negative	Total
5	Pre-test Odds +ve	0.0101	G8/(1-G8)			Test Positive	8	50	58
6	Pre-test Odds -ve	99.0000	(1-G8)/G8			Test Negative	2	940	942
7	Post-tests Odds +ve	0.1616	B5*B3			Total	10	990	1000
8	Post-tests Odds -ve	20.8421	B6*B4			Prevalence	0.01		
9	Post-test Probability +ve	0.1391	B7/(1+B7)			Sensitivity (Se)	0.8		
10	Post-test Probability -ve	0.9542	B8/(1+B8)			specificity (Sp)	0.95		
11	PPV	13.79%	G5/(G5+H5)						
12	NPV	99.79%	H6/(G6+H6)						
13									
14	LR+	16.0000	G20/(1-G21)				The "truth"		
15	LR-	0.2105	(1-G20)/G21				Disease Positive	Disease Negative	Total
16	Pre-test Odds +ve	1.0000	G19/(1-G19)			Test Positive	400	25	425
17	Pre-test Odds -ve	1.0000	(1-G19)/G19			Test Negative	100	475	575
18	Post-tests Odds +ve	16.0000	B16*B14			Total	500	500	1000
19	Post-tests Odds -ve	0.2105	B17*B15			Prevalence	0.5		
20	Post-test Probability +ve	0.9412	B18/(1+B18)			Sensitivity (Se)	0.8		
21	Post-test Probability -ve	0.1739	B19/(1+B19)			specificity (Sp)	0.95		
22	PPV	94.12%	G16/(G16+H16)						
23	NPV	82.61%	H17/(G17+H17)						

Figure 8.1 Calculating the meaning of a test result.

- The proportion of positive tests that are truly positive (PPV) = 400/425 = 94%
- The proportion of negative tests that are truly negative (NPV) = 475/575 = 83%

Under these conditions, using the same test we can be fairly confident that a positive result is correct but now we are not so sure about a negative result.

Since PPV and NPV are so much easier to calculate why do we go through this complicated process? As mentioned above PPV and NPV can be affected by the prevalence. Likelihood ratios can cope with a range of Se and Sp (think of the range of clinical severity a patient presents with), provide insight into whether you can rule in or rule out a disease using a test, and also allow for easier computing of post-test odds than PPV and NPV when using a series of diagnostic tests (Parikh et al., 2009):

$$\text{Post-test odds} = \text{pretest odds} \times \text{LR1} \times \text{LR2} \times \text{LR3} \ldots \times \text{LRn}$$

If you do not want to calculate the post-test odds, you can use Fagan's nomogram or the two-step Fagan's nomogram (Caraguel and Vanderstichel, 2013; if the paper is accessed online then you can download a potential template to use). Alternatively, you could set up a spreadsheet based on Figure 8.1.

Tests in Combination

A single test may not provide enough certainty for our requirements. Additional tests may provide more clarity. Combinations of tests can be used in an "and" or an "or" method. When used in an "and" method then the animal needs to test positive to test 1 and test 2 and test 3, and so on, to be considered positive. This is called testing in series. Using an "or" method the animal only needs to test positive to test 1 or test 2 or test 3 and so on, to be considered positive. This is called testing in parallel.

In parallel testing, multiple tests can be used at one time. It can be quick, increases Se and NPV, and decreases Sp and PPV. With serial testing, the tests are conducted sequentially with only positive animals being retested. This is slower, decreases Se and NPV, and maximizes Sp and PPV. Serial testing is a useful method as part of a disease eradication program. Be aware when using multiple testing strategies that you increase the probability of a type I error (false positive) occurring.

To Obtain an Estimation of Disease Prevalence

As previously stated, you may be able to use a suitable disease prevalence (p) based on the known disease characteristics, such as morbidity or mortality, to calculate the test characteristics. You may be able to obtain one from published scientific papers or other sources, such as expert opinion. In some cases, you will need to use your best estimate. Below is one formula to estimate disease prevalence. The example and Figure 8.2 look at two issues with using such a formula, unknown prevalence, and dealing with small populations. There is a third problem, the size of the sample, as potentially the epidemiological unit might decline on economic or welfare grounds if the test is lethal. The formula is:

	A	B	C	D
1		**Basic Sample size calculations**		
2	$n = P \times (1 - P) \times (z/e)^2$		Actual value or Excel Formula	
3	P= Prevelance 0.2	0.2	20%	
4	P= Prevelance 0.5	0.5	50%	
5	z= value of the normal etc	1.96	95% confidence	
6	e = allowable error	0.05	5%	
7	Small population	1000		
8	Result for P=0.2	245.8624	$B$3*(1-$B$3)*($B$5/$B$6)^2	
9	Result for P=0.5	384.16	$B$4*(1-$B$4)*($B$5/$B$6)^2	
10	The above works for an infinite population (with replacement) but if the population is small (e.g. we sample more than 5% of the population) then we need to adjust using the formula:			
11	$n_{finite} = (nxN)/(n+N)$			
12	where n is the sample size for an infinite population and N is the population size.			
13	For P = 0.2	197.3431	($B$8*$B$7)/($B$8+$B$7)	
14	For P = 0.5	277.5402	($B$9*$B$7)/($B$9+$B$7)	
15				
16	Obviously we cannot sample "part" of an animal so we always round up to the next whole number. So used answers would be 246, 385, 278. The formula for B8 and B9 have been made "absolute references". This can be useful if you do not want the cell reference to change. To cycle through select the formula in the formula bar and press F4.			

Figure 8.2 Basic sample size calculations.

$$n = \left(Z^2 \times p(1-p)\right)/L^2$$

Where: Z = is value of the standard normal distribution corresponding to the desired confidence (e.g. 1.96 for 95% confidence); p = the expected proportion of diseased animals in the population; n = the number to be sampled; L = the desired precision of the prevalence estimate.

Example

You would like to know the prevalence of a disease in a population. You are uncertain about the true level, so you assume that it will be there in 50% of the animals ($p = 0.5$); 50% is used as it always implies the largest sample size and if the true prevalence is greater or less than 50% then you will either have greater confidence or greater precision. You would like to be 95% confident that the true prevalence lies within 5% of 50% (i.e. between 45% and 55%, therefore the desired precision is 0.05).

$$Z = 1.96$$

$$p = 0.5$$

$$L = 0.05$$

$$n = \left(1.96^2 \times 0.5(1-0.5)\right)/0.05^2 = 384$$

This formula presumes a perfect test but gives an indication of the necessary sample size. If we used a test with an Se of 90% and an Sp of 95% the sample size increases to 531 from our population, which we assume is large. If your sample size is more than 5% of the population then you need to adjust as demonstrated in the figure below. Note that the formula used looks different but is pretty much identical. Alternatively, there are several websites which will allow you to enter the data and generate the result for you (e.g. Epitools: https://epitools.ausvet.com.au). However, you do need an understanding of the principles of modelling and provide the correct input parameters to use such websites.

As indicated below (e.g adjusting for population size) there are methodologies that can be used to decrease the number of animals tested and hence costs. The use of scenario trees is an example (Food and Agriculture Organization, 2014). However, unless you are researching a disease or working for the competent authority, it is unlikely that you will be compensated for testing for prevalence on the epidemiological unit, and it is perfectly acceptable to use average values reported in the scientific literature.

References

Bours MJ. Bayes' rule in diagnosis. *J Clin Epidemiol* 2021; 131: 158–160.

Caraguel CGB, Gardner IA, Hammell LK. Selection and interpretation of diagnostic tests in aquaculture biosecurity. *J Appl Aquacult* 2015; 27: 279–298.

Caraguel CGB, Vanderstichel R. The two-step Fagan's nomogram: ad hoc interpretation of a diagnostic test result without calculation. *Evid Based Med* 2013; 18: 125–128.

Coulthard MG. Quantifying how tests reduce diagnostic uncertainty. *Arch Dis Child* 2007; 92(5): 404–408.

Evans AF. Causation and disease – the Henle-Koch postulates revisited. *Yale J Biol Med* 1976; 49: 175–195.

Food and Agriculture Organization. *Risk-Based Disease Surveillance: A manual for veterinarians on the design and analysis of surveillance for demonstration of freedom from disease*. Animal Production and Health Manual No. 17. Rome, Italy: FAO.

MacAulay S, Ellison AR, Kille P, Cable J. Moving towards improved surveillance and earlier diagnosis of aquatic pathogens: from traditional methods to emerging technologies. *Rev Aquacult* 2022; 14: 1813–1829.

Mandel DR. The psychology of Bayesian reasoning. *Front Psychol* 2014; 5: 1144.

Parikh R, Mathai A, Parikh S, et al. Understanding and using sensitivity, specificity and predictive values. *Indian J Ophthalmol* 2008; 56: 45–50.

Parikh R, Parikh S, Arun E, Thomas R. Likelihood ratios: clinical application in day-to-day practice. *Indian J Ophthalmol* 2009; 57: 217–221.

9

Biosecurity: The Use of Risk Assessment, Surveillance, Outbreak Investigation, Modelling Disease Outbreaks

Chris Walster and Leo Foyle

Many of the elements of epidemiology are common to biosecurity, such as risk analysis, surveillance, outbreak investigation, sampling, and diagnostic testing. Observations made can be summarized by statistics and hypotheses tested. Clearly, epidemiology provides recognized tools to assist in the development, implementation, and maintenance activities of any biosecurity plan including underpinning requirements of auditing and certification.

Biosecurity implies the maintenance of a spatial separation between organisms of concern. It is a normal part of animal production and might be conceived as a modern way of thinking and talking about activities that have gone before. It is a way of formalizing disease control strategies and communicating these strategies to stakeholders. However, for the farmer, concepts are not useful or practical unless they can be shown to have a real impact on the economic viability and profitability of the enterprise. The degree of biosecurity required and how to achieve it is dependent on the type of epidemiological unit and the amount of risk present. Open epidemiological units are at more risk compared with closed ones, and a commercial epidemiological unit's biosecurity needs might differ compared with a hobby facility.

The barriers to implementing an effective biosecurity plan are:

- Attitude – both you and your client need to agree what is the right approach.
- Knowledge – fully assess the needs.
- Understanding – what is achievable; what is the purpose?
- Ownership – it must be worth something. Your client will not implement it unless they can see a value.

Risk Assessment

Disease Risk Analysis: Evaluating an Operation's Risk from Disease Hazard

$$\text{risk} = \text{probability} \times \text{consequence}$$

Risk is a simple equation, but it can be extremely difficult to decide the value of the terms. Probability is perhaps the easiest term for which to determine a numerical value (i.e. probability of introduction of disease from suppliers) but assessing consequence can be extremely

Pathology and Epidemiology of Aquatic Animal Diseases for Practitioners, First Edition.
Edited by Laura Urdes, Chris Walster, and Julius Tepper.

difficult (i.e. when loss of reputation is considered greater than economic loss or the presence of disease on the property). Perceived difficulties in conducting a quantitative risk analysis (cost, time, lack of data, knowledge of, and experience in probability distributions and methods) make qualitative risk analysis more popular. Qualitative models are subjective and the risk matrices may produce risk estimates that are little better than chance and open to interpretation. These perceived difficulties with quantitative analysis arise from the complexity of the concepts, and because they usually involve using multiple pathways and parameters. However, for a single epidemiological unit, a robust quantitative risk analysis can be carried out fairly simply using epidemiological principles (Table 9.1). An alternative to a risk matrix would be the use of a decision tree. Whether qualitative or quantitative all relevant stakeholders should be involved in what is an iterative process as people's risk perceptions vary (previous experience, reputation, pride, animal welfare etc.) and should be accommodated to help acceptance of the final list.

Regardless of the methodology used for this step, the aim is to answer three questions of the disease hazards identified in step one and create a prioritized list of diseases:

1) Are they a risk? The answer can be a yes or no based on the information assessed or prioritized by using a risk matrix, decision tree, or simply of most concern to the epidemiological unit. Remember that this risk is to epidemiological unit stock, people, or the wider environment. Diseases that are of no consequence (i.e. vector not present, incorrect water temperature, age of stock) can be removed and the reason why it was removed recorded. This information should not be discarded.
2) Is the hazard on the premises (epidemiological unit)? Again, this can be a yes or no answer. If there is doubt, steps should be taken to confirm absence or presence. It is essential that an accurate baseline of disease presence is determined. Not only does this assist in determining appropriate actions to either control or eradicate the hazard but also contributes towards accurate economic assessment of the benefits of the biosecurity plan in the future.
3) What are the consequences? In general, consequence assessment will be assessed on the economic impact of the risk. The consequence should evaluate not just the mortality and morbidity but also the likely degree of spread (within and outside the epidemiological unit), as well as the cost of control or eradication. The assessment does not have to be quantified at this stage but can be expressed qualitatively as high, medium, or low.

Table 9.1 An example of a risk matrix.

Risk		**Consequence**				
		Very low	**Low**	**Medium**	**High**	**Very high**
Score		**1**	**3**	**5**	**7**	**9**
Very Low	1	1	3	5	7	9
Low	3	3	9	15	21	27
Medium	5	5	15	25	35	45
High	7	7	21	35	49	63
Very High	9	9	27	45	63	81

Identifying an Aquaculture Operations Critical Control Points

A critical control point (CCP) is a point or operational step in a procedure that can be controlled to prevent, eliminate, or minimize the likelihood of the identified hazard occurring. Critical limits (maximum or minimum) that separate acceptable from unacceptable need to be set and a monitoring system established to ensure continuing the control of the CCPs. As an example, hand washing and disinfection of footwear prior to entering different areas of a site can decrease pathogen spread, but it is not a CCP since it would be difficult to set critical limits or monitor the effectiveness of the procedure due to variation in handwashing technique, disinfection efficacy, and avoidance of the footbath, among others. It would therefore be better to incorporate such procedures as "good hygiene practices" that staff must follow. On the other hand, a terrestrial site may identify the water intake as a CCP since it is possible to treat the water sufficiently to decrease the pathogen load, set minimum and maximum log reductions in pathogens and effectively monitor the process.

In essence, all farm inputs are potential disease entry points (water intake, contact with/presence of other epidemiological unit's, stock, feed delivery and storage, equipment, staff etc.) that need to be evaluated, and where possible identified as a CCP with a clear critical limit. Requirements for the CCP and critical limit, or some other mitigating measure, should be incorporated into the standard operating procedure covering that part of the farm's process. Specific disease prevention recommendations will depend on the aquatic species, the diseases of concern, routes of transmission, and the likelihood of exposure.

Disease Risk Management/Mitigation Options

The easiest way to prevent a disease outbreak on an epidemiological unit is to prevent the pathogen from entering. If this is not achieved, there should also be controls to prevent spread within the epidemiological unit. This is achieved by erecting barriers that might be physical (e.g. fencing), chemical (e.g. disinfection), biological (e.g. vaccines), behavioural (e.g. deterrence of contact), spatial (e.g. distance between units), social (e.g. staff not allowed to keep aquatic animals), and educational (e.g. staff training).

For a land-based closed system, these barriers can be thought of as solid and providing good (measurable) protection since it is easy to erect a fence to prevent unwanted visitors and ensure water intake is free of pathogens. A fully closed system is able to control pathogen entry and eradicate any disease present. As the system becomes more open, some of these barriers may become more porous and the ability to prevent or eradicate a disease lessens, since the epidemiological unit may not be able to isolate itself from disease reservoirs present in wild populations or in adjacent epidemiological units. Although the same barriers are used in an open or closed system, the emphasis in an open system moves more towards control through methods such as testing and surveillance (for early detection) rather than eradication, unless there is cooperation between epidemiological units in the adjacent areas or those linked epidemiologically. Cooperation between epidemiological units has been shown to be effective for many disease scenarios.

While the aim of any biosecurity plan is to prevent introduction of disease from external sources, it should also address how to prevent spread of disease already present on the epidemiological unit or disease spread if the biosecurity measures are breached. The approach to correcting the critical weak spots can be summarised with three connected considerations:

- What are the biosecurity plan requirements (i.e. control or eradication, internal, or external benefits)?
- The available resources (i.e. economic, laboratory, staff training)?

- Epidemiologically achievable (i.e. testing, surveillance, isolation)?
- All three considerations are interconnected.

From these general concepts more specific details that need to be addressed include:

- Site location and separation from adjacent epidemiological units – what biosecurity controls do they have? What diseases are present on them and how easily can they be transferred?
- Are there other facilities close by that could act as sources of disease – slaughterhouses, rendering plants, feed mills, or other concentrations of animals?
- What are the effective means of physical separation?
- Access control for people – visitor book, a requirement for changing areas and showers?
- Vehicle access control – do they need to enter the site? If so, are there facilities for washing and disinfection (prior to entry, if they have been on another epidemiological unit, and on leaving).
- Water supply – sharing, can wild populations be excluded, methods of pathogen reduction?
- Feed supply – assured or certified source and storage?
- Prevention of exposure to vectors – what are the relevant vectors, and can exposure be prevented?

To detect disease entry or spread the following needs to be considered:

- Are personnel aware of the signs and symptoms of disease?
- What might trigger an "outbreak investigation?"
- Monitoring and surveillance activities?
- Laboratories – are they accredited, are test results valid?
- How should disease occurrences be reported?
- If an outbreak occurs, will there be an effective response?

From these considerations, it will be apparent where to concentrate resources on risk mitigation and what the appropriate measures will be.

Disease Epidemiology and Surveillance Information

Below is an outline of important principles in disease epidemiology and surveillance information:

- Epidemiology asks who has what (disease), when and where (time and space), why and how (risk factors and transmission), and in this process defines the disease outbreak.
- You cannot compare disease outbreaks without the above information and hence will not be able to correctly evaluate the benefits arising from the biosecurity plan.
- Terms that you need to understand, and use include, probability, relative risk, odds ratio, prevalence, incidence, sensitivity (Se), specificity (Sp), and the difference between test Se/Sp and laboratory Se/Sp, likelihood ratios, positive and negative predictive values, and the difference between monitoring and surveillance.

The goals of surveillance for an epidemiological unit are:

- The rapid detection of disease outbreaks (to minimise control costs).
- The early identification of disease problems (including environmental causes).
- Assessment of the health status of the defined population (working towards certification/ or audit).
- Definition of priorities for disease control and prevention (from risk assessment and cost/benefit analysis).
- Identification of new and emerging diseases (as part of contingency planning).

- Evaluation of the disease control programmes.
- Confirmation of absence of a specific disease (certification, disease free status).

Elements of an 'ideal' surveillance system are:

- A pre-agreed intervention threshold (e.g. percentage mortality that triggers an investigation).
- An agreed case definition (e.g. the signs/symptoms/pattern that constitute a case or episode of a specific disease).
- Harmonised diagnostic procedures (e.g.to ensure that you are comparing like with like).
- Defined population at risk (e.g. the epidemiological unit – epidemiological unit).
- Method of recording cases (farm and veterinary records).
- Method to report data (within epidemiological unit, between epidemiological unit, veterinarian, and official services).
- Timely and competent data analysis (designed dependent on who/what will use the data – requires some foresight).
- Means to assess the effect of an intervention (measures to assess prevalence).
- It is a continuous process (iterative).
- Means to communicate findings in a timely fashion.

Determining Disease Status and Freedom – Qualitative Compared With Quantitative Approaches

A qualitative approach uses multiple sources of evidence such as laboratory records from farm diagnostic testing or structured surveys carried out by the official services, other information from farm and slaughter records, and disease information databases. Using a panel of experts, this type of approach, has been used by World Organisation for Animal Health (WOAH) and national authorities to assess claims of freedom from disease following disease eradication programmes. While it would seem to be a commonsense approach using all of the available evidence, it tends to be a subjective assessment with problems of transparency and repeatability. Further, the outcome is "likely to be free from infection or not" with the inherent uncertainty unmeasured. For an epidemiological unit, this might be an appropriate approach for internal use but may not be "convincing" for external use.

A quantitative approach could be a structured representative survey of the relevant population. The necessary number of animals to test at the design prevalence (P*) can be determined by using the Epitools epidemiological calculators (https://epitools.ausvet.com.au). If the probability of disease presence is less than the agreed P* then the population is considered free. While the cost of these surveys can be reduced by targeting animals at risk rather than the whole population (which reduces the number to be tested), they can be expensive to carry out. Other weaknesses include failing to include other relevant evidence and the fact that they are ephemeral (e.g. only relevant at the time they are carried out unless repeated).

A method which combines the advantages of both the above by using multiple sources of surveillance data (both random and non-random) is scenario tree modelling for disease freedom.

Disease Diagnostics and Monitoring

The clinical signs expressed by aquatic animals may not be pathognomonic and additionally they maybe subclinically infected (i.e. not showing signs). There is thus a requirement for some form of diagnostic testing to ensure correct pathogen/disease identification and early identification of a disease incursion. Since an effective biosecurity plan requires knowledge of the disease status of stock already on the epidemiological unit and any stock introduced, the implication is that these diagnostics will be carried out routinely over a specified period. By recording this information, we are monitoring the stock. Diagnostics will include:

- Observation of stock behaviour – this is an essential activity for any epidemiological unit.
- Clinical examination.
- Onsite diagnostic testing such as skin scrapes, gill snips, routine blood biochemistry and postmortem.
- Samples may be processed on site for culture and sensitivity or sent to an external laboratory.
- Currently, there are some pen or tankside tests available for viral or bacterial infections with others under development. Potential issues in using such tests not only revolve around the test Se and Sp, which is needed to interpret the test correctly but also variance in results due to operator technique.
- For external laboratory diagnostics it is better to use an accredited laboratory (e.g. WOAH accredited).
- The frequency of testing should be decided and recorded within the biosecurity plan.

All this information should be recorded and should form part of the farm and veterinary record. Monitoring will include:

- Carrying out and recording all the above.
- Water quality parameters.
- Stock movements and density.
- Recording of mortality.
- Recording morbidity.
- Feed usage.
- Recording movements both on and off site and also within the epidemiological unit if it is divided into separate sections or zones.
- Treatment records (often required under national legislation).
- Significant weather events.

Auditing and Certifying Biosecurity Status

Auditing is verifying that procedures are in place and working correctly against an identified standard (checking what is supposed to have been done/occurred, in the standard compared with what has been done/occurred). Auditing is often carried out by external, third parties. The process can be summarised as:

- Opening meeting
- Inspection
- Verification
- Documentation of findings
- Closing meeting
- Report.

The report should identify the epidemiological unit, set out the biosecurity risks and the actions taken, corrective actions required/suggested with a measure of the confidence the auditor has in these actions. The results could be summarised as shown in Table 9.2. The aim of auditing is to

Table 9.2 Audit results.

Criteria	Description
Excellent	Effective procedures
	Biosecurity principles applied satisfactorily
	No action necessary
Acceptable	Procedures requiring only minor correction
	Biosecurity principles generally applied satisfactorily, only minor corrections necessary
	Action advisable
Poor	Procedures inadequate
	Biosecurity principles inadequately applied
	Potentially significant implications of biosecurity failure
	Action required (and if regulated likely formal enforcement if no action taken)
Unacceptable	Immediate serious risk of biosecurity failure
	Animal health and welfare at risk
	Biosecurity principles not applied
	Immediate action necessary (and if regulated formal enforcement if no action taken)

assist the epidemiological unit achieve its objectives and when carried out by an external assessor (i.e. veterinarian) provides an independent and objective opinion based on verifiable facts.

Auditing should be carried out annually by a veterinarian, but it is best practice that the epidemiological unit carries out internal audits to ensure their own procedures are compliant with the standard, and that records are available and complete on a monthly basis.

Certifying is somewhat different to auditing and for a veterinarian is carried out within a set of strict rules which provides assurance of the validity. For example, whereas an audit evaluates the effectiveness of the biosecurity plan procedures against a standard or agreed plan, its implementation and user compliance based on records and evidence supplied. A veterinary certificate could only state that an audit has taken place since the attending veterinarian is unlikely to have personal knowledge that the procedure was carried out even though the evidence may well imply this. A veterinary certificate can only attest to an event/occurrence/test/criterion where the signing veterinarian is fully aware and conversant with all of the facts.

Certification is a procedure to ensure that a product, process or service conforms to specified criteria (requirements). It can be split in to three types:

1) First Party certification is basically a self-declaration that the producer has met a certain standard.
2) Second Party certification is basically the producer has met the requirements of a standard set by an external group (i.e. consumers, government or NGO's). The producer is externally assessed but often it is the same group that sets and assesses the standard thus there may be an issue as the standards may reflect the interests of the group that sets and assesses them.
3) Third Party certification is based upon standards created by a multi-stakeholder process. Compliance is voluntary and is assessed by an accredited, independent third party holding no vested interest in the standards, certification, product or stakeholder group. The International Organization for Standardization (ISO) defines third party certification as the highest order for proof of compliance.

The Risk of Introducing Infection

Probabilities can help us decide what the risk of introducing infection is when buying in stock, particularly from several producers. Each producer has a 95% chance of being free of infection which you feel is acceptable and you wish to buy from 4 producers and do not screen the stock yourself. What is your actual risk?

The probability that a supplier at level n in the supply chain will be free of infection is given by the formula:

$$P_n = \left(P_{n-1} + X\left(1 - P_{n-1}\right)\right)S$$

Where: P_{n-1} is the probability that a supplier in the level below will be free of infection; X is the effectiveness of screening; S is the number of suppliers in the layer below. The probability of infection is $1 - P_n$.

In this example you buy from a chain of suppliers with four levels who all have 95% confidence that their stock is not infected. Filling in the equation with these values gives:

$$P_n = \left(0.95 + 0\left(1 - 0.95\right)\right)4 = 0.954 = 0.81$$

You have a 19% probability of receiving infected stock. If you had purchased from a layer of eight producers, you would have 34% probability. That is pretty concerning. Without screening or quarantining your new stock, even when buying from "healthy" sources runs a considerable risk of introducing disease.

While the above talks about the risk from using multiple suppliers, Figure 9.1 indicates the risk using an "imperfect" test, although with realistic Se and Sp, for an individual animal and a consignment even when the disease is probably not detectable and may well be considered from a disease free source. Practical epidemiological advice like this should help convince clients of the need for quarantine.

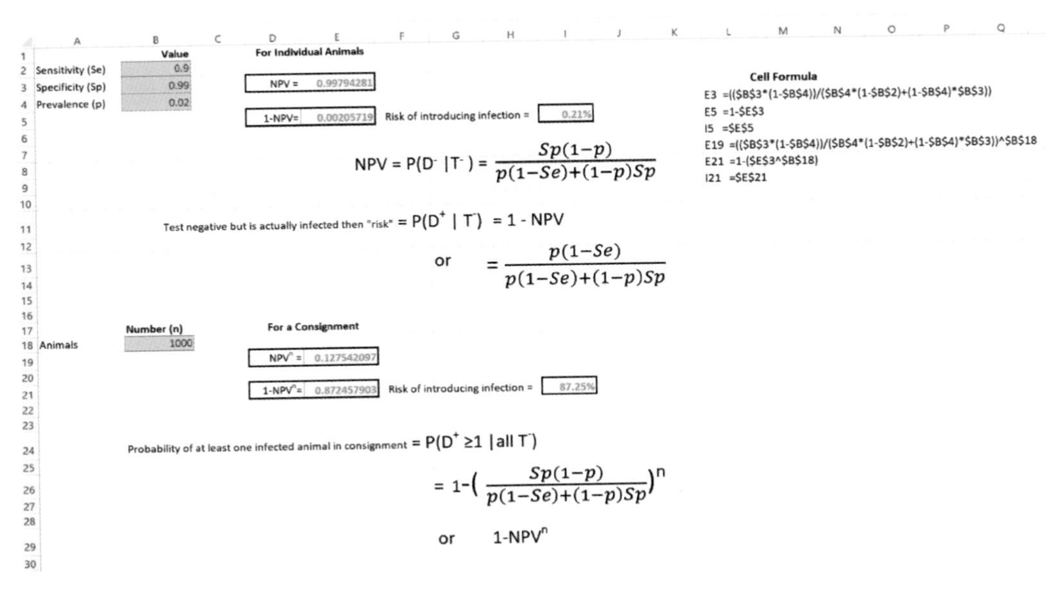

Figure 9.1 Calculating negative predictive value.

Demonstrating Freedom from Disease

How do you demonstrate that a disease is not present in the epidemiological unit? How do you detect the presence of disease in the epidemiological unit? How do you establish the prevalence of disease in the epidemiological unit? You could sample all the animals to prove it, but this is costly and time consuming. It may be acceptable that you have 95% confidence that the disease is not present at a prevalence substantially below that which would be expected if the animals in the epidemiological unit had disease. This would allow you to sample only a certain number of animals saving cost and time. The size of the sample is dependent on the size of the population in question, the likely prevalence of the disease if present and the reliability required of the conclusions. The formula is:

$$n = \left(1 - (1 - \alpha)^{1/d}\right)\left(N - \left((d-1)/2\right)\right)$$

Where: N = is the population size; d = the number of positives in the population; n = the number to be sampled; α = the desired confidence level (the probability of finding at least one positive in the sample). An example of the calculation is given below:

$$\begin{aligned} N &= 20000 \,(\text{size of population of interest}) \\ d &= 1000 \,(\text{desired prevalence} < 5\%) \\ \alpha &= 95\% \,(\text{i.e.probability of } 0.95) \end{aligned}$$

$$\begin{aligned} n &= \left(1 - (1 - 0.95)^{1/1000}\right)\left(20000 - \left((1000 - 1)/2\right)\right) \\ &= (1 - 0.997)(20000 - 499.5) \\ &= 0.003 \times 19500.5 \\ &= 58.5 \,(\text{so sample } 59) \end{aligned}$$

If there are no positives in the 59 samples then we can be 95% confident that the disease is not present at a prevalence of 5% or greater. If there are one or more positives, then we can be 95% confident that the disease is present at a prevalence of at least 5%. However, this result presumes we have used the perfect test (i.e. Se and Sp of 100%) which is unlikely. Sensitivity (Se) and specificity (Sp) are discussed in Chapter 7, but if you used a test with a diagnostic Se of 90% and an Sp of 95% then the required sample size rises to 398. If we sample 398 animals using our imperfect test and if we have up to 27 (false) positive reactors (based on an Epitools report), then we can conclude that the population is disease free (at the expected 5% prevalence) with 95% confidence. Is this sufficient to conclude that the population is completely disease free? The answer is no, although depending on the disease of interest, the value and the intended use of the animals this result may give us sufficient confidence to purchase the animals as "disease free".

With the imperfect test example, we've hit the problem of sample size again, particularly if it is part of a surveillance program and you wish to test monthly or even weekly! How can you get around this and still provide confidence that the epidemiological unit is disease free (of a specific disease)? It is beyond the scope of this summary chapter to discuss these fully and further information can be found in the references and further reading. However, you can use historical information of freedom from disease, sanitary measures introduced to protect against introduction of disease, and risk based sampling such as using Relative Risk (RR) to reduce sampling numbers by sampling from a population most at risk. A simple scenario would be to sample from moribund fish in the face of an outbreak, since they will have an RR greater than 1 for the disease of interest. This is what often happens in practice. Another example would be to use Scenario Tree modelling, which is discussed briefly later in the chapter.

Another approach could be to sample a small proportion of the population and conduct a Bayesian inference calculation or simulation. This requires that all the animals test negative, and we then model what this might mean. Figures 9.2–9.5 demonstrate this using a sample of 30 animals from a population of thousands. It is not necessary to know the exact population size. By graphing the resulting probability density and looking at the area under the curve, we can infer a likely prevalence and a probable range (confidence interval). The x axis, labelled probability, is equal to prevalence.

In Figure 9.3, we have some information that suggests the prevalence of disease is between 1% and 10%, with a most likely value of 5%. A triangular distribution has been used, as it is slightly simpler to set up than a PERT distribution, although a PERT distribution is considered the best way to model expert opinion. Of note is that, as the number of animals sampled increases and we obtain more information, the posterior distribution as graphed changes from a triangle shape to a narrower distribution. Again, by looking at the area under the curve we can see that the most likely prevalence has changed and appears to lie between 4% and 5%, although we still have a wide confidence interval.

We now repeat the process using a PERT distribution. The reason it is preferred over the triangular is that it provides for a smoother distribution and variation in the weighting of the mean. This provides for greater flexibility to model expert opinion. A standard PERT distribution uses a weighting of four times the most likely value, as used here, but could be any value (as demonstrated in the PERT distribution example in Chapter 7, Figure 7.6).

Figure 9.5 runs both the uninformed and informed PERT using a commercially available Microsoft Excel add-in. There are some advantages to using these add-ins, such as more distribution functions, and beyond the cost, there are really no disadvantages. The model uses a Monte

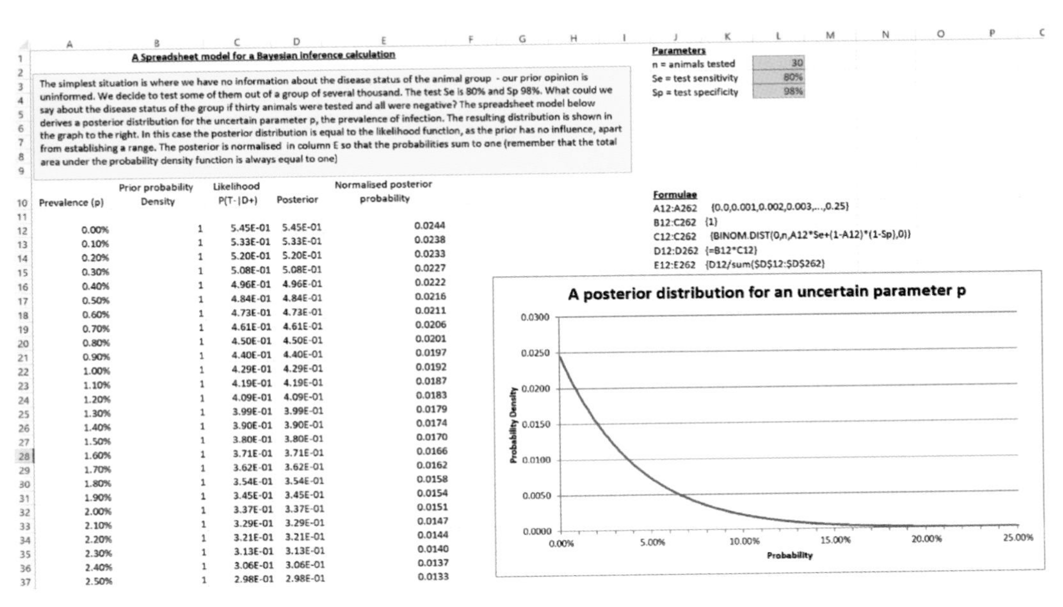

A Spreadsheet model for a Bayesian Inference calculation

The simplest situation is where we have no information about the disease status of the animal group - our prior opinion is uninformed. We decide to test some of them out of a group of several thousand. The test Se is 80% and Sp 98%. What could we say about the disease status of the group if thirty animals were tested and all were negative? The spreadsheet model below derives a posterior distribution for the uncertain parameter p, the prevalence of infection. The resulting distribution is shown in the graph to the right. In this case the posterior distribution is equal to the likelihood function, as the prior has no influence, apart from establishing a range. The posterior is normalised in column E so that the probabilities sum to one (remember that the total area under the probability density function is always equal to one)

Prevalence (p)	Prior probability Density	Likelihood P(T-|D+)	Posterior	Normalised posterior probability
0.00%	1	5.45E-01	5.45E-01	0.0244
0.10%	1	5.33E-01	5.33E-01	0.0238
0.20%	1	5.20E-01	5.20E-01	0.0233
0.30%	1	5.08E-01	5.08E-01	0.0227
0.40%	1	4.96E-01	4.96E-01	0.0222
0.50%	1	4.84E-01	4.84E-01	0.0216
0.60%	1	4.73E-01	4.73E-01	0.0211
0.70%	1	4.61E-01	4.61E-01	0.0206
0.80%	1	4.50E-01	4.50E-01	0.0201
0.90%	1	4.40E-01	4.40E-01	0.0197
1.00%	1	4.29E-01	4.29E-01	0.0192
1.10%	1	4.19E-01	4.19E-01	0.0187
1.20%	1	4.09E-01	4.09E-01	0.0183
1.30%	1	3.99E-01	3.99E-01	0.0179
1.40%	1	3.90E-01	3.90E-01	0.0174
1.50%	1	3.80E-01	3.80E-01	0.0170
1.60%	1	3.71E-01	3.71E-01	0.0166
1.70%	1	3.62E-01	3.62E-01	0.0162
1.80%	1	3.54E-01	3.54E-01	0.0158
1.90%	1	3.45E-01	3.45E-01	0.0154
2.00%	1	3.37E-01	3.37E-01	0.0151
2.10%	1	3.29E-01	3.29E-01	0.0147
2.20%	1	3.21E-01	3.21E-01	0.0144
2.30%	1	3.13E-01	3.13E-01	0.0140
2.40%	1	3.06E-01	3.06E-01	0.0137
2.50%	1	2.98E-01	2.98E-01	0.0133

Parameters

n = animals tested	30
Se = test sensitivity	80%
Sp = test specificity	98%

Formulae

A12:A262 {0.0,0.001,0.002,0.003,...,0.25}
B12:C262 {1}
C12:C262 {BINOM.DIST(0,n,A12*Se+(1-A12)*(1-Sp),0)}
D12:D262 {=B12*C12}
E12:E262 {D12/sum($D$12:$D$262)}

Figure 9.2 Bayesian inference calculation – uninformed prior.

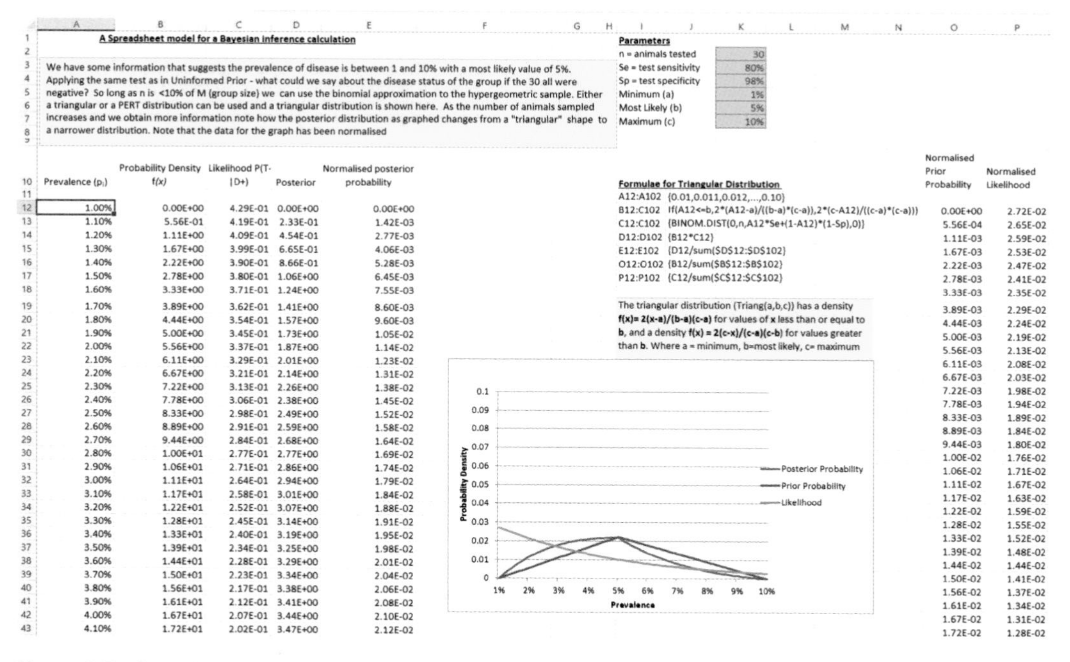

Figure 9.3 Bayesian inference calculation informed prior (triangular distribution).

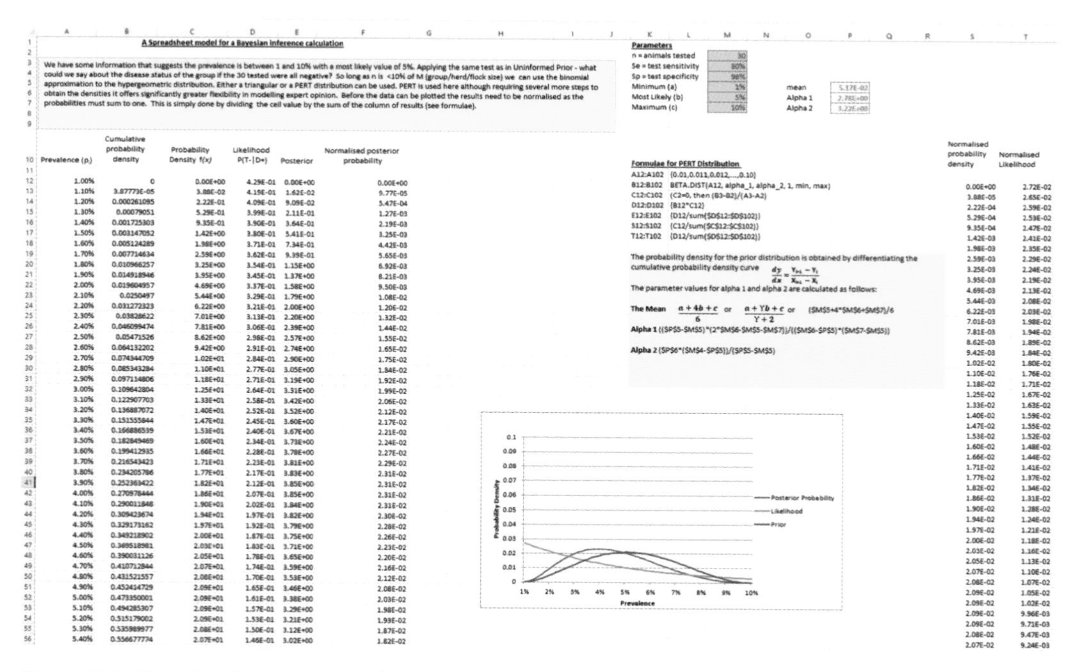

Figure 9.4 Bayesian inference calculation informed prior (PERT distribution).

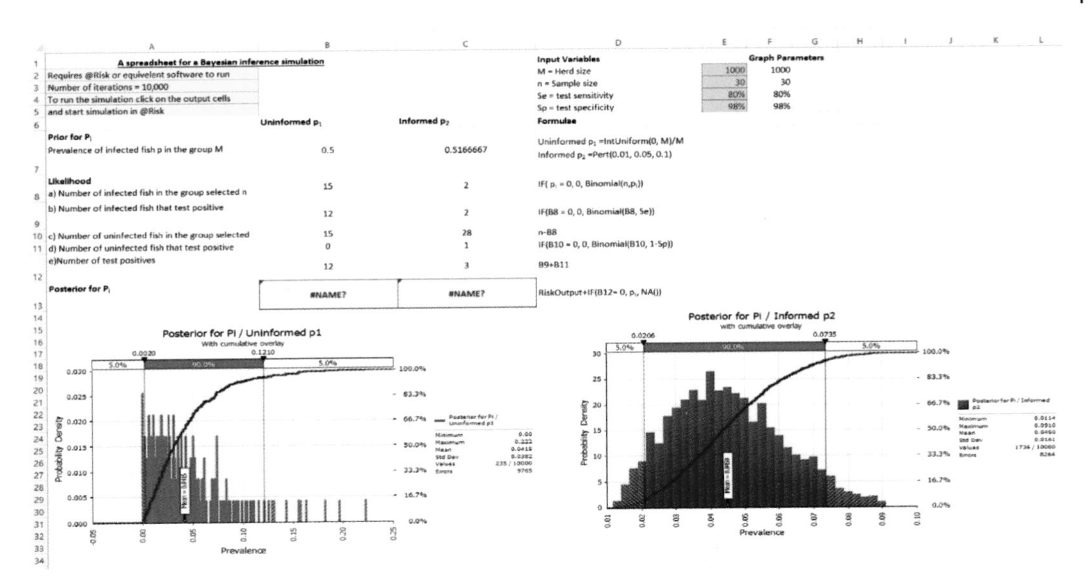

Figure 9.5 Bayesian inference simulation using Monte Carlo.

Carlo simulation and is a stochastic model whereas the previous are deterministic. You can run Monte Carlo simulations in Excel and the Excel help files demonstrate how to do this.

The model has gone through 10,000 iterations to produce the graphs shown in Figure 9.5. In this way, we can model the uncertainty around our small sample size. Each time we run the model using the same inputs we get different outputs. When these outputs are drawn together, we can have greater confidence in the results. If you look at the different graphs you can see that the actual results between each model (comparing uninformed or comparing informed) are not that dissimilar, but if you presented the uninformed graph for the deterministic model, would you be happy to state that the maximum prevalence is 22%? In the stochastic uninformed it is clearly the maximum and potentially you could claim that the likely maximum is considerably lower. In other words, you have more confidence.

What has been achieved by all this modelling? We have obtained a possible prevalence where it was not previously known, but more importantly, we have significantly reduced the number of animals tested from well over 300 to 30 and potentially we can be as certain as possible that the population is free of disease.

Basic Sampling for Presence or Absence of Disease

1) Review the literature to obtain likely prevalence, if present, or set design prevalence to WOAH recommended levels (i.e. $\leq 2\%$ if absent), or consider initial prevalence at 50% (since we have no information whether disease is present or absent), which maximises the sample size to provide the greatest confidence in any results regardless of actual/true prevalence.
2) Decide the confidence required, usually 95%.
3) Select the testing regimen. If available, use WOAH recommendations (www.woah.org).
4) Use test Se and Sp if they are known. Sometimes these values are unknown, so consider the available evidence (scientific literature) to assume a suitable Se and Sp or carry out a small

scale study with known samples. When multiple tests are used, it is often safe to assume that Sp is 100%.
5) Sample size is dependent on prevalence, confidence level, test Se and Sp, and population size. You can use either the formulas given in this chapter or sample sizes can be calculated for you by websites such as Epitools.
6) Decide on laboratory to use, dependent on expected use of results (i.e. an in-house laboratory might be applicable if the results are only to be used internally; if results are to be used to prove freedom from disease to the regulatory authorities then use an appropriately credentialed laboratory).
7) Use WOAH recommendations to collect samples, if available, or record the method used and ensure that the sample reflects the proportions of the whole population of interest and is random.
8) Ensure that the sample is preserved correctly during transportation to the laboratory.
9) Record all methodology and results (for future comparisons, transparency etc.).

Risk-Based Sampling for Presence or Absence of Disease

Risk-based sampling assumes three things:

1) There is no clustering (i.e. we are sampling at the farm level).
2) The Sp of the surveillance system is effectively 1 (i.e. any positive is followed up to ensure they are not false positives).
3) That the relative risk (RR) of the risk population is greater than 1.

The advantage of risk-based sampling is it requires a smaller sample size, thus reducing cost.

Scenario Tree Modelling

Scenario tree modelling (Martin et al., 2007) is an example of risk-based sampling and can provide good evidence of freedom, using justifiable reason, with only a small sample number. Scenario tree modelling is really only useful for detection (yes/no) of disease. It requires a binary (dichotomous) answer, but you can get around this by using case definitions to create subpopulations. A summary of the steps in a scenario tree might be:

1) Case definition → presence/absence.
2) Test to use. Use WOAH recommendation if available.
3) Surveillance units – based on the distribution of the population.
4) Output must be quantifiable.
5) Level of confidence in the testing and in freedom.
6) Quantify the value of the test, given we likely have imperfect tests.
7) Incorporate historical disease status. Remember that the epidemiological unit may not have wished to previously look "actively" for disease.
8) Using historical data that used a different unit of measurement or scale requires reanalysis using the current scale.
9) Risk levels and risk factors – the probability of being infected.
10) Risk analysis includes the consequences.

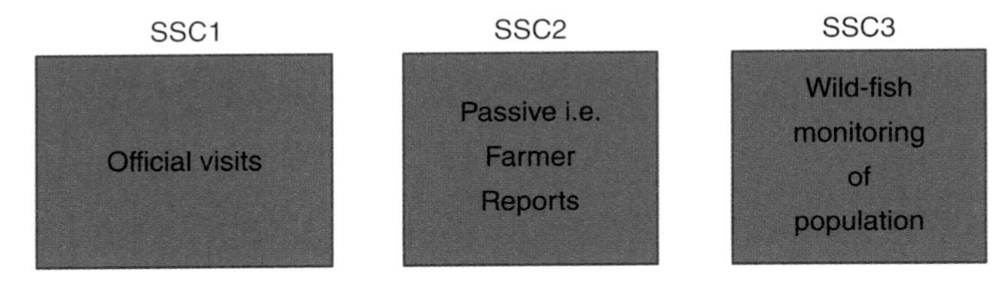

Figure 9.6 Surveillance system components.

11) Risk = probability (P).
12) Incorporate levels of ability to detect (i.e. farmers/vets recognise disease = Se).
13) Surveillance unit may be an individual animal/pen/herd that is part of the reference population.
14) Confidence of biosecurity measures should be measured, as well as the probability of freedom from disease.
15) The system must be quantitative, repeatable, transparent, understandable, and valid.
16) A surveillance system consists of surveillance system components (Figure 9.6).

Surveillance

Surveillance data is the basis of epidemiology and a key part of any continuing biosecurity plan. Surveillance can be active (looking for cases) or passive (recording cases as they occur). Within an epidemiological unit, surveillance should be designed to be active.

Why Do Surveillance?

1) To demonstrate freedom from disease.
2) To estimate population prevalence and define when to take action.
3) To determine status.
4) To monitor progress of the disease control program.
5) For early detection of new disease.
6) To determine where to apply controls.

The goals of a surveillance system are:

- The rapid detection of disease outbreaks (to minimize control costs).
- The early identification of disease problems (including environmental causes).
- Assessment of the health status of the defined population (working towards certification/audit).
- Definition of priorities for disease control and prevention (from risk assessment and cost–benefit analysis).
- Identification of new and emerging diseases (as part of contingency planning).
- Evaluation of the disease control programs.
- Confirmation of absence of a specific disease (certification, disease free status.) Additionally, one might wish to use the information to plan and conduct research.

Elements of an “ideal” surveillance system are:

- A preagreed intervention threshold (e.g. percentage mortality that triggers an investigation).
- An agreed case definition (e.g. the signs/symptoms/pattern that constitute a case or episode of a specific disease).

- Harmonized diagnostic procedures (e.g.to ensure that you are comparing like with like).
- Defined population at risk (e.g. the epidemiological unit).
- Method of recording cases (farm and veterinary records).
- Method to report data (within epidemiological unit, between epidemiological unit, veterinarian, and competent authority).
- Timely and competent data analysis (designed dependent on who/what will use the data requires some foresight).
- Means to assess the effect of an intervention (measures to assess prevalence).
- It is a continuous process (iterative).

If the surveillance system extends to a larger geographical area beyond an individual epidemiological unit or farm, then additionally you may need to consider:

- Means to communicate findings in a timely fashion.
- "Collectors" of cases.
- Central data collation.

Principles of Outbreak Investigation

The WOAH definition is "An occurrence of disease in an agricultural establishment, breeding establishment or premises, as well as adjoining premises, where animals are present." The steps of an outbreak investigation are:

- Create a case definition.
- Consider differential diagnoses/
- Identify the population at risk/
- Calculate the rate of disease (animal pattern):
  - In the overall population
  - In subgroups of the population.
- Establish the existence of an outbreak.
- Orient the outbreak in time (temporal pattern).
- Orient the outbreak in space (spatial pattern).
- Plan preventative/control measures.

Disease Contingency Plans

The WOAH code defines contingency plans as "a documented work plan designed to ensure that all needed actions, requirements and resources are provided in order to eradicate or bring under control outbreaks of specified diseases of aquatic animals." A contingency plan is initiated from the results of monitoring (i.e. a response to increased mortality) and should consider the following:

1) What triggers an outbreak investigation (i.e. increase in mortality beyond expected levels).
2) Who should this be reported to/or who to inform?
3) What diagnostic procedure will be used to confirm the suspected outbreak?
4) Specific instructions for all farm staff if a disease outbreak is confirmed and/or during confirmation.

5) These should be general for any possible disease outbreak but should include:
   a) How to handle affected animals.
   b) How to dispose of any dead animals.
   c) Deal with affected animals last.
   d) Within site movement restrictions.
   e) Additional hygiene precautions.
6) If animals are to be slaughtered how is this to be carried out, and how will they be disposed of hygienically?
7) Is emergency slaughter to market an option?
8) What disease control measures will be put in place?
9) Will the whole epidemiological unit be quarantined and how will this be achieved?
10) Any additional surveillance of unaffected stock that might be necessary?
11) Details of any disinfection procedures necessary?
12) How to establish that the outbreak is controlled or eradicated?
13) How will the epidemiological unit be restocked?
14) Will there be a need for fallowing?
15) Any necessary training for staff?
16) The objective of the contingency plan is to ensure any outbreak is minimized and localized as much as possible. Following the precautionary principle, if there are any doubts, err on the side of caution to minimize any potential disease outbreak. Key parts of the contingency plan might include rapid culling of infected populations and any contacts, speedy diagnosis and movement controls of animals, people and equipment on the premises.

By being prepared for any disease incursions, the speed with which the outbreak can be controlled or eradicated is much improved. Quantitative modelling can assist in developing strategies in preparation for an outbreak and for predicting and evaluating the effectiveness of control policies during an outbreak.

Disease Dynamics, Prevention and Control

How likely are we to get a disease outbreak in a given population? How fast will infection spread?
How many of the individuals will become infected? How can we control the spread of infection?

Threshold for Disease Transmission

The basic reproduction number, R_0, is the average number of infected individuals produced by a single infected individual introduced into a fully susceptible population.

Factors affecting R_0:

- The infectiousness of an individual>
- The period of infectiousness>
- The population density>
- The probability of making contacts with susceptible individuals>
- The probability of a contact resulting in transmission.

Disease invasion and large outbreaks are possible when R_0 is greater than 1, but when R_0 is less than 1 disease invasion is unlikely and only small outbreaks are possible. Thus, to prevent disease invasion and spread we need to manipulate the factors influencing R_0 to reduce the average number of secondary cases to less than 1.

The ability of an infected individual to contact and infect other individuals depends on the number of those contacts that are susceptible. The principle behind vaccination strategies is that a sufficient proportion of the susceptibles are rendered immune to reduce the number of secondary cases produced by an infected individual to less than 1. The critical vaccination coverage can be calculated from:

$$R_0(1 - p_{crit}) = 1 \text{ or } p_{crit} = 1 - 1/R_0$$

where p_{crit} is the critical population and R is the observed or effective reproduction ratio. This is illustrated in Table 9.3. We may only achieve partial coverage due to imperfect efficacy of the vaccine, maternal antibodies, declining immunity, or an influx of susceptibles, and these factors need to be also considered. We are able to prevent infection from invading the population by protecting not all but a critical proportion of the individuals. This is the concept behind herd immunity.

How Fast Does an Outbreak Take-Off?

R_0 does not specify how quickly an outbreak will take off, but the initial rate of increase in cases depends on R_0 and the generation time, G:

$$\frac{R_0 - 1}{G}$$

R_0 will determine the amount of control required, while G will determine how quickly control measures need to be implemented.

Observed or Effective Reproduction Ratio

The observed or effective reproduction ratio is the observed number of secondary cases produced by an infected individual. The number varies depending on whether the population is vaccinated within a population during a continuing outbreak as animals are removed due to resistance or mortality and as control measures are implemented. Successful control measures will aim to achieve $R<1$. By estimating R during the course of an outbreak, we can tell whether the outbreak has come under control.

When designing control measures, we need to understand the factors governing the spread of the disease, host, environment and pathogen. To tease apart the different influences on R_0 can require the use of mathematical models.

Table 9.3 Critical vaccination coverage.

R_0	Fraction vaccinated, p_{crit}	Fraction remaining susceptible, $1 - p_{crit}$	R_0 fraction remaining susceptible
2	$\frac{1}{2}$	$\frac{1}{2}$	1
3	$\frac{2}{3}$	$\frac{1}{3}$	1
4	$\frac{3}{4}$	$\frac{1}{4}$	1
5	$\frac{4}{5}$	$\frac{1}{5}$	1
10	$\frac{9}{10}$	$\frac{1}{10}$	1
15	$\frac{14}{15}$	$\frac{1}{15}$	1

Modeling Disease Dynamics

Models can be built for a number of reasons, including to help us understand the disease dynamics and estimate unknown parameters such as R_0 and R. Models can help us to identify where we need more data and to explore control options. Importantly, they can help us to make predictions.

Selecting the Model Structure

Models can be simple or extremely complex, depending on the scenario you are modeling, but the concept is to break down an apparently complex process into easily managed and explored steps, with each step representing a part of the process. Several models are illustrated in Figure 9.7.

Models may be deterministic, which will always give the same output for the same data set used. They give "average" behavior and are suitable for large numbers of animals. Probabilistic (or stochastic) models introduce the element of chance, providing different outputs for the same input, and giving a range of possible outcomes. Probabilistic models are suitable for small numbers of animals.

Difference Equation Models

Pick a suitable time step (e.g. a day, week, month, year) and calculate the number of infected individuals at the next time point based on the number at the current time step. Differential equation models allow the continuous updating of the number of infected (Figure 9.8). The simplest

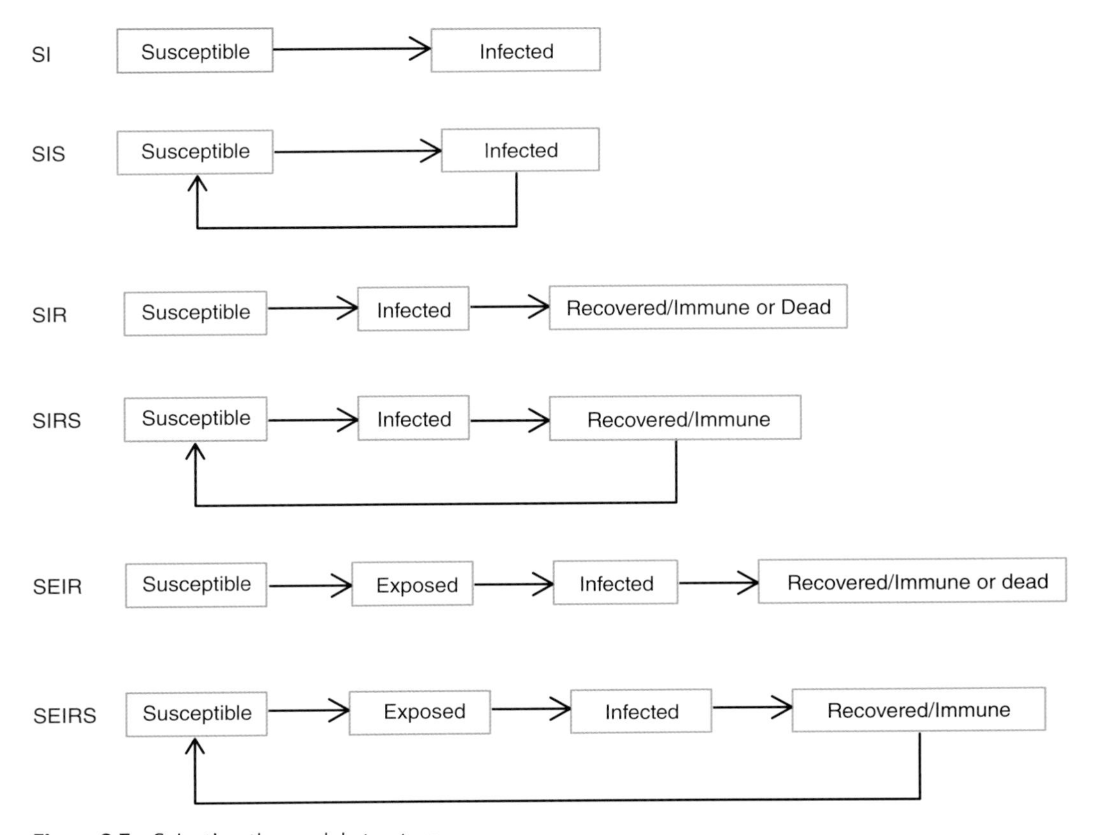

Figure 9.7 Selecting the model structure.

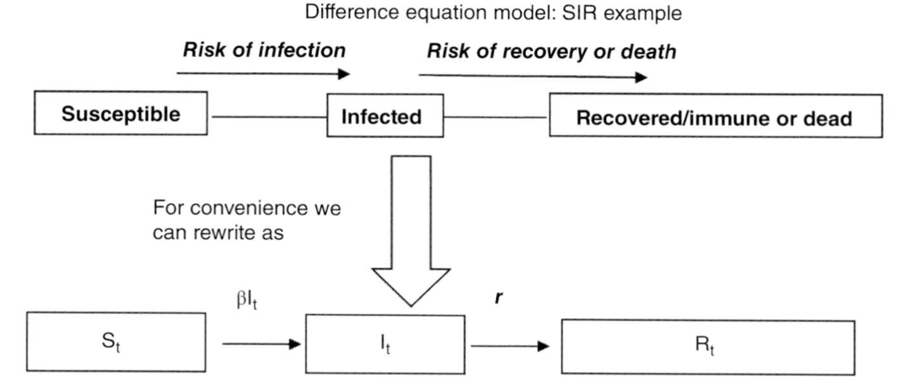

Figure 9.8 Difference equation model: SIR example.

models can be run using a calculator, although it is easier to use a spreadsheet. More complicated models may require a dedicated package or a flexible programming environment.

Model Parameters

- r is the risk of removal from the infected state – the proportion of infected individuals that will recover/die in per unit of time. Note that the risk will change as we change the unit of time from hour/day/week etc.
- β is the risk of transmission – the proportion of susceptibles that will become infected per unit of time per infected individual present (Figure 9.9).

Putting this into differential equation format:

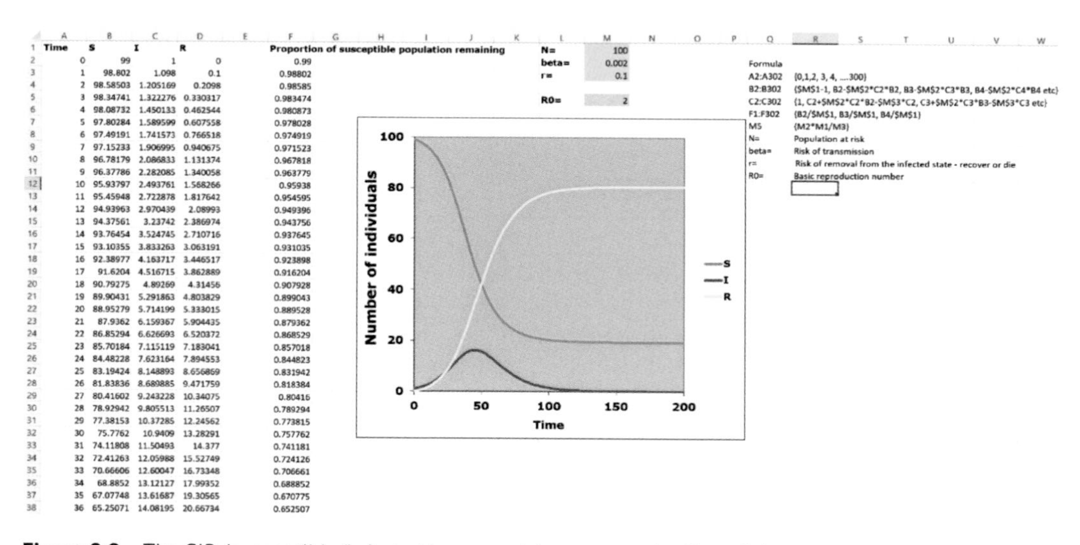

Time	S	I	R	Proportion of susceptible population remaining
0	99	1	0	0.99
1	98.802	1.098	0.1	0.98802
2	98.58503	1.205169	0.2098	0.98585
3	98.34741	1.322276	0.330317	0.983474
4	98.08732	1.450133	0.462544	0.980873
5	97.80284	1.589599	0.607558	0.978028
6	97.49191	1.741573	0.766518	0.974919
7	97.15233	1.906995	0.940675	0.971523
8	96.78179	2.086833	1.131374	0.967818
9	96.37786	2.282085	1.340058	0.963779
10	95.93797	2.493761	1.568266	0.95938
11	95.45948	2.722878	1.817642	0.954595
12	94.93963	2.970439	2.08993	0.949396
13	94.37561	3.23742	2.386974	0.943756
14	93.76454	3.524745	2.710716	0.937645
15	93.10355	3.833263	3.063191	0.931035
16	92.38977	4.163717	3.446517	0.923898
17	91.6204	4.516715	3.862889	0.916204
18	90.79275	4.89269	4.31456	0.907928
19	89.90431	5.291863	4.803829	0.899043
20	88.95279	5.714199	5.333015	0.889528
21	87.9362	6.159367	5.904435	0.879362
22	86.85294	6.626693	6.520372	0.868529
23	85.70184	7.115119	7.183041	0.857018
24	84.48228	7.623164	7.894553	0.844823
25	83.19424	8.148893	8.656869	0.831942
26	81.83836	8.689885	9.471759	0.818384
27	80.41602	9.243228	10.34075	0.80416
28	78.92942	9.805513	11.26507	0.789294
29	77.38153	10.37285	12.24562	0.773815
30	75.7762	10.9409	13.28291	0.757762
31	74.11808	11.50493	14.377	0.741181
32	72.41263	12.05988	15.52749	0.724126
33	70.66606	12.60047	16.73348	0.706661
34	68.8852	13.12127	17.99352	0.688852
35	67.07748	13.61687	19.30565	0.670775
36	65.25071	14.08195	20.66734	0.652507

N=	100
beta=	0.002
r=	0.1
R0=	2

Formula	
A2:A302	(0,1,2, 3, 4, ...300)
B2:B302	($M$1-1, B2-$M$2*C2*B2, B3-$M$2*C3*B3, B4-$M$2*C4*B4 etc)
C2:C302	(1, C2+$M$2*C2*B2-$M$3*C2, C3+$M$2*C3*B3-$M$3*C3 etc)
F1:F302	(B2/$M$1, B3/$M$1, B4/$M$1)
M5	(M2*M1/M3)
N=	Population at risk
beta=	Risk of transmission
r=	Risk of removal from the infected state - recover or die
R0=	Basic reproduction number

Figure 9.9 The SIR (susceptible/infected/recovered, immune or dead) model.

Susceptibles at t+1

S_{t+1} = number who were susceptible at time t (S_t) – number newly recovered/immune/dead between time t and t+1

S_{t+1} = $S_t - \beta I_t S_t$

Infected at t+1

I_{t+1} = number who were infected at time t (I_t) + number becoming recovered/immune/dead between time t and t+1

I_{t+1} = $I_t + \beta I_t S_t - RI_t$

Recovered/immune/dead at t+1 = number newly recovered/immune/dead at time t (R_t) + number newly recovered/immune/dead between time t and t+1

R_{t+1} = number who were infected at time t (R_t) + number newly recovered/immune/dead between time t and t+1

R_{t+1} = $R_t + rI_t$

R_0 can be calculated from this model:

R_0 = (mean number of new infections per unit time caused by introduced individual) (mean time spent infectious)

R_0 = $(\beta \times N \times 1) \times (1/r)$

or

$$R_0 = \frac{\beta N}{r}$$

Remember that although this model might represent the "average" in a population, it does not take into account variables such as the age structure or spatial structure of the population. The apparent rate of transmission may be affected by the immunity of previously exposed individuals or there may be a latent period. For a review and introduction of disease modelling see Matthews and Woodhouse (2005). Two further models are demonstrated in Figures 9.10 and 9.11.

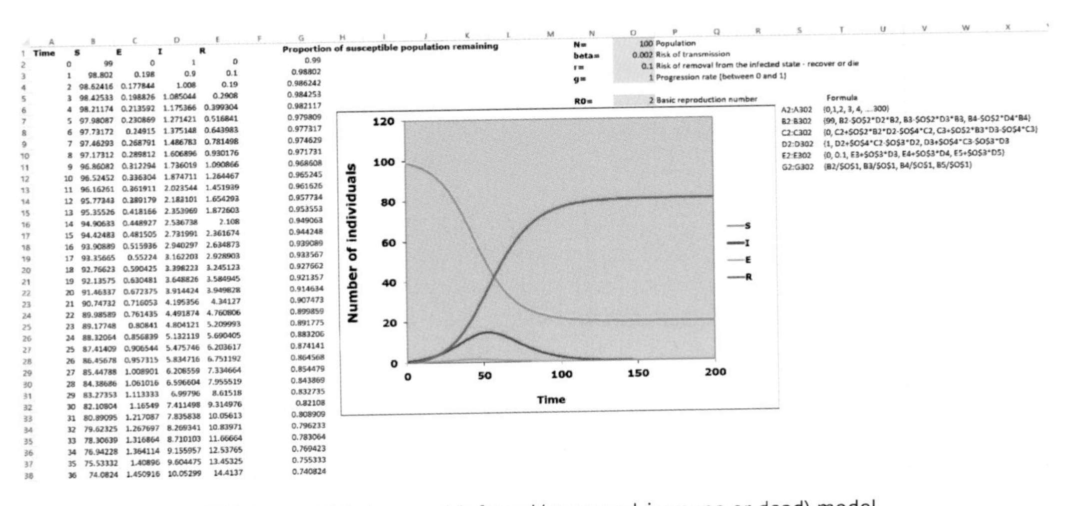

Time	S	E	I	R	Proportion of susceptible population remaining
0	99	0	1	0	0.99
1	98.802	0.198	0.9	0.1	0.98802
2	98.62416	0.177844	1.008	0.19	0.986242
3	98.42533	0.198826	1.085044	0.2908	0.984253
4	98.21174	0.213592	1.175366	0.399304	0.982117
5	97.98087	0.230869	1.271421	0.516841	0.979809
6	97.73172	0.24915	1.375148	0.643983	0.977317
7	97.46293	0.268791	1.486783	0.781498	0.974629
8	97.17312	0.289812	1.606896	0.930176	0.971731
9	96.86082	0.312294	1.736019	1.090866	0.968608
10	96.52452	0.336304	1.874711	1.264467	0.965245
11	96.16261	0.361911	2.023544	1.451939	0.961626
12	95.77343	0.389179	2.183101	1.654293	0.957734
13	95.35526	0.418166	2.353969	1.872603	0.953553
14	94.90633	0.448927	2.536738	2.108	0.949063
15	94.42483	0.481505	2.731991	2.361674	0.944248
16	93.90889	0.515936	2.940297	2.634873	0.939089
17	93.35665	0.55224	3.162203	2.928903	0.933567
18	92.76623	0.590425	3.398223	3.245123	0.927662
19	92.13575	0.630481	3.648826	3.584945	0.921357
20	91.46337	0.672375	3.914424	3.949828	0.914634
21	90.74732	0.716053	4.195356	4.34127	0.907473
22	89.98589	0.761435	4.491874	4.760806	0.899859
23	89.17748	0.80841	4.804121	5.209993	0.891775
24	88.32064	0.856839	5.132119	5.690405	0.883206
25	87.41409	0.906544	5.475746	6.203617	0.874141
26	86.45678	0.957315	5.834716	6.751192	0.864568
27	85.44788	1.008901	6.208559	7.334664	0.854479
28	84.38686	1.061016	6.596604	7.955519	0.843869
29	83.27353	1.113333	6.99796	8.61518	0.832735
30	82.10804	1.16549	7.411498	9.314976	0.82108
31	80.89095	1.217087	7.835838	10.05613	0.808909
32	79.62325	1.267697	8.269341	10.83971	0.796233
33	78.30639	1.316864	8.710103	11.66664	0.783064
34	76.94228	1.364114	9.155957	12.53765	0.769423
35	75.53332	1.40896	9.604475	13.45325	0.755333
36	74.0824	1.450916	10.05299	14.4137	0.740824

Parameter	Value	Description
N=	100	Population
beta=	0.002	Risk of transmission
r=	0.1	Risk of removal from the infected state - recover or die
g=	1	Progression rate (between 0 and 1)
R0=	2	Basic reproduction number

	Formula
A2:A302	{0,1,2, 3, 4, ...300}
B2:B302	{99, B2-$O$2*D2*B2, B3-$O$2*D3*B3, B4-$O$2*D4*B4}
C2:C302	{0, C2+$O$2*B2*D2-$O$4*C2, C3+$O$2*B3*D3-$O$4*C3}
D2:D302	{1, D2+$O$4*C2-$O$3*D2, D3+$O$4*C3-$O$3*D3
E2:E302	{0, 0.1, E3+$O$3*D3, E4+$O$3*D4, E5+$O$3*D5}
G2:G302	{B2/$O$1, B3/$O$1, B4/$O$1, B5/$O$1}

Figure 9.10 The SEIR (susceptible/exposed/infected/recovered, immune or dead) model.

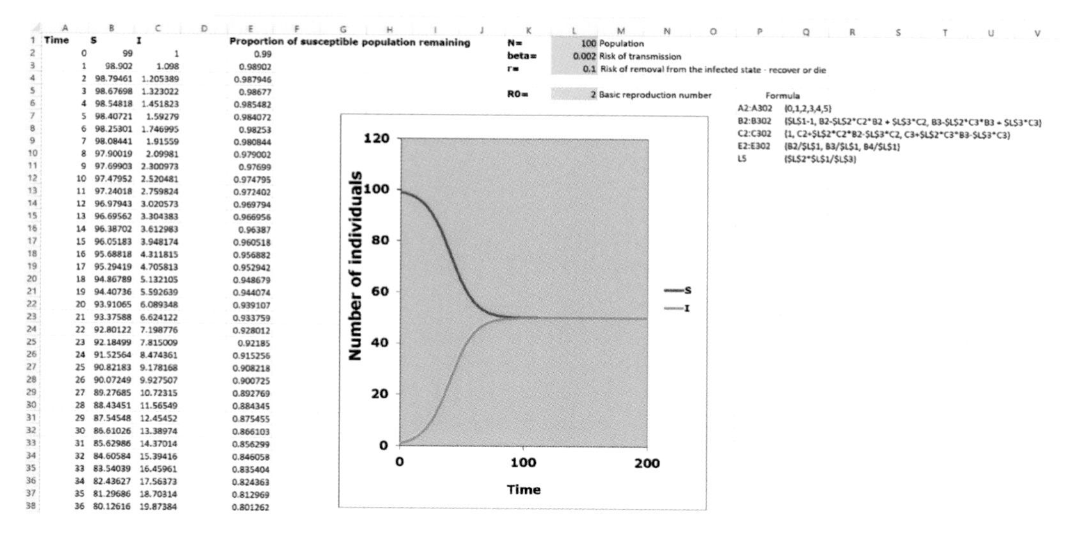

Time	S	I	Proportion of susceptible population remaining
0	99	1	0.99
1	98.902	1.098	0.98902
2	98.79461	1.205389	0.987946
3	98.67698	1.323022	0.98677
4	98.54818	1.451823	0.985482
5	98.40721	1.59279	0.984072
6	98.25301	1.746995	0.98253
7	98.08441	1.91559	0.980844
8	97.90019	2.09981	0.979002
9	97.69903	2.300973	0.97699
10	97.47952	2.520481	0.974795
11	97.24018	2.759824	0.972402
12	96.97943	3.020573	0.969794
13	96.69562	3.304383	0.966956
14	96.38702	3.612983	0.96387
15	96.05183	3.948174	0.960518
16	95.68818	4.311815	0.956882
17	95.29419	4.705813	0.952942
18	94.86789	5.132105	0.948679
19	94.40736	5.592639	0.944074
20	93.91065	6.089348	0.939107
21	93.37588	6.624122	0.933759
22	92.80122	7.198776	0.928012
23	92.18499	7.815009	0.92185
24	91.52564	8.474361	0.915256
25	90.82183	9.178168	0.908218
26	90.07249	9.927507	0.900725
27	89.27685	10.72315	0.892769
28	88.43451	11.56549	0.884345
29	87.54548	12.45452	0.875455
30	86.61026	13.38974	0.866103
31	85.62986	14.37014	0.856299
32	84.60584	15.39416	0.846058
33	83.54039	16.45961	0.835404
34	82.43627	17.56373	0.824363
35	81.29686	18.70314	0.812969
36	80.12616	19.87384	0.801262

N= 100 Population
beta= 0.002 Risk of transmission
r= 0.1 Risk of removal from the infected state - recover or die

R0= 2 Basic reproduction number

Formula
A2:A302 {0,1,2,3,4,5}
B2:B302 {$L$1-1, B2-$L$2*C2*B2 + $L$3*C2, B3-$L$2*C3*B3 + $L$3*C3}
C2:C302 {1, C2+$L$2*C2*B2-$L$3*C2, C3+$L$2*C3*B3-$L$3*C3}
E2:E302 {B2/$L$1, B3/$L$1, B4/$L$1}
L5 {$L$2*$L$1/$L$3}

Figure 9.11 The SIS (susceptible/infected) model.

References

Martin PAJ, Cameron AR, Greiner M. Demonstrating freedom from disease using multiple complex data sources: 1: a new methodology based on scenario trees. *Prev Vet Med* 2007; 79: 71–97.

Matthews L, Woolhouse M. New approaches to quantifying the spread of infection. *Nat Rev Mol Cell Biol* 2005; 3: 529–536.

Further Reading

Comin A, Grewar J, van Schaik G, et al. Development of reporting guidelines for animal health surveillance—AHSURED. *Front Vet Sci* 2019; 6: 426.

Food and Agriculture Organization. *Risk-Based Disease Surveillance: A manual for veterinarians on the design and analysis of surveillance for demonstration of freedom from disease*. FAO Animal Production and Health Manual No. 17. Rome, Italy: FAO; 2014.

Gary F, Clauss M, Bonbon E, Myers L. *Good Emergency Management Practice: The essentials. A guide to preparing for animal health emergencies*, 3rd edn. FAO Animal Production and Health Manual No. 25. Rome, Italy: FAO; 2021.

Kirkeby C, Brookes VJ, Ward MP, Dürr S, Halasa T. A practical introduction to mechanistic modelling of disease transmission in veterinary science. *Front Vet Sci* 2021; 7: 546651.

Murray AG. Existing and potential use of models in the control and prevention of disease emergencies affecting aquatic animals: changing trends in managing aquatic animal disease emergencies. *Rev Sci Tech* 2008; 2: 211–228.

Oidtmann B, Peeler E, Lyngstad T, et al. Risk-based methods for fish and terrestrial animal disease surveillance. *Prev Vet Med* 2013; 112: 13–26.

Peeler EJ, Taylor NG. The application of epidemiology in aquatic animal health: opportunities and challenges. *Vet Res* 2011; 42: 94.

Pfeiffer D. *Veterinary Epidemiology: An introduction*. Chichester, UK: Wiley-Blackwell; 2010.

Qviller L, Kristoffersen AB, Lyngstad TM, Lillehaug A. Infectious salmon anemia and farm-level culling strategies. *Front Vet Sci* 2020; 6: 481.
Stevenson MA. Sample size estimation in veterinary epidemiologic research. *Front Vet Sci* 2021; 7: 539573.
Sub-Committee on Aquatic Animal Health. *Aquaculture Farm Biosecurity Plan: Generic guidelines and template*. Canberra, Australia: Department of Agriculture and Water Resources; 2016.
Thrusfield M, Christly R. *Veterinary Epidemiology*, 4th edn. Hoboken, NJ: Wiley; 2018.
World Organisation for Animal Health. *Manual 5: Surveillance and Epidemiology*. Paris, France: WOAH; 2018.

10

Animal Health Economics

Chris Walster and Leo Foyle

Economics and Biosecurity

There are four reasons why an epidemiological unit might adopt and develop a biosecurity plan, all of which relate to economics: public good, improvement in animal welfare, increased productivity, and increased profitability:

1) A *public good* could be where an epidemiological unit decides to be the first in an area to undertake a disease control strategy of an endemic disease, such as vaccination. While the epidemiological unit gains a benefit, there is also a benefit to surrounding farms from the reduction in the prevalence of disease in the area, which leads to lower infection rates. This external benefit to surrounding farms is an example of an externality and can lead to the problem of "freeloaders". Because of this issue, public goods are often funded through public means such as taxes or producer levies.
2) Animal welfare and health are linked with improvements in one improving the other. Animal welfare criteria are often part of quality assurance schemes and consumers are said to be willing to pay a premium for a product they perceive as being produced in a "welfare friendly" fashion. Additionally, the epidemiological unit may wish to have a reputation for taking "the best care" or wants to exhibit a certain level of pride in their work. While these social benefits may be hard to quantify, they are part of any economic benefit. However, in economic terms farmers sell a homogenous product with similar appearance and quality, making it difficult for them to differentiate their product, so any increased value due to better welfare may simply be a result of the farmers' increased pride in the job.
3) Productivity is a measure of efficiency based on the variation in output as additional equal units of variable input are used. There are three types of input:
   a) Variable inputs vary with the amount of product produced and can be controlled by the epidemiological unit (e.g. health care).
   b) Fixed inputs do not vary over the period of analysis (e.g. buildings or labor costs).
   c) Random inputs are usually treated as constant and can be ignored. An example of a random input would be the weather.

   Decreasing exposure to endemic diseases improves food conversion ratio, weight gain, and organoleptic qualities, and enhances the ability to assess genetic merit correctly. All of these will increase productivity, which in turn increases profitability. But consider what happens if all

Pathology and Epidemiology of Aquatic Animal Diseases for Practitioners, First Edition.
Edited by Laura Urdes, Chris Walster, and Julius Tepper.

farmers take up measures to increase productivity, which in turn leads to sufficient increase in production: there is a decrease in the price paid for the product. This could cause a fall in profits, although in economic terms the benefit is transferred to the consumer, who now pays a lower price for the product.

4) Increased profitability would appear to be the natural outcome of any disease control strategy. "Evidence from a wide variety of studies over the last thirty years has shown that because of the substantial effects of diseases on productivity and the relatively low cost of control measures, the net economic benefit obtained from controlling animal diseases is very high, commonly in the range 200% to 1,500% return on invested funds" (Morris 1999).

From the above, it would seem that disease control strategies produce a net economic benefit with the only issues being who pays the cost and who gains the benefit. For the veterinarian working with a client, there are few if any publications to provide an economic assessment of biosecurity on an individual unit basis, although there may be information on a regional or national basis, mainly due to the numerous variables that need to be considered on a site by site or disease basis. A description of the process, admittedly for bovine viral diarrhea, is given by Stott et al. (2003) and it would seem that at the farm level there will be a need to assess the economics on a case-by-case basis. There are additional issues that affect the uptake of biosecurity plans, and these are discussed in the next section.

Opportunity Costs

An almost ubiquitous story that most veterinarians will recognize is that a farmer will increase the chance of detection of estrus by observing their animals during the evening; however, many farmers prefer to spend this time with their family. This is an example of an opportunity cost where the decision to take one action removes the option to take another action, with consequences that can be termed as costs.

Opportunity costs are not necessarily financial, they can be emotional or convenience. To evaluate the opportunity costs properly, individual producers need to know how much effort they need to invest in disease control where information is lacking, the cost of collecting that information, and ultimately how to design disease control strategies. Optimal economic strategies may not be identical for all businesses as the interpretation of what provides the greatest value in terms of "costs" will vary. In developing a biosecurity plan, consideration must be given to the needs, wishes, and aims of the epidemiological unit.

Rational Choices

An economist would say that a rational choice has been made when the decision creates the largest benefit relative to the cost. Decisions should not be made solely on epidemiological unit costs, but should also compare the likely benefits to be derived. People making rational choices know the cost and understand the value of the decision. People making poor decisions could be said to know the cost of everything and the value of nothing. In encouraging an epidemiological unit to make the rational choice, not only are we required to provide as accurate an estimate of cost as possible, but also the value of the likely returns. Rational choice focuses on the comparison of total costs with total benefits.

Marginal Costs and Benefits

A fish farm produces X^1 amount of product (output or "benefit") for Y^1 costs (inputs) but can with additional costs (such as additional labour, time, feed, vaccinating stock) produce X^2 for Y^2 costs. Is it worth adopting these additional procedures? This calculation involves assessing the marginal costs ($Y^2 - Y^1$) of the extra inputs compared with the marginal benefits ($X^2 - X^1$) that they create. Even though there may be an additional benefit, it may not warrant the additional costs.

Production Functions

Production is the process of using materials (inputs) to create goods or services (outputs). All livestock systems are production activities. Production functions are a mathematical description of the unique amount of output that can be gained from a given set of inputs. The generalized expression of a production function in equation form is:

$$Y = f\left(X_1, X_2, X_3, X_n\right)$$

Where Y = output; X_1, X_2 = inputs; f means function of. Where there are fixed costs, the equation is written as:

$$Y = f\left(X_1 \middle| X_2, X_3, X_n\right)$$

Anything before the solid line is a variable cost. There are several measures of production:

- Total output may be called the *total physical product* (TPP). In equation form, it is expressed as:

$$TPP = Y = f\left(X_1 \middle| X_2, X_n\right)$$

- *Average physical product* (APP) is the average output per unit of variable input and measures the efficiency of converting input to output:

$$APPx_1 = TPP/\left(\text{Variable input}\left(X_1\right)\right) = Y/\left(X_1\right)$$

- *Marginal physical product* (MPP) is the change in the amount of product produced over the change in the amount of input used. MPP is equal to the slope of TPP and represents the rate at which an input is transformed into an output:

$$MPPx_1 = dy/(dx_1)$$

- *Elasticity of production* (εp) is the percentage change of an output over the percentage change of an input:

$$\varepsilon_p = \left(\%\text{change in output}\right)/\left(\%\text{change in input}\right) = \left(MPPx_1\right)/\left(APPx_1\right)$$

Although the graph in Figure 10.1 is idealized, it demonstrates the three stages of production and the relationship between the measures of production (Table 10.1). To calculate the most profitable amount of variable input to use to generate the most profitable amount of product to produce, it is necessary to know the price of the input and output. To calculate this profit maximization for a single input to single output relationship (factor/product), we can calculate the profit for different levels of input use and the resultant output, graph the profit line to determine where it reaches

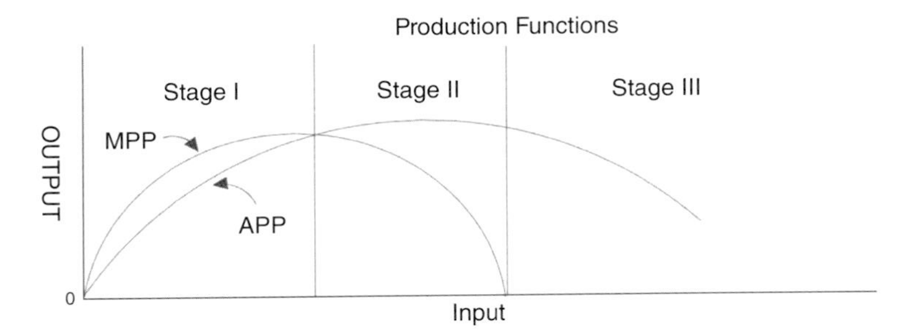

Figure 10.1 Idealized production functions.

Table 10.1 The three stages of production and the relationship between the measures of production.

Stage	Relationships
I	TPP and APP are increasing with MPP > APP. MPP reaches a maximum during this stage; εp > 1, meaning that the response to increases in input levels is elastic.
End of I and beginning of II	MPP = APP, εp = 1, APP reaches its maximum.
II	TPP is increasing at a diminishing rate and therefore productivity is decreasing. APP > MPP. The efficiency of using a variable input is at its greatest at the start of stage II whereas the efficiency of using fixed inputs is greatest at the end of stage II; εp is between 1 and 0 and the responsiveness of output to increases in input can be described as inelastic.
End of II and beginning of III	TPP reaches maximum and MPP = 0; εp is also 0.
III	TPP declines, MPP is negative, and APP is declining. εp < 0. The optimal use of inputs occurs during stage II as it is here that the farmer uses their resources in the most efficient manner. Stage II is the rational region of production.

APP, average physical product; εp, elasticity of production; MPP, marginal physical product; TPP, total physical product.

a maximum, or calculate it algebraically. This requires some further definitions, which assist in determining where this maximum profit point lies:

- *Total value product* (TVP) is the total monetary value of the production of the farm:

  $$TVP = P_y \times Y$$

  Where Y = the amount of output at any level of input; P_y = the price per unit of output.

- *Average value product* (AVP) is APP times the price per unit of Y:

  $$AVP = APP \times P_y = Y/(X) \times P_y = TVP/X$$

  Where X = the amount of variable input used.

- *Marginal value product* (MVP) is MPP times the price per unit of Y. MVP is the slope of the TVP line:

  $$MVP = MPP \times P_y = (dy/dx) \times P_y$$

- *Total variable costs* (TVC) are the total monetary costs for a variable input used for production. Variable inputs are commonly defined as those inputs the farmer has control over (i.e. the farmer can decide the amount of input they wish to use) and disease control is an obvious example.

  $$TVC = P_x \times X$$

  Where P_x = the price per unit of input.

- *Total fixed costs* (TFC) are the total monetary value of fixed inputs used for production. Fixed inputs are those inputs that the farmer has no control over. In other words, they cannot change the input. An obvious example would be the amount of land available or, in our case, the amount of water. This of course leads to the issue of what is a fixed or variable cost, which is often dependent on the length of time available. Over time a farm can buy or rent additional land or may even sell some.
- *Total costs* (TC) are the total monetary value of all costs of production:

  $$TC = TVC + TFC$$

  $$\text{Profit}\ (\pi) = TVP - TC = TVP - TVC - TFC = P_y \times Y - P_x \times X - TFC$$

Figure 10.2 summarizes the relationships between input and output with the various measures used to determine the point of maximum profit. What does this information tell us? Somewhere around 18–20 units of input give the maximum profitability and around 8 units of input the business starts to make a profit. Stage I ends and stage II starts around 16 units of input, and at 24 units of input we have reached and entered stage III.

While a table of figures looks good and assists in explaining your reasoning to the client, it is rather laborious to prepare and there may be information in it that we really do not need. The simplest way to find the point of maximum profit is algebraically. If one considers the equation for profit as a function of input, then by differentiating with respect to X:

$$\text{Profit} = P_y f(X) - P_x X - TFC$$

$$d\text{Profit}/dX = P_y (dY/dX) - P_x$$

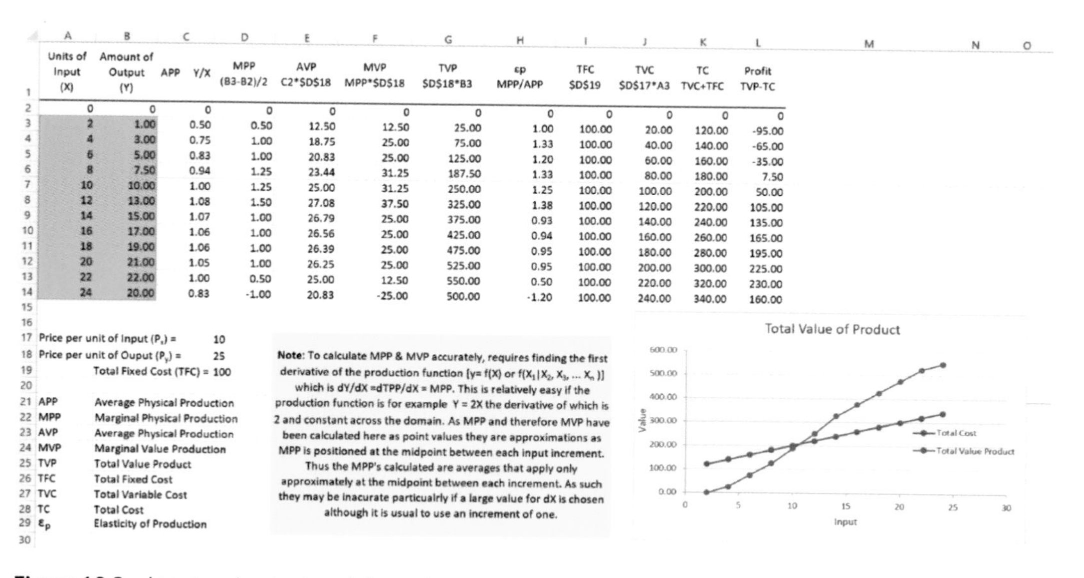

Units of Input (X)	Amount of Output (Y)	APP Y/X	MPP (B3-B2)/2	AVP C2*$D$18	MVP MPP*$D$18	TVP $D$18*B3	εp MPP/APP	TFC $D$19	TVC $D$17*A3	TC TVC+TFC	Profit TVP-TC
0	0	0	0	0	0	0	0	0	0	0	0
2	1.00	0.50	0.50	12.50	12.50	25.00	1.00	100.00	20.00	120.00	-95.00
4	3.00	0.75	1.00	18.75	25.00	75.00	1.33	100.00	40.00	140.00	-65.00
6	5.00	0.83	1.00	20.83	25.00	125.00	1.20	100.00	60.00	160.00	-35.00
8	7.50	0.94	1.25	23.44	31.25	187.50	1.33	100.00	80.00	180.00	7.50
10	10.00	1.00	1.25	25.00	31.25	250.00	1.25	100.00	100.00	200.00	50.00
12	13.00	1.08	1.50	27.08	37.50	325.00	1.38	100.00	120.00	220.00	105.00
14	15.00	1.07	1.00	26.79	25.00	375.00	0.93	100.00	140.00	240.00	135.00
16	17.00	1.06	1.00	26.56	25.00	425.00	0.94	100.00	160.00	260.00	165.00
18	19.00	1.06	1.00	26.39	25.00	475.00	0.95	100.00	180.00	280.00	195.00
20	21.00	1.05	1.00	26.25	25.00	525.00	0.95	100.00	200.00	300.00	225.00
22	22.00	1.00	0.50	25.00	12.50	550.00	0.50	100.00	220.00	320.00	230.00
24	20.00	0.83	-1.00	20.83	-25.00	500.00	-1.20	100.00	240.00	340.00	160.00

Price per unit of Input (P_x) = 10
Price per unit of Ouput (P_y) = 25
Total Fixed Cost (TFC) = 100

APP Average Physical Production
MPP Marginal Physical Production
AVP Average Physical Production
MVP Marginal Value Production
TVP Total Value Product
TFC Total Fixed Cost
TVC Total Variable Cost
TC Total Cost
ε_p Elasticity of Production

Note: To calculate MPP & MVP accurately, requires finding the first derivative of the production function [$y = f(X)$ or $f(X_1 | X_2, X_3, \ldots X_n)$] which is dY/dX =dTPP/dX = MPP. This is relatively easy if the production function is for example Y = 2X the derivative of which is 2 and constant across the domain. As MPP and therefore MVP have been calculated here as point values they are approximations as MPP is positioned at the midpoint between each input increment. Thus the MPP's calculated are averages that apply only approximately at the midpoint between each increment. As such they may be inacurate particualrly if a large value for dX is chosen although it is usual to use an increment of one.

Figure 10.2 Input and output and the various costs, profitability, and productivity measures.

Since this equation represents the slope of the profit line and the maximum point is reached when the slope is equal to zero and we wish to find for a single variable input:

$$\text{dProfit/dX} = P_y\left(\text{dY/dX}\right) - P_x = 0$$

$$= P_y\text{MPP} - P_x = 0 \text{ or } P_y\text{MPP} = P_x \text{ or } \text{MVP}/\left(\text{Px}\right) = 1$$

This implies that an input should be increased until the point is reached where the last unit of money spent on an input returns exactly its incremental cost. As disease control can be considered a single variable input then this implies that the optimum expenditure on disease control is at this point.

Economic Analysis of the Epidemiological Unit Biosecurity Plan

The above allows you to better understand the stage of production of the epidemiological unit and what money might be available for biosecurity. It does not provide you with any information on what might be the impact of the biosecurity plan in five years' time or whether you have allocated scarce resources to provide the greatest benefit. The following focuses on evaluating the marginal or additional benefit of introducing or intensifying disease control at an economically optimal level for the epidemiological unit. Readers should be aware that the economic assessment methodology varies somewhat between farm, regional, national, and international level. To obtain a fuller picture, consult the literature in the Further Reading.

Any analysis requires a baseline of disease prevalence and what is the level of production of the epidemiological unit with or without the disease. Two questions that arise regarding data: how accurate do they need to be and are they available? Carrying out a literature search of published work on a disease will often reveal a surprising amount of data on the economic impact but where data are missing then it is perfectly acceptable to use expert opinion. However, any analysis is only as good as the data used. Where there is doubt, analyzing the information generated within a couple of production cycles between productivity of animal groups with or without disease can provide a good indication of the production loss due to disease or the expected gains due to control measures. A final general consideration is whether the control measure is technically feasible and socially acceptable.

There are three methods that can be used individually or in combination to assist the economic decision at the farm or epidemiological unit level, in most cases. These are:

1) Partial budgeting.
2) Decision tree analysis.
3) Cost benefit analysis.

All three methods are relatively easy to carry out using computer spreadsheets. There are some further terms to introduce:

- *Discounting, net present value* (NPV) and *internal rate of return* (IRR): is $1000 received today the same as receiving $1000 in two years' time? The answer is no and can be calculated by the following formula:

$$\text{PV} = \text{FS}/\left(1 + \text{r}\right)^{\text{n}}$$

where: PV = present value; FS = future sum; r = periodic interest (discount) rate; n = number of periods. That is:

$$\$1000 \text{ received 2 years, hence discounted at } 7\% = 1000/\left(1+0.07\right)\hat{}\,2 = 1000/\left(1.145\right) = \$873.36$$

For a cost benefit analysis, the NPV is used, which is the sum for each period (usually one year) of the project, being the total benefits received during the period minus the total costs, discounted by the appropriate discount factor to convert each total to the present value:

$$\text{NPV} = \sum_{t=0}^{t} \frac{\left(B^t - C^t\right)}{\left(1+r\right)^t}$$

where: Bt = monetary benefits received in any year t; Ct = costs incurred in any year t; r = discount rate.

From this, the higher the discount rate used, the lower the present value of future cash flows. The discount rate to use is often debated but the real interest rate (the cost of borrowing money minus the inflation rate) is a common starting point.

The IRR is calculated by finding the discount rate that would provide an NPV of zero and can be used to compare alternative uses of the funds. To manually calculate the IRR requires a trial-and-error approach. The simplest way to calculate both the IRR and NPV is using a computer spreadsheet (Figure 10.3).

	A	B	C	D	E	F	G	H	I
1									
2				Discount rate (%) =		0.08	Yr/Qtr/Mth		
3	**Time period Yr/Qtr/Mth**	**Discount Factor (Cell F2)**	**Costs**	**Benefits**	**Net Cash Flow**	**Cumulative Cash Flow**	**Discounted Cash Flow**	**Discounted Costs**	**Discounted Benefits**
4	0	1.0000	10000	0	-10000	-10000	-10000	10000	0
5	1	0.9259	10000	4500	-5500	-15500	-5093	9259	4167
6	2	0.8573	5000	15000	10000	-5500	8573	4287	12860
7	3	0.7938	1000	13000	12000	6500	9526	794	10320
8	4	0.7350	1000	8000	7000	13500	5145	735	5880
9	5	0.6806	0	5000	5000	18500	3403	0	3403
10	**Totals**		**27000**	**45500**	**18500**	**7500**	**11555**	**25075**	**36630**
11									
12		**Formula used**				**Net Present Value (NPV) =**		**11555**	
13		B6 to B10	(NPV(B5,$F$2)			**Benefit-Cost Ratio (BCR) =**		**1.46**	
14		E6 to E10	(D4-C4)			**Internal Rate of return (IRR) =**		**33.20%**	
15		F6 to F10	(F5+E6)						
16		G5 to G10	(E5*B5)						
17		H5 to H10	(C5*B5)						
18		I5 to I10	(D5*B5)						
19		Amount Input							
20		H13	G11						
21		H14	I11/H11						
22		H15	IRR(E5:E10)						

Figure 10.3 Calculating the net present value (NPV), benefit–cost ratio (BCR) and internal rate of return (IRR) of a project (see spreadsheet in Appendix 9.3).

Partial Budgeting

For our purposes partial budgeting is only concerned with the variable cost (disease control) and the revenue affected by the proposed intervention. Partial budgeting uses four headings:

- Additional income (e.g. increased number of fish produced).
- Reduced expenses (e.g. savings in treatment costs).
- Reduced income (e.g. possible decreased market value if production increased sufficiently).
- Additional expenses, e.g. staff training, equipment net benefit = (1 + 2) – (3 + 4).

The advantage of partial budgeting is that it is quicker to carry out than a complete budget and focuses on the issues of interest. There are several disadvantages which really mean it is only useful for an initial appraisal and should a project pass this first hurdle then one of the following techniques should be used.

Decision Tree Analysis

Decision tree analysis allows you to incorporate the uncertainties inherent in any animal health decision and the economic consequences. The decision tree is a pictorial representation of the logical flow of events and can be a good way of communicating veterinary opinion to the farmer. An example is given in Figure 10.4.

The initial step in building a decision tree is to identify all the possible courses of action that might be used to address the problem. Figure 10.4 uses the example of a diseased batch of fish and the options that a veterinarian might suggest. The first node of a decision tree is always a decision node which is represented by a rectangular box. There is one separate branch for each possible decision with each branch leading to either a chance node (circle) or a terminal node (triangle). The chance nodes describe the probability of each possible outcome and the probabilities at each chance node must sum to one (or 100%). The terminal nodes provide information on the value at the end of the branch.

The preferred course of action is determined by a process called folding back. Here the monetary value of each terminal node is multiplied by the probability given at the preceding chance node. The products of the branches originating from the same node are summed to provide the expected value (EV) of the node. The folding back process is continued until a single EV is obtained for each branch originating from the decision node at the source of the decision tree. In Figure 10.4, the EV of the treat branch is calculated as follows:

$$\text{EV}\left(\text{treated and lives}\right) = 0.8 \times \left(5000 - 800\right) = 3360$$

$$\text{EV}\left(\text{treated and dies}\right) = 0.2 \times \left(1000 + 800\right) = 360$$

$$\text{EV}\left(\text{treat}\right) = 3360 - 360 = 3000$$

As can be seen in Figure 10.4 the three EVs are:

Treat = \$3000

No treatment = \$1400

Wait and see = \$1850

As the EV for treat provides the greatest value of all the options including culling then it is the preferred option. Decision tree analysis makes you look at all the available options including

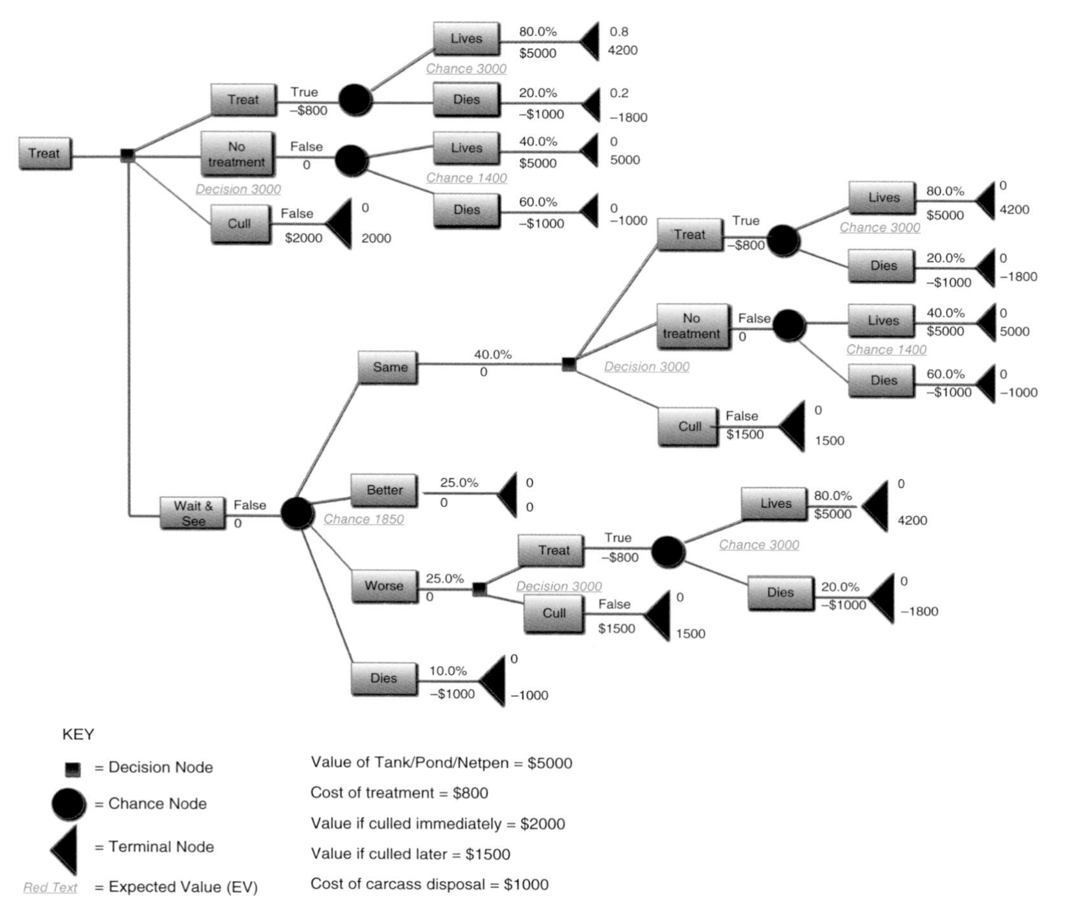

Figure 10.4 An example of a decision tree.

timing choices (e.g. when to cull), and incorporates the uncertainties involved in making the decision. Probabilities are used not only to state the likelihood that an animal or group of animals will live or die but can also be used to explore whether an epidemiological unit will experience a clinical outbreak of disease.

While a decision tree helps to ensure that you have looked at all the available options, it is probably easier to explain and use in practice when incorporated into a spreadsheet (Figure 10.5).

Cost–Benefit Analysis

Cost–benefit analysis (CBA) is used to compare different disease control strategies over a period of years, say over 5–20 years. In our case, it could simply compare no control with a proposed control program at the epidemiological unit over a period of five years (Figure 10.6). As you extend the analysis further into the future the less accurate it will become. CBAs do not mean that you know all of the figures, and they frequently involve some form of subjective judgments. If the control

	A	B	C	D	E	F	G	H	I	J
1		**Example of a Decision Tree Spreadsheet**								
2										
3			**Cost or %**	**%Live**	**% Mort**		**Initial Value=**	5000		
4	**Treat**		800	0.8	0.2					
5	**Do not treat**		0	0.4	0.6					
6	**Cull now**		2000	0	1					
7	**Cull later**		1500	0	1					
8	**Disposal**		1000							
9		Same	0.4							
10	**Wait and See**	Better	0.25							
11		Worse	0.25							
12		Dies	0.1							
13										
14		**Expected Value (EV) Treat =**	3000		EV Treat = SUM((D4*H3)-(E4*C8)-C4))					
15		**EV No Treatment =**	1400		EV No Treatment = SUM((D5*H3)-(E5*C8))					
16		**EV Wait & See =**	1850		EV wait & See = SUM((C9*C14)+(C11*C14)-(C12*C8))					

Figure 10.5 Expected values.

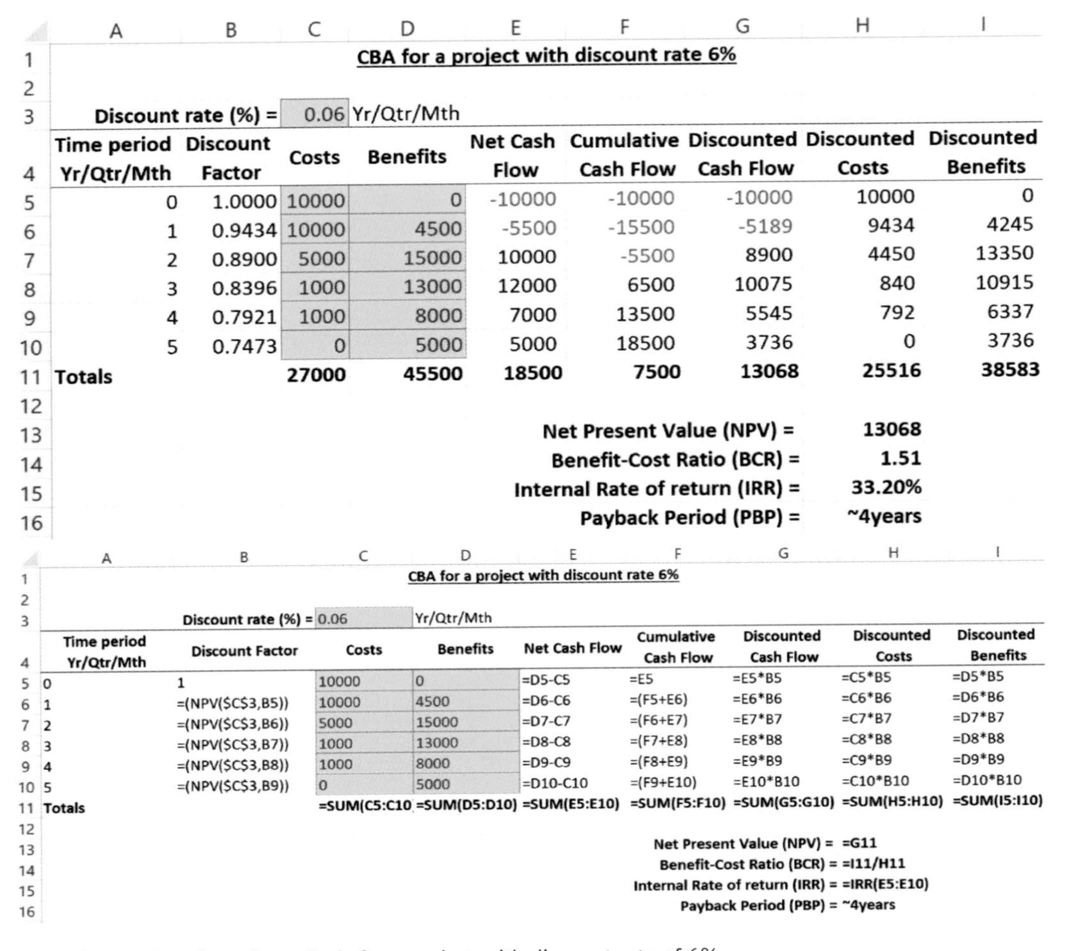

	A	B	C	D	E	F	G	H	I
1				**CBA for a project with discount rate 6%**					
2									
3	**Discount rate (%) =**		0.06	Yr/Qtr/Mth					
4	**Time period Yr/Qtr/Mth**	**Discount Factor**	**Costs**	**Benefits**	**Net Cash Flow**	**Cumulative Cash Flow**	**Discounted Cash Flow**	**Discounted Costs**	**Discounted Benefits**
5	0	1.0000	10000	0	-10000	-10000	-10000	10000	0
6	1	0.9434	10000	4500	-5500	-15500	-5189	9434	4245
7	2	0.8900	5000	15000	10000	-5500	8900	4450	13350
8	3	0.8396	1000	13000	12000	6500	10075	840	10915
9	4	0.7921	1000	8000	7000	13500	5545	792	6337
10	5	0.7473	0	5000	5000	18500	3736	0	3736
11	**Totals**		**27000**	**45500**	**18500**	**7500**	**13068**	**25516**	**38583**
12									
13							**Net Present Value (NPV) =**	**13068**	
14							**Benefit-Cost Ratio (BCR) =**	**1.51**	
15							**Internal Rate of return (IRR) =**	**33.20%**	
16							**Payback Period (PBP) =**	**~4years**	

	A	B	C	D	E	F	G	H	I
1				**CBA for a project with discount rate 6%**					
2									
3		**Discount rate (%) =**	0.06	Yr/Qtr/Mth					
4	**Time period Yr/Qtr/Mth**	**Discount Factor**	**Costs**	**Benefits**	**Net Cash Flow**	**Cumulative Cash Flow**	**Discounted Cash Flow**	**Discounted Costs**	**Discounted Benefits**
5	0	1	10000	0	=D5-C5	=E5	=E5*B5	=C5*B5	=D5*B5
6	1	=(NPV($C$3,B5))	10000	4500	=D6-C6	=(F5+E6)	=E6*B6	=C6*B6	=D6*B6
7	2	=(NPV($C$3,B6))	5000	15000	=D7-C7	=(F6+E7)	=E7*B7	=C7*B7	=D7*B7
8	3	=(NPV($C$3,B7))	1000	13000	=D8-C8	=(F7+E8)	=E8*B8	=C8*B8	=D8*B8
9	4	=(NPV($C$3,B8))	1000	8000	=D9-C9	=(F8+E9)	=E9*B9	=C9*B9	=D9*B9
10	5	=(NPV($C$3,B9))	0	5000	=D10-C10	=(F9+E10)	=E10*B10	=C10*B10	=D10*B10
11	**Totals**		**=SUM(C5:C10**	**=SUM(D5:D10)**	**=SUM(E5:E10)**	**=SUM(F5:F10)**	**=SUM(G5:G10)**	**=SUM(H5:H10)**	**=SUM(I5:I10)**
12									
13							**Net Present Value (NPV) =**	**=G11**	
14							**Benefit-Cost Ratio (BCR) =**	**=I11/H11**	
15							**Internal Rate of return (IRR) =**	**=IRR(E5:E10)**	
16							**Payback Period (PBP) =**	**~4years**	

Figure 10.6 Cost–benefit analysis for a project with discount rate of 6%.

program requires finance, then it is adequate to project over five years. CBA can be summarized as four steps specifying:

1) The flow of costs – what is the cost of the project for each period? You may need to quantify non-monetary costs into a monetary value.
2) The flow of returns – what is the monetary value of the benefits.
3) Deciding on appropriate discount rate – commonly the real interest rate.
4) The decision criterion - usually are NPV, BCR, IRR and payback period (PBP).

Decisions are based on the following:

- If NPV > zero, the return is greater than the opportunity cost (discount rate).
- If BCR > 1 – then NPV must be > 0.
- IRR (NPV = 0) allows comparison with alternative uses of the funds. It may vary over the lifetime of the project and may not exist if net cash flow is positive for each year of the project as NPV will never be zero.
- PBP = (costs – benefits = 0) is calculated ignoring the time value of money and ignores any future returns.
- Whether sufficient capital is available for the project.

References

Morris RS. The application of economics in animal health programmes: a practical guide. *Rev Sci Tech* 1999; 18: 305–314.
Stott A, Lloyd J, Humphry R, Gunn G. A linear programming approach to estimate the economic impact of bovine viral diarrhoea (BVD) at the whole-farm level in Scotland. *Prev Vet Med* 2003; 59: 51–66.

Further Reading

Chary K, Brigolin D, Callier MD. Farm-scale models in fish aquaculture: an overview of methods and applications. *Rev Aquacult* 2022; 14: 2122–2157.
Perry BD. The economics of animal disease control. *Rev Sci Tech* 1999; 18(2): doi: http://dx.doi.org/10.20506/rst.issue.18.2.11.
Rushton J. *The Economics of Animal Health and Production: Practical and theoretical guide.* Wallingford, UK: CABI; 2011.
Rushton J. The economics of animal health. *Rev Sci Tech* 2017; 36(1):11–384. doi: https://doi.org/10.20506/rst.issue.36.1.2604.

Index

Page locators in **bold** indicate tables. Page locators in *italics* indicate figures. This index uses letter-by-letter alphabetization.

a

Pathology and Epidemiology of Aquatic Animal Diseases for Practitioners, First Edition.
Edited by Laura Urdes, Chris Walster, and Julius Tepper.

u

v

w

x

y

z